Patient Assessment Practice Scenarios

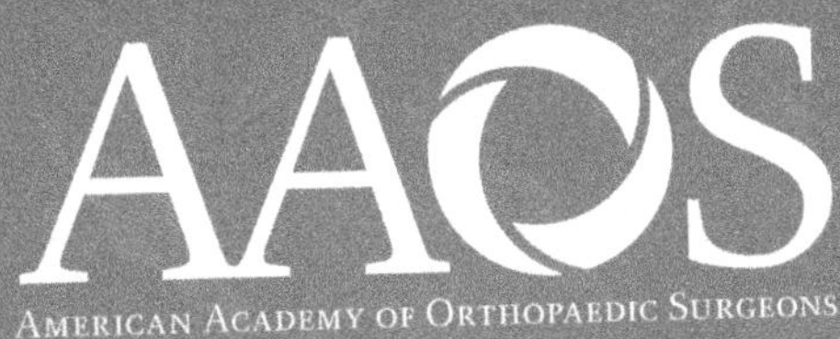

Les Hawthorne, BA, NREMT-P
Maryland Fire and Rescue Institute
University of Maryland
College Park, Maryland

JONES AND BARTLETT PUBLISHERS
Sudbury, Massachusetts
BOSTON TORONTO LONDON SINGAPORE

World Headquarters
Jones and Bartlett Publishers
40 Tall Pine Drive
Sudbury, MA 01776
978-443-5000
info@jbpub.com
www.jbpub.com

Jones and Bartlett Publishers
Canada
6339 Ormindale Way
Mississauga, Ontario L5V 1J2
Canada

Jones and Bartlett Publishers
International
Barb House, Barb Mews
London W6 7PA
United Kingdom

Jones and Bartlett's books and products are available through most bookstores and online booksellers. To contact Jones and Bartlett Publishers directly, call 800-832-0034, fax 978-443-8000, or visit our website, www.jbpub.com.

Substantial discounts on bulk quantities of Jones and Bartlett's publications are available to corporations, professional associations, and other qualified organizations. For details and specific discount information, contact the special sales department at Jones and Bartlett via the above contact information or send an email to specialsales@jbpub.com.

AAOS
AMERICAN ACADEMY OF ORTHOPAEDIC SURGEONS

Editorial Credits
Chief Education Officer: Mark W. Wieting
Director, Department of Publications: Marilyn L. Fox, PhD
Managing Editor: Barbara A. Scotese
Associate Senior Editor: Gayle Murray

Production Credits
V.P., Design and Production: Anne Spencer
V.P., Manufacturing and Inventory Control: Therese Connell
Publisher: Kimberly Brophy
Acquisitions Editor—EMS: Christine Emerton
Managing Editor: Carol B. Guerrero
Associate Editor: Nicholas Cronin
Editorial Assistant: Kara Ebrahim
Production Manager: Jenny L. Corriveau
Director of Sales, Public Safety Group: Matthew Maniscalco
Director of Marketing: Alisha Weisman
Text Design: Anne Spencer
Composition: Shepherd, Inc.
Cover and Title Page Design: Scott Moden
Cover Image: Courtesy of Les Hawthorne
Cover Printing: Courier Stoughton
Printing and Binding: Courier Stoughton

ISBN: 978-0-7637-7820-0

The procedures and protocols in this book are based on the most current recommendations of responsible medical sources. The American Academy of Orthopaedic Surgeons and the publisher, however, make no guarantee as to, and assume no responsibility for, the correctness, sufficiency, or completeness of such information or recommendations. Other or additional safety measures may be required under particular circumstances.

This textbook is intended solely as a guide to the appropriate procedures to be employed when rendering emergency care to the sick and injured. It is not intended as a statement of the standards of care required in any particular situation, because circumstances and the patient's physical condition can vary widely from one emergency to another. Nor is it intended that this textbook shall in any way advise emergency personnel concerning legal authority to perform the activities or procedures discussed. Such local determinations should be made only with the aid of legal counsel.

6048
Printed in the United States of America
14 13 12 11 10 10 9 8 7 6 5 4 3 2 1

Contents

Acknowledgments

The American Academy of Orthopaedic Surgeons, Jones and Bartlett Publishers, and the author would like to thank the reviewers of this book.

Reviewers

John G. Alexander, BS, NREMT-P
Maryland Fire and Rescue Institute
University of Maryland
College Park, Maryland

David Andrade, MS Ed, Paramedic
EMS-Instructor
Joint Hospital Planning Council EMS Programs
Central Magnet High School
Stratford, Connecticut

Steven L. Ashworth, EMT-P, BA
South Florida Community College
Avon Park, Florida

Donna Garbacz Bader, MA, MSN, RNC, CFN, D-ABMDI
Assistant Professor
BryanLGH College of Health Sciences
School of Nursing and General Education
Lincoln, Nebraska

Blance Keith Bankston, NREMT-P
LSU-Fire and Emergency Training Institute
Baton Rouge, Louisiana

Dawn Bauer
Superior, Montana

Angela L. Bennett, MS, NREMT-P
Maryland Fire and Rescue Institute
University of Maryland
College Park, Maryland

Jimmie D. Blacker, Jr, BAS, EMT-B, PHTLS
Van Buren Intermediate School District Technology Center
Lawrence, Michigan

Shawn Bowe, NREMT-P, FP-C
North Shore–Long Island Jewish Health System Center for EMS
Syosset, New York

Timothy S. Brisbin, BSN, RN, NREMT-P
The Center for Prehospital Medicine
Gastonia, North Carolina

Robert J. Brumblay, MD, FACEP
Kapiolani Community College
Honolulu, Hawaii

David A. Budde, AASPS
Emergency Services Director
Lake Land Community College
Mattoon, Illinois

Russ Christiansen, NREMT-P, CCEMTP
Paramedic Technology Program Director
Casper College
Casper, Wyoming

Michael T. Davis, EMT-B
Davis Training Center, LLC
Reynolds Station, Kentucky

Bradley Dean, BBA, NREMT-P
Alamance Community College/Wake Forest University Baptist Medical Center
Thomasville, North Carolina
Winston-Salem/Davidson County Emergency Services
Lexington, North Carolina

Bobbie Lynn Doran, RN, EMT-P, IC
Jackson State Community College
Beech Bluff, Tennessee

Skip Gelati, BA, EMSI, EMT-I, BLSI-RF, BLSI-TCF, NIMS-I, MCI-I, CEVO-I
Naugatuck Valley Community College
Waterbury, Connecticut

Amber Gisriel, MS, NREMT-P
Maryland Fire Rescue Institute
University of Maryland
College Park, Maryland

Carol Gupton, BS, NREMT-P
Program Director
Emergency Provider Instruction
Omaha, Nebraska

Eryq M. Hastings, NREMT-P
San Manuel Fire Department
San Manuel, Arizona

Victor Robert Hernandez, BA, EMT-P
Sierra College
Rocklin, California

Joseph P. Hopple, NREMT-P
Education Coordinator
Sussex County EMS
Georgetown, Delaware

Carla M. Isenberg
Program Coordinator
Emergency Health Services Federation
New Cumberland, Pennsylvania

Edward J. Kalinowski, MEd, Dr PH
Kapiolani Community College
University of Hawaii
Honolulu, Hawaii

Amy Krueger, NREMT-P
Rupert, Indiana

Richard Main, BS, NREMT-P
National Center for Technical Instruction
Las Vegas, Nevada

Kelly Marsh, Firefighter/Paramedic
Belmont Fire Department
Belmont, New Hampshire

Kevin McFarlane, RN, CEN, EMT-I I/C
New Mexico EMS Bureau
Santa Fe, New Mexico

SGT Earl K. Newman, III, NREMT-P
RIARNG Medical Detachment
North Kingstown, Rhode Island

Charles L. Parmley, NREMT-P, FFIII
Lead Instructor, Program Coordinator
North Tech High School Fire and EMS Academy
Florissant, Missouri

Christopher P. Patrello, BS, EMT-P I/C
Genesys Regional Medical Center
Flint, Michigan

Mark Podgwaite, SR, NEC EMS I/C
Vermont EMS
Northfield, Vermont

Danny W. Roach
Assistant Chief/Training Chief
Whitfield County Fire Department
Dalton, Georgia

Curt Schmittling, BS, EMT-P
Southwestern Illinois College
Belleville, Illinois

Robert F. Shields, Jr, NREMT-P
EMS Instructor/Coordinator, Training Officer
Cumberland Rescue Service
Cumberland, Rhode Island

David M. Stamey, CCEMT-P, Flight Paramedic
Western Pennsylvania Center for Emergency Medicine
Maryland Fire and Rescue Institute
University of Maryland
College Park, Maryland

Geri Strohmeyer, Paramedic
EMS Coordinator
Southwestern Illinois College
Maryville, Illinois

Robert S. Wales, BS, NREMT-P, CCEMT-P
Upstate EMS Council, Inc
Easley, South Carolina

Richard C. Wilkinson, II, NREMT-P, ILEM
HEMSI
Huntsville, Alabama

Dean Williams, EMT-I
Battalion Chief
West Valley City Fire Department
West Valley City, Utah

Eric Wilson, EMT-Paramedic, Firefighter
South Western Illinois College
Granite City, Illinois

Monroe Yancie
IHM Health Studies Center
St. Louis, Missouri

Introduction: How to Use This Book

Introduction

Proficiency with trauma and medical patient assessments is, without a doubt, the most difficult task for the EMS student to accomplish. It seems as though there is never enough time in the classroom for students to get all the practice time that they want and need. This interactive book gives the student a tool with which to practice and cement knowledge of the patient assessment process by walking the student through 150 trauma and medical case studies, most of which are based on real cases.

The cases presented here follow the steps in the relevant National Registry patient assessment skill sheet, depending on whether the case is categorized as trauma or medical:

- Patient Assessment/Management: Trauma
- Patient Assessment/Management: Medical

These National Registry skill sheets are shown at the end of this introduction for reference. Students and instructors will find these skill sheets to be a useful study tool when studying these cases and preparing for national examinations.

Structure

This book is set up as scripted proctor and student statements. The scenarios are easy to read, follow, and understand. Each case consists of scripted statements for both student and proctor. The proctor can be anyone—instructor, fellow student, and so on. The proctor does not need to be versed in EMS lingo, tactics, or treatment.

Uses

This book may be used in any of the following ways, and is relevant to both self-study and classroom use:

- *Drilling in the assessment process by rote.* Both the student and the proctor have a copy of the book. Each reads his or her portion of the case aloud, similar to a skit, to practice following the assessment process by rote.
- *Testing knowledge of the assessment process.* Only the proctor has a copy of the book. The proctor reads the dispatch information, and then the student works through the assessment process assisted by prompts from the proctor. This method tests the student's knowledge of the assessment process and pinpoints problem areas.
- *In-class use.* The book may be used in class for role plays and small-group activities. It has applications in both lab and lecture formats.
- *Continuing education and refresher training.* Using these cases for practice can help keep your skills sharp and in practice.

The reading level and overall writing style of each case are acceptable for students at both the basic life support (BLS) and advanced life support (ALS) levels. ALS-level material is identified by the labels "ALS Student" and "ALS Proctor."

Format

Each case includes the following sections:

Dispatch Information

Dispatch information is to be read by the proctor at the outset of the case. The Dispatch Information sections in this book provide varying levels of detail, to reflect the differences students may experience in the real world.

Pre-scene Action (BSI)

Pre-scene action identifies the forms of body substance isolation (BSI) the student should list as being needed for the case.

Critical Criteria

Beginning in the Pre-scene Action section, each case lists the critical criteria that apply. Critical criteria are also listed after the other main sections of the case. These are the same critical criteria listed on the National Registry patient assessment skill sheets.

Proctors may check off criteria that the student met or, conversely, circle critical criteria that the student did not meet. After concluding the case, the proctor may discuss items missed by the student to help the student focus on learning these items.

Scene Size-up

Scene Size-up covers the issues the student should address as part of the scene size-up: determining scene safety, determining the mechanism of injury or nature of the illness, determining the number of patients, assessing the need for additional resources, and deciding whether to perform cervical spine (c-spine) stabilization.

Initial Assessment

Initial assessment covers the following core components of this stage of the assessment process: forming a general impression; assessing the patient's responsiveness and level of consciousness; determining the chief complaint and apparent life threats; assessing airway, breathing, and circulation; providing initial management; identifying the patient's priority; and making the transport decision.

Focused History and Physical Examination/Rapid Trauma Assessment

This section begins with the student determining whether the patient requires a focused assessment or a rapid assessment, and provides the script for the student to walk through the appropriate assessment. Medical cases follow one of the seven lines of questioning provided in the National Registry Patient Assessment/Management—Medical skill sheet: respiratory/cardiac, altered mental status, allergic reaction, poisoning/overdose, environmental emergency, obstetrics, or behavioral. This section also includes placement of the cervical collar and backboard if applicable. Injury/wound management is covered, as well as reevaluating the transport decision, obtaining baseline vital signs, and obtaining a SAMPLE history.

Detailed Physical Examination

In real life, the detailed physical exam is usually performed en route to the hospital and if time allows. The EMS provider's time, however, may be consumed with managing life threats and supporting the patient's ABCs—airway, breathing, and circulation.

Most cases in this book include a detailed physical exam for the sake of student practice. The student may or may not opt to practice this portion, depending on his or her judgment of the patient. Practicing this portion will help solidify an understanding of the steps of the detailed physical exam.

Radio Report

Each case includes a reminder to the student to give a radio report. This item is not included on National Registry testing sheets, so students are not expected to provide this information in a national testing station. Nevertheless, the Radio Report section is included in the cases as a reminder to the student that this step should be performed.

Ongoing Assessment

Ongoing assessment includes a reassessment of the vital signs and mental status, followed by a statement as to whether the vital signs have changed significantly—called trending vital signs. Trending vital signs is not required in a national testing station for assessment, but is an important step in the assessment process in real-life situations.

The ongoing assessment also includes checking interventions. Students identify which interventions they have performed. ALS-level interventions are listed separately.

Handoff Report to Emergency Department Staff

As with the radio report, each case includes a reminder to the student to give a handoff report to the emergency department staff. Like the Radio Report step, this item is not included on National Registry testing sheets. Students are not expected to provide this information in a national testing station. Nevertheless, this section is included in the cases as a reminder to the student that this step should be performed.

Pass/Fail

This section is provided for instructors who opt to use this book for in-class testing situations. The instructor or proctor may mark whether the student passed or failed the case, note the date, and make additional notes as needed.

Case Topics

It may seem as though a disproportionate number of the scenarios in this book involves gunshot wounds and motor vehicle collisions. This is not necessarily so. Once they are practicing EMS providers, many students will receive calls involving gunshot wounds and motor vehicle collisions on a daily basis. Others will not, depending on the area where they practice. In any event, these types of cases require students to assess every part of the body; if the entire body is not assessed, critical findings may be missed. Therefore, these cases help students fine-tune their basic skills and become proficient at the full assessment process. If a student can find a puncture wound in training or practice, he or she will be ready to find the same kind of wound when the time comes for assessing real patients.

Treatment and Protocols

This book is not designed to teach a specific local protocol or to replace the assessment portion of any textbook. If a disagreement arises between the treatment rendered in this book and a local protocol, students must follow their local protocol. Local EMS protocols and systems vary greatly. This book is not intended to create local protocol, but rather supports the student in using his or her local protocols in a practice setting.

For this reason, this book cannot dictate when certain non-life-threatening treatment occurs. Of course, no EMS system would allow a medical provider to postpone treatment of a life threat, such as gurgling in the airway; treatment (in this case, suctioning the airway) must occur first. When it comes to life-or-death issues, the provider must treat the life threat as soon as it is found. For example, if the airway is not open, the provider must open it immediately with the appropriate method. If the patient has gone into cardiac arrest, the provider must begin cardiopulmonary resuscitation (CPR) immediately.

Cervical Stabilization and Immobilization

The National Registry Patient Assessment/Management skill sheets do not specify precisely where in the course of the patient assessment process a patient should be placed in a cervical collar and backboard. Local protocols on this topic vary. One EMS system may require the trauma patient to be fitted with a cervical collar as soon as the neck is assessed. A different system may require the provider to place a cervical collar after he or she has performed more of the assessment (as long as a second provider is maintaining spinal immobilization of the patient).

Because placement of the cervical collar is so important, it is included in cases in this book where applicable. The cases note several points in the assessment process when the cervical collar could be placed, depending on the local protocol. Students should state the appropriate point as dictated by their local protocol.

Backboarding is included within the rapid physical exam. Be aware that in some areas, backboarding may occur earlier in the assessment process per the local protocol. It would not occur later than the rapid physical exam, however, which explains why we have included it at this point. Again, students should state the appropriate point for backboarding per their local protocol.

CPR

Finally, this book contains very few cases that result in CPR, for the reason that providers must focus on administering CPR rather than continue the assessment process.

Conclusion

The goal of this book is to provide cases of varying difficulty and nature to help the student become the best EMS provider possible. The goal is not just to get through the class and pass the trauma and medical assessment testing stations, but rather to become a quality medical care provider.

As a student, you must buckle down and memorize the trauma and medical assessment algorithms. If you stop to think about it, the assessment process is really a logical one; it is a head-to-toe assessment. When you get flustered and do not know what to do next, orient yourself by figuring out where you are in the patient assessment process and go on from there.

The key to learning this process is practice, practice, practice, and more practice. Certainly, this book is useful in the classroom. But if a student really wants to improve his or her assessment skills, the individual will have to practice assessment at home and in study groups. By practicing outside of class, the student will be far more prepared for classroom practice sessions and much more prepared when the time comes to treat actual patients. Best of luck!

Patient Assessment/Management - Trauma

Start Time: ____________

Stop Time: ____________ Date: ____________

Candidate's Name: ____________

Evaluator's Name: ____________

		Points Possible	Points Awarded
Takes, or verbalizes, body substance isolation precautions		1	
SCENE SIZE-UP			
Determines the scene is safe		1	
Determines the mechanism of injury		1	
Determines the number of patients		1	
Requests additional help if necessary		1	
Considers stabilization of spine		1	
INITIAL ASSESSMENT			
Verbalizes general impression of the patient		1	
Determines responsiveness/level of consciousness		1	
Determines chief complaint/apparent life threats		1	
Assesses airway and breathing	Assessment	1	
	Initiates appropriate oxygen therapy	1	
	Assures adequate ventilation	1	
	Injury management	1	
Assesses circulation	Assesses/controls major bleeding	1	
	Assesses pulse	1	
	Assesses skin (color, temperature and conditions)	1	
Identifies priority patients/makes transport decision		1	
FOCUSED HISTORY AND PHYSICAL EXAMINATION/RAPID TRAUMA ASSESSMENT			
Selects appropriate assessment (**focused or rapid assessment**)		1	
Obtains, or directs assistance to obtain, baseline vital signs		1	
Obtains S.A.M.P.L.E. history		1	
DETAILED PHYSICAL EXAMINATION			
Assesses the head	Inspects and palpates the scalp and ears	1	
	Assesses the eyes	1	
	Assesses the facial areas including oral and nasal areas	1	
Assesses the neck	Inspects and palpates the neck	1	
	Assesses for JVD	1	
	Assesses for tracheal deviation	1	
Assesses the chest	Inspects	1	
	Palpates	1	
	Auscultates	1	
Assesses the abdomen/pelvis	Assesses the abdomen	1	
	Assesses the pelvis	1	
	Verbalizes assessment of genitalia/perineum as needed	1	
Assesses the extremities	1 point for each extremity includes inspection, palpation, and assessment of motor, sensory, and circulatory function	4	
Assesses the posterior	Assesses thorax	1	
	Assesses lumbar	1	
Manages secondary injuries and wounds appropriately **1 point for appropriate management of the secondary injury/wound**		1	
Verbalizes re-assessment of the vital signs		1	
	Total:	40	

Critical Criteria

____________ Did not take, or verbalize, body substance isolation precautions
____________ Did not determine scene safety
____________ Did not assess for spinal protection
____________ Did not provide for spinal protection when indicated
____________ Did not provide high concentration of oxygen
____________ Did not find, or manage, problems associated with airway, breathing, hemorrhage or shock (hypoperfusion)
____________ Did not differentiate patient's need for transportation versus continued assessment at the scene
____________ Did other detailed physical examination before assessing the airway, breathing and circulation
____________ Did not transport patient within (10)-minute time limit

Patient Assessment/Management - Medical

Start Time: ____________

Stop Time: ____________ Date: ____________

Candidate's Name: ________________________

Evaluator's Name: ________________________

		Points Possible	Points Awarded
Takes, or verbalizes, body substance isolation precautions		1	
SCENE SIZE-UP			
Determines the scene is safe		1	
Determines the mechanism of injury/nature of illness		1	
Determines the number of patients		1	
Requests additional help if necessary		1	
Considers stabilization of spine		1	
INITIAL ASSESSMENT			
Verbalizes general impression of the patient		1	
Determines responsiveness/level of consciousness		1	
Determines chief complaint/apparent life threats		1	
Assesses airway and breathing	Assessment	1	
	Indicates appropriate oxygen therapy	1	
	Assures adequate ventilation	1	
Assesses circulation	Assesses/controls major bleeding	1	
	Assesses pulse	1	
	Assesses skin (color, temperature and condition)	1	
Identifies priority patients/makes transport decisions		1	
FOCUSED HISTORY AND PHYSICAL EXAMINATION/RAPID ASSESSMENT			
Signs and symptoms (Assess history of present illness)		1	

Respiratory	Cardiac	Altered Mental Status	Allergic Reaction	Poisoning/ Overdose	Environmental Emergency	Obstetrics	Behavioral
*Onset? *Provokes? *Quality? *Radiates? *Severity? *Time? *Interventions?	*Onset? *Provokes? *Quality? *Radiates? *Severity? *Time? *Interventions?	*Description of the episode. *Onset? *Duration? *Associated Symptoms? *Evidence of Trauma? *Interventions? *Seizures? *Fever?	*History of allergies? *What were you exposed to? *How were you exposed? *Effects? *Progression? *Interventions?	*Substance? When did you ingest/become exposed? *How much did you ingest? *Over what time period? *Interventions? *Estimated weight?	*Source? *Environment? *Duration? *Loss of consciousness? *Effects-general or local?	*Are you pregnant? *How long have you been pregnant? *Pain or contractions? *Bleeding or discharge? *Do you feel the need to push? *Last menstrual period?	*How do you feel? *Determine suicidal tendencies. *Is the patient a threat to self or others? Is there a medical problem? Interventions?

	Points Possible	Points Awarded
Allergies	1	
Medications	1	
Past pertinent history	1	
Last oral intake	1	
Event leading to present illness (rule out trauma)	1	
Performs focused physical examination (assesses affected body part/system or, if indicated, completes rapid assessment)	1	
Vitals (obtains baseline vital signs)	1	
Interventions (obtains medical direction or verbalizes standing order for medication interventions and verbalizes proper additional intervention/treatment)	1	
Transport (re-evaluates the transport decision)	1	
Verbalizes the consideration for completing a detailed physical examination	1	
ONGOING ASSESSMENT (verbalized)		
Repeats initial assessment	1	
Repeats vital signs	1	
Repeats focused assessment regarding patient complaint or injuries	1	
Total:	30	

Critical Criteria

____________ Did not take, or verbalize, body substance isolation precautions when necessary

____________ Did not determine scene safety

____________ Did not obtain medical direction or verbalize standing orders for medical interventions

____________ Did not provide high concentration of oxygen

____________ Did not find or manage problems associated with airway, breathing, hemorrhage or shock (hypoperfusion)

____________ Did not differentiate patient's need for transportation versus continued assessment at the scene

____________ Did detailed or focused history/physical examination before assessing the airway, breathing and circulation

____________ Did not ask questions about the present illness

____________ Administered a dangerous or inappropriate intervention

Dispatch Information

PROCTOR: EMS 10, respond to a 24-year-old male who has been shot. He is conscious and breathing. Law enforcement has been dispatched.

Pre-scene Action (BSI)

Student: I am wearing nonlatex gloves, safety glasses, mask, and gown.
PROCTOR: Noted.

Critical Criteria:
- ❑ Did not take, or verbalize, body substance isolation (BSI) precautions when necessary

Scene Size-up

Scene Safety

Student: Is the scene safe?
PROCTOR: Yes, police are on scene and you are given clearance to enter.

Mechanism of Injury

Student: What was the mechanism of injury?
PROCTOR: Gunshot wound. The patient was holding up a store with a fake gun.

Number of Patients

Student: How many patients are there?
PROCTOR: One.

Additional Resources

Student: I would call for advanced life support (ALS) assistance.
PROCTOR: Noted.

C-Spine Stabilization

Student: On the basis of the mechanism of injury, I would stabilize the patient's cervical spine (c-spine) in a neutral in-line position.
PROCTOR: Noted.

Critical Criteria:
- ❑ Did not determine scene safety
- ❑ Did not assess for spinal protection
- ❑ Did not provide for spinal protection when indicated

Initial Assessment

Student: As I perform midline c-spine stabilization, I identify myself and ask the patient not to move.
PROCTOR: Noted.

General Impression

Student: My general impression is that the patient's condition is unstable.
PROCTOR: Noted.

Responsiveness/Level of Consciousness

Student: What is the patient's level of consciousness?
PROCTOR: Alert.

Chief Complaint/Apparent Life Threats

Student: What is the patient's chief complaint?
PROCTOR: The patient is complaining of being shot in the left chest and shortness of breath.
Student: There is an apparent life threat; the life threat is a gunshot wound.
PROCTOR: Noted.

Assess the Airway and Breathing

Assessment

Student: I am assessing the airway.
PROCTOR: Noted.
Student: What are the rate and the quality of breathing?
PROCTOR: Rate: Rapid. Quality: Guarded.

Provide Oxygen

Student: I am assisting ventilations with a bag-valve device and 100% oxygen.
PROCTOR: Noted.

Ensure Adequate Ventilation

Student: I will assist ventilation with a bag-valve device and 100% oxygen.
PROCTOR: Noted.

Injury Management

Student: I will apply an occlusive dressing to the gunshot wound on the left upper chest.
PROCTOR: Noted.
Student: I will listen to the patient's breath sounds.
PROCTOR: The patient's breath sounds are diminished on the left side of the chest.

Assess Circulation

Student: I am assessing the patient's circulation.
PROCTOR: Noted.

Assess for and Control Major Bleeding

Student: Do I find any major bleeding?
PROCTOR: Yes, to the right side of the head.
Student: I would apply direct pressure and a dressing.
PROCTOR: Noted.

Assess the Pulse

Student: What are the rate and the quality of pulses?
PROCTOR: Rate: Tachycardic. Quality: Thready.

Assess the Skin

Student: I am assessing the skin. What are the color, temperature, and condition of the skin?
PROCTOR: Color: Pale. Temperature: Cool. Condition: Moist.

Identify Priority Patients/Make Transport Decision

Student: The patient is a high priority and is a load-and-go. I will begin packaging and transport.
PROCTOR: Noted.

Critical Criteria:
- ❑ Did not provide high concentration of oxygen
- ❑ Did not find or manage problems associated with airway, breathing, hemorrhage or shock (hypoperfusion)
- ❑ Did not differentiate patient's need for transportation versus continued assessment at the scene
- ❑ Did other detailed examination before assessing the airway, breathing and circulation

Focused History and Physical Examination/Rapid Trauma Assessment

Select the Appropriate Assessment (Focused or Rapid)

Student: I am selecting the rapid physical exam to identify and treat life threats. I am checking for DCAP-BTLS. This acronym stands for deformities, contusions, abrasions, punctures, penetrations, and paradoxical motion in the chest, and burns, tenderness, lacerations, and swelling.
PROCTOR: Noted.

Head

Student: I am rapidly assessing the head.
PROCTOR: There is a graze injury involving the right temporal artery.
Student: I will apply direct pressure.
PROCTOR: The bleeding is controlled at this time.

Neck

Student: I am rapidly assessing the neck.
PROCTOR: There are no obvious injuries.
Student: I will apply a cervical collar.
PROCTOR: Noted.

▸ Chest

Student: I am rapidly inspecting and palpating the chest.
PROCTOR: The occlusive dressing is over the gunshot wound to the left upper chest.
Student: I will assess the chest for tension pneumothorax by auscultation, and assessment (jugular vein distention [JVD], tracheal deviation, and decreased lung sounds).
PROCTOR: The lung sounds appear diminished on the left, jugular vein distention is present, and the trachea is deviated to the right.
Student: I will burp the occlusive dressing on the left chest.
PROCTOR: Noted.
ALS Student: I will assess the chest for hyperresonance to percussion.
ALS Proctor: Noted. There is a tension pneumothorax on the left side.
ALS Student: I will decompress the left chest.
ALS Proctor: Noted. The decompression is effective.
ALS Student: I will continuously reassess the chest.
ALS Proctor: Noted.

▸ Abdomen/Pelvis

Student: I am rapidly assessing the abdomen.
PROCTOR: There are no obvious injuries.
Student: I am rapidly assessing the pelvis.
PROCTOR: The pelvis is stable with no obvious injuries.

▸ Extremities

Student: I am rapidly assessing the extremities.
PROCTOR: There are no obvious injuries.

▸ Assess Motor, Sensory, and Circulatory Function

Student: I am checking for DCAP-BTLS. I am also checking motor and sensory function, and pulses. Right leg?
PROCTOR: Negative DCAP-BTLS. Motor and sensory functions are present. Pulses are present.
Student: Left leg?
PROCTOR: Negative DCAP-BTLS. Motor and sensory functions are present. Pulses are present.
Student: Right arm?
PROCTOR: Negative DCAP-BTLS. Motor and sensory functions are present. Pulses are present.
Student: Left arm?
PROCTOR: Negative DCAP-BTLS. Motor and sensory functions are present. Pulses are present.

▸ Posterior

Student: I am rapidly assessing the back. We will now log roll the patient as a unit to check the back. The person at the head will count to three and we will roll the patient.
PROCTOR: Noted.

▸ Assess the Thorax

Student: I am assessing the thorax. Do I find injuries?
PROCTOR: No.

▸ Assess the Lumbar Area

Student: I am assessing the flanks and lumbar area. Do I find injuries?
PROCTOR: No.

▸ Assess the Entire Backside

Student: I am assessing the entire backside. Do I find injuries?
PROCTOR: No.

▸ Manage Secondary Injuries/Wounds

Student: We will apply a cervical collar and backboard with full immobilization per local protocol, if not yet done, at this time.
PROCTOR: Noted.
Student: Are there any changes in motor and sensory functions and pulses?
PROCTOR: No.

▸ Reevaluate Transport Decision

Student: This patient is a load-and-go due to gunshot wounds and shock.
PROCTOR: Noted.

▾ **Baseline Vital Signs**

Student: What are the patient's baseline vital signs, including blood pressure, pulse, respirations, pulse oximetry, and level of consciousness?
PROCTOR: Blood pressure, 110/72 mm Hg; pulse, 124 beats/min; respirations, 24 breaths/min; pulse oximetry reading, 91%; and the patient is alert.

▾ **SAMPLE History**

Student: At this time I will gather a SAMPLE history from the patient or family. What are the patient's signs and symptoms?
PROCTOR: Pain in the head and chest and difficulty breathing.
Student: Allergies?
PROCTOR: No allergies.
Student: Medications?
PROCTOR: No medications.
Student: Pertinent past medical history?
PROCTOR: Previously shot in the chest twice.
Student: Last oral intake?
PROCTOR: 2 hours ago.
Student: Events leading up to the injury or illness?
PROCTOR: The patient was robbing a gas station and was shot by the owner.

Critical Criteria:
- ❑ Did not differentiate patient's need for transportation versus continued assessment at the scene
- ❑ Did not provide for spinal protection when indicated

Detailed Physical Exam

Student: I am conducting the detailed physical exam. I am looking for DCAP-BTLS.
PROCTOR: Noted. The detailed physical exam will be performed during transport.

▾ **Assess the Head**

Student: I am assessing the head. Do I find any DCAP-BTLS? Do I find any evidence of Battle's sign or raccoon eyes?
PROCTOR: You note bleeding to the side of the head. Bleeding is controlled.

▸ Inspect and Palpate the Head and Ears

Student: I am assessing the head and ears.
PROCTOR: There are no obvious injuries.

▸ Assess the Eyes

Student: I am assessing the eyes. Are the pupils equal, round, and regular in size, and react properly to light (PEARRL)?
PROCTOR: They are PEARRL.

▸ Assess the Facial Area Including Oral and Nasal Areas

Student: I am assessing the face, nose, and mouth. Do I see any discharge or hear any obstructions?
PROCTOR: No.

▾ **Assess the Neck**

▸ Inspect and Palpate the Neck

Student: I am assessing the neck for DCAP-BTLS.
PROCTOR: There is no obvious DCAP-BTLS.

▸ Assess for Jugular Vein Distention

Student: Do I find any jugular vein distention (JVD)?
PROCTOR: No.

▸ Assess for Tracheal Deviation

Student: Do I see any tracheal deviation?
PROCTOR: No.

▾ **Assess the Chest**

Student: I am assessing the chest for DCAP-BTLS.
PROCTOR: Noted.

Student: I will assess the chest for tension pneumothorax by auscultation, and assessment (jugular vein distention [JVD], tracheal deviation, and decreased lung sounds).
PROCTOR: The lung sounds appear clear bilaterally, jugular vein distention is not present, and the trachea is midline.
ALS Student: I will assess the chest for hyperresonance to percussion.
ALS Proctor: Noted. There is no tension pneumothorax.
ALS Student: I will continuously reassess the chest.
ALS Proctor: Noted.

Inspect

Student: What do I see when I look at the chest?
PROCTOR: An occlusive dressing over the entrance wound to the left chest.
Student: Does the chest appear symmetric?
PROCTOR: Yes.

Palpate

Student: When I touch the chest, do I feel crepitus or a flail segment?
PROCTOR: No.

Auscultate

Student: Are they present in all fields?
PROCTOR: Yes.
Student: Do I hear any sucking sounds coming from the chest?
PROCTOR: No (if an occlusive dressing is in place).

Assess the Abdomen/Pelvis

Assess the Abdomen

Student: I am assessing the abdomen for DCAP-BTLS. I am assessing all four quadrants. Do I find any problems?
PROCTOR: No.

Assess the Pelvis

Student: I am assessing the pelvis for DCAP-BTLS. Is the pelvis stable?
PROCTOR: Yes.

Assess the Genitalia/Perineum as Needed (Verbalize in Training)

Student: I am assessing the genitalia/perineum as needed for DCAP-BTLS.
PROCTOR: The area is unremarkable.

Assess the Extremities

Inspect

Student: I am assessing the lower and upper extremities for DCAP-BTLS. Do I find anything?
PROCTOR: No.

Palpate

Student: Do I feel anything unusual?
PROCTOR: No.

Assess Motor, Sensory, and Circulatory Function

Student: I am checking for DCAP-BTLS, motor and sensory function, and pulses. Right leg?
PROCTOR: Negative DCAP-BTLS. Motor and sensory functions are present. Pulses are present.
Student: Left leg?
PROCTOR: Negative DCAP-BTLS. Motor and sensory functions are present. Pulses are present.
Student: Right arm?
PROCTOR: Negative DCAP-BTLS. Motor and sensory functions are present. Pulses are present.
Student: Left arm?
PROCTOR: Negative DCAP-BTLS. Motor and sensory functions are present. Pulses are present.

Assess the Posterior

Note: This portion of the detailed physical exam would not be done if the patient were previously backboarded per local protocol.
Student: We will not check the back since it was previously checked and the patient is backboarded.
PROCTOR: Noted.

Manage Secondary Injuries/Wounds

Student: I am covering the patient with a blanket to keep him warm.
PROCTOR: Noted.
ALS Student: I am performing basic life support (BLS) interventions, plus the following: I am starting two large-bore IVs.
ALS Proctor: Noted.
Student: Do I find any secondary injuries?
PROCTOR: No.

Reassess Vital Signs

Student: I will reassess vital signs and mental status.
PROCTOR: Blood pressure, 96/64 mm Hg; pulse, 130 beats/min; respirations, 24 breaths/min; pulse oximetry reading, 91%; and the patient is sleepy.
Student: The vital signs are deteriorating. The patient is now beginning to exhibit signs of impending decompensated shock.
PROCTOR: Noted.
ALS Student: I will administer IV fluid challenge of 20 mL/kg if necessary to maintain a minimum systolic blood pressure of 90 mm Hg.
ALS Proctor: Noted.

Reassess Interventions

Student: I will reassess my interventions: oxygen; bleeding control; occlusive dressing; burp the dressing if pneumothorax develops; and immobilization and straps.
PROCTOR: Noted.
ALS Student: I will reassess BLS interventions, plus the following: two large-bore IVs and cardiac monitoring.
ALS Proctor: Noted. The cardiac monitor shows sinus tachycardia.

Critical Criteria:
- ❑ Did not find or manage problems associated with airway, breathing, hemorrhage or shock (hypoperfusion)

Radio Report

(Provided by the student.)
PROCTOR: Noted.

Ongoing Assessment

Repeat Vital Signs

Student: I will reassess vital signs and mental status.

PROCTOR: Blood pressure, 110/62 mm Hg; pulse, 128 beats/min; respirations, 24 breaths/min; pulse oximetry reading, 91%; and the patient is sleepy.

Student: The vital signs have deteriorated.

PROCTOR: Noted.

Check Interventions

Student: I will check my interventions: oxygen; bleeding control; occlusive dressing; burp the dressing if pneumothorax develops; and immobilization and straps.

PROCTOR: Noted.

ALS Student: I will check BLS interventions, plus the following: two large-bore IVs and cardiac monitoring.

ALS Proctor: Noted. The cardiac monitor shows sinus tachycardia.

Critical Criteria:

- ❑ Did not find or manage problems associated with airway, breathing, hemorrhage or shock (hypoperfusion)

Handoff Report to Emergency Department Staff

Student: The patient's condition deteriorated during transport.

PROCTOR: Noted.

Critical Criteria:

- ❑ Did not transport patient within the (10) minute time limit

Critical Criteria

(Inform the student of items missed, if any.)

❑ Pass ❑ Fail Date: ______________________

Proctor Comments: ______________________

____

____

Dispatch Information

PROCTOR: EMS 10, respond to a 28-year-old male who has attempted suicide by slitting his wrists. His father says he is conscious and breathing and has apparently been drinking all day. Police officers are on scene.

Pre-scene Action (BSI)

Student: I am wearing nonlatex gloves, safety glasses, mask, and gown.
PROCTOR: Noted.

Critical Criteria:
- ❑ Did not take, or verbalize, body substance isolation (BSI) precautions when necessary

Scene Size-up

Scene Safety

Student: Is the scene safe?
PROCTOR: Yes, police are on scene and you are given clearance to enter.

Mechanism of Injury

Student: What was the mechanism of injury?
PROCTOR: Penetrating trauma to both arms. You find the patient ambulatory and drinking beer. The patient is depressed over a pending divorce. He admits to having been drinking all day and using a steak knife to slit his arms from the wrist to the elbow on both arms.

Number of Patients

Student: How many patients are there?
PROCTOR: One.

Additional Resources

Student: I would call for advanced life support (ALS) assistance.
PROCTOR: Noted.

C-Spine Stabilization

Student: I would not stabilize the cervical spine (c-spine).
PROCTOR: Noted.

Critical Criteria:
- ❑ Did not determine scene safety
- ❑ Did not assess for spinal protection
- ❑ Did not provide for spinal protection when indicated

Initial Assessment

Student: As I approach the patient, I identify myself and ask the patient not to move.
PROCTOR: Noted.

General Impression

Student: My general impression is that the patient's condition is unstable.
PROCTOR: Noted.

Responsiveness/Level of Consciousness

Student: What is the patient's level of consciousness?
PROCTOR: Alert.

Chief Complaint/Apparent Life Threats

Student: What is the patient's chief complaint?
PROCTOR: The patient wants to die.
Student: There are apparent life threats; the life threats are blood loss and suicidal wishes.
PROCTOR: Noted.

Assess the Airway and Breathing

Student: Is the patient breathing?
PROCTOR: Yes.

Assessment

Student: What are the rate and the quality of breathing?
PROCTOR: Rate: Tachypneic. Quality: Deep.

Provide Oxygen

Student: I am applying oxygen at 15 L/min via nonrebreathing mask.
PROCTOR: Noted.

Ensure Adequate Ventilation

Student: The patient has adequate ventilations at this time.
PROCTOR: Noted.

Injury Management

Student: I will direct my partner to control bleeding and apply direct pressure as I continue assessment.
PROCTOR: Noted.

Assess Circulation

Student: I am assessing the patient's circulation.
PROCTOR: Noted.

Assess for and Control Major Bleeding

Student: Do I find any major bleeding?
PROCTOR: Yes, heavy blood loss is evident throughout the house.
Student: I would apply direct pressure and a dressing.
PROCTOR: Noted.

Assess the Pulse

Student: What are the rate and the quality of pulses?
PROCTOR: Rate: Tachycardic. Quality: Thready.

Assess the Skin

Student: I am assessing the skin. What are the color, temperature, and condition of the skin?
PROCTOR: Color: Cyanotic. Temperature: Cold. Condition: Diaphoretic.

Identify Priority Patients/Make Transport Decision

Student: The patient is a high priority and is a load-and-go. I will begin packaging and transport.
PROCTOR: Noted.

Critical Criteria:
- ❑ Did not provide high concentration of oxygen
- ❑ Did not find or manage problems associated with airway, breathing, hemorrhage or shock (hypoperfusion)
- ❑ Did not differentiate patient's need for transportation versus continued assessment at the scene
- ❑ Did other detailed examination before assessing the airway, breathing and circulation

Focused History and Physical Examination/Rapid Trauma Assessment

Select the Appropriate Assessment (Focused or Rapid)

Student: I am selecting the rapid physical exam to identify and treat life threats. I am checking for DCAP-BTLS. This acronym stands for deformities, contusions, abrasions, punctures, penetrations, and paradoxical motion in the chest, and burns, tenderness, lacerations, and swelling.
PROCTOR: Noted.

Head

Student: I am rapidly assessing the head.
PROCTOR: There are no obvious injuries.

Neck

Student: I am rapidly assessing the neck.
PROCTOR: There are no obvious injuries.

Chest

Student: I am rapidly assessing the chest. What are the lung sounds?
PROCTOR: There are no obvious injuries. Lung sounds are clear bilaterally.

Abdomen/Pelvis

Student: I am rapidly assessing the abdomen.
PROCTOR: There are no obvious injuries.

Student: I am rapidly assessing the pelvis.

PROCTOR: There are no obvious injuries.

▸ **Extremities**

Student: I am rapidly assessing the extremities.

PROCTOR: The incisions to both arms are to the bone, with muscle tissue exposed and hanging loose prior to dressing.

▸ **Posterior**

Student: We will now check the back.

PROCTOR: Noted.

▸ **Assess the Thorax**

Student: I am assessing the thorax. Do I find injuries?

PROCTOR: No.

▸ **Assess the Lumbar Area**

Student: I am assessing the flanks and lumbar area. Do I find injuries?

PROCTOR: No.

▸ **Assess the Entire Backside**

Student: I am assessing the entire backside. Do I find injuries?

PROCTOR: No.

▸ **Manage Secondary Injuries**

ALS Student: I will establish two large-bore IVs en route to the hospital and administer a bolus of 20 mL/kg in order to maintain a systolic blood pressure of 90 mm Hg.

ALS Proctor: Noted.

▸ **Reevaluate Transport Decision**

Student: This patient is a load-and-go due to blood loss and shock.

PROCTOR: Noted.

▼ Baseline Vital Signs

Student: What are the patient's baseline vital signs, including blood pressure, pulse, respirations, pulse oximetry, and level of consciousness?

PROCTOR: Blood pressure, 88/50 mm Hg; pulse rate, 134 beats/min; respirations, 24 breaths/min; pulse oximetry reading, N/A; and the patient is tired.

▼ SAMPLE History

Student: At this time I will gather a SAMPLE history from the patient or family. What are the patient's signs and symptoms?

PROCTOR: He says he wanted to die. He does not think he has anything to live for.

Student: Allergies?

PROCTOR: No allergies.

Student: Medications?

PROCTOR: Inhaler.

Student: Pertinent past medical history?

PROCTOR: Asthma.

Student: Last oral intake?

PROCTOR: Drinking beer all afternoon.

Student: Events leading up to the incident?

PROCTOR: The patient was upset over his divorce.

Critical Criteria:

- ☐ Did not differentiate patient's need for transportation versus continued assessment at the scene
- ☐ Did not provide for spinal protection when indicated

▼ Detailed Physical Examination

Student: I am conducting the detailed physical exam. I am looking for DCAP-BTLS.

PROCTOR: Noted. The detailed physical exam will be performed during transport.

▼ Assess the Head

Student: I am assessing the head. Do I find any DCAP-BTLS? Do I find any evidence of Battle's sign or raccoon eyes?

PROCTOR: No.

▸ **Inspect and Palpate the Head and Ears**

Student: I am assessing the head and ears.

PROCTOR: There are no obvious injuries.

▸ **Assess the Eyes**

Student: I am assessing the eyes. Are the pupils equal, round, and regular in size, and react properly to light (PEARRL)?

PROCTOR: They are sluggish.

▸ **Assess the Facial Area Including Oral and Nasal Areas**

Student: I am assessing the face, nose, and mouth. Do I see any discharge or hear any obstructions?

PROCTOR: No.

▼ Assess the Neck

▸ **Inspect and Palpate the Neck**

Student: I am assessing the neck for DCAP-BTLS.

PROCTOR: There are no obvious injuries.

▸ **Assess for Jugular Vein Distention**

Student: Do I find any jugular vein distention (JVD)?

PROCTOR: No.

▸ **Assess for Tracheal Deviation**

Student: Do I see any tracheal deviation?

PROCTOR: No.

▼ Assess the Chest

Student: I am assessing the chest for DCAP-BTLS.

PROCTOR: Noted.

▸ **Inspect**

Student: What do I see when I look at the chest?

PROCTOR: There are no obvious injuries.

Student: Does the chest appear symmetric?

PROCTOR: Yes.

▸ **Palpate**

Student: When I touch the chest, do I feel crepitus or a flail segment?

PROCTOR: No.

▸ **Auscultate**

Student: Are lung sounds present in all fields?

PROCTOR: Yes.

Student: Do I hear any sucking sounds from the chest?

PROCTOR: No.

▼ Assess the Abdomen/Pelvis

▸ **Assess the Abdomen**

Student: I am assessing the abdomen for DCAP-BTLS. I am assessing all four quadrants. Do I find any problems?

PROCTOR: No.

▸ **Assess the Pelvis**

Student: I am assessing the pelvis for DCAP-BTLS. Is the pelvis stable?

PROCTOR: Yes.

▸ **Assess the Genitalia/Perineum as Needed (Verbalize in Training)**

Student: I am assessing the genitalia/perineum as necessary for DCAP-BTLS.

PROCTOR: The area is unremarkable.

▼ Assess the Extremities

▸ **Inspect**

Student: I am assessing the lower and upper extremities for DCAP-BTLS. Do I find anything?

PROCTOR: Yes.

▸ **Palpate**

Student: Do I feel anything unusual?

PROCTOR: Yes.

▸ **Assess Motor, Sensory, and Circulatory Function**

Student: I am checking for DCAP-BTLS, motor and sensory function, and pulses. Right leg?

PROCTOR: Negative DCAP-BTLS. Motor and sensory functions are present. Pulses are absent.

Student: Left leg?
PROCTOR: Negative DCAP-BTLS. Motor and sensory functions are present. Pulses are absent.
Student: Right arm?
PROCTOR: Bleeding from the wounds to the lateral arm is controlled with minimal pressure. Motor and sensory functions are present. Pulses are absent.
Student: Left arm?
PROCTOR: Bleeding from the wounds to the medial arm is controlled with minimal pressure. Motor and sensory functions are present. Pulses are absent.

▼ Assess the Posterior
Student: We will not check the back since it was checked earlier.
PROCTOR: Noted.

▼ Manage Secondary Injuries/Wounds
Student: I would direct my partner to continue with direct pressure to control bleeding.
PROCTOR: Noted.

▼ Reassess Vital Signs
Student: I will reassess vital signs and mental status.
PROCTOR: Blood pressure, 80 mm Hg by palpation; pulse rate, 140 beats/min; respirations, 24 breaths/min; pulse oximetry reading, N/A; and the patient is responsive to verbal commands.
Student: The vital signs are deteriorating.
PROCTOR: Noted.

▼ Reassess Interventions
Student: I will reassess my interventions: oxygen, bleeding control, and reassurance.
PROCTOR: Noted.
ALS Student: I will reassess basic life support (BLS) interventions, plus the following: two large-bore IVs and cardiac monitor.
ALS Proctor: Noted. The cardiac monitor shows sinus tachycardia.

Critical Criteria:
❑ Did not find or manage problems associated with airway, breathing, hemorrhage or shock (hypoperfusion)

▼ Radio Report
(Provided by the student.)
PROCTOR: Noted.

▼ Ongoing Assessment

▼ Repeat Vital Signs
Student: I will reassess vital signs and mental status.
PROCTOR: Blood pressure, 76 mm Hg by palpation; pulse rate, 136 beats/min; respirations, 24 breaths/min; pulse oximetry reading, N/A; and the patient is responsive to verbal commands.
Student: The vital signs have deteriorated.
PROCTOR: Noted.

▼ Check Interventions
Student: I will check my interventions: oxygen, bleeding control, and reassurance.
PROCTOR: Noted.
ALS Student: I will check BLS interventions, plus the following: two large-bore IVs and cardiac monitor.
ALS Proctor: Noted. The cardiac monitor shows sinus tachycardia.

Critical Criteria:
❑ Did not find or manage problems associated with airway, breathing, hemorrhage or shock (hypoperfusion)

▼ Handoff Report to Emergency Department Staff
Student: The patient's condition deteriorated during transport.
PROCTOR: Noted.

Critical Criteria:
❑ Did not transport patient within the (10) minute time limit

▼ Critical Criteria
(Inform the student of items missed, if any.)

❑ Pass ❑ Fail Date: ____________________

Proctor Comments: ____________________

CASE 2

Notes

CASE 3

Dispatch Information

PROCTOR: EMS 10, respond to a welding accident involving a 35-year-old male. The patient has been burned and crushed. He is conscious and breathing.

Pre-scene Action (BSI)

Student: I am wearing nonlatex gloves, safety glasses, mask, and gown.
PROCTOR: Noted.

Critical Criteria:
- ❑ Did not take, or verbalize, body substance isolation (BSI) precautions when necessary

Scene Size-up

Scene Safety

Student: Is the scene safe?
PROCTOR: Yes.

Mechanism of Injury

Student: What was the mechanism of injury?
PROCTOR: Burn and crush injury. You find that the patient has removed himself from under the bed of the trailer and is ambulatory. The patient was using a cutting torch to convert a truck bed into a trailer when the bed fell on his arm; the cutting torch burned his other hand.

Number of Patients

Student: How many patients are there?
PROCTOR: One.

Additional Resources

Student: I would call for advanced life support (ALS) assistance and fire/rescue.
PROCTOR: Noted.

C-Spine Stabilization

Student: I would not stabilize the cervical spine (c-spine) because the injury is isolated to the patient's arm and hand.
PROCTOR: Noted.

Critical Criteria:
- ❑ Did not determine scene safety
- ❑ Did not assess for spinal protection
- ❑ Did not provide for spinal protection when indicated

Initial Assessment

Student: As I approach the patient, I identify myself and ask the patient not to move.
PROCTOR: Noted.

General Impression

Student: My general impression is that the patient's condition is stable.
PROCTOR: Noted.

Responsiveness/Level of Consciousness

Student: What is the patient's level of consciousness?
PROCTOR: Alert.

Chief Complaint/Apparent Life Threats

Student: What is the patient's chief complaint?
PROCTOR: The patient is complaining of burns to his right hand and a broken left arm.
Student: There are no apparent life threats.
PROCTOR: Noted.

Assess the Airway and Breathing

Student: Is the patient breathing?
PROCTOR: Yes.

Assessment

Student: What are the rate and the quality of breathing?
PROCTOR: Rate: Adequate. Quality: Deep.

Provide Oxygen

Student: I am applying oxygen at 15 L/min via nonrebreathing mask.
PROCTOR: Noted.

Ensure Adequate Ventilation

Student: The patient has adequate ventilations at this time.
PROCTOR: Noted.

Injury Management

Student: I will direct my partner to continue providing oxygen.
PROCTOR: Noted.

Assess Circulation

Student: I am assessing the patient's circulation.
PROCTOR: Noted.

Assess for and Control Major Bleeding

Student: Do I find any major bleeding?
PROCTOR: No.

Assess the Pulse

Student: What are the rate and the quality of pulses?
PROCTOR: Rate: Slightly tachycardic. Quality: Strong.

Assess the Skin

Student: I am assessing the skin. What are the color, temperature, and condition of the skin?
PROCTOR: Color: Flushed. Temperature: Hot. Condition: Moist.

Identify Priority Patients/Make Transport Decision

Student: The patient is a high priority and is a load-and-go due to a burn to the hand. I will begin packaging and transport to a burn center.
PROCTOR: Noted.

Critical Criteria:
- ❑ Did not provide high concentration of oxygen
- ❑ Did not find or manage problems associated with airway, breathing, hemorrhage or shock (hypoperfusion).
- ❑ Did not differentiate patient's need for transportation versus continued assessment at the scene
- ❑ Did other detailed examination before assessing the airway, breathing and circulation

Focused History and Physical Examination/Rapid Trauma Assessment

Select the Appropriate Assessment (Focused or Rapid)

Student: I am selecting the rapid physical exam to identify and treat life threats. I am checking for DCAP-BTLS. This acronym stands for deformities, contusions, abrasions, punctures, penetrations, and paradoxical motion in the chest, and burns, tenderness, lacerations, and swelling.
PROCTOR: Noted.

Head

Student: I am rapidly assessing the head.
PROCTOR: There are no obvious injuries.

Neck

Student: I am rapidly assessing the neck.
PROCTOR: There are no obvious injuries.

Chest

Student: I am rapidly assessing the chest. What are the lung sounds?
PROCTOR: There are no obvious injuries. Lung sounds are clear bilaterally.

Abdomen/Pelvis

Student: I am rapidly assessing the abdomen.
PROCTOR: There are no obvious injuries.
Student: I am rapidly assessing the pelvis.
PROCTOR: There are no obvious injuries.

▸ **Extremities**

Student: I am rapidly assessing the extremities.

PROCTOR: There are no obvious injuries.

▸ **Assess Motor, Sensory, and Circulatory Function**

Student: I am checking for DCAP-BTLS. I am also checking motor and sensory function, and pulses. Right leg?

PROCTOR: Negative DCAP-BTLS. Motor and sensory functions are absent. Pulses are present.

Student: Left leg?

PROCTOR: Negative DCAP-BTLS. Motor and sensory functions are absent. Pulses are present.

Student: Right arm?

PROCTOR: You find that the wound is open and the bone appears to be burned. The whole hand is swollen and blistered. (This is a full-thickness burn.) Motor and sensory functions are present. Pulses are present.

Student: I would stop the burning process and dress the burn per protocol.

PROCTOR: Noted.

Student: Left arm?

PROCTOR: There is a compound fracture to the ulna/radius. Motor and sensory functions are present. Pulses are present.

Student: I would splint the arm and use a sling and swathe.

PROCTOR: Noted.

Student: Are there any changes in motor and sensory functions and pulses?

PROCTOR: No.

▸ **Posterior**

Student: We will check the back.

PROCTOR: Noted.

▸ **Assess the Thorax**

Student: I am assessing the thorax. Do I find injuries?

PROCTOR: No.

▸ **Assess the Lumbar Area**

Student: I am assessing the flanks and lumbar area. Do I find injuries?

PROCTOR: No.

▸ **Assess the Entire Backside**

Student: I am assessing the entire backside. Do I find injuries?

PROCTOR: No.

▸ **Manage Secondary Injuries**

ALS Student: I will establish two large-bore IVs en route to the hospital and administer a bolus of 20 mL/kg in order to maintain a systolic blood pressure of 90 mm Hg.

ALS Proctor: Noted.

▸ **Reevaluate Transport Decision**

Student: This patient is a high priority and requires transport to a burn center.

PROCTOR: Noted.

▾ Baseline Vital Signs

Student: What are the patient's baseline vital signs, including blood pressure, pulse, respirations, pulse oximetry, and level of consciousness?

PROCTOR: Blood pressure, 138/90 mm Hg; pulse rate, 120 beats/min; respirations, 24 breaths/min; pulse oximetry reading, 99%; and the patient is alert.

▾ SAMPLE History

Student: At this time I will gather a SAMPLE history from the patient or family. What are the patient's signs and symptoms?

PROCTOR: He has a burn to the right hand and a fracture to the left arm.

Student: Allergies?

PROCTOR: No allergies.

Student: Medications?

PROCTOR: No medications.

Student: Pertinent past medical history?

PROCTOR: No pertinent medical history.

Student: Last oral intake?

PROCTOR: 4 hours ago.

Student: Events leading up to the incident?

PROCTOR: The patient was under the bed of a truck using a cutting torch when the jack failed and the bed fell on his left arm, pinning the torch to his right hand for a moment.

Critical Criteria:

- ❑ Did not differentiate patient's need for transportation versus continued assessment at the scene
- ❑ Did not provide for spinal protection when indicated

▼ Detailed Physical Examination

Student: I am conducting the detailed physical exam. I am looking for DCAP-BTLS.

PROCTOR: Noted. The detailed physical exam will be performed during transport.

▾ Assess the Head

Student: I am assessing the head. Do I find any DCAP-BTLS? Do I find any evidence of Battle's sign or raccoon eyes?

PROCTOR: No.

▸ **Inspect and Palpate the Head and Ears**

Student: I am assessing the head and ears.

PROCTOR: There are no obvious injuries.

▸ **Assess the Eyes**

Student: I am assessing the eyes. Are the pupils equal, round, and regular in size, and react properly to light (PEARRL)?

PROCTOR: They are PEARRL.

▸ **Assess the Facial Area Including Oral and Nasal Areas**

Student: I am assessing the face, nose, and mouth. Do I see any discharge or hear any obstructions?

PROCTOR: No.

▾ Assess the Neck

▸ **Inspect and Palpate the Neck**

Student: I am assessing the neck for DCAP-BTLS.

PROCTOR: There are no obvious injuries.

▸ **Assess for Jugular Vein Distention**

Student: Do I find any jugular vein distention (JVD)?

PROCTOR: No.

▸ **Assess for Tracheal Deviation**

Student: Do I see any tracheal deviation?

PROCTOR: No.

▾ Assess the Chest

Student: I am assessing the chest for DCAP-BTLS.

PROCTOR: Noted.

▸ **Inspect**

Student: What do I see when I look at the chest?

PROCTOR: There are no obvious injuries.

Student: Does the chest appear symmetric?

PROCTOR: Yes.

▸ **Palpate**

Student: When I touch the chest, do I feel crepitus or a flail segment?

PROCTOR: No.

▸ **Auscultate**

Student: Are lung sounds present in all fields?

PROCTOR: Yes.

▾ Assess the Abdomen/Pelvis

▸ **Assess the Abdomen**

Student: I am assessing the abdomen for DCAP-BTLS. I am assessing all four quadrants. Do I find any problems?

PROCTOR: No.

▸ **Assess the Pelvis**

Student: I am assessing the pelvis for DCAP-BTLS. Is the pelvis stable?

PROCTOR: Yes.

Assess the Genitalia/Perineum as Needed (Verbalize in Training)

Student: I am assessing the genitalia/perineum as necessary for DCAP-BTLS.

PROCTOR: The area is unremarkable.

Assess the Extremities

Inspect

Student: I am assessing the lower and upper extremities for DCAP-BTLS. Do I find anything?

PROCTOR: Yes, the burn to the right hand is dressed and the deformed, swollen left arm is splinted.

Palpate

Student: Do I feel anything unusual?

PROCTOR: No.

Assess Motor, Sensory, and Circulatory Function

Student: I will recheck for DCAP-BTLS, motor and sensory function, and pulses. Right leg?

PROCTOR: Negative DCAP-BTLS. Motor and sensory functions are present. Pulses are present.

Student: Left leg?

PROCTOR: Negative DCAP-BTLS. Motor and sensory functions are present. Pulses are present.

Student: Right arm?

PROCTOR: The burn wound is dressed. Motor and sensory functions are present. Pulses are present.

Student: Left arm?

PROCTOR: The ulna/radius fracture is splinted. Motor and sensory functions are present. Pulses are present.

Assess the Posterior

Student: We will not check the back since it was checked earlier.

PROCTOR: Noted.

Manage Secondary Injuries/Wounds

Student: I would direct my partner to reassess the hand.

PROCTOR: Noted.

Reassess Vital Signs

Student: I will reassess vital signs and mental status.

PROCTOR: Blood pressure, 134/84 mm Hg; pulse rate, 112 beats/min, respirations, 20 breaths/min; pulse oximetry reading, 99%; and the patient is alert.

Student: The vital signs have not changed significantly.

PROCTOR: Noted.

Reassess Interventions

Student: I will reassess my interventions: oxygen, burn dressing, splint, and sling and swathe.

PROCTOR: Noted.

ALS Student: I will reassess basic life support (BLS) interventions, plus the following: one or two large-bore IVs and pain management per protocol.

ALS Proctor: Noted.

Critical Criteria:

❑ Did not find or manage problems associated with airway, breathing, hemorrhage or shock (hypoperfusion)

Radio Report

(Provided by the student.)

PROCTOR: Noted.

Ongoing Assessment

Repeat Vital Signs

Student: I will reassess vital signs and mental status.

PROCTOR: Blood pressure, 130/78 mm Hg; pulse rate, 108 beats/min, respirations, 20 breaths/min; pulse oximetry reading, 99%; and the patient is alert.

Student: The vital signs have not changed significantly.

PROCTOR: Noted.

Check Interventions

Student: I will check my interventions: oxygen, burn dressing, splint, and sling and swathe.

PROCTOR: Noted.

ALS Student: I will check BLS interventions, plus the following: IVs and pain management per protocol.

ALS Proctor: Noted.

Critical Criteria:

❑ Did not find or manage problems associated with airway, breathing, hemorrhage or shock (hypoperfusion)

Handoff Report to Emergency Department Staff

Student: There was no change during transport.

PROCTOR: Noted.

Critical Criteria:

❑ Did not transport patient within the (10) minute time limit

Critical Criteria

(Inform the student of items missed, if any.)

❑ Pass ❑ Fail Date: ____________________

Proctor Comments: ____________________

____

____

Notes

Dispatch Information

PROCTOR: EMS 10, respond with EMS 12 to a two-car motor vehicle collision. There are two patients.

Pre-scene Action (BSI)

Student: I am wearing a high-visibility vest, personal protective equipment, helmet, extrication gloves, nonlatex gloves, safety glasses, mask, and gown.
PROCTOR: Noted.

Critical Criteria:
- ❑ Did not take, or verbalize, body substance isolation (BSI) precautions when necessary

Scene Size-up

Scene Safety

Student: Is the scene safe?
PROCTOR: Yes.

Mechanism of Injury

Student: What was the mechanism of injury?
PROCTOR: Motor vehicle collision. The patient was driving and was struck head-on by someone making a left turn. She is complaining of a cut on her face and some pain to the arm. She was wearing a seat belt and the airbag deployed.

Number of Patients

Student: How many patients are there?
PROCTOR: One 76-year-old patient; EMS 12 will treat the other patient.

Additional Resources

Student: I would call for additional resources: fire/rescue and police.
PROCTOR: Noted.

C-Spine Stabilization

Student: On the basis of the mechanism of injury, I would stabilize the cervical spine (c-spine) in a neutral in-line position.
PROCTOR: Noted.

Critical Criteria:
- ❑ Did not determine scene safety
- ❑ Did not assess for spinal protection
- ❑ Did not provide for spinal protection when indicated

Initial Assessment

Student: As I perform midline c-spine stabilization, I identify myself and ask the patient not to move.
PROCTOR: Noted.

General Impression

Student: My general impression is that the patient's condition is stable.
PROCTOR: Noted.

Responsiveness/Level of Consciousness

Student: What is the patient's level of consciousness?
PROCTOR: Alert.

Chief Complaint/Apparent Life Threats

Student: What is the patient's chief complaint?
PROCTOR: The patient is complaining of a cut on her face and right arm pain.
Student: There are no apparent life threats.
PROCTOR: Noted.

Assess the Airway and Breathing

Student: Is the airway open? Is the patient breathing?
PROCTOR: Yes, the airway is open and the patient is breathing.

Assessment

Student: What are the rate and the quality of breathing?
PROCTOR: Rate: Within normal limits. Quality: Normal.

Provide Oxygen

Student: I am applying oxygen at 15 L/min via nonrebreathing mask.
PROCTOR: Noted.

Ensure Adequate Ventilation

Student: The patient has adequate ventilations at this time.
PROCTOR: Noted.

Injury Management

Student: I will direct my partner to take over c-spine control as I continue assessment.
PROCTOR: Noted.

Assess Circulation

Student: I am assessing the patient's circulation.
PROCTOR: Noted.

Assess for and Control Major Bleeding

Student: Do I find any major bleeding?
PROCTOR: No.

Assess the Pulse

Student: What are the rate and the quality of pulses?
PROCTOR: Rate: Within normal limits. Quality: Normal.

Assess the Skin

Student: I am assessing the skin. What are the color, temperature, and condition of the skin?
PROCTOR: Color: Normal. Temperature: Warm. Condition: Normal.

Identify Priority Patients/Make Transport Decision

Student: The patient is a low priority and does not require immediate transport.
PROCTOR: Noted.

Critical Criteria:
- ❑ Did not provide high concentration of oxygen
- ❑ Did not find or manage problems associated with airway, breathing, hemorrhage or shock (hypoperfusion)
- ❑ Did not differentiate patient's need for transportation versus continued assessment at the scene
- ❑ Did other detailed examination before assessing the airway, breathing and circulation

Focused History and Physical Examination/Rapid Trauma Assessment

Select the Appropriate Assessment (Focused or Rapid)

Student: I am selecting the rapid physical exam to identify and treat life threats. I am checking for DCAP-BTLS. This acronym stands for deformities, contusions, abrasions, punctures, penetrations, and paradoxical motion in the chest, and burns, tenderness, lacerations, and swelling.
PROCTOR: Noted.

Head

Student: I am rapidly assessing the head.
PROCTOR: There is a small cut from the patient's glasses from when the airbag deployed. The nosepiece of her glasses punctured the skin between the patient's nose and eye. Bleeding is insignificant; we will dress and bandage it while en route.

Neck

Student: I am rapidly assessing the neck.
PROCTOR: There are no obvious injuries.
Student: I will apply a cervical collar.
PROCTOR: Noted.

Chest

Student: I am rapidly assessing the chest. What are the lung sounds?
PROCTOR: There are no obvious injuries. Lung sounds are clear bilaterally.

▸ **Abdomen/Pelvis**

Student: I am rapidly assessing the abdomen.
PROCTOR: There are no obvious injuries.
Student: I am rapidly assessing the pelvis.
PROCTOR: There are no obvious injuries.

▸ **Extremities**

Student: I am rapidly assessing the extremities.
PROCTOR: There is an open fracture to the right ulna/radius. The patient is holding her right arm against her chest with her left arm.

▸ **Assess Motor, Sensory, and Circulatory Function**

Student: I am checking for DCAP-BTLS. I am also checking motor and sensory function, and pulses. Right arm?
PROCTOR: There is an open wound and deformity to the right ulna/radius. The patient is holding her right arm against her chest.
Student: I will apply a dressing to the wound on her right arm and splint it in the position of function. I will check pulse and motor and sensory function before and after splinting.
PROCTOR: Noted. Motor and sensory functions are present. Pulses are present.
Student: Left arm?
PROCTOR: Negative DCAP-BTLS. Motor and sensory functions are present. Pulses are present.
Student: Right leg?
PROCTOR: Negative DCAP-BTLS. Motor and sensory functions are present. Pulses are present.
Student: Left leg?
PROCTOR: Negative DCAP-BTLS. Motor and sensory functions are present. Pulses are present.

▸ **Posterior**

Student: We will check the patient's back while she is sitting in the car.
PROCTOR: Noted.

▸ **Assess the Thorax**

Student: I am assessing the thorax. Do I find injuries?
PROCTOR: No.

▸ **Assess the Lumbar Area**

Student: I am assessing the flanks and lumbar area. Do I find injuries?
PROCTOR: No.

▸ **Assess the Entire Backside**

Student: I am assessing the entire backside. Do I find injuries?
PROCTOR: No.

▸ **Manage Secondary Injuries/Wounds**

Student: We will use a Kendrick extrication device (KED) per protocol. We will transfer the patient to a backboard, checking pulse and motor and sensory function before and after immobilizing her. The person at the head will count to three and we will transfer the patient.
PROCTOR: Noted.
Student: Are there any changes in motor and sensory functions and pulses?
PROCTOR: No.

▸ **Reevaluate Transport Decision**

Student: The patient is a low priority and does not require immediate transport.
PROCTOR: Noted.

▾ Baseline Vital Signs

Student: What are the patient's baseline vital signs, including blood pressure, pulse, respirations, pulse oximetry, and level of consciousness?
PROCTOR: Blood pressure, 140/86 mm Hg; pulse rate, 96 beats/min; respirations, 16 breaths/min; pulse oximetry reading, 98%; and the patient is alert.

▾ SAMPLE History

Student: At this time I will gather a SAMPLE history from the patient or family. What are the patient's signs and symptoms?
PROCTOR: She has pain in the right arm.
Student: Allergies?
PROCTOR: No allergies.
Student: Medications?
PROCTOR: Calcium supplements.
Student: Pertinent past medical history?
PROCTOR: Osteoporosis.
Student: Last oral intake?
PROCTOR: 3 hours ago.
Student: Events leading up to the incident?
PROCTOR: She was a restrained driver in a near head-on collision.

Critical Criteria:
- ❑ Did not differentiate patient's need for transportation versus continued assessment at the scene
- ❑ Did not provide for spinal protection when indicated

▼ Detailed Physical Examination

Student: I am conducting the detailed physical exam. I am looking for DCAP-BTLS.
PROCTOR: Noted. The detailed physical exam will be performed during transport.

▾ Assess the Head

Student: I am assessing the head. Do I find any DCAP-BTLS? Do I find any evidence of Battle's sign or raccoon eyes?
PROCTOR: No.

▸ **Inspect and Palpate the Head and Ears**

Student: I am assessing the head and ears.
PROCTOR: There is an 8-mm laceration from the nose piece of the patient's glasses above her right eye. Bleeding is insignificant.
Student: I will dress the laceration.
PROCTOR: Noted.

▸ **Assess the Eyes**

Student: I am assessing the eyes. Are the pupils equal, round, and regular in size, and react properly to light (PEARRL)?
PROCTOR: They are PEARRL.

▸ **Assess the Facial Area Including Oral and Nasal Areas**

Student: I am assessing the face, nose, and mouth. Do I see any discharge or hear any obstructions?
PROCTOR: No.

▾ Assess the Neck

▸ **Inspect and Palpate the Neck**

Student: I am assessing the neck for DCAP-BTLS.
PROCTOR: There are no obvious injuries.

▸ **Assess for Jugular Vein Distention**

Student: Do I find any jugular vein distention (JVD)?
PROCTOR: No.

▸ **Assess for Tracheal Deviation**

Student: Do I see any tracheal deviation?
PROCTOR: No.

▾ Assess the Chest

Student: I am assessing the chest for DCAP-BTLS.
PROCTOR: Noted.

▸ **Inspect**

Student: What do I see when I look at the chest?
PROCTOR: There are no obvious injuries.
Student: Does the chest appear symmetric?
PROCTOR: Yes.

▸ **Palpate**

Student: When I touch the chest, do I feel crepitus or a flail segment?

PROCTOR: No.

▸ **Auscultate**

Student: Are lung sounds present in all fields?

PROCTOR: Yes.

Student: Do I hear any sucking sounds from the chest?

PROCTOR: No.

▾ Assess the Abdomen/Pelvis

▸ **Assess the Abdomen**

Student: I am assessing the abdomen for DCAP-BTLS. I am assessing all four quadrants. Do I find any problems?

PROCTOR: No.

▸ **Assess the Pelvis**

Student: I am assessing the pelvis for DCAP-BTLS. Is the pelvis stable?

PROCTOR: Yes.

▸ **Assess the Genitalia/Perineum as Needed (Verbalize in Training)**

Student: I am assessing the genitalia/perineum as necessary for DCAP-BTLS.

PROCTOR: The area is unremarkable.

▾ Assess the Extremities

▸ **Inspect**

Student: I am assessing the lower and upper extremities for DCAP-BTLS. Do I find anything?

PROCTOR: Yes.

▸ **Palpate**

Student: Do I feel anything unusual?

PROCTOR: Yes.

▸ **Assess Motor, Sensory, and Circulatory Function**

Student: I am checking for DCAP-BTLS, motor and sensory function, and pulses. Right arm?

PROCTOR: The arm is splinted.

Student: I will recheck pulse and motor and sensory function.

PROCTOR: Noted. Motor and sensory functions are present. Pulses are present.

Student: Left arm?

PROCTOR: Negative DCAP-BTLS. Motor and sensory functions are present. Pulses are present.

Student: Right leg?

PROCTOR: Negative DCAP-BTLS. Motor and sensory functions are present. Pulses are present.

Student: Left leg?

PROCTOR: Negative DCAP-BTLS. Motor and sensory functions are present. Pulses are present.

▾ Assess the Posterior

Note: This portion of the detailed physical exam would not be done if the patient were previously backboarded per local protocol.

Student: We will not check the back since it was previously checked and the patient is backboarded.

PROCTOR: Noted.

▾ Manage Secondary Injuries/Wounds

Student: I would direct my partner to reassure the patient.

PROCTOR: Noted.

▾ Reassess Vital Signs

Student: I will reassess vital signs and mental status.

PROCTOR: Blood pressure, 136/80 mm Hg; pulse rate, 88 beats/min; respirations, 16 breaths/min; pulse oximetry reading, 98%; and the patient is alert.

Student: The vital signs have not changed significantly.

PROCTOR: Noted.

▾ Reassess Interventions

Student: I will reassess my interventions: oxygen, bleeding control, splint to the right arm, and full immobilization.

PROCTOR: Noted.

Critical Criteria:

❑ Did not find or manage problems associated with airway, breathing, hemorrhage or shock (hypoperfusion)

▼ Radio Report

(Provided by the student.)

PROCTOR: Noted.

▼ Ongoing Assessment

▾ Repeat Vital Signs

Student: I will reassess vital signs and mental status.

PROCTOR: Blood pressure, 130/80 mm Hg; pulse rate, 86 beats/min; respirations, 16 breaths/min; pulse oximetry reading, 98%; and the patient is alert.

Student: The vital signs have not changed significantly.

PROCTOR: Noted.

▾ Check Interventions

Student: I will check my interventions: oxygen, bleeding control, splint to the right arm, and full immobilization.

PROCTOR: Noted.

Critical Criteria:

❑ Did not find or manage problems associated with airway, breathing, hemorrhage or shock (hypoperfusion)

▼ Handoff Report to Emergency Department Staff

Student: There was no change during transport.

PROCTOR: Noted.

Critical Criteria:

❑ Did not transport patient within the (10) minute time limit

▼ Critical Criteria

(Inform the student of items missed, if any.)

❑ Pass ❑ Fail Date: ____________________

Proctor Comments: ____________________

____

____

CASE 4

Notes

CASE 5

Dispatch Information

PROCTOR: EMS 10, respond to a report of a car that has fallen on a 28-year-old mechanic. It is unknown if he is conscious or breathing.

Pre-scene Action (BSI)

Student: I am wearing personal protective equipment, a helmet, extrication gloves, nonlatex gloves, safety glasses, mask, and gown.
PROCTOR: Noted.

Critical Criteria:
- ❑ Did not take, or verbalize, body substance isolation (BSI) precautions when necessary

Scene Size-up

Scene Safety

Student: Is the scene safe?
PROCTOR: Yes.

Mechanism of Injury

Student: What was the mechanism of injury?
PROCTOR: Crush injury. The patient was working under a car when the jack failed and the car fell on top of him. He is pinned under the car.

Number of Patients

Student: How many patients are there?
PROCTOR: One.

Additional Resources

Student: I would call for advanced life support (ALS) assistance and fire/rescue. I will first have the fire department responders lift the car.
PROCTOR: Noted.

C-Spine Stabilization

Student: On the basis of the mechanism of injury, I would stabilize the cervical spine (c-spine) in a neutral in-line position.
PROCTOR: Noted.

Critical Criteria:
- ❑ Did not determine scene safety
- ❑ Did not assess for spinal protection
- ❑ Did not provide for spinal protection when indicated

Initial Assessment

Student: As I perform midline c-spine stabilization, I identify myself and ask the patient not to move.
PROCTOR: Noted.

General Impression

Student: My general impression is that the patient's condition is unstable.
PROCTOR: Noted.

Responsiveness/Level of Consciousness

Student: What is the patient's level of consciousness?
PROCTOR: Alert.

Chief Complaint/Apparent Life Threats

Student: What is the patient's chief complaint?
PROCTOR: The patient is complaining of chest, abdominal, and left arm pain.
Student: There is an apparent life threat; the mechanism of injury (MOI) indicates possible life-threatening injuries to the chest and abdomen.
PROCTOR: Noted.

Assess the Airway and Breathing

Student: The patient is talking to me, so his airway is open. Is it clear? Is the patient breathing?
PROCTOR: Yes, the airway is clear and the patient is breathing.

Assessment

Student: What are the rate and the quality of breathing?
PROCTOR: Rate: Rapid. Quality: Shallow.

Provide Oxygen

Student: I am assisting ventilations with a bag-valve device with 100% oxygen.
PROCTOR: Noted.

Ensure Adequate Ventilation

Student: I am assisting ventilations with the bag-valve device.
PROCTOR: Noted.

Injury Management

Student: I will direct my partner to take over c-spine control and ventilation as I continue assessment.
PROCTOR: Noted.

Assess Circulation

Student: I am assessing the patient's circulation.
PROCTOR: Noted.

Assess for and Control Major Bleeding

Student: Do I find any major bleeding?
PROCTOR: No.

Assess the Pulse

Student: What are the rate and the quality of pulses?
PROCTOR: Rate: Tachycardic. Quality: Bounding.

Assess the Skin

Student: I am assessing the skin. What are the color, temperature, and condition of the skin?
PROCTOR: Color: Mottled. Temperature: Cool. Condition: Diaphoretic.

Identify Priority Patients/Make Transport Decision

Student: The patient is a high priority and is a load-and-go. I will begin packaging and transport.
PROCTOR: Noted.

Critical Criteria:
- ❑ Did not provide high concentration of oxygen
- ❑ Did not find or manage problems associated with airway, breathing, hemorrhage or shock (hypoperfusion)
- ❑ Did not differentiate patient's need for transportation versus continued assessment at the scene
- ❑ Did other detailed examination before assessing the airway, breathing and circulation

Focused History and Physical Examination/Rapid Trauma Assessment

Select the Appropriate Assessment (Focused or Rapid)

Student: I am selecting the rapid physical exam to identify and treat life threats. I am checking for DCAP-BTLS. This acronym stands for deformities, contusions, abrasions, punctures, penetrations, and paradoxical motion in the chest, and burns, tenderness, lacerations, and swelling.
PROCTOR: Noted.

Head

Student: I am rapidly assessing the head.
PROCTOR: There are no obvious injuries.

Neck

Student: I am rapidly assessing the neck.
PROCTOR: Jugular vein distention (JVD) and mottling are noted. The trachea is deviated to the right.

Student: I will apply a cervical collar.
PROCTOR: Noted.

- Chest

Student: I am rapidly palpating the chest and listening for lung sounds.
PROCTOR: There is an obvious crush injury to the chest with mottling noted. Lung sounds are diminished on the left.
Student: I will assess the chest for tension pneumothorax by auscultation, and assessment (jugular vein distention [JVD], tracheal deviation, and decreased lung sounds).
PROCTOR: The lung sounds appear diminished on the left, jugular vein distention is present, and the trachea is deviated to the right.
Student: I will continue with bag-valve ventilations to stabilize the chest. I will also stabilize the chest with a bulky dressing or with a pillow and tape.
PROCTOR: Noted.
ALS Student: I will assess the chest for hyperresonance to percussion.
ALS Proctor: Noted. There is a tension pneumothorax on the left side.
ALS Student: I will decompress the left chest.
ALS Proctor: Noted. The decompression is effective.
ALS Student: I will continuously reassess the chest.
ALS Proctor: Noted.

- Abdomen/Pelvis

Student: I am rapidly assessing the abdomen.
PROCTOR: Rigidity is noted.
Student: I am rapidly assessing the pelvis.
PROCTOR: There are no obvious injuries.

- Extremities

Student: I am rapidly assessing the extremities.
PROCTOR: The left arm is shattered, with bone protruding through the skin in several locations.

- Assess Motor, Sensory, and Circulatory Function

Student: I am checking for DCAP-BTLS. I am also checking motor and sensory function, and pulses. Right leg?
PROCTOR: Negative DCAP-BTLS. Motor and sensory functions are present. Pulses are present.
Student: Left leg?
PROCTOR: Negative DCAP-BTLS. Motor and sensory functions are present. Pulses are present.
Student: Right arm?
PROCTOR: Negative DCAP-BTLS. Motor and sensory functions are present. Pulses are present.
Student: Left arm?
PROCTOR: The arm is splintered from the direct impact of the weight. Motor and sensory functions are present. Pulses are present.
Student: I will have another EMT control bleeding and splint the arm.
PROCTOR: Noted.

- Posterior

Student: We will now log roll the patient as a unit to check the back. The person at the head will count to three and we will roll the patient.
PROCTOR: Noted.

  - Assess the Thorax

Student: I am assessing the thorax. Do I find injuries?
PROCTOR: No.

  - Assess the Lumbar Area

Student: I am assessing the flanks and lumbar area. Do I find injuries?
PROCTOR: You see pooling in the flanks.

  - Assess the Entire Backside

Student: I am assessing the entire backside. Do I find injuries?
PROCTOR: No.

- Manage Secondary Injuries/Wounds

Student: We will apply a cervical collar and backboard with full immobilization per local protocol, if not yet done, at this time.
PROCTOR: Noted.
Student: Are there any changes in motor and sensory functions and pulses?
PROCTOR: No.
ALS Student: I will establish two large-bore IVs en route to the hospital and administer a bolus of 20 mL/kg in order to maintain a systolic blood pressure of 90 mm Hg.
ALS Proctor: Noted.

- Reevaluate Transport Decision

Student: This patient is a load-and-go due to multiple trauma.
PROCTOR: Noted.

Baseline Vital Signs

Student: What are the patient's baseline vital signs, including blood pressure, pulse, respirations, pulse oximetry, and level of consciousness?
PROCTOR: Blood pressure, 90/70 mm Hg; pulse, 130 beats/min; respirations per bag-valve device; pulse oximetry reading, 86%; and the patient is oriented to verbal instructions.

SAMPLE History

Student: At this time I will gather a SAMPLE history from the patient or family. What are the patient's signs and symptoms?
PROCTOR: He is not speaking (decreased level of consciousness).
Student: Allergies?
PROCTOR: Unknown.
Student: Medications?
PROCTOR: Unknown.
Student: Pertinent past medical history?
PROCTOR: Unknown.
Student: Last oral intake?
PROCTOR: Unknown.
Student: Events leading up to the incident?
PROCTOR: The patient was working under a car when the jack failed. His left arm was upright and splintered through the skin. Fire/rescue responders lifted the car.

Critical Criteria:
- ❑ Did not differentiate patient's need for transportation versus continued assessment at the scene
- ❑ Did not provide for spinal protection when indicated

Detailed Physical Examination

Student: I am conducting the detailed physical exam. I am looking for DCAP-BTLS.
PROCTOR: Noted. The detailed physical exam will be performed during transport.

Assess the Head

Student: I am assessing the head. Do I find any DCAP-BTLS? Do I find any evidence of Battle's sign or raccoon eyes?
PROCTOR: No.

- Inspect and Palpate the Head and Ears

Student: I am assessing the head and ears.
PROCTOR: There are no obvious injuries.

- Assess the Eyes

Student: I am assessing the eyes. Are the pupils equal, round, and regular in size, and react properly to light (PEARRL)?
PROCTOR: There is bleeding around the eyes and the eyes are bloodshot.

- Assess the Facial Area Including Oral and Nasal Areas

Student: I am assessing the face, nose, and mouth. Do I see any discharge or hear any obstructions?
PROCTOR: No.
ALS Student: I will intubate (rapid sequence intubation [RSI] per protocol), confirming my tube placement with end-tidal CO_2 levels and by checking lung sounds.
ALS Proctor: Noted. End-tidal CO_2 and lung sounds confirm endotracheal (ET) tube placement.

▼ Assess the Neck

► **Inspect and Palpate the Neck**

Student: I am assessing the neck for DCAP-BTLS.
PROCTOR: There are no obvious injuries.

► **Assess for Jugular Vein Distention**

Student: Do I find any jugular vein distention (JVD)?
PROCTOR: No, if treated by ALS.

► **Assess for Tracheal Deviation**

Student: Do I see any tracheal deviation?
PROCTOR: No, if treated by ALS.

▼ Assess the Chest

Student: I am assessing the chest for DCAP-BTLS.
PROCTOR: Noted.

► **Inspect**

Student: What do I see when I look at the chest?
PROCTOR: You see a bruising imprint of the frame of the car on his chest. There are no open wounds.
Student: Does the chest appear symmetric?
PROCTOR: No, but it was treated with a bulky dressing.

► **Palpate**

Student: When I touch the chest, do I feel crepitus or a flail segment?
PROCTOR: Yes, there is a large flail segment on the left side.
Student: I would stabilize the flail segment with a bulky dressing or a pillow and tape (if not previously done).
PROCTOR: Noted.

► **Auscultate**

Student: Are lung sounds present in all fields?
PROCTOR: Yes.
Student: Do I hear any sucking sounds from the chest?
PROCTOR: No.

▼ Assess the Abdomen/Pelvis

► **Assess the Abdomen**

Student: I am assessing the abdomen for DCAP-BTLS. I am assessing all four quadrants. Do I find any problems?
PROCTOR: You see bruising and the abdomen is rigid.

► **Assess the Pelvis**

Student: I am assessing the pelvis for DCAP-BTLS. Is the pelvis stable?
PROCTOR: Yes.

► **Assess the Genitalia/Perineum as Needed (Verbalize in Training)**

Student: I am assessing the genitalia/perineum as necessary for DCAP-BTLS.
PROCTOR: He is incontinent of urine and stool.

▼ Assess the Extremities

► **Inspect**

Student: I am assessing the lower and upper extremities for DCAP-BTLS. Do I find anything?
PROCTOR: Yes, the left arm was shattered with bone protruding through the skin in several locations, but is now splinted.

► **Palpate**

Student: Do I feel anything unusual?
PROCTOR: No.

► **Assess Motor, Sensory, and Circulatory Function**

Student: I am checking for DCAP-BTLS, motor and sensory function, and pulses. Right leg?
PROCTOR: Negative DCAP-BTLS. Motor and sensory functions are present. Pulses are present.
Student: Left leg?
PROCTOR: Negative DCAP-BTLS. Motor and sensory functions are present. Pulses are present.
Student: Right arm?
PROCTOR: Negative DCAP-BTLS. Motor and sensory functions are present. Pulses are present.
Student: Left arm?
PROCTOR: The arm is splinted. Motor and sensory functions are present. Pulses are present.

▼ Assess the Posterior

Note: This portion of the detailed physical exam would not be done if the patient were previously backboarded per local protocol.
Student: We will not check the back since it was previously checked and the patient is backboarded.
PROCTOR: Noted.

▼ Manage Secondary Injuries/Wounds

Student: I would direct my partner to continue to manage the airway.
PROCTOR: Noted.

▼ Reassess Vital Signs

Student: I will reassess vital signs and mental status.
PROCTOR: Blood pressure, 86/72 mm Hg; pulse, 120 beats/min; respirations per bag-valve device; pulse oximetry reading, 85%; and the patient is oriented to pain.
Student: The vital signs are deteriorating.
PROCTOR: Noted.

▼ Reassess Interventions

Student: I will reassess my interventions: airway, breathing, bag-valve device, oral airway, and oxygen; circulation and bleeding control; and splints, immobilization, and straps.
PROCTOR: Noted.
ALS Student: I will reassess basic life support (BLS) interventions, plus the following: two large-bore IVs, cardiac monitor, and confirmation of tube placement. Monitor for tension pneumothorax.
ALS Proctor: Noted. The cardiac monitor shows sinus tachycardia. End tidal CO_2 confirms ET tube placement.

Critical Criteria:
- ❑ Did not find or manage problems associated with airway, breathing, hemorrhage or shock (hypoperfusion)

▼ Radio Report

(Provided by the student.)
PROCTOR: Noted.

▼ Ongoing Assessment

▼ Repeat Vital Signs

Student: I will reassess vital signs and mental status.
PROCTOR: Blood pressure, 0/0 mm Hg; pulse, 0 beats/min; respirations per bag-valve device; pulse oximetry, N/A; and the patient is unresponsive.
Student: The vital signs have deteriorated. We will begin CPR.
PROCTOR: Noted.

▼ Check Interventions

Student: I will check my interventions: CPR, airway, breathing, bag-valve device, oral airway, and oxygen; circulation and bleeding control; splints, immobilization, and straps; and transport to a trauma center.
PROCTOR: Noted.

CASE 5

ALS Student: I will check BLS interventions, plus the following: intubation, two large-bore IVs, cardiac monitoring, confirmation of tube placement, and advanced cardiac life support (ACLS) and regional protocol. Monitor needle decompression to the left chest.

ALS Proctor: Noted. The cardiac monitor shows pulseless electrical activity. End-tidal CO_2 and lung sounds confirm ET tube placement.

Critical Criteria:
- ❑ Did not find or manage problems associated with airway, breathing, hemorrhage or shock (hypoperfusion)

Handoff Report to Emergency Department Staff

Student: The patient's condition deteriorated during transport.
PROCTOR: Noted.

Critical Criteria:
- ❑ Did not transport patient within the (10) minute time limit

Critical Criteria

(Inform the student of items missed, if any.)

❑ Pass ❑ Fail Date: ____________________

Proctor Comments: ____________________

____

____

CASE 6

Dispatch Information

PROCTOR: EMS 10, respond to a 42-year-old male who has been struck with a machete while working in his yard. He is conscious and breathing.

Pre-scene Action (BSI)

Student: I am wearing nonlatex gloves, safety glasses, mask, and gown.
PROCTOR: Noted.

> **Critical Criteria:**
> ❑ Did not take, or verbalize, body substance isolation (BSI) precautions when necessary

Scene Size-up

Scene Safety

Student: Is the scene safe?
PROCTOR: Yes.

Mechanism of Injury

Student: What was the mechanism of injury?
PROCTOR: Soft-tissue injury. The patient was clearing brush in his yard and hit himself in the groin with a very sharp machete. Extreme blood loss is evident.
Student: I would apply direct pressure and a dressing as soon as possible.
PROCTOR: Noted.

Number of Patients

Student: How many patients are there?
PROCTOR: One.

Additional Resources

Student: I would call for advanced life support (ALS) assistance.
PROCTOR: Noted.

C-Spine Stabilization

Student: I would not stabilize the cervical spine (c-spine).
PROCTOR: Noted.

> **Critical Criteria:**
> ❑ Did not determine scene safety
> ❑ Did not assess for spinal protection
> ❑ Did not provide for spinal protection when indicated

Initial Assessment

Student: I identify myself and ask the patient not to move.
PROCTOR: Noted.

General Impression

Student: My general impression is that the patient's condition is unstable.
PROCTOR: Noted.

Responsiveness/Level of Consciousness

Student: What is the patient's level of consciousness?
PROCTOR: Alert.

Chief Complaint/Apparent Life Threats

Student: What is the patient's chief complaint?
PROCTOR: The patient is saying he is going to die.
Student: There are apparent life threats; the life threats are shock and the mechanism of injury.
PROCTOR: Noted.

Assess the Airway and Breathing

Student: Is the airway open? Is the patient breathing?
PROCTOR: Yes, the airway is open and the patient is breathing.

Assessment

Student: What are the rate and the quality of breathing?
PROCTOR: Rate: Rapid. Quality: Deep.

Provide Oxygen

Student: I am applying oxygen at 15 L/min via nonrebreathing mask.
PROCTOR: Noted.

Ensure Adequate Ventilation

Student: The patient has adequate ventilations at this time.
PROCTOR: Noted.

Injury Management

Student: I will direct my partner to take over direct pressure as I continue assessment.
PROCTOR: Noted.

Assess Circulation

Student: I am assessing the patient's circulation.
PROCTOR: Noted.

Assess for and Control Major Bleeding

Student: Do I find any major bleeding?
PROCTOR: Yes.
Student: My partner will apply manual pressure and a bulky dressing.
PROCTOR: Noted.

Assess the Pulse

Student: What are the rate and the quality of pulses?
PROCTOR: Rate: Fast. Quality: Thready.

Assess the Skin

Student: I am assessing the skin. What are the color, temperature, and condition of the skin?
PROCTOR: Color: Pasty white. Temperature: Cool. Condition: Diaphoretic.

Identify Priority Patients/Make Transport Decision

Student: The patient is a high priority and is a load-and-go. I will begin packaging and transport.
PROCTOR: Noted.

> **Critical Criteria:**
> ❑ Did not provide high concentration of oxygen
> ❑ Did not find or manage problems associated with airway, breathing, hemorrhage or shock (hypoperfusion)
> ❑ Did not differentiate patient's need for transportation versus continued assessment at the scene
> ❑ Did other detailed examination before assessing the airway, breathing and circulation

Focused History and Physical Examination/Rapid Trauma Assessment

Select the Appropriate Assessment (Focused or Rapid)

Student: I am selecting the rapid physical exam to identify and treat life threats. I am checking for DCAP-BTLS. This acronym stands for deformities, contusions, abrasions, punctures, penetrations, and paradoxical motion in the chest, and burns, tenderness, lacerations, and swelling.
PROCTOR: Noted.

Head

Student: I am rapidly assessing the head.
PROCTOR: There are no obvious injuries.

Neck

Student: I am rapidly assessing the neck.
PROCTOR: There are no obvious injuries.

Chest

Student: I am rapidly assessing the chest. What are the lung sounds?
PROCTOR: There are no obvious injuries. Lung sounds are clear bilaterally.

Abdomen/Pelvis

Student: I am rapidly assessing the abdomen.
PROCTOR: There are no obvious injuries.

Student: I am rapidly assessing the pelvis.
PROCTOR: The scrotum is lacerated and bleeding heavily.
Student: My partner is applying manual pressure and a bulky dressing to control bleeding.
PROCTOR: Noted.

▸ **Extremities**

Student: I am rapidly assessing the extremities.
PROCTOR: There are no obvious injuries.

▸ **Posterior**

Student: We will now check the back.
PROCTOR: Noted.

▸ **Assess the Thorax**

Student: I am assessing the thorax. Do I find injuries?
PROCTOR: No.

▸ **Assess the Lumbar Area**

Student: I am assessing the flanks and lumbar area. Do I find injuries?
PROCTOR: No.

▸ **Assess the Entire Backside**

Student: I am assessing the entire backside. Do I find injuries?
PROCTOR: No.

▸ **Manage Secondary Injuries**

ALS Student: I will establish two large-bore IVs en route to the hospital and administer a bolus of 20 mL/kg in order to maintain a systolic blood pressure of 90 mm Hg.
ALS Proctor: Noted.

▸ **Reevaluate Transport Decision**

Student: This patient is a load-and-go due to shock.
PROCTOR: Noted.

▾ Baseline Vital Signs

Student: What are the patient's baseline vital signs, including blood pressure, pulse, respirations, pulse oximetry, and level of consciousness?
PROCTOR: Blood pressure, 100/60 mm Hg; pulse, 140 beats/min; respirations, 20 breaths/min; pulse oximetry reading, 94%; and the patient is alert but anxious.

▾ Interventions

Student: We will monitor blood loss and treat for shock.
PROCTOR: Noted.
ALS Student: I will establish two large-bore IVs and administer 20 mL/kg en route to the hospital, if necessary, to maintain a minimum systolic blood pressure of 90 mm Hg.
ALS Proctor: Noted.

▾ SAMPLE History

Student: At this time I will gather a SAMPLE history from the patient or family. What are the patient's signs and symptoms?
PROCTOR: Pain in scrotum and feels faint.
Student: Allergies?
PROCTOR: Penicillin (PCN).
Student: Medications?
PROCTOR: No medications.
Student: Pertinent past medical history?
PROCTOR: No pertinent medical history.
Student: Last oral intake?
PROCTOR: 3 hours ago.
Student: Events leading up to the incident?
PROCTOR: The patient was working in the yard clearing brush. He took a downward swing with the machete and missed the branch. He struck himself in the groin.
Student: Interventions?
PROCTOR: The patient and his wife attempted to stop the bleeding with a towel.

Critical Criteria:
- ❑ Did not differentiate patient's need for transportation versus continued assessment at the scene
- ❑ Did not provide for spinal protection when indicated

▾ Detailed Physical Examination

Student: I am conducting the detailed physical exam. I am looking for DCAP-BTLS. This acronym stands for deformities, contusions, abrasions, punctures, penetrations, paradoxical motion in the chest, and burns, tenderness, lacerations, and swelling.
PROCTOR: Noted. The detailed physical exam will be performed during transport.

▾ Assess the Head

Student: I am assessing the head. Do I find any DCAP-BTLS? Do I find any evidence of Battle's sign or raccoon eyes?
PROCTOR: No.

▸ **Inspect and Palpate the Head and Ears**

Student: I am assessing the head and ears.
PROCTOR: There are no obvious injuries.

▸ **Assess the Eyes**

Student: I am assessing the eyes. Are the pupils equal, round, and regular in size, and react properly to light (PEARRL)?
PROCTOR: They are sluggish (they are slow to react).

▸ **Assess the Facial Area Including Oral and Nasal Areas**

Student: I am assessing the face, nose, and mouth. Do I see any discharge or hear any obstructions?
PROCTOR: No.

▾ Assess the Neck

▸ **Inspect and Palpate the Neck**

Student: I am assessing the neck for DCAP-BTLS.
PROCTOR: There are no obvious injuries.

▸ **Assess for Jugular Vein Distention**

Student: Do I find any jugular vein distention (JVD)?
PROCTOR: No.

▸ **Assess for Tracheal Deviation**

Student: Do I see any tracheal deviation?
PROCTOR: No.

▾ Assess the Chest

Student: I am assessing the chest for DCAP-BTLS.
PROCTOR: Noted.

▸ **Inspect**

Student: What do I see when I look at the chest?
PROCTOR: There are no obvious injuries.
Student: Does the chest appear symmetric?
PROCTOR: Yes.

▸ **Palpate**

Student: When I touch the chest, do I feel crepitus or a flail segment?
PROCTOR: No.

▸ **Auscultate**

Student: Are lung sounds present in all fields?
PROCTOR: Yes.
Student: Do I hear any sucking sounds from the chest?
PROCTOR: No.

▾ Assess the Abdomen/Pelvis

▸ **Assess the Abdomen**

Student: I am assessing the abdomen for DCAP-BTLS. I am assessing all four quadrants. Do I find any problems?
PROCTOR: No.

▸ **Assess the Pelvis**

Student: I am assessing the pelvis for DCAP-BTLS. Is the pelvis stable?
PROCTOR: Yes.

▾ Assess the Genitalia/Perineum as Needed (Verbalize in Training)

Student: I am assessing the genitalia/perineum as necessary for DCAP-BTLS.
PROCTOR: The scrotum is lacerated and bleeding is controlled.

Assess the Extremities

Inspect

Student: I am assessing the lower and upper extremities for DCAP-BTLS. Do I find anything?

PROCTOR: No.

Palpate

Student: Do I feel anything unusual?

PROCTOR: No.

Assess Motor, Sensory, and Circulatory Function

Student: I am checking for DCAP-BTLS, motor and sensory function, and pulses. Right leg?

PROCTOR: Negative DCAP-BTLS. Motor and sensory functions are absent. Pulses are weak.

Student: Left leg?

PROCTOR: Negative DCAP-BTLS. Motor and sensory functions are absent. Pulses are weak.

Student: Right arm?

PROCTOR: Negative DCAP-BTLS. Motor and sensory functions are absent. Pulses are weak.

Student: Left arm?

PROCTOR: Negative DCAP-BTLS. Motor and sensory functions are absent. Pulses are weak.

Assess the Posterior

Student: We will not check the back since it was checked earlier.

PROCTOR: Noted.

Manage Secondary Injuries/Wounds

Student: I would direct my partner to continue bleeding control with direct pressure.

PROCTOR: Noted.

Reassess Vital Signs

Student: I will reassess vital signs and mental status.

PROCTOR: Blood pressure, 94/54 mm Hg; pulse, 136 beats/min; respirations, 20 breaths/min; pulse oximetry reading, 94%; and the patient is tired.

Student: The vital signs are deteriorating.

PROCTOR: Noted.

Reassess Interventions

Student: I will reassess my interventions: oxygen, circulation and bleeding control, and treatment for shock (keep the patient still and warm and cover him with a blanket).

PROCTOR: Noted.

ALS Student: I will reassess basic life support (BLS) interventions, plus the following: two large-bore IVs, 20 mL/kg bolus to maintain a blood pressure of 90 mm/Hg, and cardiac monitoring.

ALS Proctor: Noted. The cardiac monitor shows sinus tachycardia.

Critical Criteria:
- ❑ Did not find or manage problems associated with airway, breathing, hemorrhage or shock (hypoperfusion)

Radio Report

(Provided by the student.)

PROCTOR: Noted.

Ongoing Assessment

Repeat Vital Signs

Student: I will reassess vital signs and mental status.

PROCTOR: Blood pressure, 90/50 mm Hg; pulse, 140 beats/min; respirations, 20 breaths/min; pulse oximetry reading, 94%; and the patient is faint.

Student: The vital signs have deteriorated.

PROCTOR: Noted.

Check Interventions

Student: I will check my interventions: oxygen, circulation and bleeding control, and treatment for shock (keep the patient still and warm and cover him with a blanket).

PROCTOR: Noted.

ALS Student: I will check BLS interventions, plus the following: two large-bore IVs, 20 mL/kg bolus to maintain a blood pressure of 90 mm/Hg, and cardiac monitoring.

ALS Proctor: Noted. The cardiac monitor shows sinus tachycardia.

Critical Criteria:
- ❑ Did not find or manage problems associated with airway, breathing, hemorrhage or shock (hypoperfusion)

Handoff Report to Emergency Department Staff

Student: The patient's condition deteriorated during transport.

PROCTOR: Noted.

Critical Criteria:
- ❑ Did not transport patient within the (10) minute time limit

Critical Criteria

(Inform the student of items missed, if any.)

❑ Pass ❑ Fail Date: ____________________

Proctor Comments: ____________________

____

____

Notes

Dispatch Information

PROCTOR: EMS 10, respond to a 22-year-old male who was sleeping with a gun on the nightstand when, according to his wife, the phone rang; he shot himself in the head instead of answering the phone. He is unconscious and having a seizure. Police are en route.

Pre-scene Action (BSI)

Student: I am wearing nonlatex gloves, safety glasses, mask, and gown.
PROCTOR: Noted.

> **Critical Criteria:**
> - ❑ Did not take, or verbalize, body substance isolation (BSI) precautions when necessary

Scene Size-up

Scene Safety

Student: Is the scene safe?
PROCTOR: Yes, police are on scene and you are given clearance to enter.

Mechanism of Injury

Student: What was the mechanism of injury?
PROCTOR: Gunshot wound. The patient was sleeping when the phone rang and he shot himself.

Number of Patients

Student: How many patients are there?
PROCTOR: One.

Additional Resources

Student: I would call for advanced life support (ALS) assistance.
PROCTOR: Noted.

C-Spine Stabilization

Student: On the basis of the mechanism of injury, I would stabilize the cervical spine (c-spine) in a neutral in-line position.
PROCTOR: Noted.

> **Critical Criteria:**
> - ❑ Did not determine scene safety
> - ❑ Did not assess for spinal protection
> - ❑ Did not provide for spinal protection when indicated

Initial Assessment

Student: As I perform midline c-spine stabilization, I identify myself and ask the patient not to move.
PROCTOR: Noted.

General Impression

Student: My general impression is that the patient's condition is unstable.
PROCTOR: Noted.

Responsiveness/Level of Consciousness

Student: What is the patient's level of consciousness?
PROCTOR: Unresponsive.

Chief Complaint/Apparent Life Threats

Student: What is the patient's chief complaint?
PROCTOR: The patient is unresponsive.
Student: There is an apparent life threat; the life threat is the gunshot wound to the head.
PROCTOR: Noted.

Assess the Airway and Breathing

Student: I am opening the airway using the jaw-thrust maneuver. Is the patient breathing?
PROCTOR: Yes.

Assessment

Student: What are the rate and the quality of breathing?
PROCTOR: Rate: 4 breaths/min. Quality: Gasping.

Provide Oxygen

Student: I am assisting ventilations with a bag-valve device with 100% oxygen and an oral airway, and I will suction the airway as needed.
PROCTOR: Noted.
ALS Student: I will apply basic life support (BLS) interventions, plus the following: intubation and confirm end tidal CO_2 and lung sounds.
ALS Proctor: Noted. End tidal CO_2 and lung sounds confirm placement of the endotracheal (ET) tube.

Ensure Adequate Ventilation

Student: I am assisting ventilations with a bag-valve device.
PROCTOR: Noted.

Injury Management

Student: I will direct my partner to take over c-spine control as I continue assessment.
PROCTOR: Noted.

Assess Circulation

Student: I am assessing the patient's circulation.
PROCTOR: Noted.

Assess for and Control Major Bleeding

Student: Do I find any major bleeding?
PROCTOR: Yes, from the right side of the head.
Student: I would treat the head injury per local protocol.
PROCTOR: Noted.

Assess the Pulse

Student: What are the rate and the quality of pulses?
PROCTOR: Rate: Within normal limits. Quality: Bounding.

Assess the Skin

Student: I am assessing the skin. What are the color, temperature, and condition of the skin?
PROCTOR: Color: Normal. Temperature: Cool. Condition: Moist.

Identify Priority Patients/Make Transport Decision

Student: The patient is a high priority and is a load-and-go. I will begin packaging and transport to a trauma center.
PROCTOR: Noted.

> **Critical Criteria:**
> - ❑ Did not provide high concentration of oxygen
> - ❑ Did not find or manage problems associated with airway, breathing, hemorrhage or shock (hypoperfusion)
> - ❑ Did not differentiate patient's need for transportation versus continued assessment at the scene
> - ❑ Did other detailed examination before assessing the airway, breathing and circulation

Focused History and Physical Examination/Rapid Trauma Assessment

Select the Appropriate Assessment (Focused or Rapid)

Student: I am selecting the rapid physical exam to identify and treat life threats. I am checking for DCAP-BTLS. This acronym stands for deformities, contusions, abrasions, punctures, penetrations, and paradoxical motion in the chest, and burns, tenderness, lacerations, and swelling.
PROCTOR: Noted.

Head

Student: I am rapidly assessing the head.
PROCTOR: You see the bulging of brain matter on the right side of the head. There is cerebrospinal fluid (CSF) present in a halo test.

Student: As noted, I would treat the head injury per local protocol.
PROCTOR: Noted.

► **Neck**

Student: I am rapidly assessing the neck.
PROCTOR: There are no obvious injuries.
Student: I will apply a cervical collar.
PROCTOR: Noted.

► **Chest**

Student: I am rapidly assessing the chest. What are the lung sounds?
PROCTOR: There are no obvious injuries. Lung sounds are clear bilaterally.

► **Abdomen/Pelvis**

Student: I am rapidly assessing the abdomen.
PROCTOR: There are no obvious injuries.
Student: I am rapidly assessing the pelvis.
PROCTOR: There are no obvious injuries.

► **Extremities**

Student: I am rapidly assessing the extremities.
PROCTOR: There are no obvious injuries.

► **Assess Motor, Sensory, and Circulatory Function**

Student: I am checking for DCAP-BTLS. I am also checking motor and sensory function, and pulses. Right leg?
PROCTOR: Negative DCAP-BTLS. Motor and sensory functions are absent. Pulses are present.
Student: Left leg?
PROCTOR: Negative DCAP-BTLS. Motor and sensory functions are absent. Pulses are present.
Student: Right arm?
PROCTOR: Negative DCAP-BTLS. Motor and sensory functions are absent. Pulses are present.
Student: Left arm?
PROCTOR: Negative DCAP-BTLS. Motor and sensory functions are absent. Pulses are present.

► **Posterior**

Student: I will rapidly assess the back. We will now log roll the patient as a unit to check the back. The person at the head will count to three and we will roll the patient.
PROCTOR: Noted.

► **Assess the Thorax**

Student: I am assessing the thorax. Do I find injuries?
PROCTOR: Yes, a puncture wound to the right upper back.
Student: I would apply an occlusive dressing and reassess the chest.
PROCTOR: Noted.

► **Assess the Lumbar Area**

Student: I am assessing the flanks and lumbar area. Do I find injuries?
PROCTOR: No.

► **Assess the Entire Backside**

Student: I am assessing the entire backside. Do I find injuries?
PROCTOR: No.

► **Manage Secondary Injuries/Wounds**

Student: We will apply a cervical collar and backboard with full immobilization per local protocol, if not yet done, at this time.
PROCTOR: Noted.
Student: Are there any changes in motor and sensory functions or pulses?
PROCTOR: No.
ALS Student: I will establish two large-bore IVs en route to the hospital and administer a bolus of 20 mL/kg in order to maintain a systolic blood pressure of 90 mm Hg.
ALS Proctor: Noted.

► **Reevaluate Transport Decision**

Student: This patient is a high priority and a load-and-go due to the gunshot wound in his head and the puncture in his upper right back.
PROCTOR: Noted.

▼ **Baseline Vital Signs**

Student: What are the patient's baseline vital signs, including blood pressure, pulse, respirations, pulse oximetry, and level of consciousness?
PROCTOR: Blood pressure, 150/100 mm Hg; pulse rate, 72 beats/min; respirations per bag-valve device; pulse oximetry reading, 94%; and the patient is unresponsive.

▼ **SAMPLE History**

Student: At this time I will gather a SAMPLE history from the patient or family. What are the patient's signs and symptoms?
PROCTOR: You see just the head wound and puncture wound to the right upper back.
Student: Allergies?
PROCTOR: Unknown.
Student: Medications?
PROCTOR: Medications for HIV as well as cocaine, methamphetamine, heroin, and other unknown drugs.
Student: Pertinent past medical history?
PROCTOR: HIV positive.
Student: Last oral intake?
PROCTOR: 7 hours ago.
Student: Events leading up to the incident?
PROCTOR: The patient was sleeping when the phone rang and he shot himself, according to his wife.

Critical Criteria:
- ❑ Did not differentiate patient's need for transportation versus continued assessment at the scene
- ❑ Did not provide for spinal protection when indicated

▼ Detailed Physical Examination

Student: I am conducting the detailed physical exam. I am looking for DCAP-BTLS.
PROCTOR: Noted. The detailed physical exam will be performed during transport.

▼ **Assess the Head**

Student: I am assessing the head. Do I find any DCAP-BTLS? Do I find any evidence of Battle's sign or raccoon eyes?
PROCTOR: Yes, you see Battle's sign and instability to the skull.

► **Inspect and Palpate the Head and Ears**

Student: I am assessing the head and ears.
PROCTOR: You see the bulging of brain matter on the right side of the head. There is CSF present in a halo test and bleeding is controlled.

► **Assess the Eyes**

Student: I am assessing the eyes. Are the pupils equal, round, and regular in size, and react properly to light (PEARRL)?
PROCTOR: The right pupil is dilated.

► **Assess the Facial Area Including Oral and Nasal Areas**

Student: I am assessing the face, nose, and mouth. Do I see any discharge or hear any obstructions?
PROCTOR: No.

▼ **Assess the Neck**

► **Inspect and Palpate the Neck**

Student: I am assessing the neck for DCAP-BTLS.
PROCTOR: There are no obvious injuries.

▸ **Assess for Jugular Vein Distention**

Student: Do I find any jugular vein distention (JVD)?

PROCTOR: No.

▸ **Assess for Tracheal Deviation**

Student: Do I see any tracheal deviation?

PROCTOR: No.

▾ Assess the Chest

Student: I am assessing the chest for DCAP-BTLS.

PROCTOR: Noted.

▸ **Inspect**

Student: What do I see when I look at the chest?

PROCTOR: There are no obvious injuries.

Student: Does the chest appear symmetric?

PROCTOR: Yes.

▸ **Palpate**

Student: When I touch the chest, do I feel crepitus or a flail segment?

PROCTOR: No.

▸ **Auscultate**

Student: Are lung sounds present in all fields?

PROCTOR: Yes.

Student: Do I hear any sucking sounds from the chest?

PROCTOR: No.

▾ Assess the Abdomen/Pelvis

▸ **Assess the Abdomen**

Student: I am assessing the abdomen for DCAP-BTLS. I am assessing all four quadrants. Do I find any problems?

PROCTOR: No.

▸ **Assess the Pelvis**

Student: I am assessing the pelvis for DCAP-BTLS. Is the pelvis stable?

PROCTOR: Yes.

▾ Assess the Genitalia/Perineum as Needed (Verbalize in Training)

Student: I am assessing the genitalia/perineum as necessary for DCAP-BTLS.

PROCTOR: The area is unremarkable.

▾ Assess the Extremities

▸ **Inspect**

Student: I am assessing the lower and upper extremities for DCAP-BTLS. Do I find anything?

PROCTOR: No.

▸ **Palpate**

Student: Do I feel anything unusual?

PROCTOR: No.

▸ **Assess Motor, Sensory, and Circulatory Function**

Student: I am checking for DCAP-BTLS, motor and sensory function, and pulses. Right leg?

PROCTOR: Negative DCAP-BTLS. Motor and sensory functions are absent. Pulses are present.

Student: Left leg?

PROCTOR: Negative DCAP-BTLS. Motor and sensory functions are absent. Pulses are present.

Student: Right arm?

PROCTOR: Negative DCAP-BTLS. Motor and sensory functions are absent. Pulses are present.

Student: Left arm?

PROCTOR: Negative DCAP-BTLS. Motor and sensory functions are absent. Pulses are present.

▾ Assess the Posterior

Note: This portion of the detailed physical exam would not be done if the patient were previously backboarded per local protocol.

Student: We will not check the back because it was previously checked and the patient is backboarded.

PROCTOR: Noted.

▾ Manage Secondary Injuries/Wounds

Student: I would direct my partner to manage the airway.

PROCTOR: Noted.

▾ Reassess Vital Signs

Student: I will reassess vital signs and mental status.

PROCTOR: Blood pressure, 130/70 mm Hg; pulse rate, 84 beats/min; respirations per bag-valve device; pulse oximetry reading, 92%; and the patient is unresponsive.

Student: The vital signs are deteriorating.

PROCTOR: Noted.

▾ Reassess Interventions

Student: I will reassess my interventions: airway, suction, breathing, bag-valve device, and oxygen; circulation and bleeding control; occlusive dressing; immobilization and straps; and treatment for shock.

PROCTOR: Noted.

ALS Student: I will reassess BLS interventions, plus the following: intubation, confirm end tidal CO_2, check lung sounds, two large-bore IVs, and cardiac monitor.

ALS Proctor: Noted. The cardiac monitor shows normal sinus rhythm and end tidal CO_2 and lung sounds confirm placement of the ET tube.

Critical Criteria:

- ❑ Did not find or manage problems associated with airway, breathing, hemorrhage or shock (hypoperfusion)

Radio Report

(Provided by the student.)

PROCTOR: Noted.

Ongoing Assessment

▾ Repeat Vital Signs

Student: I will reassess vital signs and mental status.

PROCTOR: Blood pressure, 110/50 mm Hg; pulse rate, 94 beats/min; respirations per bag-valve device; pulse oximetry reading, 90%; and the patient is unresponsive.

Student: The vital signs have deteriorated.

PROCTOR: Noted.

▾ Check Interventions

Student: I will check my interventions: airway, suction, breathing, bag-valve device, and oxygen; circulation and bleeding control; occlusive dressing; immobilization and straps; and treatment for shock.

PROCTOR: Noted.

ALS Student: I will check BLS interventions, plus the following: intubation, confirm end tidal CO_2, check lung sounds, two large-bore IVs, and cardiac monitor.

ALS Proctor: Noted. The cardiac monitor shows normal sinus rhythm and end tidal CO_2 and lung sounds confirm placement of the ET tube.

Critical Criteria:

❑ Did not find or manage problems associated with airway, breathing, hemorrhage or shock (hypoperfusion)

Handoff Report to Emergency Department Staff

Student: The patient's condition deteriorated during transport.

PROCTOR: Noted.

Student: I would contact police and notify them of the gunshot wound in the back.

PROCTOR: Noted.

Critical Criteria:

❑ Did not transport patient within the (10) minute time limit

Critical Criteria

(Inform the student of items missed, if any.)

❑ Pass ❑ Fail Date: ______________________________

Proctor Comments: ______________________________

____

____

Dispatch Information

PROCTOR: EMS 10, respond to a domestic disturbance with a 24-year-old female shot. She is conscious and breathing. Police have been dispatched.

Pre-scene Action (BSI)

Student: I am wearing nonlatex gloves, safety glasses, mask, and gown.
PROCTOR: Noted.

Critical Criteria:
- ❑ Did not take, or verbalize, body substance isolation (BSI) precautions when necessary

Scene Size-up

Scene Safety

Student: Is the scene safe?
PROCTOR: Yes, police are on scene and you are given clearance to enter.

Mechanism of Injury

Student: What was the mechanism of injury?
PROCTOR: Gunshot wound. The patient was fighting with her boyfriend and he shot her in the chest.

Number of Patients

Student: How many patients are there?
PROCTOR: One.

Additional Resources

Student: I would call for advanced life support (ALS) assistance.
PROCTOR: Noted.

C-Spine Stabilization

Student: On the basis of the mechanism of injury, I would stabilize the cervical spine (c-spine) in a neutral in-line position.
PROCTOR: Noted.

Critical Criteria:
- ❑ Did not determine scene safety
- ❑ Did not assess for spinal protection
- ❑ Did not provide for spinal protection when indicated

Initial Assessment

Student: As I perform midline c-spine stabilization, I identify myself and ask the patient not to move.
PROCTOR: Noted.

General Impression

Student: My general impression is that the patient's condition is unstable.
PROCTOR: Noted.

Responsiveness/Level of Consciousness

Student: What is the patient's level of consciousness?
PROCTOR: Alert.

Chief Complaint/Apparent Life Threats

Student: What is the patient's chief complaint?
PROCTOR: The patient is complaining of difficulty breathing (shot to the chest).
Student: There is an apparent life threat; the life threat is a gunshot wound to the chest.
PROCTOR: Noted.

Assess the Airway and Breathing

Student: Is the airway open? Is the patient breathing?
PROCTOR: Yes, the airway is open and the patient is breathing.

▸ Assessment

Student: What are the rate and the quality of breathing?
PROCTOR: Rate: Rapid. Quality: Shallow.

▸ Provide Oxygen

Student: I am assisting ventilations with a bag-valve device with 100% oxygen.
PROCTOR: Noted.

▸ Ensure Adequate Ventilation

Student: I will continue assisting ventilations with the bag-valve device.
PROCTOR: Noted.

▸ Injury Management

Student: I will apply an occlusive dressing to the gunshot wound to the chest.
PROCTOR: Noted.

Assess Circulation

Student: I am assessing the patient's circulation.
PROCTOR: Noted.

▸ Assess for and Control Major Bleeding

Student: Do I find any major bleeding?
PROCTOR: No. There is only minor bleeding from the gunshot wound to the chest.

▸ Assess the Pulse

Student: What are the rate and the quality of pulses?
PROCTOR: Rate: Tachycardic. Quality: Thready.

▸ Assess the Skin

Student: I am assessing the skin. What are the color, temperature, and condition of the skin?
PROCTOR: Color: Pasty white. Temperature: Cool. Condition: Diaphoretic.

Identify Priority Patients/Make Transport Decision

Student: The patient is a high priority and is a load-and-go. I will begin packaging and transport.
PROCTOR: Noted.

Critical Criteria:
- ❑ Did not provide high concentration of oxygen
- ❑ Did not find or manage problems associated with airway, breathing, hemorrhage or shock (hypoperfusion)
- ❑ Did not differentiate patient's need for transportation versus continued assessment at the scene
- ❑ Did other detailed examination before assessing the airway, breathing and circulation

Focused History and Physical Examination/Rapid Trauma Assessment

Select the Appropriate Assessment (Focused or Rapid)

Student: I am selecting the rapid physical exam to identify and treat life threats. I am checking for DCAP-BTLS. This acronym stands for deformities, contusions, abrasions, punctures, penetrations, and paradoxical motion in the chest, and burns, tenderness, lacerations, and swelling.
PROCTOR: Noted.

▸ Head

Student: I am rapidly assessing the head.
PROCTOR: There are no obvious injuries.

▸ Neck

Student: I am rapidly assessing the neck.
PROCTOR: There are no obvious injuries.
Student: I will apply a cervical collar.
PROCTOR: Noted.

▸ Chest

Student: I am rapidly assessing the chest.
PROCTOR: There is an occlusive dressing over the open wound to the left chest.
Student: I will assess the chest for tension pneumothorax by auscultation, and assessment (jugular vein distention [JVD], tracheal deviation, and decreased lung sounds).
PROCTOR: The lung sounds appear diminished on the left, jugular vein distention is present, and the trachea is deviated to the right.

Student: I will burp the occlusive dressing on the left chest.
PROCTOR: Noted.
ALS Student: I will assess the chest for hyperresonance to percussion.
ALS Proctor: Noted. There is a tension pneumothorax on the left side.
ALS Student: I will decompress the left chest.
ALS Proctor: Noted. The decompression is effective.
ALS Student: I will continuously reassess the chest.
ALS Proctor: Noted.

▸ **Abdomen/Pelvis**

Student: I am rapidly assessing the abdomen.
PROCTOR: There are no obvious injuries.
Student: I am rapidly assessing the pelvis.
PROCTOR: There are no obvious injuries.

▸ **Extremities**

Student: I am rapidly assessing the extremities.
PROCTOR: There are no obvious injuries.

▸ **Assess Motor, Sensory, and Circulatory Function**

Student: I am checking for DCAP-BTLS. I am also checking motor and sensory function, and pulses. Right leg?
PROCTOR: Negative DCAP-BTLS. Motor and sensory functions are present. Pulses are weak.
Student: Left leg?
PROCTOR: Negative DCAP-BTLS. Motor and sensory functions are present. Pulses are weak.
Student: Right arm?
PROCTOR: Negative DCAP-BTLS. Motor and sensory functions are present. Pulses are weak.
Student: Left arm?
PROCTOR: Negative DCAP-BTLS. Motor and sensory functions are present. Pulses are weak.

▸ **Posterior**

Student: We will now log roll the patient as a unit to check the back. The person at the head will count to three and we will roll the patient.
PROCTOR: Noted.

▸ **Assess the Thorax**

Student: I am assessing the thorax. Do I find injuries?
PROCTOR: Yes, an exit wound.
Student: I would apply another occlusive dressing.
PROCTOR: Noted.

▸ **Assess the Lumbar Area**

Student: I am assessing the flanks and lumbar area. Do I find injuries?
PROCTOR: No.

▸ **Assess the Entire Backside**

Student: I am assessing the entire backside. Do I find injuries?
PROCTOR: No.

▸ **Manage Secondary Injuries/Wounds**

Student: We will apply a cervical collar and backboard with full immobilization per local protocol, if not yet done, at this time.
PROCTOR: Noted.
Student: Are there any changes in motor and sensory functions and pulses?
PROCTOR: No.
ALS Student: I will establish two large-bore IVs en route to the hospital and administer a bolus of 20 mL/kg in order to maintain a systolic blood pressure of 90 mm Hg.
ALS Proctor: Noted.

▸ **Reevaluate Transport Decision**

Student: This patient is a load-and-go due to the gunshot wound to the left chest.
PROCTOR: Noted.

▾ Baseline Vital Signs

Student: What are the patient's baseline vital signs, including blood pressure, pulse, respirations, pulse oximetry, and level of consciousness?
PROCTOR: Blood pressure, 88/60 mm Hg; pulse, 120 breaths/min; respirations per bag-valve device; pulse oximetry reading, 80%; and the patient is tired.

▾ SAMPLE History

Student: At this time I will gather a sample history from the patient or family. What are the patient's signs and symptoms?
PROCTOR: Pain in the chest.
Student: Allergies?
PROCTOR: No allergies.
Student: Medications?
PROCTOR: No medications.
Student: Pertinent past medical history?
PROCTOR: No pertinent medical history.
Student: Last oral intake?
PROCTOR: 8 hours ago.
Student: Events leading up to the incident?
PROCTOR: The patient was fighting with her boyfriend and he shot her.

Critical Criteria:
- ❑ Did not differentiate patient's need for transportation versus continued assessment at the scene
- ❑ Did not provide for spinal protection when indicated

Detailed Physical Examination

Student: I am conducting the detailed physical exam. I am looking for DCAP-BTLS.
PROCTOR: Noted. The detailed physical exam will be performed during transport.

▾ Assess the Head

Student: I am assessing the head. Do I find any DCAP-BTLS? Do I find any evidence of Battle's sign or raccoon eyes?
PROCTOR: No.

▸ **Inspect and Palpate the Head and Ears**

Student: I am assessing the head and ears.
PROCTOR: There are no obvious injuries.

▸ **Assess the Eyes**

Student: I am assessing the eyes. Are the pupils equal, round, and regular in size, and react properly to light (PEARRL)?
PROCTOR: They are PEARRL.

▸ **Assess the Facial Area Including Oral and Nasal Areas**

Student: I am assessing the face, nose, and mouth. Do I see or hear any discharge or obstructions?
PROCTOR: No.

▾ Assess the Neck

▸ **Inspect and Palpate the Neck**

Student: I am assessing the neck for DCAP-BTLS.
PROCTOR: There are no obvious injuries.

▸ **Assess for Jugular Vein Distention**

Student: Do I find any jugular vein distention (JVD)?
PROCTOR: No.

▸ **Assess for Tracheal Deviation**

Student: Do I see any tracheal deviation?
PROCTOR: Yes.

▾ Assess the Chest

Student: I am assessing the chest for DCAP-BTLS.
PROCTOR: Noted.

▸ **Inspect**

Student: What do I see when I look at the chest?
PROCTOR: An open wound to the left chest treated with an occlusive dressing.
Student: Does the chest appear symmetric?
PROCTOR: Yes.

▸ **Palpate**

Student: When I touch the chest, do I feel crepitus or a flail segment?
PROCTOR: No.

▸ Auscultate

Student: Are lung sounds present in all fields?

PROCTOR: No, they are diminished on the left side. Yes, if treated by ALS.

Student: Do I hear any sucking sounds from the chest?

PROCTOR: No.

Student: I would burp the occlusive dressing.

PROCTOR: Noted.

▾ **Assess the Abdomen/Pelvis**

▸ **Assess the Abdomen**

Student: I am assessing the abdomen for DCAP-BTLS. I am assessing all four quadrants. Do I find any problems?

PROCTOR: No.

▸ **Assess the Pelvis**

Student: I am assessing the pelvis for DCAP-BTLS. Is the pelvis stable?

PROCTOR: Yes.

▸ **Assess the Genitalia/Perineum as Needed (Verbalize in Training)**

Student: I am assessing the genitalia/perineum as necessary for DCAP-BTLS.

PROCTOR: The area is unremarkable.

▾ **Assess the Extremities**

▸ **Inspect**

Student: I am assessing the lower and upper extremities for DCAP-BTLS. Do I find anything?

PROCTOR: No.

▸ **Palpate**

Student: Do I feel anything unusual?

PROCTOR: No.

▸ **Assess Motor, Sensory, and Circulatory Function**

Student: I am checking for DCAP-BTLS, motor and sensory function, and pulses. Right leg?

PROCTOR: Negative DCAP-BTLS. Motor and sensory functions are present. Pulses are weak.

Student: Left leg?

PROCTOR: Negative DCAP-BTLS. Motor and sensory functions are present. Pulses are weak.

Student: Right arm?

PROCTOR: Negative DCAP-BTLS. Motor and sensory functions are present. Pulses are weak.

Student: Left arm?

PROCTOR: Negative DCAP-BTLS. Motor and sensory functions are present. Pulses are weak.

▾ **Assess the Posterior**

Note: This portion of the detailed physical exam would not be done if the patient were previously backboarded per local protocol.

Student: We will not check the back since it was previously checked and the patient is backboarded.

PROCTOR: Noted.

▾ **Manage Secondary Injuries/Wounds**

Student: I would direct my partner to apply direct pressure as needed.

PROCTOR: Noted.

▾ **Reassess Vital Signs**

Student: At this time I will reassess vital signs and mental status.

PROCTOR: Blood pressure, 80/56 mm Hg; pulse, 126 beats/min; respirations per bag-valve device; pulse oximetry reading, 78%; and the patient is tired.

Student: The vital signs are deteriorating.

PROCTOR: Noted.

▾ **Reassess Interventions**

Student: I will reassess my interventions: bag-valve device with 100% oxygen, occlusive dressing with bleeding control, and full immobilization.

PROCTOR: Noted.

ALS Student: I will reassess basic life support (BLS) interventions, plus the following: establish two large-bore IVs and administer 20 mL/kg to maintain a blood pressure of 90 mm Hg, and cardiac monitor.

ALS Proctor: Noted. The cardiac monitor shows sinus tachycardia.

Critical Criteria:
- ❑ Did not find or manage problems associated with airway, breathing, hemorrhage or shock (hypoperfusion)

Radio Report

(Provided by student.)

PROCTOR: Noted.

Ongoing Assessment

▾ **Repeat Vital Signs**

Student: I will reassess vital signs and mental status.

PROCTOR: Blood pressure, 78/56 mm Hg; pulse, 130 beats/min; respirations per bag-valve device; pulse oximetry reading, 74%; and the patient is tired.

Student: The vital signs have deteriorated.

PROCTOR: Noted.

▾ **Check Interventions**

Student: I will check my interventions: bag-valve device with 100% oxygen, occlusive dressing with bleeding control, and full immobilization.

PROCTOR: Noted.

ALS Student: I will check BLS interventions, plus the following: two large-bore IVs and administer 20 mL/kg to maintain a blood pressure of 90 mm Hg, and cardiac monitor.

ALS Proctor: Noted. The cardiac monitor shows sinus tachycardia.

Critical Criteria:
- ❑ Did not find or manage problems associated with airway, breathing, hemorrhage or shock (hypoperfusion)

Handoff Report to Emergency Department Staff

Student: The patient's condition deteriorated during transport.

PROCTOR: Noted.

Critical Criteria:
- ❑ Did not transport patient within the (10) minute time limit

Critical Criteria

(Inform the student of items missed, if any.)

❑ Pass ❑ Fail Date: ______________________

Proctor Comments: ______________________

____

____

CASE 8

Notes

CASE 9

Dispatch Information

PROCTOR: EMS 10, respond to a 45-year-old electrician who has been shocked by a high-voltage electrical line. He is conscious and breathing.

Pre-scene Action (BSI)

Student: I am wearing nonlatex gloves and safety glasses.
PROCTOR: Noted.

Critical Criteria:
- ❑ Did not take, or verbalize, body substance isolation (BSI) precautions when necessary

Scene Size-up

Scene Safety

Student: Is the scene safe?
PROCTOR: Yes.

Mechanism of Injury

Student: What was the mechanism of injury?
PROCTOR: Electrical shock. The patient was shocked by a high-voltage line.

Number of Patients

Student: How many patients are there?
PROCTOR: One.

Additional Resources

Student: I would call for advanced life support (ALS) assistance.
PROCTOR: Noted.

C-Spine Stabilization

Student: On the basis of the mechanism of injury, I would stabilize the cervical spine (c-spine) in a neutral in-line position.
PROCTOR: Noted.

Critical Criteria:
- ❑ Did not determine scene safety
- ❑ Did not assess for spinal protection
- ❑ Did not provide for spinal protection when indicated

Initial Assessment

Student: As I perform midline c-spine stabilization, I identify myself and ask the patient not to move.
PROCTOR: Noted.

General Impression

Student: My general impression is that the patient's condition is unstable.
PROCTOR: Noted.

Responsiveness/Level of Consciousness

Student: What is the patient's level of consciousness?
PROCTOR: Alert.

Chief Complaint/Apparent Life Threats

Student: What is the patient's chief complaint?
PROCTOR: The patient is complaining of burns to the hands and foot, and chest pain.
Student: There are apparent life threats; the life threats are the mechanism of injury and chest pain.
PROCTOR: Noted.

Assess the Airway and Breathing

Student: Is the airway open? Is the patient breathing?
PROCTOR: Yes, the airway is open and the patient is breathing.

Assessment

Student: What are the rate and the quality of breathing?
PROCTOR: Rate: Rapid. Quality: Normal.

Provide Oxygen

Student: I am applying oxygen at 15 L/min via nonrebreathing mask.
PROCTOR: Noted.

Ensure Adequate Ventilation

Student: The patient has adequate ventilations at this time.
PROCTOR: Noted.

Injury Management

Student: I will direct my partner to remove the patient's clothes as I continue assessment.
PROCTOR: Noted.

Assess Circulation

Student: I am assessing the patient's circulation.
PROCTOR: Noted.

Assess for and Control Major Bleeding

Student: Do I find any major bleeding?
PROCTOR: No.

Assess the Pulse

Student: What are the rate and the quality of pulses?
PROCTOR: Rate: Fast. Quality: Bounding.

Assess the Skin

Student: I am assessing the skin. What are the color, temperature, and condition of the skin?
PROCTOR: Color: Pale. Temperature: Warm. Condition: Moist.

Identify Priority Patients/Make Transport Decision

Student: The patient is a high priority and is a load-and-go. I will begin packaging and transport.
PROCTOR: Noted.

Critical Criteria:
- ❑ Did not provide high concentration of oxygen
- ❑ Did not find or manage problems associated with airway, breathing, hemorrhage or shock (hypoperfusion)
- ❑ Did not differentiate patient's need for transportation versus continued assessment at the scene
- ❑ Did other detailed examination before assessing the airway, breathing and circulation

Focused History and Physical Examination/Rapid Trauma Assessment

Select the Appropriate Assessment (Focused or Rapid)

Student: I am selecting the rapid physical exam to identify and treat life threats. I am checking for DCAP-BTLS. This acronym stands for deformities, contusions, abrasions, punctures, penetrations, and paradoxical motion in the chest, and burns, tenderness, lacerations, and swelling.
PROCTOR: Noted.

Head

Student: I am rapidly assessing the head.
PROCTOR: There are no obvious injuries.

Neck

Student: I am rapidly assessing the neck.
PROCTOR: There are no obvious injuries.
Student: I will apply a cervical collar.
PROCTOR: Noted.

Chest

Student: I am rapidly assessing the chest.
PROCTOR: There is an exit wound to the left chest at the bottom of the ribs.
Student: I will treat with an occlusive dressing.
PROCTOR: Noted.
Student: I will assess the chest for tension pneumothorax by auscultation, and assessment (jugular vein distention [JVD], tracheal deviation, and decreased lung sounds).
PROCTOR: The lung sounds appear clear bilaterally, jugular vein distention is not present, and the trachea is midline.

ALS Student: I will assess the chest for hyperresonance to percussion.
ALS Proctor: Noted. There is no tension pneumothorax.
ALS Student: I will continuously reassess the chest.
ALS Proctor: Noted.

▸ **Abdomen/Pelvis**

Student: I am rapidly assessing the abdomen.
PROCTOR: There are no obvious injuries.

▸ **Extremities**

Student: I am rapidly assessing the extremities.
PROCTOR: There are entrance wounds to both hands, and an exit wound to the left foot at the bottom of the toes.
Student: I will dress these wounds later.
PROCTOR: Noted.

▸ **Assess Motor, Sensory, and Circulatory Function**

Student: I am checking for DCAP-BTLS. I am also checking motor and sensory function, and pulses. Right leg?
PROCTOR: Negative DCAP-BTLS. Motor and sensory functions are present. Pulses are present.
Student: Left leg?
PROCTOR: There are exit wounds to the bottoms of the toes. Motor and sensory functions are present. Pulses are present.
Student: Right arm?
PROCTOR: There are entrance wounds to the hands. Motor and sensory functions are present. Pulses are present.
Student: Left arm?
PROCTOR: There are entrance wounds to the hands. Motor and sensory functions are present. Pulses are present.

▸ **Posterior**

Student: I am rapidly checking the back. We will now log roll the patient as a unit to check the back. The person at the head will count to three and we will roll the patient.
PROCTOR: Noted.

▸ **Assess the Thorax**

Student: I am assessing the thorax. Do I find injuries?
PROCTOR: No.

▸ **Assess the Lumbar Area**

Student: I am assessing the flanks and lumbar area. Do I find injuries?
PROCTOR: No.

▸ **Assess the Entire Backside**

Student: I am assessing the entire backside. Do I find injuries?
PROCTOR: No.

▸ **Manage Secondary Injuries**

Student: We will apply a cervical collar and backboard with full immobilization per local protocol, if not yet done, at this time.
PROCTOR: Noted.
Student: Are there any changes in motor and sensory functions and pulses?
PROCTOR: No.
ALS Student: I will establish two large-bore IVs en route to the hospital and administer a bolus of 20 mL/kg in order to maintain a systolic blood pressure of 90 mm Hg.
ALS Proctor: Noted.

▸ **Reevaluate Transport Decision**

Student: This patient is a load-and-go due to the mechanism of injury.
PROCTOR: Noted.

▾ Baseline Vital Signs

Student: What are the patient's baseline vital signs, including blood pressure, pulse, respirations, pulse oximetry, and level of consciousness?
PROCTOR: Blood pressure, 190/90 mm Hg; pulse, 160 beats/min; respirations, 24 breaths/min; pulse oximetry reading, 97%; and the patient is alert.

▾ SAMPLE History

Student: At this time I will gather a SAMPLE history from the patient or family. What are the patient's signs and symptoms?
PROCTOR: Pain in shoulders, chest, hands, and left foot.
Student: Allergies?
PROCTOR: No allergies.
Student: Medications?
PROCTOR: No medications.
Student: Pertinent past medical history?
PROCTOR: No pertinent medical history.
Student: Last oral intake?
PROCTOR: 3 hours ago.
Student: Events leading up to the incident?
PROCTOR: He was working on a high-voltage electrical line when he was shocked. A coworker just approached you with a suicide note signed by the patient.

Critical Criteria:
- ❑ Did not differentiate patient's need for transportation versus continued assessment at the scene
- ❑ Did not provide for spinal protection when indicated

▾ Detailed Physical Examination

Student: I am conducting the detailed physical exam. I am looking for DCAP-BTLS.
PROCTOR: Noted. The detailed physical exam will be performed during transport.

▾ Assess the Head

Student: I am assessing the head. Do I find any DCAP-BTLS? Do I find any evidence of Battle's sign or raccoon eyes?
PROCTOR: No.

▸ **Inspect and Palpate the Head and Ears**

Student: I am assessing the head and ears.
PROCTOR: There are no obvious injuries.

▸ **Assess the Eyes**

Student: I am assessing the eyes. Are the pupils equal, round, and regular in size, and react properly to light (PEARRL)?
PROCTOR: They are PEARRL.

▸ **Assess the Facial Area Including Oral and Nasal Areas**

Student: I am assessing the face, nose, and mouth. Do I see any discharge or hear any obstructions?
PROCTOR: No.

▾ Assess the Neck

▸ **Inspect and Palpate the Neck**

Student: I am assessing the neck for DCAP-BTLS.
PROCTOR: There are no obvious injuries.

▸ **Assess for Jugular Vein Distention**

Student: Do I find any jugular vein distention (JVD)?
PROCTOR: Yes.

▸ **Assess for Tracheal Deviation**

Student: Do I see any tracheal deviation?
PROCTOR: No.

▾ Assess the Chest

Student: I am assessing the chest for DCAP-BTLS.
PROCTOR: Noted.

▸ **Inspect**

Student: What do I see when I look at the chest?
PROCTOR: There is a small round exit wound to the bottom rib of the left chest with the smell of burnt flesh treated with an occlusive dressing.
Student: Does the chest appear symmetric?
PROCTOR: Yes.

▸ **Palpate**

Student: When I touch the chest, do I feel crepitus or a flail segment?
PROCTOR: No.

▸ **Auscultate**

Student: Are lung sounds present in all fields?

PROCTOR: Yes.

Student: Do I hear any sucking sounds from the chest?

PROCTOR: No.

▾ Assess the Abdomen/Pelvis

▸ **Assess the Abdomen**

Student: I am assessing the abdomen for DCAP-BTLS. I am assessing all four quadrants. Do I find any problems?

PROCTOR: No.

▸ **Assess the Pelvis**

Student: I am assessing the pelvis for DCAP-BTLS. Is the pelvis stable?

PROCTOR: Yes.

▸ **Assess the Genitalia/Perineum as Needed (Verbalize in Training)**

Student: I am assessing the genitalia/perineum as necessary for DCAP-BTLS.

PROCTOR: The area is unremarkable.

▾ Assess the Extremities

▸ **Inspect**

Student: I am assessing the lower and upper extremities for DCAP-BTLS. Do I find anything?

PROCTOR: Yes, you find the entrance and exit wounds.

▸ **Palpate**

Student: Do I feel anything unusual?

PROCTOR: No.

▸ **Assess Motor, Sensory, and Circulatory Function**

Student: I am checking for DCAP-BTLS, motor and sensory function, and pulses. Right leg?

PROCTOR: Negative DCAP-BTLS. Motor and sensory functions are present. Pulses are present.

Student: Left leg?

PROCTOR: There are exit wounds to the bottoms of the toes. Motor and sensory functions are present. Pulses are present.

Student: Right arm?

PROCTOR: There are entrance wounds to the hands. Motor and sensory functions are present. Pulses are present.

Student: Left arm?

PROCTOR: There are entrance wounds to the hands. Motor and sensory functions are present. Pulses are present.

▾ Assess the Posterior

Note: This portion of the detailed physical exam would not be done if the patient were previously backboarded per local protocol.

Student: We will not check the back since it was previously checked and the patient is backboarded.

PROCTOR: Noted.

▾ Manage Secondary Injuries/Wounds

Student: I would direct my partner to apply dressings to the burn wounds.

PROCTOR: Noted.

▾ Reassess Vital Signs

Student: I will reassess vital signs and mental status.

PROCTOR: Blood pressure, 180/86 mm Hg; pulse, 154 beats/min; respirations, 24 breaths/min; pulse oximetry reading, 97%; and the patient is alert.

Student: The vital signs have not significantly changed.

PROCTOR: Noted.

▾ Reassess Interventions

Student: I will reassess my interventions: oxygen; dressings to the hands, left chest, and left toes per local protocol; reassurance; and full immobilization.

PROCTOR: Noted.

ALS Student: I will reassess basic life support (BLS) interventions, plus the following: two large-bore IVs, 12-lead ECG and cardiac monitoring, and local protocol, including pain management.

ALS Proctor: Noted. The cardiac monitor shows supraventricular tachycardia.

> **Critical Criteria:**
> ❑ Did not find or manage problems associated with airway, breathing, hemorrhage or shock (hypoperfusion)

Radio Report

(Provided by the student.)

PROCTOR: Noted.

Ongoing Assessment

▾ Repeat Vital Signs

Student: I will reassess vital signs and mental status.

PROCTOR: Blood pressure, 174/82 mm Hg; pulse, 148 beats/min; respirations, 22 breaths/min; pulse oximetry reading, 97%; and the patient is alert.

Student: The vital signs have not significantly changed.

PROCTOR: Noted.

▾ Check Interventions

Student: I will check my interventions: oxygen; dressings to the hands, left chest, and left toes per local protocol; reassurance; and full immobilization.

PROCTOR: Noted.

ALS Student: I will check BLS interventions, plus the following: two large-bore IVs, 12-lead ECG and cardiac monitoring, and local protocol.

ALS Proctor: Noted. The cardiac monitor shows sinus tachycardia.

> **Critical Criteria:**
> ❑ Did not find or manage problems associated with airway, breathing, hemorrhage or shock (hypoperfusion)

Handoff Report to Emergency Department Staff

Student: There was no change during transport. I will notify nursing staff about the signed suicide note.

PROCTOR: Noted.

> **Critical Criteria:**
> ❑ Did not transport patient within the (10) minute time limit

Critical Criteria

(Inform the student of items missed, if any.)

❑ Pass ❑ Fail Date: ____________________

Proctor Comments: ____________________

____

____

CASE 9

Notes

Dispatch Information

PROCTOR: EMS 10, respond to a 16-year-old male who has been shot. The patient is conscious and breathing. The police have been dispatched.

Pre-scene Action (BSI)

Student: I am wearing nonlatex gloves, safety glasses, mask, and gown.
PROCTOR: Noted.

> **Critical Criteria:**
> ❑ Did not take, or verbalize, body substance isolation (BSI) precautions when necessary

Scene Size-up

Scene Safety

Student: Is the scene safe?
PROCTOR: Yes, police are on scene and you are given clearance to enter.

Mechanism of Injury

Student: What was the mechanism of injury?
PROCTOR: Gunshot wound. The patient was stealing food from a farmer and was shot in the buttocks and foot.

Number of Patients

Student: How many patients are there?
PROCTOR: One.

Additional Resources

Student: I would not call for additional resources.
PROCTOR: Noted.

C-Spine Stabilization

Student: On the basis of the mechanism of injury, I would stabilize the cervical spine (c-spine) in a neutral in-line position.
PROCTOR: Noted.

> **Critical Criteria:**
> ❑ Did not determine scene safety
> ❑ Did not assess for spinal protection
> ❑ Did not provide for spinal protection when indicated

Initial Assessment

Student: As I perform midline c-spine stabilization, I identify myself and ask the patient not to move.
PROCTOR: Noted.

General Impression

Student: My general impression is that the patient's condition is stable.
PROCTOR: Noted.

Responsiveness/Level of Consciousness

Student: What is the patient's level of consciousness?
PROCTOR: Alert.

Chief Complaint/Apparent Life Threats

Student: What is the patient's chief complaint?
PROCTOR: The patient is complaining of pain in his buttocks and foot.
Student: There are no apparent life threats.
PROCTOR: Noted.

Assess the Airway and Breathing

Student: Is the airway open? Is the patient breathing?
PROCTOR: Yes, the airway is open and the patient is breathing.

Assessment

Student: What are the rate and the quality of breathing?
PROCTOR: Rate: Within normal limits. Quality: Normal.

Provide Oxygen

Student: I am applying oxygen at 15 L/min via nonrebreathing mask.
PROCTOR: Noted.

Ensure Adequate Ventilation

Student: The patient has adequate ventilations at this time.
PROCTOR: Noted.

Injury Management

Student: I will direct my partner to take over c-spine control as I continue the assessment.
PROCTOR: Noted.

Assess Circulation

Student: I am assessing the patient's circulation.
PROCTOR: Noted.

Assess for and Control Major Bleeding

Student: Do I find any major bleeding?
PROCTOR: No. There is only minor bleeding from gunshot wounds to the buttocks and top of the right foot.

Assess the Pulse

Student: What are the rate and the quality of pulses?
PROCTOR: Rate: Within normal limits. Quality: Bounding.

Assess the Skin

Student: I am assessing the skin. What are the color, temperature, and condition of the skin?
PROCTOR: Color: Flushed. Temperature: Warm. Condition: Moist.

Identify Priority Patients/Make Transport Decision

Student: The patient is a low priority and does not require immediate transport.
PROCTOR: Noted.

> **Critical Criteria:**
> ❑ Did not provide high concentration of oxygen
> ❑ Did not find or manage problems associated with airway, breathing, hemorrhage or shock (hypoperfusion)
> ❑ Did not differentiate patient's need for transportation versus continued assessment at the scene
> ❑ Did other detailed examination before assessing the airway, breathing and circulation

Focused History and Physical Examination/Rapid Trauma Assessment

Select the Appropriate Assessment (Focused or Rapid)

Student: I am selecting the rapid physical exam to identify and treat life threats. I am checking for DCAP-BTLS. This acronym stands for deformities, contusions, abrasions, punctures, penetrations, and paradoxical motion in the chest, and burns, tenderness, lacerations, and swelling.
PROCTOR: Noted.

Head

Student: I am rapidly assessing the head.
PROCTOR: There are no obvious injuries.

Neck

Student: I am rapidly assessing the neck.
PROCTOR: There are no obvious injuries.
Student: I will apply a cervical collar.
PROCTOR: Noted.

Chest

Student: I am rapidly assessing the chest. What are the lung sounds?
PROCTOR: There are no obvious injuries. Lung sounds are clear bilaterally.

Abdomen/Pelvis

Student: I am rapidly assessing the abdomen.
PROCTOR: There are no obvious injuries.
Student: I am rapidly assessing the pelvis.
PROCTOR: The pelvis is intact.

▸ **Extremities**

Student: I am rapidly assessing the extremities.

PROCTOR: There is a gunshot wound to the top of the right foot with minimal bleeding.

▸ **Assess Motor, Sensory, and Circulatory Function**

Student: I am checking for DCAP-BTLS. I am also checking motor and sensory function, and pulses. Right leg?

PROCTOR: Slight bleeding from the right foot is noted. Motor and sensory functions are present. Pulses are present.

Student: I would treat it with direct pressure, a bandage, and splint.

PROCTOR: Noted.

Student: Are there any changes in motor and sensory functions and pulses?

PROCTOR: No.

Student: Left leg?

PROCTOR: Negative DCAP-BTLS. Motor and sensory functions are present. Pulses are present.

Student: Right arm?

PROCTOR: Negative DCAP-BTLS. Motor and sensory functions are present. Pulses are present.

Student: Left arm?

PROCTOR: Negative DCAP-BTLS. Motor and sensory functions are present. Pulses are present.

▸ **Posterior**

Student: We will now log roll the patient as a unit to check the back. The person at the head will count to three and we will roll the patient.

PROCTOR: Noted.

▸ **Assess the Thorax**

Student: I am assessing the thorax. Do I find injuries?

PROCTOR: No.

▸ **Assess the Lumbar Area**

Student: I am assessing the flanks and lumbar area. Do I find injuries?

PROCTOR: No.

▸ **Assess the Entire Backside**

Student: I am assessing the entire backside. Do I find injuries?

PROCTOR: Yes, a small puncture wound to the right buttocks.

Student: I would treat it with a dressing and a bandage.

PROCTOR: Noted.

▸ **Manage Secondary Injuries/Wounds**

Student: We will apply a cervical collar and backboard with full immobilization per local protocol, if not yet done, at this time.

PROCTOR: Noted.

Student: Are there any changes in motor and sensory functions and pulses?

PROCTOR: No.

ALS Student: I will establish two large-bore IVs en route to the hospital and administer a bolus of 20 mL/kg in order to maintain a systolic blood pressure of 90 mm Hg.

ALS Proctor: Noted.

▸ **Reevaluate Transport Decision**

Student: This patient is a low priority and does not require immediate transport.

PROCTOR: Noted.

▾ **Baseline Vital Signs**

Student: What are the patient's baseline vital signs, including blood pressure, pulse, respirations, pulse oximetry, and level of consciousness?

PROCTOR: Blood pressure, 160/92 mm Hg; pulse, 100 beats/min; respirations, 20 breaths/min; pulse oximetry reading, 99%; and the patient is alert.

▾ **SAMPLE History**

Student: At this time I will gather a SAMPLE history from the patient or family. What are the patient's signs and symptoms?

PROCTOR: Pain in the buttocks and foot.

Student: Allergies?

PROCTOR: No allergies.

Student: Medications?

PROCTOR: No medications.

Student: Pertinent past medical history?

PROCTOR: No pertinent medical history.

Student: Last oral intake?

PROCTOR: 2 hours ago.

Student: Events leading up to the incident?

PROCTOR: The patient was stealing food when the farmer shot at him.

Critical Criteria:

- ❑ Did not differentiate patient's need for transportation versus continued assessment at the scene
- ❑ Did not provide for spinal protection when indicated

▾ Detailed Physical Exam

Student: I am conducting the detailed physical exam. I am looking for DCAP-BTLS.

PROCTOR: Noted. The detailed physical exam will be performed during transport.

▸ **Assess the Head**

Student: I am assessing the head. Do I find any DCAP-BTLS? Do I find any evidence of Battle's sign or raccoon eyes?

PROCTOR: No.

▸ **Inspect and Palpate the Head and Ears**

Student: I am assessing the head and ears.

PROCTOR: There are no obvious injuries.

▸ **Assess the Eyes**

Student: I am assessing the eyes. Are the pupils equal, round, and regular in size, and react properly to light (PEARRL)?

PROCTOR: They are PEARRL.

▸ **Assess the Facial Area Including Oral and Nasal Areas**

Student: I am assessing the face, nose, and mouth. Do I see any discharge or hear obstructions?

PROCTOR: No.

▾ **Assess the Neck**

▸ **Inspect and Palpate the Neck**

Student: I am assessing the neck for DCAP-BTLS.

PROCTOR: There are no obvious injuries.

▸ **Assess for Jugular Vein Distention**

Student: Do I find any jugular vein distention (JVD)?

PROCTOR: No.

▸ **Assess for Tracheal Deviation**

Student: Do I see any tracheal deviation?

PROCTOR: No.

▾ **Assess the Chest**

Student: I am assessing the chest for DCAP-BTLS.

PROCTOR: Noted.

▸ **Inspect**

Student: What do I see when I look at the chest?

PROCTOR: There are no obvious injuries.

Student: Does the chest appear symmetric?

PROCTOR: Yes.

▸ **Palpate**

Student: When I touch the chest, do I feel crepitus or a flail segment?

PROCTOR: No.

▸ **Auscultate**

Student: Are lung sounds present in all fields?

PROCTOR: Yes.

▾ **Assess the Abdomen/Pelvis**

▸ **Assess the Abdomen**

Student: I am assessing the abdomen for DCAP-BTLS. I am assessing all four quadrants. Do I find any problems?

PROCTOR: No.

▸ **Assess the Pelvis**

Student: I am assessing the pelvis for DCAP-BTLS. Is the pelvis stable?
PROCTOR: Yes.

▸ **Assess the Genitalia/Perineum as Needed (Verbalize in Training)**

Student: I am assessing the genitalia/perineum as necessary for DCAP-BTLS.
PROCTOR: The area is unremarkable.

▾ **Assess the Extremities**

▸ **Inspect**

Student: I am assessing the lower and upper extremities for DCAP-BTLS. Do I find anything?
PROCTOR: Bleeding is controlled in the right foot.

▸ **Palpate**

Student: Do I feel anything unusual?
PROCTOR: No.

▸ **Assess Motor, Sensory, and Circulatory Function**

Student: I am checking for DCAP-BTLS, motor and sensory function, and pulses. Right leg?
PROCTOR: Bleeding from the right foot is controlled. Motor and sensory functions are present. Pulses are present.
Student: Left leg?
PROCTOR: Negative DCAP-BTLS. Motor and sensory functions are present. Pulses are present.
Student: Right arm?
PROCTOR: Negative DCAP-BTLS. Motor and sensory functions are present. Pulses are present.
Student: Left arm?
PROCTOR: Negative DCAP-BTLS. Motor and sensory functions are present. Pulses are present.

▾ **Assess the Posterior**

Note: This portion of the detailed physical exam would not be done if the patient were previously backboarded per local protocol.
Student: We will not check the back since it was previously checked and the patient is backboarded.
PROCTOR: Noted.

▾ **Manage Secondary Injuries/Wounds**

Student: I would direct my partner to continue providing oxygen.
PROCTOR: Noted.

▾ **Reassess Vital Signs**

Student: At this time I will reassess vital signs and mental status.
PROCTOR: Blood pressure, 150/86 mm Hg; pulse, 96 beats/min; respirations, 16 breaths/min; pulse oximetry reading, 99%; and the patient is alert.
Student: The vital signs are improving.
PROCTOR: Noted.

▾ **Reassess Interventions**

Student: I will reassess my interventions: airway, breathing, and oxygenation; circulation and bleeding control; and immobilization and straps.
PROCTOR: Noted.
ALS Student: I will reassess basic life support (BLS) interventions, plus the following: one or two large-bore IVs (per local protocol).
ALS Proctor: Noted.

Critical Criteria:
❑ Did not find or manage problems associated with airway, breathing, hemorrhage or shock (hypoperfusion)

Radio Report

(Provided by student.)
PROCTOR: Noted.

Ongoing Assessment

▾ **Repeat Vital Signs**

Student: I will reassess vital signs and mental status.
PROCTOR: Blood pressure, 140/74 mm Hg; pulse, 94 beats/min; respirations, 16 breaths/min; pulse oximetry reading, 99%; and the patient is alert.
Student: The vital signs have improved.
PROCTOR: Noted.

▾ **Check Interventions**

Student: I will check my interventions: airway, breathing, and oxygenation; circulation and bleeding control; and immobilization and straps.
PROCTOR: Noted.
ALS Student: I will check BLS interventions, plus the following: large-bore IV(s) (per local protocol).
ALS Proctor: Noted.

Critical Criteria:
❑ Did not find or manage problems associated with airway, breathing, hemorrhage or shock (hypoperfusion)

Handoff Report to Emergency Department Staff

Student: The patient's condition improved during transport.
PROCTOR: Noted.

Critical Criteria:
❑ Did not transport patient within the (10) minute time limit

Critical Criteria

(Inform the student of items missed, if any.)

❑ Pass ❑ Fail Date: ______________________

Proctor Comments: ______________________

____

____

Notes

Dispatch Information

PROCTOR: EMS 10, respond to a motor vehicle collision. There is one 25-year-old patient who has struck a tree. She is conscious and breathing. She is complaining of an eye injury.

Pre-scene Action (BSI)

Student: I am wearing nonlatex gloves and safety glasses.
PROCTOR: Noted.

Critical Criteria:
- ❑ Did not take, or verbalize, body substance isolation (BSI) precautions when necessary

Scene Size-up

Scene Safety

Student: Is the scene safe?
PROCTOR: Yes.

Mechanism of Injury

Student: What was the mechanism of injury?
PROCTOR: Motor vehicle collision and burn injury. The patient was smoking a cigarette while driving. She lost control on a curve and struck a tree. She was wearing a seat belt. Her airbag deployed and put her cigarette out in her eye. She does have a burn to the eye.

Number of Patients

Student: How many patients are there?
PROCTOR: One.

Additional Resources

Student: I would call for additional resources: fire/rescue and police.
PROCTOR: Noted.

C-Spine Stabilization

Student: On the basis of the mechanism of injury, I would stabilize the cervical spine (c-spine) in a neutral in-line position.
PROCTOR: Noted.

Critical Criteria:
- ❑ Did not determine scene safety
- ❑ Did not assess for spinal protection
- ❑ Did not provide for spinal protection when indicated

Initial Assessment

Student: As I perform midline c-spine stabilization, I identify myself and ask the patient not to move.
PROCTOR: Noted.

General Impression

Student: My general impression is that the patient's condition is stable.
PROCTOR: Noted.

Responsiveness/Level of Consciousness

Student: What is the patient's level of consciousness?
PROCTOR: Alert.

Chief Complaint/Apparent Life Threats

Student: What is the patient's chief complaint?
PROCTOR: The patient is complaining of a cigarette burn to her left eye.
Student: There are no apparent life threats.
PROCTOR: Noted.

Assess the Airway and Breathing

Student: Is the airway open? Is the patient breathing?
PROCTOR: Yes, the airway is open and the patient is breathing.

Assessment

Student: What are the rate and the quality of breathing?
PROCTOR: Rate: Tachypneic. Quality: Crying.

Provide Oxygen

Student: I am applying oxygen at 15 L/min via nonrebreathing mask.
PROCTOR: Noted.

Ensure Adequate Ventilation

Student: The patient has adequate ventilations at this time.
PROCTOR: Noted.

Injury Management

Student: I will direct my partner to take over c-spine control as I continue assessment.
PROCTOR: Noted.

Assess Circulation

Student: I am assessing the patient's circulation.
PROCTOR: Noted.

Assess for and Control Major Bleeding

Student: Do I find any major bleeding?
PROCTOR: No.

Assess the Pulse

Student: What are the rate and the quality of pulses?
PROCTOR: Rate: Tachycardic. Quality: Strong.

Assess the Skin

Student: I am assessing the skin. What are the color, temperature, and condition of the skin?
PROCTOR: Color: Flushed. Temperature: Warm. Condition: Moist.

Identify Priority Patients/Make Transport Decision

Student: The patient is a low priority and does not require immediate transport.
PROCTOR: Noted.

Critical Criteria:
- ❑ Did not provide high concentration of oxygen
- ❑ Did not find or manage problems associated with airway, breathing, hemorrhage or shock (hypoperfusion)
- ❑ Did not differentiate patient's need for transportation versus continued assessment at the scene
- ❑ Did other detailed examination before assessing the airway, breathing and circulation

Focused History and Physical Examination/Rapid Trauma Assessment

Select the Appropriate Assessment (Focused or Rapid)

Student: I am selecting the rapid physical exam to identify and treat life threats. I am checking for DCAP-BTLS. This acronym stands for deformities, contusions, abrasions, punctures, penetrations, and paradoxical motion in the chest, and burns, tenderness, lacerations, and swelling.
PROCTOR: Noted.

Head

Student: I am rapidly assessing the head.
PROCTOR: There is a burn to the left eye.
Student: I will flush the eye with saline; I will flush with an IV of saline solution without a needle, directing the tubing to the eye through a nasal cannula. I will apply a moist dressing to the eye.
PROCTOR: Noted.

Neck

Student: I am rapidly assessing the neck.
PROCTOR: There are no obvious injuries.
Student: I will apply a cervical collar.
PROCTOR: Noted.

Chest

Student: I am rapidly assessing the chest. What are the lung sounds?
PROCTOR: The patient has bruising from a seat belt injury to her left shoulder. The lung sounds are clear bilaterally.

▸ **Abdomen/Pelvis**

Student: I am rapidly assessing the abdomen.
PROCTOR: There are no obvious injuries.
Student: I am rapidly assessing the pelvis.
PROCTOR: There are no obvious injuries.

▸ **Extremities**

Student: I am rapidly assessing the extremities.
PROCTOR: The patient has bruising to both wrists from the steering wheel.

▸ **Assess Motor, Sensory, and Circulatory Function**

Student: I am checking for DCAP-BTLS. I am also checking motor and sensory function, and pulses. Right leg?
PROCTOR: Negative DCAP-BTLS. Motor and sensory functions are present. Pulses are present.
Student: Left leg?
PROCTOR: Negative DCAP-BTLS. Motor and sensory functions are present. Pulses are present.
Student: Right arm?
PROCTOR: There are superficial friction burns to the wrist from the steering wheel. Motor and sensory functions are present. Pulses are present.
Student: Left arm?
PROCTOR: There are superficial friction burns to the wrist from the steering wheel. Motor and sensory functions are present. Pulses are present.

▸ **Posterior**

Student: I am rapidly assessing the back. We will now log roll the patient as a unit to check the back. The person at the head will count to three and we will roll the patient.
PROCTOR: Noted.

▸ **Assess the Thorax**

Student: I am assessing the thorax. Do I find injuries?
PROCTOR: No.

▸ **Assess the Lumbar Area**

Student: I am assessing the flanks and lumbar area. Do I find injuries?
PROCTOR: No.

▸ **Assess the Entire Backside**

Student: I am assessing the entire backside. Do I find injuries?
PROCTOR: No.

▸ **Manage Secondary Injuries/Wounds**

Student: We will apply a cervical collar and vest-type immobilization device. The person at the head will count to three and we will position the patient. We will then position her on a backboard with full immobilization per local protocol at this time.
PROCTOR: Noted.
Student: Are there any changes in motor and sensory functions or pulses?
PROCTOR: No.

▸ **Reevaluate Transport Decision**

Student: This patient is a low priority and does not require immediate transport.
PROCTOR: Noted.

▼ Baseline Vital Signs

Student: What are the patient's baseline vital signs, including blood pressure, pulse, respirations, pulse oximetry, and level of consciousness?
PROCTOR: Blood pressure, 142/86 mm Hg; pulse, 128 beats/min; respirations, 20 breaths/min; pulse oximetry reading, 100%; and the patient is alert.

▼ SAMPLE History

Student: At this time I will gather a SAMPLE history from the patient or family. What are the patient's signs and symptoms?
PROCTOR: She has pain in the left eye.
Student: Allergies?
PROCTOR: No allergies.
Student: Medications?
PROCTOR: Seizure medications.
Student: Pertinent past medical history?
PROCTOR: Seizures.
Student: Last oral intake?
PROCTOR: 4 hours ago.
Student: Events leading up to the incident?
PROCTOR: The patient was smoking a cigarette while driving. She lost control of her car on a curve and struck a tree. She was wearing a seat belt. Her airbag deployed and put her cigarette out in her eye. She has a burn to the eye.

Critical Criteria:
- ❑ Did not differentiate patient's need for transportation versus continued assessment at the scene
- ❑ Did not provide for spinal protection when indicated

▼ Detailed Physical Examination

Student: I am conducting the detailed physical exam. I am looking for DCAP-BTLS.
PROCTOR: Noted. The detailed physical exam will be performed during transport.

▼ Assess the Head

Student: I am assessing the head. Do I find any DCAP-BTLS? Do I find any evidence of Battle's sign or raccoon eyes?
PROCTOR: There is a cigarette burn to the left eye that is dressed.

▸ **Inspect and Palpate the Head and Ears**

Student: I am assessing the head and ears.
PROCTOR: There is a cigarette burn to the left eye that is dressed.

▸ **Assess the Eyes**

Student: I am assessing the eyes. Are the pupils equal, round, and regular in size, and react properly to light (PEARRL)?
PROCTOR: The left eye is covered with the dressing.
Student: I will recheck the dressing.
PROCTOR: Noted.

▸ **Assess the Facial Area Including Oral and Nasal Areas**

Student: I am assessing the face, nose, and mouth. Do I see any discharge or hear any obstructions?
PROCTOR: No.

▼ Assess the Neck

▸ **Inspect and Palpate the Neck**

Student: I am assessing the neck for DCAP-BTLS.
PROCTOR: There are no obvious injuries.

▸ **Assess for Jugular Vein Distention**

Student: Do I find any jugular vein distention (JVD)?
PROCTOR: No.

▸ **Assess for Tracheal Deviation**

Student: Do I see any tracheal deviation?
PROCTOR: No.

▼ Assess the Chest

Student: I am assessing the chest for DCAP-BTLS.
PROCTOR: Noted.

▸ **Inspect**

Student: What do I see when I look at the chest?
PROCTOR: There is bruising from a seat belt injury to the left shoulder.
Student: Does the chest appear symmetric?
PROCTOR: Yes.

▸ **Palpate**

Student: When I touch the chest, do I feel crepitus or a flail segment?
PROCTOR: No.

▸ Auscultate

Student: Are lung sounds present in all fields?

PROCTOR: Yes.

Student: Do I hear any sucking sounds from the chest?

PROCTOR: No.

▼ Assess the Abdomen/Pelvis

▸ Assess the Abdomen

Student: I am assessing the abdomen for DCAP-BTLS. I am assessing all four quadrants. Do I find any problems?

PROCTOR: No.

▸ Assess the Pelvis

Student: I am assessing the pelvis for DCAP-BTLS. Is the pelvis stable?

PROCTOR: Yes.

▼ Assess the Genitalia/Perineum as Needed (Verbalize in Training)

Student: I am assessing the genitalia/perineum as necessary for DCAP-BTLS.

PROCTOR: The area is unremarkable.

▼ Assess the Extremities

▸ Inspect

Student: I am assessing the lower and upper extremities for DCAP-BTLS. Do I find anything?

PROCTOR: Yes, there is bruising to the left shoulder and bilateral wrist burns.

▸ Palpate

Student: Do I feel anything unusual?

PROCTOR: No.

▸ Assess Motor, Sensory, and Circulatory Function

Student: I am checking for DCAP-BTLS, motor and sensory function, and pulses. Right leg?

PROCTOR: Negative DCAP-BTLS. Motor and sensory functions are present. Pulses are present.

Student: Left leg?

PROCTOR: Negative DCAP-BTLS. Motor and sensory functions are present. Pulses are present.

Student: Right arm?

PROCTOR: There are minor friction burns to the wrist from the steering wheel. Motor and sensory functions are present. Pulses are present.

Student: Left arm?

PROCTOR: There are minor friction burns to the wrist from the steering wheel. Motor and sensory functions are present. Pulses are present.

▼ Assess the Posterior

Note: This portion of the detailed physical exam would not be done if the patient were previously backboarded per local protocol.

Student: We will not check the back since it was previously checked and the patient is backboarded.

PROCTOR: Noted.

▼ Manage Secondary Injuries/Wounds

Student: I would continue to monitor the patient.

PROCTOR: Noted.

▼ Reassess Vital Signs

Student: I will reassess vital signs and mental status.

PROCTOR: Blood pressure, 136/84 mm Hg; pulse, 122 beats/min; respirations, 20 breaths/min; pulse oximetry reading, 100%; and the patient is alert.

Student: The vital signs have not changed significantly.

PROCTOR: Noted.

▼ Reassess Interventions

Student: I will reassess my interventions: oxygen, flush the eye with saline, full immobilization, and saline flushed through an IV bag through a nasal cannula.

PROCTOR: Noted.

Critical Criteria:

❑ Did not find or manage problems associated with airway, breathing, hemorrhage or shock (hypoperfusion)

▼ Radio Report

(Provided by the student.)

PROCTOR: Noted.

▼ Ongoing Assessment

▼ Repeat Vital Signs

Student: I will reassess vital signs and mental status.

PROCTOR: Blood pressure, 128/80 mm Hg; pulse, 112 beats/min; respirations, 20 breaths/min; pulse oximetry reading, 100%; and the patient is alert.

Student: The vital signs have not changed significantly.

PROCTOR: Noted.

▼ Check Interventions

Student: I will check my interventions: oxygen, flush the eye with saline, full immobilization, and saline flushed through an IV bag through a nasal cannula.

PROCTOR: Noted.

Critical Criteria:

❑ Did not find or manage problems associated with airway, breathing, hemorrhage or shock (hypoperfusion)

▼ Handoff Report to Emergency Department Staff

Student: There was no change during transport.

PROCTOR: Noted.

Critical Criteria:

❑ Did not transport patient within the (10) minute time limit

▼ Critical Criteria

(Inform the student of items missed, if any.)

❑ Pass ❑ Fail Date: ______________________

Proctor Comments: ______________________

____

____

Notes

Dispatch Information

PROCTOR: EMS 10, respond to a 17-year-old cheerleader who was struck in the back by a football player's helmet. She is conscious and breathing.

Pre-scene Action (BSI)

Student: I am wearing nonlatex gloves, safety glasses, mask, and gown.
PROCTOR: Noted.

Critical Criteria:
- ❑ Did not take, or verbalize, body substance isolation (BSI) precautions when necessary

Scene Size-up

Scene Safety

Student: Is the scene safe?
PROCTOR: Yes.

Mechanism of Injury

Student: What was the mechanism of injury?
PROCTOR: Blunt trauma. The patient was cheerleading and was struck by a football player.

Number of Patients

Student: How many patients are there?
PROCTOR: One.

Additional Resources

Student: I would not call for advanced life support (ALS) assistance.
PROCTOR: Noted.

C-Spine Stabilization

Student: On the basis of the mechanism of injury, I would stabilize the cervical spine (c-spine) in a neutral in-line position.
PROCTOR: Noted.

Critical Criteria:
- ❑ Did not determine scene safety
- ❑ Did not assess for spinal protection
- ❑ Did not provide for spinal protection when indicated

Initial Assessment

Student: As I perform midline c-spine stabilization, I identify myself and ask the patient not to move.
PROCTOR: Noted.

General Impression

Student: My general impression is that the patient's condition is stable.
PROCTOR: Noted.

Responsiveness/Level of Consciousness

Student: What is the patient's level of consciousness?
PROCTOR: Alert.

Chief Complaint/Apparent Life Threats

Student: What is the patient's chief complaint?
PROCTOR: The patient is complaining of pain in the lower left back.
Student: There are no apparent life threats.
PROCTOR: Noted.

Assess the Airway and Breathing

Student: Is the airway open? Is the patient breathing?
PROCTOR: Yes, the airway is open and the patient is breathing.

Assessment

Student: What are the rate and the quality of breathing?
PROCTOR: Rate: Rapid. Quality: Crying.

Provide Oxygen

Student: I am applying oxygen at 15 L/min via nonrebreathing mask.
PROCTOR: Noted.

Ensure Adequate Ventilation

Student: The patient has adequate ventilations at this time.
PROCTOR: Noted.

Injury Management

Student: I will direct my partner to take over c-spine control as I continue assessment.
PROCTOR: Noted.

Assess Circulation

Student: I am assessing the patient's circulation.
PROCTOR: Noted.

Assess for and Control Major Bleeding

Student: Do I find any major bleeding?
PROCTOR: No.

Assess the Pulse

Student: What are the rate and the quality of pulses?
PROCTOR: Rate: Within normal limits. Quality: Strong.

Assess the Skin

Student: I am assessing the skin. What are the color, temperature, and condition of the skin?
PROCTOR: Color: Flushed. Temperature: Warm. Condition: Moist.

Identify Priority Patients/Make Transport Decision

Student: The patient is a low priority and does not require immediate transport.
PROCTOR: Noted.

Critical Criteria:
- ❑ Did not provide high concentration of oxygen
- ❑ Did not find or manage problems associated with airway, breathing, hemorrhage or shock (hypoperfusion)
- ❑ Did not differentiate patient's need for transportation versus continued assessment at the scene
- ❑ Did other detailed examination before assessing the airway, breathing and circulation

Focused History and Physical Examination/Rapid Trauma Assessment

Select the Appropriate Assessment (Focused or Rapid)

Student: I am selecting the rapid physical exam to identify and treat life threats. I am checking for DCAP-BTLS. This acronym stands for deformities, contusions, abrasions, punctures, penetrations, and paradoxical motion in the chest, and burns, tenderness, lacerations, and swelling.
PROCTOR: Noted.

Head

Student: I am rapidly assessing the head.
PROCTOR: There are no obvious injuries.

Neck

Student: I am rapidly assessing the neck.
PROCTOR: There are no obvious injuries.
Student: I will apply a cervical collar.
PROCTOR: Noted.

Chest

Student: I am rapidly assessing the chest. What are the lung sounds?
PROCTOR: There are no obvious injuries. The lung sounds are clear bilaterally.

Abdomen/Pelvis

Student: I am rapidly assessing the abdomen.
PROCTOR: There are no obvious injuries.
Student: I am rapidly assessing the pelvis.
PROCTOR: There are no obvious injuries.

▸ **Extremities**

Student: I am rapidly assessing the extremities.

PROCTOR: There are no obvious injuries.

▸ **Assess Motor, Sensory, and Circulatory Function**

Student: I am checking for DCAP-BTLS. I am also checking motor and sensory function, and pulses. Right leg?

PROCTOR: Negative DCAP-BTLS. Motor and sensory functions are present. Pulses are present.

Student: Left leg?

PROCTOR: Negative DCAP-BTLS. Motor and sensory functions are present. Pulses are present.

Student: Right arm?

PROCTOR: Negative DCAP-BTLS. Motor and sensory functions are present. Pulses are present.

Student: Left arm?

PROCTOR: Negative DCAP-BTLS. Motor and sensory functions are present. Pulses are present.

▸ **Posterior**

Student: I am rapidly assessing the back. We will now log roll the patient as a unit to check the back. The person at the head will count to three and we will roll the patient.

PROCTOR: Noted.

▸ **Assess the Thorax**

Student: I am assessing the thorax. Do I find injuries?

PROCTOR: No.

▸ **Assess the Lumbar Area**

Student: I am assessing the flanks and lumbar area. Do I find injuries?

PROCTOR: You see an abrasion consistent with an impact of a helmet to the left flank area.

▸ **Assess the Entire Backside**

Student: I am assessing the entire backside. Do I find injuries?

PROCTOR: No.

▸ **Manage Secondary Injuries/Wounds**

Student: We will apply a cervical collar and backboard with full immobilization per local protocol, if not yet done, at this time.

PROCTOR: Noted.

Student: Are there any changes in motor and sensory functions or pulses?

PROCTOR: No.

ALS Student: I will establish two large-bore IVs en route to the hospital and administer a bolus of 20 mL/kg in order to maintain a systolic blood pressure of 90 mm Hg.

ALS Proctor: Noted.

▸ **Reevaluate Transport Decision**

Student: The patient is a low priority and does not require immediate transport.

PROCTOR: Noted.

▾ Baseline Vital Signs

Student: What are the patient's baseline vital signs, including blood pressure, pulse, respirations, pulse oximetry, and level of consciousness?

PROCTOR: Blood pressure, 120/72 mm Hg; pulse, 100 beats/min; respirations, 24 breaths/min; pulse oximetry reading, 99%; and the patient is alert.

▾ SAMPLE History

Student: At this time I will gather a SAMPLE history from the patient or family. What are the patient's signs and symptoms?

PROCTOR: Pain in the back on the left side just below the ribs.

Student: Allergies?

PROCTOR: No allergies.

Student: Medications?

PROCTOR: No medications.

Student: Pertinent past medical history?

PROCTOR: No pertinent medical history.

Student: Last oral intake?

PROCTOR: 3 hours ago.

Student: Events leading up to the incident?

PROCTOR: The patient was cheerleading when she was struck by a football player.

Critical Criteria:
- ❑ Did not differentiate patient's need for transportation versus continued assessment at the scene
- ❑ Did not provide for spinal protection when indicated

▾ Detailed Physical Examination

Student: I am conducting the detailed physical exam. I am looking for DCAP-BTLS.

PROCTOR: Noted. The detailed physical exam will be performed during transport.

▾ Assess the Head

Student: I am assessing the head. Do I find any DCAP-BTLS? Do I find any evidence of Battle's sign or raccoon eyes?

PROCTOR: No.

▸ **Inspect and Palpate the Head and Ears**

Student: I am assessing the head and ears.

PROCTOR: There are no obvious injuries.

▸ **Assess the Eyes**

Student: I am assessing the eyes. Are the pupils equal, round, and regular in size, and react properly to light (PEARRL)?

PROCTOR: They are PEARRL.

▸ **Assess the Facial Area Including Oral and Nasal Areas**

Student: I am assessing the face, nose, and mouth. Do I see any discharge or hear any obstructions?

PROCTOR: No.

▾ Assess the Neck

▸ **Inspect and Palpate the Neck**

Student: I am assessing the neck for DCAP-BTLS.

PROCTOR: There are no obvious injuries.

▸ **Assess for Jugular Vein Distention**

Student: Do I find any jugular vein distention (JVD)?

PROCTOR: No.

▸ **Assess for Tracheal Deviation**

Student: Do I see any tracheal deviation?

PROCTOR: No.

▾ Assess the Chest

Student: I am assessing the chest for DCAP-BTLS.

PROCTOR: Noted.

▸ **Inspect**

Student: What do I see when I look at the chest?

PROCTOR: There are no obvious injuries.

Student: Does the chest appear symmetric?

PROCTOR: Yes.

▸ **Palpate**

Student: When I touch the chest, do I feel crepitus or a flail segment?

PROCTOR: No.

▸ **Auscultate**

Student: Are lung sounds present in all fields?

PROCTOR: Yes.

Student: Do I hear any sucking sounds from the chest?

PROCTOR: No.

▾ Assess the Abdomen/Pelvis

▸ **Assess the Abdomen**

Student: I am assessing the abdomen for DCAP-BTLS. I am assessing all four quadrants. Do I find any problems?

PROCTOR: No. The abdomen is soft and nontender.

▸ **Assess the Pelvis**

Student: I am assessing the pelvis for DCAP-BTLS. Is the pelvis stable?

PROCTOR: Yes.

▾ Assess the Genitalia/Perineum as Needed (Verbalize in Training)

Student: I am assessing the genitalia/perineum as necessary for DCAP-BTLS.

PROCTOR: She is incontinent of urine.

▾ Assess the Extremities

▸ **Inspect**

Student: I am assessing the lower and upper extremities for DCAP-BTLS. Do I find anything?

PROCTOR: No.

▸ **Palpate**

Student: Do I feel anything unusual?

PROCTOR: No.

▸ **Assess Motor, Sensory, and Circulatory Function**

Student: I am checking for DCAP-BTLS, pulses, and motor and sensory function. Right leg?

PROCTOR: Negative DCAP-BTLS. Motor and sensory functions are present. Pulses are present.

Student: Left leg?

PROCTOR: Negative DCAP-BTLS. Motor and sensory functions are present. Pulses are present.

Student: Right arm?

PROCTOR: Negative DCAP-BTLS. Motor and sensory functions are present. Pulses are present.

Student: Left arm?

PROCTOR: Negative DCAP-BTLS. Motor and sensory functions are present. Pulses are present.

▾ Assess the Posterior

Note: This portion of the detailed physical exam would not be done if the patient were previously backboarded per local protocol.

Student: We will not check the back since it was previously checked and the patient is backboarded.

PROCTOR: Noted.

▾ Manage Secondary Injuries/Wounds

Student: I would direct my partner to monitor the patient.

PROCTOR: Noted.

▾ Reassess Vital Signs

Student: I will reassess vital signs and mental status.

PROCTOR: Blood pressure, 118/68 mm Hg; pulse, 110 beats/min; respirations, 20 breaths/min; pulse oximetry reading, 99%; and the patient is alert.

Student: The vital signs have not changed significantly.

PROCTOR: Noted.

▾ Reassess Interventions

Student: I will reassess my interventions: airway, oxygen, immobilization, and straps.

PROCTOR: Noted.

ALS Student: I will reassess basic life support (BLS) interventions, plus the following: two large-bore IVs and cardiac monitor or other local protocol.

ALS Proctor: Noted. The cardiac monitor shows sinus tachycardia.

Critical Criteria:
- ❑ Did not find or manage problems associated with airway, breathing, hemorrhage or shock (hypoperfusion)

Radio Report

(Provided by the student.)

PROCTOR: Noted.

Ongoing Assessment

▾ Repeat Vital Signs

Student: I will reassess vital signs and mental status.

PROCTOR: Blood pressure, 112/64 mm Hg; pulse, 104 beats/min; respirations, 20 breaths/min; pulse oximetry reading, 99%; and the patient is alert.

Student: The vital signs have not changed significantly.

PROCTOR: Noted.

▾ Check Interventions

Student: I will check my interventions: airway, oxygen, immobilization, and straps.

PROCTOR: Noted.

ALS Student: I will check BLS interventions, plus the following: two large-bore IVs and cardiac monitor or other local protocol.

ALS Proctor: Noted. The cardiac monitor shows sinus tachycardia.

Critical Criteria:
- ❑ Did not find or manage problems associated with airway, breathing, hemorrhage or shock (hypoperfusion)

Handoff Report to Emergency Department Staff

Student: There was no change during transport.

PROCTOR: Noted.

Critical Criteria:
- ❑ Did not transport patient within the (10) minute time limit

Critical Criteria

(Inform the student of items missed, if any.)

❑ Pass ❑ Fail Date: ______________________

Proctor Comments: ______________________

____

____

CASE 12

Notes

CASE 13

Dispatch Information

PROCTOR: EMS 10, respond to a 32-year-old male patient who has been burned by a radiator. He is conscious and breathing.

Pre-scene Action (BSI)

Student: I am wearing nonlatex gloves, safety glasses, mask, and gown.
PROCTOR: Noted.

Critical Criteria:
- ❑ Did not take, or verbalize, body substance isolation (BSI) precautions when necessary

Scene Size-up

Scene Safety

Student: Is the scene safe?
PROCTOR: Yes.

Mechanism of Injury

Student: What was the mechanism of injury?
PROCTOR: Burn injury. The patient was checking his overheated car and the radiator cap popped off. He has burns to his face, eyes, and hands.

Number of Patients

Student: How many patients are there?
PROCTOR: One.

Additional Resources

Student: I would call for advanced life support (ALS) assistance.
PROCTOR: Noted.

C-Spine Stabilization

Student: I would not stabilize the cervical spine (c-spine).
PROCTOR: Noted.

Critical Criteria:
- ❑ Did not determine scene safety
- ❑ Did not assess for spinal protection
- ❑ Did not provide for spinal protection when indicated

Initial Assessment

Student: I identify myself and ask the patient not to move.
PROCTOR: Noted.

General Impression

Student: My general impression is that the patient's condition is unstable.
PROCTOR: Noted.

Responsiveness/Level of Consciousness

Student: What is the patient's level of consciousness?
PROCTOR: Alert.

Chief Complaint/Apparent Life Threats

Student: What is the patient's chief complaint?
PROCTOR: The patient is complaining of difficulty breathing.
Student: There are apparent life threats; the life threats are the airway and breathing problems.
PROCTOR: Noted.

Assess the Airway and Breathing

Student: I am opening the airway. Is the patient breathing?
PROCTOR: Yes.

Assessment

Student: What are the rate and the quality of breathing?
PROCTOR: Rate: Tachypneic. Quality: Deep.

Provide Oxygen

Student: I am applying oxygen at 15 L/min via nonrebreathing mask.
PROCTOR: Noted.

Ensure Adequate Ventilation

Student: The patient has adequate ventilations at this time.
PROCTOR: Noted.

Injury Management

Student: I will direct my partner to stop the burning process as I continue assessment.
PROCTOR: Noted.

Assess Circulation

Student: I am assessing the patient's circulation.
PROCTOR: Noted.

Assess for and Control Major Bleeding

Student: Do I find any major bleeding?
PROCTOR: No.

Assess the Pulse

Student: What are the rate and the quality of pulses?
PROCTOR: Rate: Tachycardic. Quality: Strong.

Assess the Skin

Student: I am assessing the skin. What are the color, temperature, and condition of the skin?
PROCTOR: Color: Red and blistered in places. Temperature: Hot. Condition: Diaphoretic.

Identify Priority Patients/Make Transport Decision

Student: The patient is a high priority and is a load-and-go. I will begin packaging and transport.
PROCTOR: Noted.

Critical Criteria:
- ❑ Did not provide high concentration of oxygen
- ❑ Did not find or manage problems associated with airway, breathing, hemorrhage or shock (hypoperfusion)
- ❑ Did not differentiate patient's need for transportation versus continued assessment at the scene
- ❑ Did other detailed examination before assessing the airway, breathing and circulation

Focused History and Physical Examination/Rapid Trauma Assessment

Select the Appropriate Assessment (Focused or Rapid)

Student: I am selecting the rapid physical exam to identify and treat life threats. I am checking for DCAP-BTLS. This acronym stands for deformities, contusions, abrasions, punctures, penetrations, and paradoxical motion in the chest, and burns, tenderness, lacerations, and swelling.
PROCTOR: Noted.

Head

Student: I am rapidly assessing the head.
PROCTOR: There are blisters and skin sloughing noted to the skin in varying degrees. His tongue and the roof of his mouth are burned but the oral pharynx is not burned. Skin is dripping from his nose. His eyelids are burned.
Student: I would rapidly assess and protect the airway. I will notify the emergency department of the patient. I will stop the burning process and use dry dressings.
PROCTOR: Noted.
ALS Student: I will be ready with advanced airway techniques per local protocol.
ALS Proctor: Noted.

Neck

Student: I am rapidly assessing the neck.
PROCTOR: Some redness is noted.

▸ **Chest**

Student: I am rapidly assessing the chest. What are the lung sounds?

PROCTOR: Some redness is noted up high on the chest, from the nipples up, covering about 3% of his body surface area. The lung sounds are clear bilaterally.

▸ **Abdomen/Pelvis**

Student: I am rapidly assessing the abdomen.

PROCTOR: There are no obvious injuries.

Student: I am rapidly assessing the pelvis.

PROCTOR: There are no obvious injuries.

▸ **Extremities**

Student: I am rapidly assessing the extremities.

PROCTOR: The patient also has partial-thickness burns to the palms of his hands.

▸ **Posterior**

Student: I will now check the back.

PROCTOR: There are no obvious injuries.

▸ **Manage Secondary Injuries**

ALS Student: I will establish two large-bore IVs en route to the hospital and administer a bolus of 20 mL/kg in order to maintain a systolic blood pressure of 90 mm Hg.

ALS Proctor: Noted.

▸ **Reevaluate Transport Decision**

Student: This patient is a load-and-go due to airway compromise.

PROCTOR: Noted.

▼ Baseline Vital Signs

Student: What are the patient's baseline vital signs, including blood pressure, pulse, respirations, pulse oximetry, and level of consciousness?

PROCTOR: Blood pressure, 140/82 mm Hg; pulse, 120 beats/min; respirations, 24 breaths/min; pulse oximetry reading, 94%; and the patient is alert.

▼ SAMPLE History

Student: At this time I will gather a SAMPLE history from the patient or family. What are the patient's signs and symptoms?

PROCTOR: He is now having difficulty swallowing.

Student: I will rapidly transport.

PROCTOR: Noted.

Student: Allergies?

PROCTOR: Penicillin (PCN).

Student: Medications?

PROCTOR: Asthma.

Student: Pertinent past medical history?

PROCTOR: Asthma.

Student: Last oral intake?

PROCTOR: 2 hours ago.

Student: Events leading up to the incident?

PROCTOR: The patient's car was overheating when he bent over and loosened the radiator cap with a thick rag. The hot fluid blew up into his face.

Critical Criteria:
- ❑ Did not differentiate patient's need for transportation versus continued assessment at the scene
- ❑ Did not provide for spinal protection when indicated

▼ Detailed Physical Examination

Student: I am conducting the detailed physical exam. I am looking for DCAP-BTLS.

PROCTOR: Noted. The detailed physical exam will be performed during transport.

▼ Assess the Head

Student: I am assessing the head. Do I find any DCAP-BTLS? Do I find any evidence of Battle's sign or raccoon eyes?

PROCTOR: No.

▸ **Inspect and Palpate the Head and Ears**

Student: I am assessing the head and ears.

PROCTOR: You see burns in varying degrees (superficial and partial thickness).

▸ **Assess the Eyes**

Student: I am assessing the eyes. Are the pupils equal, round, and regular in size, and react properly to light (PEARRL)?

PROCTOR: They are PEARRL.

▸ **Assess the Facial Area Including Oral and Nasal Areas**

Student: I am assessing the face, nose, and mouth. Do I see any discharge or hear any obstructions?

PROCTOR: You hear hoarseness in his voice and see skin sloughing to the exterior nose.

▼ Assess the Neck

▸ **Inspect and Palpate the Neck**

Student: I am assessing the neck for DCAP-BTLS.

PROCTOR: You see redness.

▸ **Assess for Jugular Vein Distention**

Student: Do I find any jugular vein distention (JVD)?

PROCTOR: No.

▸ **Assess for Tracheal Deviation**

Student: Do I see any tracheal deviation?

PROCTOR: No.

▼ Assess the Chest

Student: I am assessing the chest for DCAP-BTLS.

PROCTOR: Noted.

▸ **Inspect**

Student: What do I see when I look at the chest?

PROCTOR: Redness above the nipples, covering approximately 3% of his body surface area.

Student: I will apply a dry dressing. Does the chest appear symmetric?

PROCTOR: Yes.

▸ **Palpate**

Student: When I touch the chest, do I feel crepitus or a flail segment?

PROCTOR: No.

▸ **Auscultate**

Student: Are lung sounds present in all fields?

PROCTOR: Yes. Lungs appear clear bilaterally with hoarseness noted to his voice.

Student: Do I hear any sucking sounds from the chest?

PROCTOR: No.

▼ Assess the Abdomen/Pelvis

▸ **Assess the Abdomen**

Student: I am assessing the abdomen for DCAP-BTLS. I am assessing all four quadrants. Do I find any problems?

PROCTOR: No.

▸ **Assess the Pelvis**

Student: I am assessing the pelvis for DCAP-BTLS. Is the pelvis stable?

PROCTOR: Yes.

▼ Assess the Genitalia/Perineum as Needed (Verbalize in Training)

Student: I am assessing the genitalia/perineum as necessary for DCAP-BTLS.

PROCTOR: The area is unremarkable.

▼ Assess the Extremities

▸ **Inspect**

Student: I am assessing the lower and upper extremities for DCAP-BTLS. Do I find anything?

PROCTOR: Yes, there are burns to the palms of the hands, with blisters on both palms and fingers.

▸ **Palpate**

Student: Do I feel anything unusual?

PROCTOR: No.

▸ **Assess Motor, Sensory, and Circulatory Function**

Student: I am checking for DCAP-BTLS, motor and sensory function, and pulses. Right leg?
PROCTOR: Negative DCAP-BTLS. Motor and sensory functions are present. Pulses are present.
Student: Left leg?
PROCTOR: Negative DCAP-BTLS. Motor and sensory functions are present. Pulses are present.
Student: Right arm?
PROCTOR: Blisters noted to the palm and fingers. Motor and sensory functions are present. Pulses are present.
Student: Left arm?
PROCTOR: Blisters noted to the palm and fingers. Motor and sensory functions are present. Pulses are present.
Student: I will dress the hands per protocol.
PROCTOR: Noted.

▾ **Assess the Posterior**

Student: I will now check the back.
PROCTOR: Noted.

▸ **Assess the Thorax**

Student: I am assessing the thorax. Do I find injuries?
PROCTOR: No.

▸ **Assess the Lumbar Area**

Student: I am assessing the flanks and lumbar area. Do I find injuries?
PROCTOR: No.

▸ **Assess the Entire Backside**

Student: I am assessing the entire backside. Do I find injuries?
PROCTOR: No.

▾ **Manage Secondary Injuries/Wounds**

Student: I would direct my partner to maintain the airway.
PROCTOR: Noted.

▾ **Reassess Vital Signs**

Student: I will reassess vital signs and mental status.
PROCTOR: Blood pressure, 138/78 mm Hg; pulse, 124 beats/min; respirations, 22 breaths/min; pulse oximetry reading, 98%; and the patient is alert.
Student: The vital signs have not changed significantly.
PROCTOR: Noted.

▾ **Reassess Interventions**

Student: I will reassess my interventions: airway, breathing, oxygen, stopping the burning process, and burn care per local protocol.
PROCTOR: Noted.
ALS Student: I will reassess basic life support (BLS) interventions, plus the following: two large-bore IVs, cardiac monitor, and advanced airway per protocol (intubate, confirm with end tidal CO_2 and lung sounds, needle cricothyrotomy [last resort]).
ALS Proctor: Noted. The cardiac monitor shows normal sinus rhythm and end tidal CO_2 and lung sounds confirm placement of the ET tube.

Critical Criteria:
❑ Did not find or manage problems associated with airway, breathing, hemorrhage or shock (hypoperfusion)

Radio Report

(Provided by the student.)
PROCTOR: Noted.

Ongoing Assessment

▾ **Repeat Vital Signs**

Student: I will reassess vital signs and mental status.
PROCTOR: Blood pressure, 140/80 mm Hg; pulse, 126 beats/min; respirations, 24 breaths/min; pulse oximetry reading, 98%; and the patient is anxious.
Student: The vital signs have not changed significantly.
PROCTOR: Noted.

▾ **Check Interventions**

Student: I will check my interventions: airway, breathing, oxygen, stopping the burning process, and burn care per local protocol.
PROCTOR: Noted.
ALS Student: I will check BLS interventions, plus the following: two large-bore IVs, cardiac monitor, and advanced airway per protocol (intubate, confirm with end tidal CO_2 and lung sounds, needle cricothyrotomy [last resort]).
ALS Proctor: Noted. The cardiac monitor shows normal sinus rhythm and end tidal CO_2 and lung sounds confirm placement of the ET tube.

Critical Criteria:
❑ Did not find or manage problems associated with airway, breathing, hemorrhage or shock (hypoperfusion)

Handoff Report to Emergency Department Staff

Student: The patient became more anxious during transport.
PROCTOR: Noted.

Critical Criteria:
❑ Did not transport patient within the (10) minute time limit

Critical Criteria

(Inform the student of items missed, if any.)

❑ Pass ❑ Fail Date: ____________________

Proctor Comments: ____________________

____

____

CASE 13

Notes

Dispatch Information

PROCTOR: EMS 10, respond to an 18-year-old male who has been stabbed just above his left clavicle and is bleeding profusely. Police are on scene and the scene is safe to enter.

Pre-scene Action (BSI)

Student: I am wearing nonlatex gloves, safety glasses, mask, and gown.
PROCTOR: Noted.

Critical Criteria:
- ❑ Did not take, or verbalize, body substance isolation (BSI) precautions when necessary

Scene Size-up

Scene Safety

Student: Is the scene safe?
PROCTOR: Yes, police are on scene and you are given clearance to enter.

Mechanism of Injury

Student: What was the mechanism of injury?
PROCTOR: Soft-tissue injury. The patient was in a fist fight and was stabbed by his girlfriend.

Number of Patients

Student: How many patients are there?
PROCTOR: One.

Additional Resources

Student: I would call for advanced life support (ALS) assistance.
PROCTOR: Noted.

C-Spine Stabilization

Student: On the basis of the mechanism of injury, I would stabilize the cervical spine (c-spine) in a neutral in-line position.
PROCTOR: Noted.

Critical Criteria:
- ❑ Did not determine scene safety
- ❑ Did not assess for spinal protection
- ❑ Did not provide for spinal protection when indicated

Initial Assessment

Student: As I perform midline c-spine stabilization, I identify myself and ask the patient not to move.
PROCTOR: Noted.

General Impression

Student: My general impression is that the patient's condition is unstable.
PROCTOR: Noted.

Responsiveness/Level of Consciousness

Student: What is the patient's level of consciousness?
PROCTOR: Conscious and alert.

Chief Complaint/Apparent Life Threats

Student: What is the patient's chief complaint?
PROCTOR: The patient says he is going to die.
Student: There is an apparent life threat; the life threat is the stab wound.
PROCTOR: Noted.

Assess the Airway and Breathing

Student: Is the airway open? Is the patient breathing?
PROCTOR: Yes, the airway is open and the patient is breathing.

Assessment

Student: What are the rate and the quality of breathing?
PROCTOR: Rate: Tachypneic. Quality: Guarded due to pain.

Provide Oxygen

Student: I am applying oxygen at 15 L/min via nonrebreathing mask.
PROCTOR: Noted.

Ensure Adequate Ventilation

Student: The patient has adequate ventilations at this time.
PROCTOR: Noted.

Injury Management

Student: I will direct my partner to take over c-spine control as I continue assessment.
PROCTOR: Noted.

Assess Circulation

Student: I am assessing the patient's circulation.
PROCTOR: Noted.

Assess for and Control Major Bleeding

Student: Do I find any major bleeding?
PROCTOR: Yes, you see evidence of blood everywhere, and blood is spurting from the area superior to the patient's left collarbone.
Student: I would apply direct pressure and a dressing.
PROCTOR: Noted.

Assess the Pulse

Student: What are the rate and the quality of pulses?
PROCTOR: Rate: Tachycardic. Quality: Thready.

Assess the Skin

Student: I am assessing the skin. What are the color, temperature, and condition of the skin?
PROCTOR: Color: Pale. Temperature: Cold. Condition: Diaphoretic.

Identify Priority Patients/Make Transport Decision

Student: The patient is a high priority and is a load-and-go. I will begin packaging and transport.
PROCTOR: Noted.

Critical Criteria:
- ❑ Did not provide high concentration of oxygen
- ❑ Did not find or manage problems associated with airway, breathing, hemorrhage or shock (hypoperfusion)
- ❑ Did not differentiate patient's need for transportation versus continued assessment at the scene
- ❑ Did other detailed examination before assessing the airway, breathing and circulation

Focused History and Physical Examination/Rapid Trauma Assessment

Select the Appropriate Assessment (Focused or Rapid)

Student: I am selecting the rapid physical exam to identify and treat life threats. I am checking for DCAP-BTLS. This acronym stands for deformities, contusions, abrasions, punctures, penetrations, and paradoxical motion in the chest, and burns, tenderness, lacerations, and swelling.
PROCTOR: Noted.

Head

Student: I am rapidly assessing the head.
PROCTOR: There are no obvious injuries.

Neck

Student: I am rapidly assessing the neck.
PROCTOR: There are no obvious injuries.
Student: I will apply a cervical collar.
PROCTOR: Noted.

Chest

Student: I am rapidly assessing the chest. What are the lung sounds?
PROCTOR: There is a ¾-inch laceration above the left clavicle. The lung sounds are clear bilaterally.

Student: I would assess the pressure dressing, continuing to apply direct pressure if the wound continues to bleed.
PROCTOR: Noted.

- **Abdomen/Pelvis**

Student: I am rapidly assessing the abdomen.
PROCTOR: There are no obvious injuries.
Student: I am rapidly assessing the pelvis.
PROCTOR: There are no obvious injuries.

- **Extremities**

Student: I am rapidly assessing the extremities.
PROCTOR: There are no obvious injuries.

- **Assess Motor, Sensory, and Circulatory Function**

Student: I am checking for DCAP-BTLS. I am also checking motor and sensory function, and pulses. Right leg?
PROCTOR: Negative DCAP-BTLS. Motor and sensory functions are present. Pulses are thready.
Student: Left leg?
PROCTOR: Negative DCAP-BTLS. Motor and sensory functions are present. Pulses are thready.
Student: Right arm?
PROCTOR: Negative DCAP-BTLS. Motor and sensory functions are present. Pulses are thready.
Student: Left arm?
PROCTOR: Negative DCAP-BTLS. Motor and sensory functions are present. Pulses are thready.

- **Posterior**

Student: I am rapidly assessing the back. We will now log roll the patient as a unit to check the back. The person at the head will count to three and we will roll the patient.
PROCTOR: Noted.

- **Assess the Thorax**

Student: I am assessing the thorax. Do I find injuries?
PROCTOR: No.

- **Assess the Lumbar Area**

Student: I am assessing the flanks and lumbar area. Do I find injuries?
PROCTOR: No.

- **Assess the Entire Backside**

Student: I am assessing the entire backside. Do I find injuries?
PROCTOR: No.

- **Manage Secondary Injuries/Wounds**

Student: We will apply a cervical collar and backboard with full immobilization per local protocol, if not yet done, at this time.
PROCTOR: Noted.
Student: Are there any changes in motor and sensory functions or pulses?
PROCTOR: No.
ALS Student: I will establish two large-bore IVs and administer 20 mL/kg and maintain a blood pressure of 90 mm Hg en route to the hospital.
ALS Proctor: Noted.

- **Reevaluate Transport Decision**

Student: This patient is a load-and-go due to shock.
PROCTOR: Noted.

Baseline Vital Signs

Student: What are the patient's baseline vital signs, including blood pressure, pulse, respirations, pulse oximetry, and level of consciousness?
PROCTOR: Blood pressure, 80/52 mm Hg; pulse rate, 144 beats/min; respirations, 28 breaths/min; pulse oximetry reading, N/A; and the patient is tired.

SAMPLE History

Student: At this time I will gather a SAMPLE history from the patient or family. What are the patient's signs and symptoms?
PROCTOR: Pain in the left chest.
Student: Allergies?
PROCTOR: Unknown.
Student: Medications?
PROCTOR: Unknown.
Student: Pertinent past medical history?
PROCTOR: No pertinent medical history.
Student: Last oral intake?
PROCTOR: 2 hours ago.
Student: Events leading up to the incident?
PROCTOR: The patient was fighting with his girlfriend and she stabbed him.
Student: Interventions?
PROCTOR: The patient ran around in anger, causing more blood loss.

Critical Criteria:
- ❑ Did not differentiate patient's need for transportation versus continued assessment at the scene
- ❑ Did not provide for spinal protection when indicated

Detailed Physical Examination

Student: I am conducting the detailed physical exam. I am looking for DCAP-BTLS.
PROCTOR: Noted. The detailed physical exam will be performed during transport.

Assess the Head

- **Inspect and Palpate the Head and Ears**

Student: I am assessing the head. Do I find any DCAP-BTLS? Do I find any evidence of Battle's sign or raccoon eyes?
PROCTOR: No.

Student: I am assessing the head and ears.
PROCTOR: There are no obvious injuries.

- **Assess the Eyes**

Student: I am assessing the eyes. Are the pupils equal, round, and regular in size, and react properly to light (PEARRL)?
PROCTOR: They are sluggish.

- **Assess the Facial Area Including Oral and Nasal Areas**

Student: I am assessing the face, nose, and mouth. Do I see any discharge or hear any obstructions?
PROCTOR: No.

Assess the Neck

- **Inspect and Palpate the Neck**

Student: I am assessing the neck for DCAP-BTLS.
PROCTOR: There are no obvious injuries.

- **Assess for Jugular Vein Distention**

Student: Do I find any jugular vein distention (JVD)?
PROCTOR: No, the veins are flat.

- **Assess for Tracheal Deviation**

Student: Do I see any tracheal deviation?
PROCTOR: No.

Assess the Chest

Student: I am assessing the chest for DCAP-BTLS.
PROCTOR: Noted.

- **Inspect**

Student: What do I see when I look at the chest?
PROCTOR: Bleeding is controlled.
Student: Does the chest appear symmetric?
PROCTOR: Yes.

- **Palpate**

Student: When I touch the chest, do I feel crepitus or a flail segment?
PROCTOR: No.

- **Auscultate**

Student: Are lung sounds present in all fields?
PROCTOR: Yes.

Student: Do I hear any sucking sounds from the chest?
PROCTOR: No.

▼ Assess the Abdomen/Pelvis

► Assess the Abdomen

Student: I am assessing the abdomen for DCAP-BTLS. I am assessing all four quadrants. Do I find any problems?
PROCTOR: No.

► Assess the Pelvis

Student: I am assessing the pelvis for DCAP-BTLS. Is the pelvis stable?
PROCTOR: Yes.

▼ Assess the Genitalia/Perineum as Needed (Verbalize in Training)

Student: I am assessing the genitalia/perineum as necessary for DCAP-BTLS.
PROCTOR: The area is unremarkable.

▼ Assess the Extremities

► Inspect

Student: I am assessing the lower and upper extremities for DCAP-BTLS. Do I find anything?
PROCTOR: No.

► Palpate

Student: Do I feel anything unusual?
PROCTOR: No.

► Assess Motor, Sensory, and Circulatory Function

Student: I am checking for DCAP-BTLS, motor and sensory function, and pulses. Right leg?
PROCTOR: Negative DCAP-BTLS. Motor and sensory functions are present. Pulses are absent.
Student: Left leg?
PROCTOR: Negative DCAP-BTLS. Motor and sensory functions are present. Pulses are absent.
Student: Right arm?
PROCTOR: Negative DCAP-BTLS. Motor and sensory functions are present. Pulses are absent.
Student: Left arm?
PROCTOR: Negative DCAP-BTLS. Motor and sensory functions are present. Pulses are absent.

▼ Assess the Posterior

Note: This portion of the detailed physical exam would not be done if the patient were previously backboarded per local protocol.
Student: We will not check the back since it was previously checked and the patient is backboarded.
PROCTOR: Noted.

▼ Manage Secondary Injuries/Wounds

Student: I would direct my partner to maintain pressure on the wound as I treat for shock.
PROCTOR: Noted.

▼ Reassess Vital Signs

Student: I will reassess vital signs and mental status.
PROCTOR: Blood pressure, 70 by palpation; pulse rate, 138 beats/min; respirations, 32 breaths/min; pulse oximetry reading, N/A; and the patient is responsive to pain only.
Student: The vital signs are deteriorating. I would begin bag-valve ventilations on this patient.
PROCTOR: Noted.

▼ Reassess Interventions

Student: I will reassess my interventions: airway, breathing, bag-valve device, and oxygen; circulation and bleeding control; and immobilization and straps.
PROCTOR: Noted.
ALS Student: I will reassess basic life support (BLS) interventions, plus the following: establish two large-bore IVs, maintain a blood pressure of 90 mm Hg, and perform cardiac monitoring.
ALS Proctor: Noted. The cardiac monitor shows sinus tachycardia.

Critical Criteria:
❑ Did not find or manage problems associated with airway, breathing, hemorrhage or shock (hypoperfusion)

Radio Report

(Provided by the student.)
PROCTOR: Noted.

Ongoing Assessment

▼ Repeat Vital Signs

Student: I will reassess vital signs and mental status.
PROCTOR: Blood pressure, none; pulse rate, 0 beats/min; respirations, 0 breaths/min; pulse oximetry reading, N/A; and the patient is unresponsive.
Student: The vital signs have deteriorated. I will begin CPR.
PROCTOR: Noted.

▼ Check Interventions

Student: I will check my interventions: CPR, airway, oral/advanced airway, breathing, bag-valve device, and oxygen; circulation and bleeding control; and immobilization and straps.
PROCTOR: Noted.
ALS Student: I will check BLS interventions, plus the following: intubate, confirm tube placement with end tidal CO_2 and lung sounds, two large-bore IVs, cardiac monitor, fluid challenge, and ACLS protocol.
ALS Proctor: Noted. The cardiac monitor shows pulseless electrical activity, end tidal CO_2 and lung sounds confirm tube placement.

Critical Criteria:
❑ Did not find or manage problems associated with airway, breathing, hemorrhage or shock (hypoperfusion)

Handoff Report to Emergency Department Staff

Student: The patient's condition deteriorated during transport.
PROCTOR: Noted.

Critical Criteria:
❑ Did not transport patient within the (10) minute time limit

Critical Criteria

(Inform the student of items missed, if any.)

❑ Pass ❑ Fail Date: ____________________

Proctor Comments: ____________________

____

____

Notes

CASE 15

Dispatch Information

PROCTOR: EMS 10, respond to a motor vehicle crash involving a 31-year-old male. A small pick-up struck the rear of a dump truck.

Pre-scene Action (BSI)

Student: I am wearing appropriate high-visibility personal protective equipment suitable for extrication, a helmet, extrication gloves, nonlatex gloves, safety glasses, mask, and gown.
PROCTOR: Noted.

Critical Criteria:
- ❑ Did not take, or verbalize, body substance isolation (BSI) precautions when necessary

Scene Size-up

Scene Safety

Student: Is the scene safe?
PROCTOR: Yes.

Mechanism of Injury

Student: What was the mechanism of injury?
PROCTOR: Motor vehicle collision. The patient was the driver of a small pick-up that rear-ended the back of a dump truck. He was not wearing a seat belt. He has severe chest pain. He is found sitting in the driver's seat of the pick-up truck. The steering wheel is deformed, and the windshield intact.

Number of Patients

Student: How many patients are there?
PROCTOR: One.

Additional Resources

Student: I would call for additional resources: advanced life support (ALS), fire/rescue, and police.
PROCTOR: Noted.

C-Spine Stabilization

Student: On the basis of the mechanism of injury, I would stabilize the cervical spine (c-spine) in a neutral in-line position.
PROCTOR: Noted.

Critical Criteria:
- ❑ Did not determine scene safety
- ❑ Did not assess for spinal protection
- ❑ Did not provide for spinal protection when indicated

Initial Assessment

Student: As I perform midline c-spine stabilization, I identify myself and ask the patient not to move.
PROCTOR: Noted.

General Impression

Student: My general impression is that the patient's condition is unstable.
PROCTOR: Noted.

Responsiveness/Level of Consciousness

Student: What is the patient's level of consciousness?
PROCTOR: Alert.

Chief Complaint/Apparent Life Threats

Student: What is the patient's chief complaint?
PROCTOR: The patient is complaining of chest pain and feeling like he is going to die.
Student: There is an apparent life threat; the life threat is the chest trauma.
PROCTOR: Noted.

Assess the Airway and Breathing

Student: I am assessing the airway. Is the patient breathing?
PROCTOR: Yes.

Assessment

Student: What are the rate and the quality of breathing?
PROCTOR: Rate: Tachypneic. Quality: Labored.

Provide Oxygen

Student: I am applying oxygen at 15 L/min via nonrebreathing mask.
PROCTOR: Noted.

Ensure Adequate Ventilation

Student: The patient has adequate ventilations at this time.
PROCTOR: Noted.

Injury Management

Student: I will direct my partner to take over c-spine control as I continue assessment.
PROCTOR: Noted.

Assess Circulation

Student: I am assessing the patient's circulation.
PROCTOR: Noted.

Assess for and Control Major Bleeding

Student: Do I find any major bleeding?
PROCTOR: No.

Assess the Pulse

Student: What are the rate and the quality of pulses?
PROCTOR: Rate: Tachycardic. Quality: Thready.

Assess the Skin

Student: I am assessing the skin. What are the color, temperature, and condition of the skin?
PROCTOR: Color: Pasty white. Temperature: Cold. Condition: Diaphoretic.

Identify Priority Patients/Make Transport Decision

Student: The patient is a high priority and is a load-and-go. I will begin rapid extrication, then package and transport.
PROCTOR: Noted.

Critical Criteria:
- ❑ Did not provide high concentration of oxygen
- ❑ Did not find or manage problems associated with airway, breathing, hemorrhage or shock (hypoperfusion)
- ❑ Did not differentiate patient's need for transportation versus continued assessment at the scene
- ❑ Did other detailed examination before assessing the airway, breathing and circulation

Focused History and Physical Examination/Rapid Trauma Assessment

Select the Appropriate Assessment (Focused or Rapid)

Student: I am selecting the rapid physical exam to identify and treat life threats. I am checking for DCAP-BTLS. This acronym stands for deformities, contusions, abrasions, punctures, penetrations, and paradoxical motion in the chest, and burns, tenderness, lacerations, and swelling.
PROCTOR: Noted.

Head

Student: I am rapidly assessing the head.
PROCTOR: There are no obvious injuries.

Neck

Student: I am rapidly assessing the neck.
PROCTOR: There are no obvious injuries.
Student: I will apply a cervical collar.
PROCTOR: Noted.

▸ Chest

Student: I am rapidly assessing the chest. What are the lung sounds?
PROCTOR: There is a large bruise across the chest that is consistent with the shape of the steering wheel. The steering wheel is deformed. The lung sounds are clear bilaterally. His heart tones are muffled.
Student: I will assess the chest for tension pneumothorax by auscultation, and assessment (jugular vein distention [JVD], tracheal deviation, and decreased lung sounds).
PROCTOR: The lung sounds appear clear bilaterally, jugular vein distention is not present, and the trachea is midline.
ALS Student: I will assess the chest for hyperresonance to percussion.
ALS Proctor: Noted. There is no tension pneumothorax.
ALS Student: I will continuously reassess the chest.
ALS Proctor: Noted.

▸ Abdomen/Pelvis

Student: I am rapidly assessing the abdomen.
PROCTOR: There are no obvious injuries.
Student: I am rapidly assessing the pelvis.
PROCTOR: There are no obvious injuries.

▸ Extremities

Student: I am rapidly assessing the extremities.
PROCTOR: There are no obvious injuries.

▸ Assess Motor, Sensory, and Circulatory Function

Student: I am checking for DCAP-BTLS. I am also checking motor and sensory function, and pulses. Right leg?
PROCTOR: Negative DCAP-BTLS. Motor and sensory functions are present. Pulses are present.
Student: Left leg?
PROCTOR: Negative DCAP-BTLS. Motor and sensory functions are present. Pulses are present.
Student: Right arm?
PROCTOR: There is bruising from the steering wheel. Motor and sensory functions are present. Pulses are present.
Student: Left arm?
PROCTOR: There is bruising from the steering wheel. Motor and sensory functions are present. Pulses are present.

▸ Posterior

Student: We will now log roll the patient as a unit to check the back. The person at the head will count to three and we will roll the patient.
PROCTOR: Noted.

▸ Assess the Thorax

Student: I am assessing the thorax. Do I find injuries?
PROCTOR: No.

▸ Assess the Lumbar Area

Student: I am assessing the flanks and lumbar area. Do I find injuries?
PROCTOR: No.

▸ Assess the Entire Backside

Student: I am assessing the entire backside. Do I find injuries?
PROCTOR: No.

▸ Manage Secondary Injuries/Wounds

Student: We will apply a cervical collar and backboard with full immobilization per local protocol, if not yet done, at this time.
PROCTOR: Noted.
Student: Are there any changes in motor and sensory functions or pulses?
PROCTOR: No.
Student: We will rapidly extricate the patient.
PROCTOR: Noted.
ALS Student: I will establish two large-bore IVs en route to the hospital and administer a bolus of 20 mL/kg in order to maintain a systolic blood pressure of 90 mm Hg.
ALS Proctor: Noted.

▸ Reevaluate Transport Decision

Student: This patient is a load-and-go due to chest trauma and shock.
PROCTOR: Noted.

▾ **Baseline Vital Signs**

Student: What are the patient's baseline vital signs, including blood pressure, pulse, respirations, pulse oximetry, and level of consciousness?
PROCTOR: Blood pressure, 100/60 mm Hg; pulse, 140 beats/min; respirations, 28 breaths/min; pulse oximetry reading, N/A; and the patient is anxious.

▾ **SAMPLE History**

Student: At this time I will gather a SAMPLE history from the patient or family. What are the patient's signs and symptoms?
PROCTOR: Pain in the chest.
Student: Allergies?
PROCTOR: No allergies.
Student: Medications?
PROCTOR: An inhaler.
Student: Pertinent past medical history?
PROCTOR: Asthma.
Student: Last oral intake?
PROCTOR: 2 hours ago.
Student: Events leading up to the incident?
PROCTOR: He was passing a car on the right and ran into the back of a dump truck.

Critical Criteria:
- ❑ Did not differentiate patient's need for transportation versus continued assessment at the scene
- ❑ Did not provide for spinal protection when indicated

Detailed Physical Examination

Student: I am conducting the detailed physical exam. I am looking for DCAP-BTLS.
PROCTOR: Noted. The detailed physical exam will be performed during transport.

▾ **Assess the Head**

Student: I am assessing the head. Do I find any DCAP-BTLS? Do I find any evidence of Battle's sign or raccoon eyes?
PROCTOR: No.

▸ Inspect and Palpate the Head and Ears

Student: I am assessing the head and ears.
PROCTOR: There are no obvious injuries.

▸ Assess the Eyes

Student: I am assessing the eyes. Are the pupils equal, round, and regular in size, and react properly to light (PEARRL)?
PROCTOR: They are sluggish.

▸ Assess the Facial Area Including Oral and Nasal Areas

Student: I am assessing the face, nose, and mouth. Do I see any discharge or hear any obstructions?
PROCTOR: No.

▾ **Assess the Neck**

▸ Inspect and Palpate the Neck

Student: I am assessing the neck for DCAP-BTLS.
PROCTOR: There are no obvious injuries.

▸ Assess for Jugular Vein Distention

Student: Do I find any jugular vein distention (JVD)?
PROCTOR: No. The neck veins are flat.

▸ Assess for Tracheal Deviation

Student: Do I see any tracheal deviation?
PROCTOR: No.

▾ **Assess the Chest**

Student: I am assessing the chest for DCAP-BTLS.
PROCTOR: Noted.

▸ Inspect

Student: What do I see when I look at the chest?
PROCTOR: There is a large bruise across the patient's chest.

Student: Does the chest appear symmetric?

PROCTOR: Yes.

▸ **Palpate**

Student: When I touch the chest, do I feel crepitus or a flail segment?

PROCTOR: No.

▸ **Auscultate**

Student: Are lung sounds present in all fields?

PROCTOR: Yes.

Student: Do I hear any sucking sounds from the chest?

PROCTOR: No.

▾ Assess the Abdomen/Pelvis

▸ **Assess the Abdomen**

Student: I am assessing the abdomen for DCAP-BTLS. I am assessing all four quadrants. Do I find any problems?

PROCTOR: No.

▸ **Assess the Pelvis**

Student: I am assessing the pelvis for DCAP-BTLS. Is the pelvis stable?

PROCTOR: Yes.

▸ **Assess the Genitalia/Perineum as Needed (Verbalize in Training)**

Student: I am assessing the genitalia/perineum for DCAP-BTLS.

PROCTOR: The area is unremarkable.

▾ Assess the Extremities

▸ **Inspect**

Student: I am assessing the lower and upper extremities for DCAP-BTLS. Do I find anything?

PROCTOR: Both arms are bruised from the steering wheel.

▸ **Palpate**

Student: Do I feel anything unusual?

PROCTOR: No.

▸ **Assess Motor, Sensory, and Circulatory Function**

Student: I am checking for DCAP-BTLS, motor and sensory function, and pulses. Right leg?

PROCTOR: Negative DCAP-BTLS. Motor and sensory functions are present. Pulses are present.

Student: Left leg?

PROCTOR: Negative DCAP-BTLS. Motor and sensory functions are present. Pulses are present.

Student: Right arm?

PROCTOR: There is bruising from the steering wheel. Motor and sensory functions are present. Pulses are present.

Student: Left arm?

PROCTOR: There is bruising from the steering wheel. Motor and sensory functions are present. Pulses are present.

▾ Assess the Posterior

Note: This portion of the detailed physical exam would not be done if the patient were previously backboarded per local protocol.

Student: We will not check the back since it was previously checked and the patient is backboarded.

PROCTOR: Noted.

▾ Manage Secondary Injuries/Wounds

Student: I would direct my partner to continue providing oxygen.

PROCTOR: Noted.

▾ Reassess Vital Signs

Student: I will reassess vital signs and mental status.

PROCTOR: The patient has just gone into cardiac arrest. Blood pressure, 0/0 mm Hg; pulse, 0 beats/min; respirations, 0 breaths/min; pulse oximetry reading, N/A; and the patient is unresponsive.

Student: I will begin CPR with an oral airway/advanced airway, a bag-valve device, and 100% oxygen.

PROCTOR: Noted.

ALS Student: I will apply basic life support (BLS) interventions, plus the following: intubation, confirm end tidal CO_2, check lung sounds, two large-bore IVs, cardiac monitoring, and advanced cardiac life support (ACLS) and regional protocol.

ALS Proctor: Noted. The cardiac monitor shows pulseless electrical activity and end tidal CO_2 and lung sounds confirm placement of the ET tube.

▾ Reassess Interventions

Student: I will reassess my interventions: CPR, oral airway/advanced airway, bag-valve device, oxygen, and full immobilization.

PROCTOR: Noted.

ALS Student: I will reassess BLS interventions, plus the following: intubation, confirm end tidal CO_2, check lung sounds, two large-bore IVs, cardiac monitoring, and ACLS protocol.

ALS Proctor: Noted. The cardiac monitor shows pulseless electrical activity and end tidal CO_2 and lung sounds confirm placement of the ET tube.

Critical Criteria:

❑ Did not find or manage problems associated with airway, breathing, hemorrhage or shock (hypoperfusion)

Radio Report

(Provided by the student.)

PROCTOR: Noted.

Ongoing Assessment

▾ Repeat Vital Signs

Student: I will reassess vital signs and mental status.

PROCTOR: Blood pressure, 0/0 mm Hg; pulse, 0 beats/min; respirations, 0 breaths/min; pulse oximetry reading, N/A; and the patient is unresponsive.

▾ Check Interventions

Student: I will check my interventions: CPR, and an oral airway/advanced airway, bag-valve device, and 100% oxygen.

PROCTOR: Noted.

ALS Student: I will check BLS interventions, plus the following: intubation, confirm end tidal CO_2, check lung sounds, two large-bore IVs, cardiac monitoring, and ACLS and regional protocol.

ALS Proctor: Noted. The cardiac monitor shows pulseless electrical activity and end tidal CO_2 and lung sounds confirm placement of the ET tube.

Critical Criteria:

❑ Did not find or manage problems associated with airway, breathing, hemorrhage or shock (hypoperfusion)

Handoff Report to Emergency Department Staff

Student: The patient's condition deteriorated during transport.

PROCTOR: Noted.

Critical Criteria:

❑ Did not transport patient within the (10) minute time limit

Critical Criteria

(Inform the student of items missed, if any.)

❑ Pass ❑ Fail Date:

Proctor Comments:

Notes

Dispatch Information

PROCTOR: EMS 10, respond to a 23-year-old male who has been involved in a parachute crash. He is conscious and breathing.

Pre-scene Action (BSI)

Student: I am wearing nonlatex gloves, safety glasses, mask, and gown.
PROCTOR: Noted.

Critical Criteria:
- ❑ Did not take, or verbalize, body substance isolation (BSI) precautions when necessary

Scene Size-up

Scene Safety

Student: Is the scene safe?
PROCTOR: Yes.

Mechanism of Injury

Student: What was the mechanism of injury?
PROCTOR: Fall. The patient was parachuting and crashed into the ground.

Number of Patients

Student: How many patients are there?
PROCTOR: One.

Additional Resources

Student: I would call for advanced life support (ALS) assistance and additional resources: fire/rescue.
PROCTOR: Noted.

C-Spine Stabilization

Student: On the basis of the mechanism of injury, I would stabilize the cervical spine (c-spine) in a neutral in-line position.
PROCTOR: Noted.

Critical Criteria:
- ❑ Did not determine scene safety
- ❑ Did not assess for spinal protection
- ❑ Did not provide for spinal protection when indicated

Initial Assessment

Student: As I perform midline c-spine stabilization, I identify myself and ask the patient not to move.
PROCTOR: Noted.

General Impression

Student: My general impression is that the patient's condition is unstable.
PROCTOR: Noted.

Responsiveness/Level of Consciousness

Student: What is the patient's level of consciousness?
PROCTOR: Alert.

Chief Complaint/Apparent Life Threats

Student: What is the patient's chief complaint?
PROCTOR: The patient is complaining of pain to both legs.
Student: There are apparent life threats; the life threats are due to the mechanism of injury.
PROCTOR: Noted.

Assess the Airway and Breathing

Student: I am opening the airway. Is the patient breathing?
PROCTOR: Yes.

Assessment

Student: What are the rate and the quality of breathing?
PROCTOR: Rate: Tachypneic. Quality: Deep.

Provide Oxygen

Student: I am applying oxygen at 15 L/min via nonrebreathing mask.
PROCTOR: Noted.

Ensure Adequate Ventilation

Student: The patient has adequate ventilations at this time.
PROCTOR: Noted.

Injury Management

Student: I will direct my partner to take over c-spine control as I continue assessment.
PROCTOR: Noted.

Assess Circulation

Student: I am assessing the circulation.
PROCTOR: Noted.

Assess for and Control Major Bleeding

Student: Do I find any major bleeding?
PROCTOR: No.

Assess the Pulse

Student: What are the rate and the quality of pulses?
PROCTOR: Rate: Tachycardic. Quality: Bounding.

Assess the Skin

Student: I am assessing the skin. What are the color, temperature, and condition of the skin?
PROCTOR: Color: Flushed. Temperature: Warm. Condition: Moist.

Identify Priority Patients/Make Transport Decision

Student: The patient is a high priority and is a load-and-go. I will begin packaging and transport.
PROCTOR: Noted.

Critical Criteria:
- ❑ Did not provide high concentration of oxygen
- ❑ Did not find or manage problems associated with airway, breathing, hemorrhage or shock (hypoperfusion)
- ❑ Did not differentiate patient's need for transportation versus continued assessment at the scene
- ❑ Did other detailed examination before assessing the airway, breathing and circulation

Focused History and Physical Examination/Rapid Trauma Assessment

Select the Appropriate Assessment (Focused or Rapid)

Student: I am selecting the rapid physical exam to identify and treat life threats. I am checking for DCAP-BTLS. This acronym stands for deformities, contusions, abrasions, punctures, penetrations, and paradoxical motion in the chest, and burns, tenderness, lacerations, and swelling.
PROCTOR: Noted.

Head

Student: I am rapidly assessing the head.
PROCTOR: There are no obvious injuries.

Neck

Student: I am rapidly assessing the neck.
PROCTOR: There are no obvious injuries.
Student: I will apply a cervical collar.
PROCTOR: Noted.

Chest

Student: I am rapidly assessing the chest. What are the lung sounds?
PROCTOR: There are no obvious injuries. The lung sounds are clear bilaterally.

Abdomen/Pelvis

Student: I am rapidly assessing the abdomen.
PROCTOR: There are no obvious injuries.
Student: I am rapidly assessing the pelvis.
PROCTOR: There are no obvious injuries.

▸ Extremities

Student: I am rapidly assessing the extremities.
PROCTOR: There are open fractures to both lower legs.
Student: I would direct my partner to apply dressings and splint the legs.
PROCTOR: Noted.

▸ Assess Motor, Sensory, and Circulatory Function

Student: I am checking for DCAP-BTLS. I am also checking motor and sensory function, and pulses. Right Leg?
PROCTOR: There is an open fracture to the lower leg. Motor and sensory functions are present. Pulses are present.
Student: Left leg?
PROCTOR: There is an open fracture to the lower leg. Motor and sensory functions are present. Pulses are present.
Student: Right arm?
PROCTOR: Negative DCAP-BTLS. Motor and sensory functions are present. Pulses are present.
Student: Left arm?
PROCTOR: Negative DCAP-BTLS. Motor and sensory functions are present. Pulses are present.

▸ Posterior

Student: I am rapidly assessing the back. We will now log roll the patient as a unit to check the back. The person at the head will count to three and we will roll the patient.
PROCTOR: Noted.

▸ Assess the Thorax

Student: I am assessing the thorax. Do I find injuries?
PROCTOR: No.

▸ Assess the Lumbar Area

Student: I am assessing the flanks and lumbar area. Do I find injuries?
PROCTOR: No.

▸ Assess the Entire Backside

Student: I am assessing the entire backside. Do I find injuries?
PROCTOR: No.

▸ Manage Secondary Injuries/Wounds

Student: We will apply a cervical collar and backboard with full immobilization per local protocol, if not yet done, at this time.
PROCTOR: Noted.
Student: Are there any changes in motor and sensory functions or pulses?
PROCTOR: No.
ALS Student: I will establish two large-bore IVs en route to the hospital and administer a bolus of 20 mL/kg in order to maintain a systolic blood pressure of 90 mm Hg.
ALS Proctor: Noted.

▸ Reevaluate Transport Decision

Student: This patient is a load-and-go due to the mechanism of injury.
PROCTOR: Noted.

▾ Baseline Vital Signs

Student: What are the patient's baseline vital signs, including blood pressure, pulse, respirations, pulse oximetry, and level of consciousness?
PROCTOR: Blood pressure, 138/78 mm Hg; pulse, 136 beats/min; respirations, 24 breaths/min; pulse oximetry reading, 97%; and the patient is alert.

▾ SAMPLE History

Student: At this time I will gather a SAMPLE history from the patient or family. What are the patient's signs and symptoms?
PROCTOR: Pain in both lower legs.
Student: Allergies?
PROCTOR: No allergies.
Student: Medications?
PROCTOR: No medications.
Student: Pertinent past medical history?
PROCTOR: No pertinent medical history.
Student: Last oral intake?
PROCTOR: 2 hours ago.
Student: Events leading up to the incident?
PROCTOR: The patient came in too fast and crashed while parachuting.

Critical Criteria:
- ❑ Did not differentiate patient's need for transportation versus continued assessment at the scene
- ❑ Did not provide for spinal protection when indicated

▾ Detailed Physical Examination

Student: I am conducting the detailed physical exam. I am looking for DCAP-BTLS.
PROCTOR: Noted. The detailed physical exam will be performed during transport.

▾ Assess the Head

Student: I am assessing the head. Do I find any DCAP-BTLS? Do I find any evidence of Battle's sign or raccoon eyes?
PROCTOR: No.

▸ Inspect and Palpate the Head and Ears

Student: I am assessing the head and ears.
PROCTOR: There are no obvious injuries.

▸ Assess the Eyes

Student: I am assessing the eyes. Are the pupils equal, round, and regular in size, and react properly to light (PEARRL)?
PROCTOR: They are PEARRL.

▸ Assess the Facial Area Including Oral and Nasal Areas

Student: I am assessing the face, nose, and mouth. Do I see any discharge or hear any obstructions?
PROCTOR: No.

▾ Assess the Neck

▸ Inspect and Palpate the Neck

Student: I am assessing the neck for DCAP-BTLS.
PROCTOR: There are no obvious injuries.

▸ Assess for Jugular Vein Distention

Student: Do I find any jugular vein distention (JVD)?
PROCTOR: No.

▸ Assess for Tracheal Deviation

Student: Do I see any tracheal deviation?
PROCTOR: No.

▾ Assess the Chest

Student: I am assessing the chest for DCAP-BTLS.
PROCTOR: Noted.

▸ Inspect

Student: What do I see when I look at the chest?
PROCTOR: There are no obvious injuries.
Student: Does the chest appear symmetric?
PROCTOR: Yes.

▸ Palpate

Student: When I touch the chest, do I feel crepitus or a flail segment?
PROCTOR: No.

▸ Auscultate

Student: Are lung sounds present in all fields?
PROCTOR: Yes.
Student: Do I hear any sucking sounds from the chest?
PROCTOR: No.

▾ Assess the Abdomen/Pelvis

▸ Assess the Abdomen

Student: I am assessing the abdomen for DCAP-BTLS. I am assessing all four quadrants. Do I find any problems?
PROCTOR: No.

▸ **Assess the Pelvis**

Student: I am assessing the pelvis for DCAP-BTLS. Is the pelvis stable?
PROCTOR: Yes.

▾ Assess the Genitalia/Perineum as Needed (Verbalize in Training)

Student: I am assessing the genitalia/perineum as necessary for DCAP-BTLS.
PROCTOR: The area is unremarkable.

▾ Assess the Extremities

▸ **Inspect**

Student: I am assessing the lower and upper extremities for DCAP-BTLS. Do I find anything?
PROCTOR: Yes, there are open fractures to both lower legs.

▸ **Palpate**

Student: Do I feel anything unusual?
PROCTOR: Yes.

▸ **Assess Motor, Sensory, and Circulatory Function**

Student: I am checking for DCAP-BTLS, motor and sensory function, and pulses. Right leg?
PROCTOR: There is an open fracture to the lower leg that is now splinted. Motor and sensory functions are present. Pulses are present.
Student: Left leg?
PROCTOR: There is an open fracture to the lower leg that is now splinted. Motor and sensory functions are present. Pulses are present.
Student: Right arm?
PROCTOR: Negative DCAP-BTLS. Motor and sensory functions are present. Pulses are present.
Student: Left arm?
PROCTOR: Negative DCAP-BTLS. Motor and sensory functions are present. Pulses are present.

▾ Assess the Posterior

Note: This portion of the detailed physical exam would not be done if the patient were previously backboarded per local protocol.
Student: We will not check the back since it was previously checked and the patient is backboarded.
PROCTOR: Noted.

▾ Manage Secondary Injuries/Wounds

Student: I would direct my partner to check the dressings and splints to the legs.
PROCTOR: Noted.

▾ Reassess Vital Signs

Student: I will reassess vital signs and mental status.
PROCTOR: Blood pressure, 124/74 mm Hg; pulse, 122 beats/min; respirations, 20 breaths/min; pulse oximetry reading, 98%; and the patient is alert.
Student: The vital signs have not changed significantly.
PROCTOR: Noted.

▾ Reassess Interventions

Student: I will reassess my interventions: oxygen; circulation and bleeding control; and splints, immobilization, and straps.
PROCTOR: Noted.
ALS Student: I will reassess basic life support (BLS) interventions, plus the following: two large-bore IVs, cardiac monitoring, and pain management per local protocol.
ALS Proctor: Noted. The cardiac monitor shows normal sinus rhythm.

Critical Criteria:
❑ Did not find or manage problems associated with airway, breathing, hemorrhage or shock (hypoperfusion)

Radio Report

(Provided by the student.)
PROCTOR: Noted.

Ongoing Assessment

▾ Repeat Vital Signs

Student: I will reassess vital signs and mental status.
PROCTOR: Blood pressure, 120/68 mm Hg; pulse, 110 beats/min; respirations, 16 breaths/min; pulse oximetry reading, 98%; and the patient is alert.
Student: The vital signs have not changed significantly.
PROCTOR: Noted.

▾ Check Interventions

Student: I will check my interventions: oxygen; circulation and bleeding control; and splints, immobilization, and straps.
PROCTOR: Noted.
ALS Student: I will check BLS interventions, plus the following: two large-bore IVs, cardiac monitoring, and pain management per local protocol.
ALS Proctor: Noted. The cardiac monitor shows normal sinus rhythm.

Critical Criteria:
❑ Did not find or manage problems associated with airway, breathing, hemorrhage or shock (hypoperfusion)

Handoff Report to Emergency Department Staff

Student: There was no change during transport.
PROCTOR: Noted.

Critical Criteria:
❑ Did not transport patient within the (10) minute time limit

Critical Criteria

(Inform the student of items missed, if any.)

❑ Pass ❑ Fail Date: ______________________

Proctor Comments: ______________________

____

____

Notes

Dispatch Information

PROCTOR: EMS 10, respond to a 19-year-old male patient who has his hand caught in a meat grinder. He is conscious and breathing.

Pre-scene Action (BSI)

Student: I am wearing nonlatex gloves, safety glasses, mask, and gown.
PROCTOR: Noted.

Critical Criteria:
- ❑ Did not take, or verbalize, body substance isolation (BSI) precautions when necessary

Scene Size-up

Scene Safety

Student: Is the scene safe?
PROCTOR: Yes.

Mechanism of Injury

Student: What was the mechanism of injury?
PROCTOR: Blunt/crushing trauma to the hand. The patient was grinding meat when his hand became caught in the grinder. His hand is still trapped in the grinder.

Number of Patients

Student: How many patients are there?
PROCTOR: One.

Additional Resources

Student: I would call for advanced life support (ALS) assistance and additional resources: fire/rescue.
PROCTOR: Noted.

C-Spine Stabilization

Student: I would not stabilize the cervical spine (c-spine).
PROCTOR: Noted.

Critical Criteria:
- ❑ Did not determine scene safety
- ❑ Did not assess for spinal protection
- ❑ Did not provide for spinal protection when indicated

Initial Assessment

Student: I identify myself and ask the patient not to move.
PROCTOR: Noted.

General Impression

Student: My general impression is that the patient's condition is unstable.
PROCTOR: Noted.

Responsiveness/Level of Consciousness

Student: What is the patient's level of consciousness?
PROCTOR: Alert, but feels like he could pass out.

Chief Complaint/Apparent Life Threats

Student: What is the patient's chief complaint?
PROCTOR: The patient is complaining of his right hand being caught in the grinder, and is in pain.
Student: There is an apparent life threat; the life threat is the loss of blood.
PROCTOR: Noted.

Assess the Airway and Breathing

Student: I am opening the airway. Is the patient breathing?
PROCTOR: Yes.

Assessment

Student: What are the rate and the quality of breathing?
PROCTOR: Rate: Rapid. Quality: Crying.

Provide Oxygen

Student: I am applying oxygen at 15 L/min via nonrebreathing mask.
PROCTOR: Noted.

Ensure Adequate Ventilation

Student: The patient has adequate ventilation at this time.
PROCTOR: Noted.

Injury Management

Student: I will direct my partner to hold the patient up as I continue assessment.
PROCTOR: Noted.

Assess Circulation

Student: I am assessing the patient's circulation.
PROCTOR: Noted.

Assess for and Control Major Bleeding

Student: Do I find any major bleeding?
PROCTOR: Yes. Blood is evident coming out of the machine.
Student: I will apply a tourniquet to the arm above the machine.
PROCTOR: Noted.

Assess the Pulse

Student: What are the rate and the quality of pulses?
PROCTOR: Rate: Tachycardic. Quality: Faint on the noninjured hand.

Assess the Skin

Student: I am assessing the skin. What are the color, temperature, and condition of the skin?
PROCTOR: Color: Pasty-white. Temperature: Cold. Condition: Diaphoretic.

Identify Priority Patients/Make Transport Decision

Student: The patient is a high priority and is a load-and-go. I will begin packaging and transport.
PROCTOR: Noted.

Critical Criteria:
- ❑ Did not provide high concentration of oxygen
- ❑ Did not find or manage problems associated with airway, breathing, hemorrhage or shock (hypoperfusion)
- ❑ Did not differentiate patient's need for transportation versus continued assessment at the scene
- ❑ Did other detailed examination before assessing the airway, breathing and circulation

Focused History and Physical Examination/Rapid Trauma Assessment

Select the Appropriate Assessment (Focused or Rapid)

Student: I am selecting the focused assessment.
PROCTOR: Noted.

Extremities

Student: I am rapidly assessing the extremities.
PROCTOR: The patient's hand is stuck in a meat grinder.
Student: I will get the patient into a comfortable position as the fire department removes the meat grinder from the table and will transport the grinder with the patient to the hospital.
PROCTOR: Noted.
ALS Student: I will establish two large-bore IVs en route to the hospital and administer a bolus of 20 mL/kg in order to maintain a systolic blood pressure of 90 mm Hg. I will administer pain management per local protocol.
ALS Proctor: Noted.

Reevaluate Transport Decision

Student: This patient is a load-and-go due to the mechanism of injury and possible shock. I will transport to a trauma center per local protocol.
PROCTOR: Noted.

Baseline Vital Signs

Student: What are the patient's baseline vital signs, including blood pressure, pulse, respirations, pulse oximetry, and level of consciousness?

PROCTOR: Blood pressure, 110/68 mm Hg; pulse rate, 130 beats/min; respirations, 20 breaths/min; pulse oximetry reading, 98%; and the patient is alert.

SAMPLE History

Student: At this time I will gather a SAMPLE history from the patient or family. What are the patient's signs and symptoms?

PROCTOR: Pain in the arm and hand, plus he feels like he will pass out.

Student: Allergies?

PROCTOR: No allergies.

Student: Medications?

PROCTOR: No medications.

Student: Pertinent past medical history?

PROCTOR: No pertinent medical history.

Student: Last oral intake?

PROCTOR: 1 hour ago.

Student: Events leading up to the incident?

PROCTOR: The patient was grinding meat when his hand was caught and ground all the way into the machine.

Critical Criteria:

- ❑ Did not differentiate patient's need for transportation versus continued assessment at the scene
- ❑ Did not provide for spinal protection when indicated

Detailed Physical Examination

Student: I am conducting the detailed physical exam. I am looking for DCAP-BTLS. This acronym stands for deformities, contusions, abrasions, punctures, penetrations, paradoxical motion in the chest, and burns, tenderness, lacerations, and swelling.

PROCTOR: Noted. The detailed physical exam will be performed during transport.

Assess the Head

Student: I am assessing the head. Do I find any DCAP-BTLS? Do I find evidence of any Battle's sign or raccoon eyes?

PROCTOR: No.

Inspect and Palpate the Head and Ears

Student: I am assessing the head and ears.

PROCTOR: There are no obvious injuries.

Assess the Eyes

Student: I am assessing the eyes. Are the pupils equal, round, and regular in size, and react properly to light (PEARRL)?

PROCTOR: They are PEARRL.

Assess the Facial Area Including Oral and Nasal Areas

Student: I am assessing the face, nose, and mouth. Do I see any discharge or hear any obstructions?

PROCTOR: No.

Assess the Neck

Inspect and Palpate the Neck

Student: I am assessing the neck for DCAP-BTLS.

PROCTOR: There are no obvious injuries.

Assess for Jugular Vein Distention

Student: Do I find any jugular vein distention (JVD)?

PROCTOR: No.

Assess for Tracheal Deviation

Student: Do I see any tracheal deviation?

PROCTOR: No.

Assess the Chest

Student: I am assessing the chest for DCAP-BTLS.

PROCTOR: Noted.

Inspect

Student: What do I see when I look at the chest?

PROCTOR: There are no obvious injuries.

Student: Does the chest appear symmetric?

PROCTOR: Yes.

Palpate

Student: When I touch the chest, do I feel crepitus or a flail segment?

PROCTOR: No.

Auscultate

Student: Are lung sounds present in all fields?

PROCTOR: Yes.

Student: Do I hear any sucking sounds from the chest?

PROCTOR: No.

Assess the Abdomen/Pelvis

Assess the Abdomen

Student: I am assessing the abdomen for DCAP-BTLS. I am assessing all four quadrants. Do I find any problems?

PROCTOR: No.

Assess the Pelvis

Student: I am assessing the pelvis for DCAP-BTLS. Is the pelvis stable?

PROCTOR: Yes.

Assess the Genitalia/Perineum as Needed (Verbalize in Training)

Student: I am assessing the genitalia/perineum as necessary for DCAP-BTLS.

PROCTOR: The area is unremarkable.

Assess the Extremities

Inspect

Student: I am assessing the lower and upper extremities for DCAP-BTLS. Do I find anything?

PROCTOR: Yes, his hand is in the meat grinder.

Palpate

Student: Do I feel anything unusual?

PROCTOR: No.

Assess Motor, Sensory, and Circulatory Function

Student: I am checking for DCAP-BTLS, motor and sensory function, and pulses. Right leg?

PROCTOR: Negative DCAP-BTLS. Motor and sensory functions are present. Pulses are present.

Student: Left leg?

PROCTOR: Negative DCAP-BTLS. Motor and sensory functions are present. Pulses are present.

Student: Right arm?

PROCTOR: The patient's arm is in the machine up to the elbow. Bleeding appears to be minimal. Motor and sensory functions and pulses are unobtainable. I will secure the meat grinder on its side on the CPR seat in the ambulance for transport.

Student: Left arm?

PROCTOR: Negative DCAP-BTLS. Motor and sensory functions are present. Pulses are present.

Assess the Posterior

Student: We will check the back.

PROCTOR: Noted.

Assess the Thorax

Student: I am assessing the thorax. Do I find injuries?

PROCTOR: No.

Assess the Lumbar Area

Student: I am assessing the flanks and lumbar area. Do I find injuries?

PROCTOR: No.

Assess the Entire Backside

Student: I am assessing the entire backside. Do I find injuries?

PROCTOR: No.

▼ **Manage Secondary Injuries/Wounds**

Student: I would direct my partner to make the patient as comfortable as possible.

PROCTOR: Noted.

▼ **Reassess Vital Signs**

Student: I will reassess vital signs and mental status.

PROCTOR: Blood pressure, 114/72 mm Hg; pulse rate, 122 beats/min; respirations, 20 breaths/min; pulse oximetry reading, 98%; and the patient is alert.

Student: The vital signs have not changed significantly.

PROCTOR: Noted.

▼ **Reassess Interventions**

Student: I will reassess my interventions: oxygen and bleeding control. I will bring the patient and the meat grinder to the hospital.

PROCTOR: Noted.

ALS Student: I will reassess basic life support (BLS) interventions, plus the following: establish two large-bore IVs and administer pain management per local protocol.

ALS Proctor: Noted.

Critical Criteria:

❑ Did not find or manage problems associated with airway, breathing, hemorrhage or shock (hypoperfusion)

Radio Report

(Provided by the student.)

PROCTOR: Noted.

Ongoing Assessment

▼ **Repeat Vital Signs**

Student: I will reassess vital signs and mental status.

PROCTOR: Blood pressure, 120/68 mm Hg; pulse rate, 120 beats/min; respirations, 20 breaths/min; pulse oximetry reading, 98%; and the patient is alert.

Student: The vital signs have not changed significantly.

PROCTOR: Noted.

▼ **Check Interventions**

Student: I will check my interventions: oxygen and bleeding control. I will bring the patient and the meat grinder to the hospital.

PROCTOR: Noted.

ALS Student: I will check BLS interventions, plus the following: IVs and administer pain management per local protocol.

ALS Proctor: Noted.

Critical Criteria:

❑ Did not find or manage problems associated with airway, breathing, hemorrhage or shock (hypoperfusion)

Handoff Report to Emergency Department Staff

Student: There was no change in the patient's condition during transport.

PROCTOR: Noted.

Critical Criteria:

❑ Did not transport patient within the (10) minute time limit

Critical Criteria

(Inform the student of items missed, if any.)

❑ Pass ❑ Fail Date: ____________________

Proctor Comments: ____________________

____

____

Notes

Dispatch Information

PROCTOR: EMS 10, respond to a domestic dispute with a 23-year-old male patient shot. He is conscious and breathing. Police are on the scene. The patient is on the third floor and weighs 375 lb.

Pre-scene Action (BSI)

Student: I am wearing nonlatex gloves, safety glasses, mask, and gown.
PROCTOR: Noted.

Critical Criteria:
- ❑ Did not take, or verbalize, body substance isolation (BSI) precautions when necessary

Scene Size-up

Scene Safety

Student: Is the scene safe?
PROCTOR: Yes. Police have secured the scene and you are given clearance to enter.

Mechanism of Injury

Student: What was the mechanism of injury?
PROCTOR: Gunshot wound. The patient was fighting with his girlfriend when he was shot.

Number of Patients

Student: How many patients are there?
PROCTOR: One.

Additional Resources

Student: I would call for advanced life support (ALS) assistance and additional resources: fire/rescue to help lift the patient.
PROCTOR: Noted.

C-Spine Stabilization

Student: On the basis of the mechanism of injury, I would stabilize the cervical spine (c-spine) in a neutral in-line position.
PROCTOR: Noted.

Critical Criteria:
- ❑ Did not determine scene safety
- ❑ Did not assess for spinal protection
- ❑ Did not provide for spinal protection when indicated

Initial Assessment

Student: As I perform midline c-spine stabilization, I identify myself and ask the patient not to move.
PROCTOR: Noted.

General Impression

Student: My general impression is that the patient's condition is unstable.
PROCTOR: Noted.

Responsiveness/Level of Consciousness

Student: What is the patient's level of consciousness?
PROCTOR: Alert.

Chief Complaint/Apparent Life Threats

Student: What is the patient's chief complaint?
PROCTOR: The patient is complaining of not being able to move his legs. He has been shot in the abdomen.
Student: There is an apparent life threat; the life threat is a gunshot wound to the abdomen.
PROCTOR: Noted.

Assess the Airway and Breathing

Student: Is the airway open? Is the patient breathing?
PROCTOR: Yes, the airway is open and the patient is breathing.

Assessment

Student: What are the rate and the quality of breathing?
PROCTOR: Rate: Within normal limits. Quality: Normal.

Provide Oxygen

Student: I am applying oxygen at 15 L/min via nonrebreathing mask.
PROCTOR: Noted.

Ensure Adequate Ventilation

Student: The patient has adequate ventilations at this time.
PROCTOR: Noted.

Injury Management

Student: I will direct my partner to take over c-spine control as I continue assessment.
PROCTOR: Noted.

Assess Circulation

Student: I am assessing the patient's circulation.
PROCTOR: Noted.

Assess for and Control Major Bleeding

Student: Do I find any major bleeding?
PROCTOR: No, only minor bleeding from the abdomen.
Student: I will apply an occlusive dressing.
PROCTOR: Noted.

Assess the Pulse

Student: What are the rate and the quality of pulses?
PROCTOR: Rate: Within normal limits. Quality: Thready.

Assess the Skin

Student: I am assessing the skin. What are the color, temperature, and condition of the skin?
PROCTOR: Color: Normal. Temperature: Normal. Condition: Dry.

Identify Priority Patients/Make Transport Decision

Student: The patient is a high priority and is a load-and-go. I will begin packaging and transport.
PROCTOR: Noted.

Critical Criteria:
- ❑ Did not provide high concentration of oxygen
- ❑ Did not find or manage problems associated with airway, breathing, hemorrhage or shock (hypoperfusion)
- ❑ Did not differentiate patient's need for transportation versus continued assessment at the scene
- ❑ Did other detailed examination before assessing the airway, breathing and circulation

Focused History and Physical Examination/Rapid Trauma Assessment

Select the Appropriate Assessment (Focused or Rapid)

Student: I am selecting the rapid physical exam to identify and treat life threats. I am checking for DCAP-BTLS. This acronym stands for deformities, contusions, abrasions, punctures, penetrations, and paradoxical motion in the chest, and burns, tenderness, lacerations, and swelling.
PROCTOR: Noted.

Head

Student: I am rapidly assessing the head.
PROCTOR: There are no obvious injuries.

Neck

Student: I am rapidly assessing the neck.
PROCTOR: There are no obvious injuries.
Student: I will apply a cervical collar.
PROCTOR: Noted.

Chest

Student: I am rapidly assessing the chest. What are the lung sounds?
PROCTOR: There are no obvious injuries. The lung sounds are clear bilaterally.

▸ **Abdomen/Pelvis**

Student: I am rapidly assessing the abdomen.

PROCTOR: The abdomen is distended, discolored, and pooling to the flanks is noted, indicating internal bleeding.

Student: I am rapidly assessing the pelvis.

PROCTOR: There are no obvious injuries.

▸ **Extremities**

Student: I am rapidly assessing the extremities.

PROCTOR: There are no obvious injuries.

▸ **Assess Motor, Sensory, and Circulatory Function**

Student: I am checking for DCAP-BTLS. I am also checking motor and sensory function, and pulses. Right leg?

PROCTOR: No motor or sensory function found. Pulses are weak.

Student: Left leg?

PROCTOR: No motor or sensory function found. Pulses are weak.

Student: Right arm?

PROCTOR: Negative DCAP-BTLS. Motor and sensory functions are present. Pulses are present.

Student: Left arm?

PROCTOR: Negative DCAP-BTLS. Motor and sensory functions are present. Pulses are present.

▸ **Posterior**

Student: I am rapidly assessing the back. We will now log roll the patient as a unit to check the back. The person at the head will count to three and we will roll the patient.

PROCTOR: Noted.

▸ **Assess the Thorax**

Student: I am assessing the thorax. Do I find injuries?

PROCTOR: No.

▸ **Assess the Lumbar Area**

Student: I am assessing the flanks and lumbar area. Do I find injuries?

PROCTOR: You see the pooling of blood in the flank area.

▸ **Assess the Entire Backside**

Student: I am assessing the entire backside. Do I find injuries?

PROCTOR: No.

▸ **Manage Secondary Injuries/Wounds**

Student: We will apply a cervical collar and backboard with full immobilization per local protocol, if not yet done, at this time.

PROCTOR: Noted.

Student: Are there any changes in motor and sensory functions or pulses?

PROCTOR: No.

ALS Student: I will establish two large-bore IVs en route to the hospital and administer a bolus of 20 mL/kg in order to maintain a systolic blood pressure of 90 mm Hg.

ALS Proctor: Noted.

▸ **Reevaluate Transport Decision**

Student: This patient is a load-and-go due to shock and neurovascular deficit.

PROCTOR: Noted.

▾ Baseline Vital Signs

Student: What are the patient's baseline vital signs, including blood pressure, pulse, respirations, pulse oximetry, and level of consciousness?

PROCTOR: Blood pressure, 100/72 mm Hg; pulse, 88 beats/min; respirations, 16 breaths/min; pulse oximetry reading, 95%; and the patient is alert.

▾ SAMPLE History

Student: At this time I will gather a SAMPLE history from the patient or family. What are the patient's signs and symptoms?

PROCTOR: Pain in the abdomen and can't move his legs.

Student: Allergies?

PROCTOR: No allergies.

Student: Medications?

PROCTOR: No medications.

Student: Pertinent past medical history?

PROCTOR: He was shot a few years ago in the chest.

Student: Last oral intake?

PROCTOR: 2 hours ago.

Student: Events leading up to the incident?

PROCTOR: The patient was fighting with his girlfriend when she shot him.

Critical Criteria:

- ❑ Did not differentiate patient's need for transportation versus continued assessment at the scene
- ❑ Did not provide for spinal protection when indicated

▼ Detailed Physical Examination

Student: I am conducting the detailed physical exam. I am looking for DCAP-BTLS.

PROCTOR: Noted. The detailed physical exam will be performed during transport.

▾ Assess the Head

Student: I am assessing the head. Do I find any DCAP-BTLS? Do I find any evidence of Battle's sign or raccoon eyes?

PROCTOR: No.

▸ **Inspect and Palpate the Head and Ears**

Student: I am assessing the head and ears.

PROCTOR: There are no obvious injuries.

▸ **Assess the Eyes**

Student: I am assessing the eyes. Are the pupils equal, round, and regular in size, and react properly to light (PEARRL)?

PROCTOR: They are PEARRL.

▸ **Assess the Facial Area Including Oral and Nasal Areas**

Student: I am assessing the face, nose, and mouth. Do I see any discharge or hear any obstructions?

PROCTOR: No.

▾ Assess the Neck

▸ **Inspect and Palpate the Neck**

Student: I am assessing the neck for DCAP-BTLS.

PROCTOR: There are no obvious injuries.

▸ **Assess for Jugular Vein Distention**

Student: Do I find any jugular vein distention (JVD)?

PROCTOR: No.

▸ **Assess for Tracheal Deviation**

Student: Do I see any tracheal deviation?

PROCTOR: No.

▾ Assess the Chest

Student: I am assessing the chest for DCAP-BTLS.

PROCTOR: Noted.

▸ **Inspect**

Student: What do I see when I look at the chest?

PROCTOR: There are no obvious injuries.

Student: Does the chest appear symmetric?

PROCTOR: Yes.

▸ **Palpate**

Student: When I touch the chest, do I feel crepitus or a flail segment?

PROCTOR: No.

▸ **Auscultate**

Student: Are lung sounds present in all fields?

PROCTOR: Yes.

Student: Do I hear any sucking sounds from the chest?

PROCTOR: No.

▾ Assess the Abdomen/Pelvis

▸ **Assess the Abdomen**

Student: I am assessing the abdomen for DCAP-BTLS. I am assessing all four quadrants. Do I find any problems?

PROCTOR: You find a gunshot wound and distention, discoloration, and pooling to the flanks indicating internal bleeding.

Student: I would apply an occlusive dressing to the entrance wound (if not already done).
PROCTOR: Noted.

► **Assess the Pelvis**

Student: I am assessing the pelvis for DCAP-BTLS. Is the pelvis stable?
PROCTOR: Yes.

► **Assess the Genitalia/Perineum as Needed (Verbalize in Training)**

Student: I am assessing the genitalia/perineum as necessary for DCAP-BTLS.
PROCTOR: The area is unremarkable.

▼ Assess the Extremities

► **Inspect**

Student: I am assessing the lower and upper extremities for DCAP-BTLS. Do I find anything?
PROCTOR: Yes, there is pooling to the flanks.

► **Palpate**

Student: Do I feel anything unusual?
PROCTOR: No.

► **Assess Motor, Sensory, and Circulatory Function**

Student: I am checking for DCAP-BTLS, pulses, and motor and sensory function. Right leg?
PROCTOR: No motor or sensory function found. Pulses are weak.
Student: Left leg?
PROCTOR: No motor or sensory function found. Pulses are weak.
Student: Right arm?
PROCTOR: Negative DCAP-BTLS. Motor and sensory functions are present. Pulses are present.
Student: Left arm?
PROCTOR: Negative DCAP-BTLS. Motor and sensory functions are present. Pulses are present.

▼ Assess the Posterior

Note: This portion of the detailed physical exam would not be done if the patient were previously backboarded per local protocol.
Student: We will not check the back since it was previously checked and the patient is backboarded.
PROCTOR: Noted.

▼ Manage Secondary Injuries/Wounds

Student: No secondary wounds were found.
PROCTOR: Noted.

▼ Reassess Vital Signs

Student: At this time I will reassess vital signs and mental status.
PROCTOR: Blood pressure, 94/66 mm Hg; pulse, 84 beats/min; respirations, 16 breaths/min; pulse oximetry reading, 93%; and the patient is alert.
Student: The vital signs are deteriorating.
PROCTOR: Noted.

▼ Reassess Interventions

Student: I will reassess my interventions: airway, breathing, and oxygen; circulation and bleeding control; and immobilization and straps.
PROCTOR: Noted.

ALS Student: I will reassess basic life support (BLS) interventions, plus the following: two large-bore IVs, normal saline bolus of 20 mL/kg to maintain a blood pressure of 90 mm Hg, and cardiac monitor.
ALS Proctor: Noted. The cardiac monitor shows normal sinus rhythm.

Critical Criteria:
❑ Did not find or manage problems associated with airway, breathing, hemorrhage or shock (hypoperfusion)

▼ Radio Report

(Provided by the student.)
PROCTOR: Noted.

▼ Ongoing Assessment

▼ Repeat Vital Signs

Student: I will reassess vital signs and mental status.
PROCTOR: Blood pressure, 88/60 mm Hg; pulse, 80 beats/min; respirations, 16 breaths/min; pulse oximetry reading, 90%; and the patient is drowsy.
Student: The vital signs have deteriorated.
PROCTOR: Noted.

▼ Check Interventions

Student: I will check my interventions: airway, breathing, and oxygen; circulation and bleeding control; and immobilization and straps.
PROCTOR: Noted.
ALS Student: I will check BLS interventions, plus the following: two large-bore IVs, normal saline bolus of 20 mL/kg to maintain a blood pressure of 90 mm Hg, and cardiac monitor.
ALS Proctor: Noted. The cardiac monitor shows normal sinus rhythm.

Critical Criteria:
❑ Did not find or manage problems associated with airway, breathing, hemorrhage or shock (hypoperfusion)

▼ Handoff Report to Emergency Department Staff

Student: The patient's condition deteriorated during transport.
PROCTOR: Noted.

Critical Criteria:
❑ Did not transport patient within the (10) minute time limit

▼ Critical Criteria

(Inform the student of items missed, if any.)

❑ Pass ❑ Fail Date: ____________________

Proctor Comments: ____________________

Notes

Dispatch Information

PROCTOR: EMS 10, respond to a 44-year-old male who has dislocated his shoulder during an aerobics class. He is conscious and breathing but in a lot of pain.

Pre-scene Action (BSI)

Student: I am wearing nonlatex gloves and safety glasses.
PROCTOR: Noted.

Critical Criteria:
- ❑ Did not take, or verbalize, body substance isolation (BSI) precautions when necessary

Scene Size-up

Scene Safety

Student: Is the scene safe?
PROCTOR: Yes.

Mechanism of Injury

Student: What was the mechanism of injury?
PROCTOR: Dislocation. The patient was doing exercises in a class when his shoulder popped out of its socket.

Number of Patients

Student: How many patients are there?
PROCTOR: One.

Additional Resources

Student: I would hold off on calling for advanced life support (ALS) assistance.
PROCTOR: Noted.

C-Spine Stabilization

Student: I would not stabilize the cervical spine (c-spine).
PROCTOR: Noted.

Critical Criteria:
- ❑ Did not determine scene safety
- ❑ Did not assess for spinal protection
- ❑ Did not provide for spinal protection when indicated

Initial Assessment

Student: As I hold the patient in a position of comfort, I identify myself and ask the patient not to move.
PROCTOR: Noted.

General Impression

Student: My general impression is that the patient's condition is stable.
PROCTOR: Noted.

Responsiveness/Level of Consciousness

Student: What is the patient's level of consciousness?
PROCTOR: Alert.

Chief Complaint/Apparent Life Threats

Student: What is the patient's chief complaint?
PROCTOR: The patient is complaining of a dislocated shoulder.
Student: There are no apparent life threats.
PROCTOR: Noted.

Assess the Airway and Breathing

Student: I am opening the airway. Is the patient breathing?
PROCTOR: Yes.

Assessment

Student: What are the rate and the quality of breathing?
PROCTOR: Rate: Within normal limits. Quality: Normal.

Provide Oxygen

Student: I am applying oxygen at 15 L/min via nonrebreathing mask.
PROCTOR: Noted.

Ensure Adequate Ventilation

Student: The patient has adequate ventilations at this time.
PROCTOR: Noted.

Injury Management

Student: I will direct my partner to take over holding the patient as I continue assessment.
PROCTOR: Noted.

Assess Circulation

Student: I am assessing the patient's circulation.
PROCTOR: Noted.

Assess for and Control Major Bleeding

Student: Do I find any major bleeding?
PROCTOR: No.

Assess the Pulse

Student: What are the rate and the quality of pulses?
PROCTOR: Rate: Within normal limits. Quality: Strong.

Assess the Skin

Student: I am assessing the skin. What are the color, temperature, and condition of the skin?
PROCTOR: Color: Flushed. Temperature: Hot. Condition: Moist.

Identify Priority Patients/Make Transport Decision

Student: The patient is a low priority and does not require immediate transport.
PROCTOR: Noted.

Critical Criteria:
- ❑ Did not provide high concentration of oxygen
- ❑ Did not find or manage problems associated with airway, breathing, hemorrhage or shock (hypoperfusion)
- ❑ Did not differentiate patient's need for transportation versus continued assessment at the scene
- ❑ Did other detailed examination before assessing the airway, breathing and circulation

Focused History and Physical Examination/Rapid Trauma Assessment

Select the Appropriate Assessment (Focused or Rapid)

Student: I am selecting the focused assessment.
PROCTOR: Noted.

Extremities

Student: I am rapidly assessing the extremities.
PROCTOR: The right shoulder is dislocated and the arm is positioned above the patient's head. The right arm has a pins-and-needles sensation.
Student: I will stabilize the shoulder with a pillow splint.
PROCTOR: Noted.

Manage Secondary Injuries

ALS Student: I will establish an IV and administer pain management per local protocol.
ALS Proctor: Noted.

Reevaluate Transport Decision

Student: This patient does not require immediate transport.
PROCTOR: Noted.

Baseline Vital Signs

Student: What are the patient's baseline vital signs, including blood pressure, pulse, respirations, pulse oximetry, and level of consciousness?
PROCTOR: Blood pressure, 140/84 mm Hg; pulse, 128 beats/min; respirations, 20 breaths/min; pulse oximetry reading, 98%; and the patient is alert.

SAMPLE History

Student: At this time I will gather a SAMPLE history from the patient or family. What are the patient's signs and symptoms?
PROCTOR: Pain in the shoulder.

Student: Allergies?
PROCTOR: No allergies.
Student: Medications?
PROCTOR: No medications.
Student: Pertinent past medical history?
PROCTOR: This has happened many times since high school when he dislocated it playing football.
Student: Last oral intake?
PROCTOR: 3 hours ago.
Student: Events leading up to the incident?
PROCTOR: The patient was exercising when he raised his arm above his head and his right shoulder became dislocated.

Critical Criteria:
- ❑ Did not differentiate patient's need for transportation versus continued assessment at the scene
- ❑ Did not provide for spinal protection when indicated

Detailed Physical Examination

Student: I am conducting the detailed physical exam. I am looking for DCAP-BTLS. This acronym stands for deformities, contusions, abrasions, punctures, penetrations, paradoxical motion in the chest, and burns, tenderness, lacerations, and swelling.
PROCTOR: Noted. The detailed physical exam will be performed during transport.

Assess the Head

Student: I am assessing the head. Do I find any DCAP-BTLS? Do I find any evidence of Battle's sign or raccoon eyes?
PROCTOR: No.

Inspect and Palpate the Head and Ears

Student: I am assessing the head and ears.
PROCTOR: There are no obvious injuries.

Assess the Eyes

Student: I am assessing the eyes. Are the pupils equal, round, and regular in size, and react properly to light (PEARRL)?
PROCTOR: They are PEARRL.

Assess the Facial Area Including Oral and Nasal Areas

Student: I am assessing the face, nose, and mouth. Do I see any discharge or hear any obstructions?
PROCTOR: No.

Assess the Neck

Inspect and Palpate the Neck

Student: I am assessing the neck for DCAP-BTLS.
PROCTOR: There are no obvious injuries.

Assess for Jugular Vein Distention

Student: Do I find any jugular vein distention (JVD)?
PROCTOR: No.

Assess for Tracheal Deviation

Student: Do I see any tracheal deviation?
PROCTOR: No.

Assess the Chest

Student: I am assessing the chest for DCAP-BTLS.
PROCTOR: Noted.

Inspect

Student: What do I see when I look at the chest?
PROCTOR: There are no obvious injuries.
Student: Does the chest appear symmetric?
PROCTOR: Yes.

Palpate

Student: When I touch the chest, do I feel crepitus or a flail segment?
PROCTOR: No.

Auscultate

Student: Are lung sounds present in all fields?
PROCTOR: Yes.
Student: Do I hear any sucking sounds from the chest?
PROCTOR: No.

Assess the Abdomen/Pelvis

Assess the Abdomen

Student: I am assessing the abdomen for DCAP-BTLS. I am assessing all four quadrants. Do I find any problems?
PROCTOR: No.

Assess the Pelvis

Student: I am assessing the pelvis for DCAP-BTLS. Is the pelvis stable?
PROCTOR: Yes.

Assess the Genitalia/Perineum as Needed (Verbalize in Training)

Student: I am assessing the genitalia/perineum as necessary for DCAP-BTLS.
PROCTOR: The area is unremarkable.

Assess the Extremities

Inspect

Student: I am assessing the lower and upper extremities for DCAP-BTLS. Do I find anything?
PROCTOR: Yes. The right shoulder is dislocated and the arm is positioned above the head.

Palpate

Student: Do I feel anything unusual?
PROCTOR: Yes, the right shoulder is dislocated.

Assess Motor, Sensory, and Circulatory Function

Student: I am checking for DCAP-BTLS, motor and sensory function, and pulses. Right leg?
PROCTOR: Negative DCAP-BTLS. Motor and sensory functions are present. Pulses are present.
Student: Left leg?
PROCTOR: Negative DCAP-BTLS. Motor and sensory functions are present. Pulses are present.
Student: Right arm?
PROCTOR: The right arm is positioned above the patient's head and has a pins-and-needles sensation. Motor and sensory functions are present. Pulses are present.
Student: Left arm?
PROCTOR: Negative DCAP-BTLS. Motor and sensory functions are present. Pulses are present.

Assess the Posterior

Student: We will check the back.
PROCTOR: Noted.

Assess the Thorax

Student: I am assessing the thorax. Do I find injuries?
PROCTOR: No.

Assess the Lumbar Area

Student: I am assessing the flanks and lumbar area. Do I find injuries?
PROCTOR: No.

Assess the Entire Backside

Student: I am assessing the entire backside. Do I find injuries?
PROCTOR: No.

Manage Secondary Injuries/Wounds

Student: I would direct my partner to hold the patient in the position of comfort, and immobilize the right arm and shoulder.
PROCTOR: Noted.

Reassess Vital Signs

Student: I will reassess vital signs and mental status.
PROCTOR: Blood pressure, 132/84 mm Hg; pulse, 120 beats/min; respirations, 20 breaths/min; pulse oximetry reading, 98%; and the patient is alert.

Student: The vital signs have not changed significantly.
PROCTOR: Noted.

▾ Reassess Interventions

Student: I will reassess my interventions: oxygen and use of a pillow splint above the head to transport the patient.
PROCTOR: Noted.
ALS Student: I will reassess basic life support (BLS) interventions, plus the following: pain control per local protocol.
ALS Proctor: Noted.

Critical Criteria:
❑ Did not find or manage problems associated with airway, breathing, hemorrhage or shock (hypoperfusion)

Radio Report

(Provided by the student.)
PROCTOR: Noted.

Ongoing Assessment

▾ Repeat Vital Signs

Student: I will reassess vital signs and mental status.
PROCTOR: Blood pressure, 140/82 mm Hg; pulse, 120 beats/min, respirations, 20 breaths/min; pulse oximetry reading, 98%; and the patient is alert.

Student: The vital signs have not changed significantly.
PROCTOR: Noted.

▾ Check Interventions

Student: I will check my interventions: oxygen and use of a pillow splint above the head to transport the patient.
PROCTOR: Noted.
ALS Student: I will check BLS interventions, plus the following: pain control per local protocol.
ALS Proctor: Noted.

Critical Criteria:
❑ Did not find or manage problems associated with airway, breathing, hemorrhage or shock (hypoperfusion)

Handoff Report to Emergency Department Staff

Student: There was no change during transport.
PROCTOR: Noted.

Critical Criteria:
❑ Did not transport patient within the (10) minute time limit

Critical Criteria

(Inform the student of items missed, if any.)

❑ Pass ❑ Fail Date: ____________________

Proctor Comments: ____________________

____

____

Notes

Dispatch Information

PROCTOR: EMS 10, respond to a reported 37-year-old fire fighter down after coming in contact with electricity. He is conscious and breathing.

Pre-scene Action (BSI)

Student: I am wearing nonlatex gloves and safety glasses.
PROCTOR: Noted.

Critical Criteria:
- ❑ Did not take, or verbalize, body substance isolation (BSI) precautions when necessary

Scene Size-up

Scene Safety

Student: Is the scene safe?
PROCTOR: Yes.

Mechanism of Injury

Student: What was the mechanism of injury?
PROCTOR: Electric shock. The patient was in the interior of a structure fighting a fire when he came in contact with a 220-volt line on his left arm through his wet turnout gear. He felt the shock come in his arm and go out through his toes. He has chest pain.

Number of Patients

Student: How many patients are there?
PROCTOR: One.

Additional Resources

Student: I would call for advanced life support (ALS) assistance and additional resources: the electrical utility company.
PROCTOR: Noted.

C-Spine Stabilization

Student: On the basis of the mechanism of injury, I would stabilize the cervical spine (c-spine) in a neutral in-line position.
PROCTOR: Noted.

Critical Criteria:
- ❑ Did not determine scene safety
- ❑ Did not assess for spinal protection
- ❑ Did not provide for spinal protection when indicated

Initial Assessment

Student: As I perform midline c-spine stabilization, I identify myself and ask the patient not to move.
PROCTOR: Noted.

General Impression

Student: My general impression is that the patient's condition is unstable.
PROCTOR: Noted.

Responsiveness/Level of Consciousness

Student: What is the patient's level of consciousness?
PROCTOR: Alert.

Chief Complaint/Apparent Life Threats

Student: What is the patient's chief complaint?
PROCTOR: The patient is complaining of chest pain.
Student: There is an apparent life threat; the life threat is the mechanism of injury with chest pain.
PROCTOR: Noted.

Assess the Airway and Breathing

Student: Is the airway open? Is the patient breathing?
PROCTOR: Yes, the airway is open and the patient is breathing.

Assessment

Student: What are the rate and the quality of breathing?
PROCTOR: Rate: Tachypneic. Quality: Deep.

Provide Oxygen

Student: I am applying oxygen at 15 L/min via nonrebreathing mask.
PROCTOR: Noted.

Ensure Adequate Ventilation

Student: The patient has adequate ventilations at this time.
PROCTOR: Noted.

Injury Management

Student: I will direct my partner to remove the patient's gear as I continue assessment.
PROCTOR: Noted.

Assess Circulation

Student: I am assessing the patient's circulation.
PROCTOR: Noted.

Assess for and Control Major Bleeding

Student: Do I find any major bleeding?
PROCTOR: No.

Assess the Pulse

Student: What are the rate and the quality of pulses?
PROCTOR: Rate: Tachycardic. Quality: Bounding.

Assess the Skin

Student: I am assessing the skin. What are the color, temperature, and condition of the skin?
PROCTOR: Color: Flushed. Temperature: Hot. Condition: Diaphoretic.

Identify Priority Patients/Make Transport Decision

Student: The patient is a high priority and is a load-and-go. I will begin packaging and transport.
PROCTOR: Noted.

Critical Criteria:
- ❑ Did not provide high concentration of oxygen
- ❑ Did not find or manage problems associated with airway, breathing, hemorrhage or shock (hypoperfusion)
- ❑ Did not differentiate patient's need for transportation versus continued assessment at the scene
- ❑ Did other detailed examination before assessing the airway, breathing and circulation

Focused History and Physical Examination/Rapid Trauma Assessment

Select the Appropriate Assessment (Focused or Rapid)

Student: I am selecting the rapid physical exam to identify and treat life threats. I am checking for DCAP-BTLS. This acronym stands for deformities, contusions, abrasions, punctures, penetrations, and paradoxical motion in the chest, and burns, tenderness, lacerations, and swelling.
PROCTOR: Noted.

Head

Student: I am rapidly assessing the head.
PROCTOR: There are no obvious injuries.

Neck

Student: I am rapidly assessing the neck.
PROCTOR: There are no obvious injuries.
Student: I will apply a cervical collar.
PROCTOR: Noted.

Chest

Student: I am rapidly assessing the chest. What are the lung sounds?
PROCTOR: There are no obvious injuries. The lung sounds are clear bilaterally.

Abdomen/Pelvis

Student: I am rapidly assessing the abdomen.
PROCTOR: There are no obvious injuries.

Student: I am rapidly assessing the pelvis.
PROCTOR: There are no obvious injuries.

► **Extremities**

Student: I am rapidly assessing the extremities.
PROCTOR: The left arm has a red area and the toes are very red but without explosive entrance or exit wounds.

► **Assess Motor, Sensory, and Circulatory Function**

Student: I am checking for DCAP-BTLS. I am also checking motor and sensory function, and pulses. Right leg?
PROCTOR: Possible first-degree burns to the toes. Motor and sensory functions are present. Pulses are present.
Student: Left leg?
PROCTOR: Possible first-degree burns to the toes. Motor and sensory functions are present. Pulses are present.
Student: Right arm?
PROCTOR: Negative DCAP-BTLS. Motor and sensory functions are present. Pulses are present.
Student: Left arm?
PROCTOR: Possible first-degree burns to the upper arm. Motor and sensory functions are present. Pulses are present.

► **Posterior**

Student: I am rapidly assessing the back. We will now log roll the patient as a unit to check the back. The person at the head will count to three and we will roll the patient.
PROCTOR: Noted.

► **Assess the Thorax**

Student: I am assessing the thorax. Do I find injuries?
PROCTOR: No.

► **Assess the Lumbar Area**

Student: I am assessing the flanks and lumbar area. Do I find injuries?
PROCTOR: No.

► **Assess the Entire Backside**

Student: I am assessing the entire backside. Do I find injuries?
PROCTOR: No.

► **Manage Secondary Injuries/Wounds**

Student: We will apply a cervical collar and backboard with full immobilization per local protocol, if not yet done, at this time.
PROCTOR: Noted.
Student: Are there any changes in motor and sensory functions or pulses?
PROCTOR: No.
ALS Student: I will establish two large-bore IVs en route to the hospital and administer a bolus of 20 mL/kg in order to maintain a systolic blood pressure of 90 mm Hg. I will also connect the patient to a cardiac monitor and perform a 12-lead ECG.
ALS Proctor: Noted. The cardiac monitor shows sinus tachycardia with premature ventricular complexes.

► **Reevaluate Transport Decision**

Student: This patient is a load-and-go due to the mechanism of injury.
PROCTOR: Noted.

▼ Baseline Vital Signs

Student: What are the patient's baseline vital signs, including blood pressure, pulse, respirations, pulse oximetry, and level of consciousness?
PROCTOR: Blood pressure, 220/100 mm Hg; pulse rate, 140 beats/min; respirations, 24 breaths/min; pulse oximetry reading, 98%; and the patient is alert.

▼ SAMPLE History

Student: At this time I will gather a SAMPLE history from the patient or family. What are the patient's signs and symptoms?
PROCTOR: Pain in the left arm, shoulder, and chest, and burning in the toes.
Student: Allergies?
PROCTOR: No allergies.
Student: Medications?
PROCTOR: No medications.
Student: Pertinent past medical history?
PROCTOR: No pertinent medical history.
Student: Last oral intake?
PROCTOR: 8 hours ago.
Student: Events leading up to the incident?
PROCTOR: The patient was fighting a fire and came in contact with a 220-volt line (the resident was stealing electricity from a neighbor).

Critical Criteria:
- ❑ Did not differentiate patient's need for transportation versus continued assessment at the scene
- ❑ Did not provide for spinal protection when indicated

▼ Detailed Physical Examination

Student: I am conducting the detailed physical exam. I am looking for DCAP-BTLS.
PROCTOR: Noted. The detailed physical exam will be performed during transport.

▼ Assess the Head

Student: I am assessing the head. Do I find any DCAP-BTLS? Do I find any evidence of Battle's sign or raccoon eyes?
PROCTOR: No.

► **Inspect and Palpate the Head and Ears**

Student: I am assessing the head and ears.
PROCTOR: There are no obvious injuries.

► **Assess the Eyes**

Student: I am assessing the eyes. Are the pupils equal, round, and regular in size, and react properly to light (PEARRL)?
PROCTOR: They are PEARRL.

► **Assess the Facial Area Including Oral and Nasal Areas**

Student: I am assessing the face, nose, and mouth. Do I see any discharge or hear any obstructions?
PROCTOR: No.

▼ Assess the Neck

► **Inspect and Palpate the Neck**

Student: I am assessing the neck for DCAP-BTLS.
PROCTOR: There are no obvious injuries.

► **Assess for Jugular Vein Distention**

Student: Do I find any jugular vein distention (JVD)?
PROCTOR: Yes.

► **Assess for Tracheal Deviation**

Student: Do I see any tracheal deviation?
PROCTOR: No.

▼ Assess the Chest

Student: I am assessing the chest for DCAP-BTLS.
PROCTOR: Noted.

► **Inspect**

Student: What do I see when I look at the chest?
PROCTOR: There are no obvious injuries.
Student: Does the chest appear symmetric?
PROCTOR: Yes.

► **Palpate**

Student: When I touch the chest, do I feel crepitus or a flail segment?
PROCTOR: No.

► **Auscultate**

Student: Are lung sounds present in all fields?
PROCTOR: Yes.

Student: Do I hear any sucking sounds from the chest?
PROCTOR: No.

▼ Assess the Abdomen/Pelvis

► **Assess the Abdomen**

Student: I am assessing the abdomen for DCAP-BTLS. I am assessing all four quadrants. Do I find any problems?
PROCTOR: No.

► **Assess the Pelvis**

Student: I am assessing the pelvis for DCAP-BTLS. Is the pelvis stable?
PROCTOR: Yes.

▼ Assess the Genitalia/Perineum as Needed (Verbalize in Training)

Student: I am assessing the genitalia/perineum as necessary for DCAP-BTLS.
PROCTOR: The area is unremarkable.

▼ Assess the Extremities

► **Inspect**

Student: I am assessing the lower and upper extremities for DCAP-BTLS. Do I find anything?
PROCTOR: Yes, minor burns to the toes and left upper arm.

► **Palpate**

Student: Do I feel anything unusual?
PROCTOR: No.

► **Assess Motor, Sensory, and Circulatory Function**

Student: I am checking for DCAP-BTLS, motor and sensory function, and pulses. Right leg?
PROCTOR: Possible first-degree burns to the toes. Motor and sensory functions are present. Pulses are present.
Student: Left leg?
PROCTOR: Possible first-degree burns to the toes. Motor and sensory functions are present. Pulses are present.
Student: Right arm?
PROCTOR: Negative DCAP-BTLS. Motor and sensory functions are present. Pulses are present.
Student: Left arm?
PROCTOR: Possible first-degree burns to the upper arm. Motor and sensory functions are present. Pulses are present.

▼ Assess the Posterior

Note: This portion of the detailed physical exam would not be done if the patient were previously backboarded per local protocol.
Student: We will not check the back since it was previously checked and the patient is backboarded.
PROCTOR: Noted.

▼ Manage Secondary Injuries/Wounds

Student: I would direct my partner to further assess and possibly treat for chest pain.
PROCTOR: Noted.

▼ Reassess Vital Signs

Student: I will reassess vital signs and mental status.
PROCTOR: Blood pressure, 210/100 mm Hg; pulse rate, 136 beats/min; respirations, 24 breaths/min; pulse oximetry reading, 98%; and the patient is alert.
Student: The vital signs have not changed significantly.
PROCTOR: Noted.

▼ Reassess Interventions

Student: I will reassess my interventions: airway, breathing, and oxygen; and immobilization and straps.
PROCTOR: Noted.
ALS Student: I will reassess basic life support (BLS) interventions, plus the following: two large-bore IVs, cardiac monitoring with a 12-lead ECG, chest pain treatment per local protocol, and pain management for burns per local protocol.
ALS Proctor: Noted. The cardiac monitor shows sinus tachycardia with premature ventricular complexes.

Critical Criteria:
- ❑ Did not find or manage problems associated with airway, breathing, hemorrhage or shock (hypoperfusion)

Radio Report

(Provided by the student.)
PROCTOR: Noted.

Ongoing Assessment

▼ Repeat Vital Signs

Student: I will reassess vital signs and mental status.
PROCTOR: Blood pressure, 208/100 mm Hg; pulse rate, 130 beats/min; respirations, 24 breaths/min; pulse oximetry reading, 98%; and the patient is alert.
Student: The vital signs have not changed significantly.
PROCTOR: Noted.

▼ Check Interventions

Student: I will check my interventions: airway, breathing, and oxygen; and immobilization and straps.
PROCTOR: Noted.
ALS Student: I will check BLS interventions, plus the following: monitor the two large-bore IVs, cardiac monitoring, chest pain treatment per local protocol, and pain management for burns per local protocol.
ALS Proctor: Noted. The cardiac monitor shows sinus tachycardia with premature ventricular complexes.

Critical Criteria:
- ❑ Did not find or manage problems associated with airway, breathing, hemorrhage or shock (hypoperfusion)

Handoff Report to Emergency Department Staff

Student: There was no change during transport.
PROCTOR: Noted.

Critical Criteria:
- ❑ Did not transport patient within the (10) minute time limit

Critical Criteria

(Inform the student of items missed, if any.)

❑ Pass ❑ Fail Date: ______________________

Proctor Comments: ______________________

Notes

Dispatch Information

PROCTOR: EMS 10, respond to a 27-year-old female who has an impaled object in her eye. She is conscious and breathing.

Pre-scene Action (BSI)

Student: I am wearing nonlatex gloves, safety glasses, mask, and gown.
PROCTOR: Noted.

Critical Criteria:
- ❑ Did not take, or verbalize, body substance isolation (BSI) precautions when necessary

Scene Size-up

Scene Safety

Student: Is the scene safe?
PROCTOR: Yes.

Mechanism of Injury

Student: What was the mechanism of injury?
PROCTOR: Penetrating trauma. The patient was watering a rose bush when a twig broke off in her eye.

Number of Patients

Student: How many patients are there?
PROCTOR: One.

Additional Resources

Student: I would call for advanced life support (ALS) assistance (for pain management).
PROCTOR: Noted.

C-Spine Stabilization

Student: I would not stabilize the cervical spine (c-spine).
PROCTOR: Noted.

Critical Criteria:
- ❑ Did not determine scene safety
- ❑ Did not assess for spinal protection
- ❑ Did not provide for spinal protection when indicated

Initial Assessment

Student: As I identify myself, I ask the patient not to move.
PROCTOR: Noted.

General Impression

Student: My general impression is that the patient's condition is stable.
PROCTOR: Noted.

Responsiveness/Level of Consciousness

Student: What is the patient's level of consciousness?
PROCTOR: Alert but very restless.

Chief Complaint/Apparent Life Threats

Student: What is the patient's chief complaint?
PROCTOR: The patient is complaining of extreme pain in the left eye.
Student: There are no apparent life threats.
PROCTOR: Noted.

Assess the Airway and Breathing

Student: Is the airway open? Is the patient breathing?
PROCTOR: Yes, the airway is open and the patient is breathing.

Assessment

Student: What are the rate and the quality of breathing?
PROCTOR: Rate: Rapid. Quality: Normal.

Provide Oxygen

Student: I am applying oxygen at 15 L/min via nonrebreathing mask.
PROCTOR: Noted.

Ensure Adequate Ventilation

Student: The patient has adequate ventilations at this time.
PROCTOR: Noted.

Injury Management

Student: I will direct my partner to help the patient lie down as I continue assessment.
PROCTOR: Noted.

Assess Circulation

Student: I am assessing the patient's circulation.
PROCTOR: Noted.

Assess for and Control Major Bleeding

Student: Do I find any major bleeding?
PROCTOR: No.

Assess the Pulse

Student: What are the rate and the quality of pulses?
PROCTOR: Rate: Tachycardic. Quality: Normal.

Assess the Skin

Student: I am assessing the skin. What are the color, temperature, and condition of the skin?
PROCTOR: Color: Flushed. Temperature: Warm. Condition: Moist.

Identify Priority Patients/Make Transport Decision

Student: The patient is a high priority and is a load-and-go. I will begin packaging and transport.
PROCTOR: Noted.

Critical Criteria:
- ❑ Did not provide high concentration of oxygen
- ❑ Did not find or manage problems associated with airway, breathing, hemorrhage or shock (hypoperfusion)
- ❑ Did not differentiate patient's need for transportation versus continued assessment at the scene
- ❑ Did other detailed examination before assessing the airway, breathing and circulation

Focused History and Physical Examination/Rapid Trauma Assessment

Select the Appropriate Assessment (Focused or Rapid)

Student: I am selecting the focused assessment; I would focus on the isolated injury.
PROCTOR: Noted.
Student: As I assess her eye, what do I see?
PROCTOR: You see the lid of the left eye closed but tented with the shape of a small stick obvious beneath.
Student: I would dress and cover both eyes, and call for ALS for pain management.
PROCTOR: Noted.
ALS Student: I will establish an IV and administer pain control per local protocol.
ALS Proctor: Noted.

Reevaluate Transport Decision

Student: This patient will be rapidly transported to the most appropriate hospital.
PROCTOR: Noted.

Baseline Vital Signs

Student: What are the patient's baseline vital signs, including blood pressure, pulse, respirations, pulse oximetry, and level of consciousness?
PROCTOR: Blood pressure, 130/78 mm Hg; pulse rate, 122 beats/min; respirations, 28 breaths/min; pulse oximetry reading, 99%; and the patient is alert.

SAMPLE History

Student: At this time I will gather a SAMPLE history from the patient or family. What are the patient's signs and symptoms?
PROCTOR: Pain in the left eye.

Student: Allergies?
PROCTOR: No allergies.
Student: Medications?
PROCTOR: Asthma medications and an inhaler.
Student: Pertinent past medical history?
PROCTOR: Asthma.
Student: Last oral intake?
PROCTOR: 2 hours ago.
Student: Events leading up to the incident?
PROCTOR: The patient was watering a rose bush from her porch when the branch broke off in her eye.

Critical Criteria:
- ❑ Did not differentiate patient's need for transportation versus continued assessment at the scene
- ❑ Did not provide for spinal protection when indicated

Detailed Physical Examination

Student: I am conducting the detailed physical exam. I am looking for DCAP-BTLS. This acronym stands for deformities, contusions, abrasions, punctures, penetrations, paradoxical motion in the chest, and burns, tenderness, lacerations, and swelling.
PROCTOR: Noted. The detailed physical exam will be performed during transport.

Assess the Head

Student: I am assessing the head. Do I find any DCAP-BTLS? Do I find any evidence of Battle's sign or raccoon eyes?
PROCTOR: No.

Inspect and Palpate the Head and Ears

Student: I am assessing the head and ears.
PROCTOR: There are no obvious injuries.

Assess the Eyes

Student: I am assessing the eyes. Are the pupils equal, round, and regular in size, and react properly to light (PEARRL)?
PROCTOR: The left eye is shut and the right eye is uninjured. The right eye reacts normally.
Student: I will apply a protective dressing over the injured eye and dress the uninjured eye as well.
PROCTOR: Noted.

Assess the Facial Area Including Oral and Nasal Areas

Student: I am assessing the face, nose, and mouth. Do I see any discharge or hear any obstructions?
PROCTOR: No.

Assess the Neck

Inspect and Palpate the Neck

Student: I am assessing the neck for DCAP-BTLS.
PROCTOR: There are no obvious injuries.

Assess for Jugular Vein Distention

Student: Do I find any jugular vein distention (JVD)?
PROCTOR: No.

Assess for Tracheal Deviation

Student: Do I see any tracheal deviation?
PROCTOR: No.

Assess the Chest

Student: I am assessing the chest for DCAP-BTLS.
PROCTOR: Noted.

Inspect

Student: What do I see when I look at the chest?
PROCTOR: There are no obvious injuries.
Student: Does the chest appear symmetric?
PROCTOR: Yes.

Palpate

Student: When I touch the chest, do I feel crepitus or a flail segment?
PROCTOR: No.

Auscultate

Student: Are lung sounds present in all fields?
PROCTOR: Yes.
Student: Do I hear any sucking sounds from the chest?
PROCTOR: No.

Assess the Abdomen/Pelvis

Assess the Abdomen

Student: I am assessing the abdomen for DCAP-BTLS. I am assessing all four quadrants. Do I find any problems?
PROCTOR: No.

Assess the Pelvis

Student: I am assessing the pelvis for DCAP-BTLS. Is the pelvis stable?
PROCTOR: Yes.

Assess the Genitalia/Perineum as Needed (Verbalize in Training)

Student: I will not assess the genitalia/perineum for DCAP-BTLS.
PROCTOR: Noted.

Assess the Extremities

Inspect

Student: I am assessing the lower and upper extremities for DCAP-BTLS. Do I find anything?
PROCTOR: No.

Palpate

Student: Do I feel anything unusual?
PROCTOR: No.

Assess Motor, Sensory, and Circulatory Function

Student: I am checking for DCAP-BTLS, motor and sensory function, and pulses. Right leg?
PROCTOR: Negative DCAP-BTLS. Motor and sensory functions are present. Pulses are present.
Student: Left leg?
PROCTOR: Negative DCAP-BTLS. Motor and sensory functions are present. Pulses are present.
Student: Right arm?
PROCTOR: Negative DCAP-BTLS. Motor and sensory functions are present. Pulses are present.
Student: Left arm?
PROCTOR: Negative DCAP-BTLS. Motor and sensory functions are present. Pulses are present.

Assess the Posterior

Student: We will now check the back.
PROCTOR: Noted.

Assess the Thorax

Student: I am assessing the thorax. Do I find injuries?
PROCTOR: No.

Assess the Lumbar Area

Student: I am assessing the flanks and lumbar area. Do I find injuries?
PROCTOR: No.

Assess the Entire Backside

Student: I am assessing the entire backside. Do I find injuries?
PROCTOR: No.

Manage Secondary Injuries/Wounds

Student: We will constantly reassure the patient.
PROCTOR: Noted.

Reassess Vital Signs

Student: I will reassess vital signs and mental status.
PROCTOR: Blood pressure, 134/78 mm Hg; pulse rate, 112 beats/min; respirations, 24 breaths/min; pulse oximetry reading, 99%; and the patient is alert.

Student: The vital signs have not changed significantly.
PROCTOR: Noted.

Reassess Interventions

Student: I will reassess my interventions: oxygen, reassurance, and eye dressings.
PROCTOR: Noted.
ALS Student: I will reassess basic life support (BLS) interventions, plus the following: establish an IV and administer pain control per local protocol.
ALS Proctor: Noted.

Critical Criteria:
- ❑ Did not find or manage problems associated with airway, breathing, hemorrhage or shock (hypoperfusion)

Radio Report

(Provided by the student.)
PROCTOR: Noted.

Ongoing Assessment

Repeat Vital Signs

Student: I will reassess vital signs and mental status.
PROCTOR: Blood pressure, 124/72 mm Hg; pulse rate, 102 beats/min; respirations, 20 breaths/min; pulse oximetry reading, 99%; and the patient is alert.
Student: The vital signs have not changed significantly.
PROCTOR: Noted.

Check Interventions

Student: I will check my interventions: oxygen, reassurance, and eye dressings.
PROCTOR: Noted.
ALS Student: I will check BLS interventions, plus the following: check IV and check pain level.
ALS Proctor: Noted.

Critical Criteria:
- ❑ Did not find or manage problems associated with airway, breathing, hemorrhage or shock (hypoperfusion)

Handoff Report to Emergency Department Staff

Student: There was no change during transport.
PROCTOR: Noted.

Critical Criteria:
- ❑ Did not transport patient within the (10) minute time limit

Critical Criteria

(Inform the student of items missed, if any.)

❑ Pass ❑ Fail Date: ______________________________

Proctor Comments: ______________________________

____

____

Notes

Dispatch Information

PROCTOR: EMS 10, respond to a 28-year-old male who has struck a guard rail on his motorcycle. He is conscious and breathing. Police are on the scene and traffic is controlled.

Pre-scene Action (BSI)

Student: I am wearing appropriate high-visibility personal protective equipment suitable for extrication, a helmet, extrication gloves, nonlatex gloves, safety glasses, mask, and gown.
PROCTOR: Noted.

Critical Criteria:
- ❑ Did not take, or verbalize, body substance isolation (BSI) precautions when necessary

Scene Size-up

Scene Safety

Student: Is the scene safe?
PROCTOR: Yes, police are on scene and you are given clearance to enter.

Mechanism of Injury

Student: What was the mechanism of injury?
PROCTOR: Motorcycle collision. The patient was driving his motorcycle at high speed when he lost control and hit a guard rail. His left leg is under his body; his left foot is behind his neck.

Number of Patients

Student: How many patients are there?
PROCTOR: One.

Additional Resources

Student: I would call for advanced life support (ALS) assistance.
PROCTOR: Noted.

C-Spine Stabilization

Student: On the basis of the mechanism of injury, I would stabilize the cervical spine (c-spine) in a neutral in-line position.
PROCTOR: Noted.

Critical Criteria:
- ❑ Did not determine scene safety
- ❑ Did not assess for spinal protection
- ❑ Did not provide for spinal protection when indicated

Initial Assessment

Student: As I perform midline c-spine stabilization, I identify myself and ask the patient not to move.
PROCTOR: Noted.

General Impression

Student: My general impression is that the patient's condition is unstable.
PROCTOR: Noted.

Responsiveness/Level of Consciousness

Student: What is the patient's level of consciousness?
PROCTOR: Alert.

Chief Complaint/Apparent Life Threats

Student: What is the patient's chief complaint?
PROCTOR: The patient is complaining of chest pain and a broken arm and leg.
Student: There is an apparent life threat; the life threat is the mechanism of injury.
PROCTOR: Noted.

Assess the Airway and Breathing

Student: I am opening the airway. Is the patient breathing?
PROCTOR: Yes.

Assessment

Student: What are the rate and the quality of breathing?
PROCTOR: Rate: Tachypneic. Quality: Shallow.

Provide Oxygen

Student: I am applying oxygen at 15 L/min via nonrebreathing mask.
PROCTOR: Noted.

Ensure Adequate Ventilation

Student: The patient has adequate ventilations at this time.
PROCTOR: Noted.

Injury Management

Student: I will direct my partner to take over c-spine control as I continue assessment.
PROCTOR: Noted.

Assess Circulation

Student: I am assessing the patient's circulation.
PROCTOR: Noted.

Assess for and Control Major Bleeding

Student: Do I find any major bleeding?
PROCTOR: No.

Assess the Pulse

Student: What are the rate and the quality of pulses?
PROCTOR: Rate: Tachycardic. Quality: Bounding.

Assess the Skin

Student: I am assessing the skin. What are the color, temperature, and condition of the skin?
PROCTOR: Color: Flushed. Temperature: Warm. Condition: Moist.

Identify Priority Patients/Make Transport Decision

Student: The patient is a high priority and is a load-and-go. I will begin packaging and transport.
PROCTOR: Noted.

Critical Criteria:
- ❑ Did not provide high concentration of oxygen
- ❑ Did not find or manage problems associated with airway, breathing, hemorrhage or shock (hypoperfusion)
- ❑ Did not differentiate patient's need for transportation versus continued assessment at the scene
- ❑ Did other detailed examination before assessing the airway, breathing and circulation

Focused History and Physical Examination/Rapid Trauma Assessment

Select the Appropriate Assessment (Focused or Rapid)

Student: I am selecting the rapid physical exam to identify and treat life threats. I am checking for DCAP-BTLS. This acronym stands for deformities, contusions, abrasions, punctures, penetrations, and paradoxical motion in the chest, and burns, tenderness, lacerations, and swelling.
PROCTOR: Noted.

Head

Student: I am rapidly assessing the head.
PROCTOR: There are no obvious injuries (the patient was wearing a helmet). The patient denies any loss of consciousness.

Neck

Student: I am rapidly assessing the neck.
PROCTOR: There are no obvious injuries.
Student: I will apply a cervical collar.
PROCTOR: Noted.

Chest

Student: I am rapidly assessing the chest.
PROCTOR: The left side is depressed with a flail segment.
Student: I will stabilize the chest with bulky dressings and listen to lung sounds.
PROCTOR: Noted. Lung sounds are diminished on the left.

Student: I will assess the chest for tension pneumothorax by auscultation, and assessment (jugular vein distention [JVD], tracheal deviation, and decreased lung sounds).
PROCTOR: The lung sounds appear clear bilaterally, jugular vein distention is not present, and the trachea is midline.
ALS Student: I will assess the chest for hyperresonance to percussion.
ALS Proctor: Noted. There is no tension pneumothorax.
ALS Student: I will continuously reassess the chest.
ALS Proctor: Noted.

▸ **Abdomen/Pelvis**

Student: I am rapidly assessing the abdomen.
PROCTOR: There are no obvious injuries.
Student: I am rapidly assessing the pelvis.
PROCTOR: There are no obvious injuries.

▸ **Extremities**

Student: I am rapidly assessing the extremities.
PROCTOR: There are obvious fractures to the left arm and left leg.

▸ **Assess Motor, Sensory, and Circulatory Function**

Student: I am checking for DCAP-BTLS. I am also checking motor and sensory function, and pulses. Right leg?
PROCTOR: Negative DCAP-BTLS. Motor and sensory functions are present. Pulses are present.
Student: Left leg?
PROCTOR: There are multiple fractures. The leg is under the body, with the foot up near the neck. Motor and sensory functions are present. Pulses are present.
Student: Right arm?
PROCTOR: Negative DCAP-BTLS. Motor and sensory functions are present. Pulses are present.
Student: Left arm?
PROCTOR: There are multiple fractures noted. Motor and sensory functions are present. Pulses are present.

▸ **Posterior**

Student: I will rapidly assess the back. We will now log roll the patient as a unit to check the back. The person at the head will count to three and we will roll the patient. We will move the leg around to normal anatomical position and will maintain manual immobilization of the left leg.
PROCTOR: Noted.

▸ **Assess the Thorax**

Student: I am assessing the thorax. Do I find injuries?
PROCTOR: No.

▸ **Assess the Lumbar Area**

Student: I am assessing the flanks and lumbar area. Do I find injuries?
PROCTOR: No.

▸ **Assess the Entire Backside**

Student: I am assessing the entire backside. Do I find injuries?
PROCTOR: No.

▸ **Manage Secondary Injuries/Wounds**

Student: We will apply a cervical collar and backboard with full immobilization per local protocol, if not yet done, at this time. The left leg is brought into anatomical position while log rolling and placing the patient on the long backboard. The arm and leg will be treated during the rapid transport to the trauma center.
PROCTOR: Noted.
Student: Are there any changes in motor and sensory functions or pulses?
PROCTOR: No.
ALS Student: I will establish two large-bore IVs en route to the hospital and a bolus of 20 mL/kg in order to maintain a systolic blood pressure of 90 mm Hg.
ALS Proctor: Noted.

▸ **Reevaluate Transport Decision**

Student: This patient is a load-and-go due to multitrauma and the mechanism of injury.
PROCTOR: Noted.

▾ Baseline Vital Signs

Student: What are the patient's baseline vital signs, including blood pressure, pulse, respirations, pulse oximetry, and level of consciousness?
PROCTOR: Blood pressure, 140/86 mm Hg; pulse rate, 130 beats/min; respirations, 28 breaths/min; pulse oximetry reading, 96%; and the patient is alert.

▾ SAMPLE History

Student: At this time I will gather a SAMPLE history from the patient or family. What are the patient's signs and symptoms?
PROCTOR: Pain in the left arm, leg, and chest.
Student: Allergies?
PROCTOR: No allergies.
Student: Medications?
PROCTOR: No medications.
Student: Pertinent past medical history?
PROCTOR: No pertinent medical history.
Student: Last oral intake?
PROCTOR: The patient had been drinking beer.
Student: Events leading up to the incident?
PROCTOR: The patient was street racing when he lost control of his motorcycle and hit a guard rail.

Critical Criteria:
- ❑ Did not differentiate patient's need for transportation versus continued assessment at the scene
- ❑ Did not provide for spinal protection when indicated

Detailed Physical Examination

Student: I am conducting the detailed physical exam. I am looking for DCAP-BTLS.
PROCTOR: Noted. The detailed physical exam will be performed during transport.

▾ Assess the Head

Student: I am assessing the head. Do I find any DCAP-BTLS? Do I find any evidence of Battle's sign or raccoon eyes?
PROCTOR: No.

▸ **Inspect and Palpate the Head and Ears**

Student: I am assessing the head and ears.
PROCTOR: There are no obvious injuries.

▸ **Assess the Eyes**

Student: I am assessing the eyes. Are the pupils equal, round, and regular in size, and react properly to light (PEARRL)?
PROCTOR: They are PEARRL.

▸ **Assess the Facial Area Including Oral and Nasal Areas**

Student: I am assessing the face, nose, and mouth. Do I see any discharge or hear any obstructions?
PROCTOR: No.

▾ Assess the Neck

▸ **Inspect and Palpate the Neck**

Student: I am assessing the neck for DCAP-BTLS.
PROCTOR: There are no obvious injuries.

▸ **Assess for Jugular Vein Distention**

Student: Do I find any jugular vein distention (JVD)?
PROCTOR: No.

▸ Assess for Tracheal Deviation

Student: Do I see any tracheal deviation?
PROCTOR: No.

▾ Assess the Chest

Student: I am assessing the chest for DCAP-BTLS.
PROCTOR: The left chest is depressed, but was stabilized earlier.
Student: I will reassess the chest.
PROCTOR: Noted. There is no change.

▸ Inspect

Student: What do I see when I look at the chest?
PROCTOR: The left chest is depressed, but has been previously treated during the rapid trauma assessment.
Student: Does the chest appear symmetric?
PROCTOR: No, but it was treated per local protocol.

▸ Palpate

Student: When I touch the chest, do I feel crepitus or a flail segment?
PROCTOR: Yes, on the left, but it was stabilized earlier.
Student: I will ventilate this patient, if necessary.
PROCTOR: Noted.

▸ Auscultate

Student: Are lung sounds present in all fields?
PROCTOR: Yes.
Student: Do I hear any sucking sounds from the chest?
PROCTOR: No.

▾ Assess the Abdomen/Pelvis

▸ Assess the Abdomen

Student: I am assessing the abdomen for DCAP-BTLS. I am assessing all four quadrants. Do I find any problems?
PROCTOR: No.

▸ Assess the Pelvis

Student: I am assessing the pelvis for DCAP-BTLS. Is the pelvis stable?
PROCTOR: Yes.

▾ Assess the Genitalia/Perineum as Needed (Verbalize in Training)

Student: I am assessing the genitalia/perineum as necessary for DCAP-BTLS.
PROCTOR: The area is unremarkable.

▾ Assess the Extremities

▸ Inspect

Student: I am assessing the lower and upper extremities for DCAP-BTLS. Do I find anything?
PROCTOR: Yes, you find an obvious injury and deformities to the left arm and left leg.

▸ Palpate

Student: Do I feel anything unusual?
PROCTOR: Yes, multiple fractures were noted to the left arm and left leg.

▸ Assess Motor, Sensory, and Circulatory Function

Student: I am checking for DCAP-BTLS, motor and sensory function, and pulses. Right leg?
PROCTOR: Negative DCAP-BTLS. Motor and sensory functions are present. Pulses are present.
Student: Left leg?
PROCTOR: There are multiple fractures. Motor and sensory functions are present. Pulses are present but weak.
Student: Right arm?
PROCTOR: Negative DCAP-BTLS. Motor and sensory functions are present. Pulses are present.
Student: Left arm?
PROCTOR: There are multiple fractures noted. Motor and sensory functions are present. Pulses are present.
Student: The left arm and left leg will be treated per local protocol and reassessed for motor and sensory function and pulse changes.
PROCTOR: Noted. The pulse is now stronger in the left leg.

▾ Assess the Posterior

Note: This portion of the detailed physical exam would not be done if the patient were previously backboarded per local protocol.
Student: We will not check the back since it was previously checked and the patient is backboarded.
PROCTOR: Noted.

▾ Manage Secondary Injuries/Wounds

Student: I would direct my partner to monitor the airway and chest.
PROCTOR: Noted.

▾ Reassess Vital Signs

Student: I will reassess vital signs and mental status.
PROCTOR: Blood pressure, 136/82 mm Hg; pulse rate, 122 beats/min; respirations, 24 breaths/min; pulse oximetry reading, 97%; and the patient is alert.
Student: The vital signs have not changed significantly.
PROCTOR: Noted.

▾ Reassess Interventions

Student: I will reassess my interventions: airway, oxygen, bleeding control, full immobilization, splints to the arm and leg, and stabilization of the flail segment.
PROCTOR: Noted.
ALS Student: I will reassess basic life support (BLS) interventions, plus the following: two large-bore IVs and cardiac monitoring.
ALS Proctor: Noted. The cardiac monitor shows sinus tachycardia.

Critical Criteria:
❑ Did not find or manage problems associated with airway, breathing, hemorrhage or shock (hypoperfusion)

Radio Report

(Provided by the student.)
PROCTOR: Noted.

Ongoing Assessment

▾ Repeat Vital Signs

Student: I will reassess vital signs and mental status.
PROCTOR: Blood pressure, 132/86 mm Hg; pulse rate, 126 beats/min; respirations, 22 breaths/min; pulse oximetry reading, 98%; and the patient is alert.
Student: The vital signs have improved.
PROCTOR: Noted.

Check Interventions

Student: I will check my interventions: airway, oxygen, bleeding control, full immobilization, splints to the arm and leg, stabilization of the flail segment, and ventilate if necessary.

PROCTOR: Noted.

ALS Student: I will check BLS interventions, plus the following: two large-bore IVs and cardiac monitoring.

ALS Proctor: Noted. The cardiac monitor shows sinus tachycardia.

Critical Criteria:
- ☐ Did not find or manage problems associated with airway, breathing, hemorrhage or shock (hypoperfusion)

Handoff Report to Emergency Department Staff

Student: The patient's condition improved during transport.

PROCTOR: Noted.

Critical Criteria:
- ☐ Did not transport patient within the (10) minute time limit

Critical Criteria

(Inform the student of items missed, if any.)

☐ Pass ☐ Fail Date: ______________________

Proctor Comments: ______________________

____

____

Dispatch Information

PROCTOR: EMS 10, respond to a shooting with a 24-year-old male subject down with difficulty breathing. Police are on scene.

Pre-scene Action (BSI)

Student: I am wearing nonlatex gloves, safety glasses, mask, and gown.

PROCTOR: Noted.

Critical Criteria:
- ❑ Did not take, or verbalize, body substance isolation (BSI) precautions when necessary

Scene Size-up

Scene Safety

Student: Is the scene safe?

PROCTOR: Yes, police are on scene and you are given clearance to enter.

Mechanism of Injury

Student: What was the mechanism of injury?

PROCTOR: Gunshot wound, plus a fall. The patient was fleeing the homeowner during a burglary attempt. He fell down the stairs after being shot.

Number of Patients

Student: How many patients are there?

PROCTOR: One.

Additional Resources

Student: I would call for advanced life support (ALS) assistance.

PROCTOR: Noted.

C-Spine Stabilization

Student: On the basis of the mechanism of injury, I would stabilize the cervical spine (c-spine) in a neutral in-line position.

PROCTOR: Noted.

Critical Criteria:
- ❑ Did not determine scene safety
- ❑ Did not assess for spinal protection
- ❑ Did not provide for spinal protection when indicated

Initial Assessment

Student: As I perform midline c-spine stabilization, I identify myself and ask the patient not to move.

PROCTOR: Noted.

General Impression

Student: My general impression is that the patient's condition is unstable.

PROCTOR: Noted.

Responsiveness/Level of Consciousness

Student: What is the patient's level of consciousness?

PROCTOR: Alert.

Chief Complaint/Apparent Life Threats

Student: What is the patient's chief complaint?

PROCTOR: The patient is complaining that he cannot breathe and he cannot move his legs.

Student: There are apparent life threats; the life threats are a gunshot wound and difficulty breathing.

PROCTOR: Noted.

Assess the Airway and Breathing

Student: Is the airway open? Is the patient breathing?

PROCTOR: Yes, the airway is open and the patient is breathing.

Assessment

Student: What are the rate and the quality of breathing?

PROCTOR: Rate: Slow. Quality: Diaphragmatic.

Provide Oxygen

Student: I am assisting ventilations with a bag-valve device with 100% oxygen.

PROCTOR: Noted.

Ensure Adequate Ventilation

Student: I will constantly reassess the airway and the adequacy of the bag-valve ventilations.

PROCTOR: Noted.

Injury Management

Student: I will direct my partner to take over c-spine control as I continue assessment.

PROCTOR: Noted.

Assess Circulation

Student: I am assessing the patient's circulation.

PROCTOR: Noted.

Assess for and Control Major Bleeding

Student: Do I find any major bleeding?

PROCTOR: No.

Assess the Pulse

Student: What are the rate and the quality of pulses?

PROCTOR: Rate: Within normal limits. Quality: Thready.

Assess the Skin

Student: I am assessing the skin. What are the color, temperature, and condition of the skin?

PROCTOR: Color: Normal. Temperature: Normal. Condition: Dry.

Identify Priority Patients/Make Transport Decision

Student: The patient is a high priority and is a load-and-go. I will begin packaging and transport.

PROCTOR: Noted.

Critical Criteria:
- ❑ Did not provide high concentration of oxygen
- ❑ Did not find or manage problems associated with airway, breathing, hemorrhage or shock (hypoperfusion)
- ❑ Did not differentiate patient's need for transportation versus continued assessment at the scene
- ❑ Did other detailed examination before assessing the airway, breathing and circulation

Focused History and Physical Examination/Rapid Trauma Assessment

Select the Appropriate Assessment (Focused or Rapid)

Student: I am selecting the rapid physical exam to identify and treat life threats. I am checking for DCAP-BTLS. This acronym stands for deformities, contusions, abrasions, punctures, penetrations, and paradoxical motion in the chest, and burns, tenderness, lacerations, and swelling.

PROCTOR: Noted.

Head

Student: I am rapidly assessing the head.

PROCTOR: There are no obvious injuries.

Neck

Student: I am rapidly assessing the neck.

PROCTOR: There are no obvious injuries.

Student: I will apply a cervical collar.

PROCTOR: Noted.

Chest

Student: I am rapidly assessing the chest. What are the lung sounds?

PROCTOR: There are no obvious injuries. Lung sounds are clear bilaterally.

▸ **Abdomen/Pelvis**

Student: I am rapidly assessing the abdomen.
PROCTOR: There are no obvious injuries.
Student: I am rapidly assessing the pelvis.
PROCTOR: There are no obvious injuries.

▸ **Extremities**

Student: I am rapidly assessing the extremities.
PROCTOR: There are no obvious injuries.

▸ **Assess Motor, Sensory, and Circulatory Function**

Student: I am checking for DCAP-BTLS. I am also checking motor and sensory function, and pulses. Right leg?
PROCTOR: Negative DCAP-BTLS. Motor and sensory functions are absent. Pulses are weak.
Student: Left leg?
PROCTOR: Negative DCAP-BTLS. Motor and sensory functions are absent. Pulses are weak.
Student: Right arm?
PROCTOR: Negative DCAP-BTLS. Motor and sensory functions are present. Pulses are weak.
Student: Left arm?
PROCTOR: Negative DCAP-BTLS. Motor and sensory functions are present. Pulses are weak.

▸ **Posterior**

Student: I will rapidly assess the back. We will now log roll the patient as a unit to check the back. The person at the head will count to three and we will roll the patient.
PROCTOR: Noted.

▸ **Assess the Thorax**

Student: I am assessing the thorax. Do I find injuries?
PROCTOR: There is a gunshot wound in the high center of the back at the base of the neck.
Student: I will apply an occlusive dressing to the wound.
PROCTOR: Noted.

▸ **Assess the Lumbar Area**

Student: I am assessing the flanks and lumbar area. Do I find injuries?
PROCTOR: No.

▸ **Assess the Entire Backside**

Student: I am assessing the entire backside. Do I find injuries?
PROCTOR: No.

▸ **Manage Secondary Injuries/Wounds**

Student: We will apply a cervical collar and backboard with full immobilization per local protocol, if not yet done, at this time.
PROCTOR: Noted.
Student: Are there any changes in motor and sensory functions or pulses?
PROCTOR: No.
ALS Student: I will establish two large-bore IVs en route to the hospital and administer a bolus of 20 mL/kg in order to maintain a systolic blood pressure of 90 mm Hg, and perform cardiac monitoring. I will intubate (or rapid sequence intubation [RSI] depending on local protocol), and confirm with end tidal CO_2 and lung sounds.
ALS Proctor: Noted. The cardiac monitor shows normal sinus rhythm. End tidal CO_2 and lung sounds confirm placement of the endotracheal (ET) tube.

▸ **Reevaluate Transport Decision**

Student: This patient is a load-and-go due to difficulty breathing, the mechanism of injury, and shock.
PROCTOR: Noted.

▾ **Baseline Vital Signs**

Student: What are the patient's baseline vital signs, including blood pressure, pulse, respirations, pulse oximetry, and level of consciousness?
PROCTOR: Blood pressure, 78/50 mm Hg; pulse rate, 80 beats/min; respirations, per bag-valve device; pulse oximetry reading, 94%; and the patient is alert.

▾ **SAMPLE History**

Student: At this time I will gather a SAMPLE history from the patient or family. What are the patient's signs and symptoms?
PROCTOR: Pain in back, difficulty breathing, and he cannot move his legs.
Student: Allergies?
PROCTOR: No allergies.
Student: Medications?
PROCTOR: No medications.
Student: Pertinent past medical history?
PROCTOR: No pertinent medical history.
Student: Last oral intake?
PROCTOR: 3 hours ago.
Student: Events leading up to the incident?
PROCTOR: The patient was running from a homeowner during a burglary attempt.

Critical Criteria:
- ❑ Did not differentiate patient's need for transportation versus continued assessment at the scene
- ❑ Did not provide for spinal protection when indicated

Detailed Physical Examination

Student: I am conducting the detailed physical exam. I am looking for DCAP-BTLS.
PROCTOR: Noted. The detailed physical exam will be performed during transport.

▾ **Assess the Head**

Student: I am assessing the head. Do I find any DCAP-BTLS? Do I find any evidence of Battle's sign or raccoon eyes?
PROCTOR: No.

▸ **Inspect and Palpate the Head and Ears**

Student: I am assessing the head and ears.
PROCTOR: There are no obvious injuries.

▸ **Assess the Eyes**

Student: I am assessing the eyes. Are the pupils equal, round, and regular in size, and react properly to light (PEARRL)?
PROCTOR: They are PEARRL.

▸ **Assess the Facial Area Including Oral and Nasal Areas**

Student: I am assessing the face, nose, and mouth. Do I see any discharge or hear any obstructions?
PROCTOR: No.

▾ **Assess the Neck**

▸ **Inspect and Palpate the Neck**

Student: I am assessing the neck for DCAP-BTLS.
PROCTOR: There are no obvious injuries.

▸ **Assess for Jugular Vein Distention**

Student: Do I find any jugular vein distention (JVD)?
PROCTOR: No.

▸ **Assess for Tracheal Deviation**

Student: Do I see any tracheal deviation?
PROCTOR: No.

Assess the Chest

Student: I am assessing the chest for DCAP-BTLS.

PROCTOR: Noted.

Inspect

Student: What do I see when I look at the chest?

PROCTOR: The breathing appears to be diaphragmatic.

Student: Does the chest appear symmetric?

PROCTOR: Yes.

Palpate

Student: When I touch the chest, do I feel crepitus or a flail segment?

PROCTOR: No.

Auscultate

Student: Are lung sounds present in all fields?

PROCTOR: Yes.

Student: Do I hear any sucking sounds from the chest?

PROCTOR: No.

Assess the Abdomen/Pelvis

Assess the Abdomen

Student: I am assessing the abdomen for DCAP-BTLS. I am assessing all four quadrants. Do I find any problems?

PROCTOR: No.

Assess the Pelvis

Student: I am assessing the pelvis for DCAP-BTLS. Is the pelvis stable?

PROCTOR: Yes.

Assess the Genitalia/Perineum as Needed (Verbalize in Training)

Student: I am assessing the genitalia/perineum as necessary for DCAP-BTLS.

PROCTOR: The area is unremarkable.

Assess the Extremities

Inspect

Student: I am assessing the lower and upper extremities for DCAP-BTLS. Do I find anything?

PROCTOR: No.

Palpate

Student: Do I feel anything unusual?

PROCTOR: No.

Assess Motor, Sensory, and Circulatory Function

Student: I am checking for DCAP-BTLS, motor and sensory function, and pulses. Right leg?

PROCTOR: Negative DCAP-BTLS. Motor and sensory functions are absent. Pulses are weak.

Student: Left leg?

PROCTOR: Negative DCAP-BTLS. Motor and sensory functions are absent. Pulses are weak.

Student: Right arm?

PROCTOR: Negative DCAP-BTLS. Motor and sensory functions are present. Pulses are weak.

Student: Left arm?

PROCTOR: Negative DCAP-BTLS. Motor and sensory functions are present. Pulses are weak.

Assess the Posterior

Note: This portion of the detailed physical exam would not be done if the patient were previously backboarded per local protocol.

Student: We will not check the back since it was previously checked and the patient is backboarded.

PROCTOR: Noted.

Manage Secondary Injuries/Wounds

Student: I would direct my partner to monitor the patient.

PROCTOR: Noted.

Reassess Vital Signs

Student: I will reassess vital signs and mental status.

PROCTOR: Blood pressure, 70/48 mm Hg; pulse rate, 78 beats/min; respirations, per bag-valve device; pulse oximetry reading, 92%; and the patient's mental status is altered. He now only responds to pain.

Student: The vital signs are deteriorating.

PROCTOR: Noted.

Reassess Interventions

Student: I will reassess my interventions: airway, breathing, and oxygen; circulation and bleeding control; immobilization and straps; and treatment for shock.

PROCTOR: Noted.

ALS Student: I will reassess basic life support (BLS) interventions, plus the following: establish two large-bore IVs and administer a bolus of normal saline at 20 mL/kg to maintain a systolic blood pressure of 90 mm Hg, and perform cardiac monitoring. Intubate (or rapid sequence intubation [RSI] depending on local protocol), and confirm with end tidal CO_2 and lung sounds.

ALS Proctor: Noted. The cardiac monitor shows normal sinus rhythm. End tidal CO_2 and lung sounds confirm placement of the ET tube.

Critical Criteria:

- ❑ Did not find or manage problems associated with airway, breathing, hemorrhage or shock (hypoperfusion)

Radio Report

(Provided by the student.)

PROCTOR: Noted.

Ongoing Assessment

Repeat Vital Signs

Student: I will reassess vital signs and mental status.

PROCTOR: Blood pressure, 68 by palpation; pulse rate, 76 beats/min; respirations, per bag-valve device; pulse oximetry reading, 99%; and the patient only responds to pain.

Student: The vital signs have deteriorated.

PROCTOR: Noted.

Check Interventions

Student: I will check my interventions: airway, breathing, and oxygen; circulation and bleeding control; immobilization and straps; and treatment for shock.

PROCTOR: Noted. Be ready to administer CPR.

ALS Student: I will check BLS interventions, plus the following: two large-bore IVs; maintain a systolic blood pressure of 90 mm Hg; be ready to perform CPR and advanced cardiac life support (ACLS) as needed; and cardiac monitoring. Confirm end tidal CO_2 and lung sounds.

ALS Proctor: Noted. The cardiac monitor shows normal sinus rhythm. End tidal CO_2 and lung sounds confirm placement of the ET tube.

Critical Criteria:
❑ Did not find or manage problems associated with airway, breathing, hemorrhage or shock (hypoperfusion)

Handoff Report to Emergency Department Staff

Student: The patient's condition deteriorated during transport.
PROCTOR: Noted.

Critical Criteria:
❑ Did not transport patient within the (10) minute time limit

Critical Criteria

(Inform the student of items missed, if any.)

❑ Pass ❑ Fail Date: ______________________

Proctor Comments: ______________________

Dispatch Information

PROCTOR: EMS 10, respond to a 35-year-old male who was attacked; his throat was slit with a hand saw. He is conscious and breathing. He is holding a towel on the injury. The scene is safe.

Pre-scene Action (BSI)

Student: I am wearing nonlatex gloves, safety glasses, mask, and gown.
PROCTOR: Noted.

> **Critical Criteria:**
> - ❑ Did not take, or verbalize, body substance isolation (BSI) precautions when necessary

Scene Size-up

Scene Safety

Student: Is the scene safe?
PROCTOR: Yes.

Mechanism of Injury

Student: What was the mechanism of injury?
PROCTOR: Penetrating trauma. The patient was attacked with a hand saw to the throat.

Number of Patients

Student: How many patients are there?
PROCTOR: One.

Additional Resources

Student: I would call for advanced life support (ALS) assistance.
PROCTOR: Noted.

C-Spine Stabilization

Student: On the basis of the mechanism of injury, I would stabilize the cervical spine (c-spine) in a neutral in-line position and immediately apply direct pressure and a dressing to the wound. I will treat the patient for shock and put him in the shock position.
PROCTOR: Noted.

> **Critical Criteria:**
> - ❑ Did not determine scene safety
> - ❑ Did not assess for spinal protection
> - ❑ Did not provide for spinal protection when indicated

Initial Assessment

Student: As I perform midline c-spine stabilization, I identify myself and ask the patient not to move.
PROCTOR: Noted.

General Impression

Student: My general impression is that the patient's condition is unstable.
PROCTOR: Noted.

Responsiveness/Level of Consciousness

Student: What is the patient's level of consciousness?
PROCTOR: Alert.

Chief Complaint/Apparent Life Threats

Student: What is the patient's chief complaint?
PROCTOR: The patient is complaining of feeling like he will pass out.
Student: There is an apparent life threat; the life threat is an open neck wound.
PROCTOR: Noted.

Assess the Airway and Breathing

Student: Is the airway open? Is the patient breathing?
PROCTOR: Yes, the airway is open and the patient is breathing.

Assessment

Student: What are the rate and the quality of breathing?
PROCTOR: Rate: Tachypneic/anxious. Quality: Deep.

Provide Oxygen

Student: I am applying oxygen at 15 L/min via nonrebreathing mask.
PROCTOR: Noted.

Ensure Adequate Ventilation

Student: The patient has adequate ventilations at this time.
PROCTOR: Noted.

Injury Management

Student: I will direct my partner to take over c-spine control and direct pressure as I continue assessment.
PROCTOR: Noted.

Assess Circulation

Student: I am assessing the patient's circulation.
PROCTOR: Noted.

Assess for and Control Major Bleeding

Student: Do I find any major bleeding?
PROCTOR: Yes, direct pressure is being used to control the bleeding from the neck wound.
Student: I will continue to apply direct pressure and apply more dressings as needed.
PROCTOR: Noted.

Assess the Pulse

Student: What are the rate and the quality of pulses?
PROCTOR: Rate: Tachycardic. Quality: Thready.

Assess the Skin

Student: I am assessing the skin. What are the color, temperature, and condition of the skin?
PROCTOR: Color: Pale. Temperature: Cool. Condition: Diaphoretic.

Identify Priority Patients/Make Transport Decision

Student: The patient is a high priority and is a load-and-go. I will begin packaging and transport to a trauma center.
PROCTOR: Noted.

> **Critical Criteria:**
> - ❑ Did not provide high concentration of oxygen
> - ❑ Did not find or manage problems associated with airway, breathing, hemorrhage or shock (hypoperfusion)
> - ❑ Did not differentiate patient's need for transportation versus continued assessment at the scene
> - ❑ Did other detailed examination before assessing the airway, breathing and circulation

Focused History and Physical Examination/Rapid Trauma Assessment

Select the Appropriate Assessment (Focused or Rapid)

Student: I am selecting the rapid physical exam to identify and treat life threats. I am checking for DCAP-BTLS. This acronym stands for deformities, contusions, abrasions, punctures, penetrations, and paradoxical motion in the chest, and burns, tenderness, lacerations, and swelling.
PROCTOR: Noted.

Head

Student: I am rapidly assessing the head.
PROCTOR: There are no obvious injuries.

Neck

Student: I am rapidly assessing the neck.
PROCTOR: You previously noted the 3-inch gaping laceration to the left side of the neck. The bulky dressing and manual direct pressure prevent you from placing a cervical collar on this patient.
Student: I would constantly assess and treat the neck.
PROCTOR: Noted.

Student: I will keep the patient still and transport on a backboard, minimizing patient movement.
PROCTOR: Noted.

▸ **Chest**

Student: I am rapidly assessing the chest. What are the lung sounds?
PROCTOR: There are no obvious injuries. Lung sounds are clear bilaterally.

▸ **Abdomen/Pelvis**

Student: I am rapidly assessing the abdomen.
PROCTOR: There are no obvious injuries.
Student: I am rapidly assessing the pelvis.
PROCTOR: There are no obvious injuries.

▸ **Extremities**

Student: I am rapidly assessing the extremities.
PROCTOR: There are no obvious injuries.

▸ **Assess Motor, Sensory, and Circulatory Function**

Student: I am checking for DCAP-BTLS. I am also checking motor and sensory function, and pulses. Right leg?
PROCTOR: Negative DCAP-BTLS. Motor and sensory functions are present. Pulses are weak.
Student: Left leg?
PROCTOR: Negative DCAP-BTLS. Motor and sensory functions are present. Pulses are weak.
Student: Right arm?
PROCTOR: Negative DCAP-BTLS. Motor and sensory functions are present. Pulses are weak.
Student: Left arm?
PROCTOR: Negative DCAP-BTLS. Motor and sensory functions are present. Pulses are weak.

▸ **Posterior**

Student: I will rapidly assess the back. We will now log roll the patient as a unit to check the back. The person at the head will count to three and we will roll the patient.
PROCTOR: Noted.

▸ **Assess the Thorax**

Student: I am assessing the thorax. Do I find injuries?
PROCTOR: No.

▸ **Assess the Lumbar Area**

Student: I am assessing the flanks and lumbar area. Do I find injuries?
PROCTOR: No.

▸ **Assess the Entire Backside**

Student: I am assessing the entire backside. Do I find injuries?
PROCTOR: No.

▸ **Manage Secondary Injuries/Wounds**

Student: We will apply a backboard and immobilization per local protocol, but I am unable to apply a cervical collar due to wound control.
PROCTOR: Noted.
ALS Student: I will establish two large-bore IVs en route to the hospital and administer a bolus of 20 mL/kg in order to maintain a systolic blood pressure of 90 mm Hg.
ALS Proctor: Noted.
Student: Are there any changes in motor and sensory functions or pulses?
PROCTOR: No.

▸ **Reevaluate Transport Decision**

Student: This patient is a load-and-go due to shock and an open neck injury.
PROCTOR: Noted.

▾ Baseline Vital Signs

Student: What are the patient's baseline vital signs, including blood pressure, pulse, respirations, pulse oximetry, and level of consciousness?
PROCTOR: Blood pressure, 102/72 mm Hg; pulse rate, 130 beats/min; respirations, 26 breaths/min; pulse oximetry reading, 96%; and the patient is alert.

▾ SAMPLE History

Student: At this time I will gather a SAMPLE history from the patient or family. What are the patient's signs and symptoms?
PROCTOR: Pain and bleeding from the neck, and the patient feels faint and weak.
Student: Allergies?
PROCTOR: No allergies.
Student: Medications?
PROCTOR: No medications.
Student: Pertinent past medical history?
PROCTOR: No pertinent medical history.
Student: Last oral intake?
PROCTOR: 2 hours ago.
Student: Events leading up to the incident?
PROCTOR: The patient was jumped from behind some bushes and attacked in a park.
Student: Interventions?
PROCTOR: The patient covered his neck with his hand and police officers assisted with towels.

Critical Criteria:
- ❑ Did not differentiate patient's need for transportation versus continued assessment at the scene
- ❑ Did not provide for spinal protection when indicated

▾ Detailed Physical Examination

Student: I am conducting the detailed physical exam. I am looking for DCAP-BTLS.
PROCTOR: Noted. The detailed physical exam will be performed during transport.

▾ Assess the Head

Student: I am assessing the head. Do I find any DCAP-BTLS? Do I find any evidence of Battle's sign or raccoon eyes?
PROCTOR: No.

▸ **Inspect and Palpate the Head and Ears**

Student: I am assessing the head and ears.
PROCTOR: There are no obvious injuries.

▸ **Assess the Eyes**

Student: I am assessing the eyes. Are the pupils equal, round, and regular in size, and react properly to light (PEARRL)?
PROCTOR: They are PEARRL.

▸ **Assess the Facial Area Including Oral and Nasal Areas**

Student: I am assessing the face, nose, and mouth. Do I see any discharge or hear any obstructions?
PROCTOR: No.

▾ Assess the Neck

▸ **Inspect and Palpate the Neck**

Student: I am assessing the neck for DCAP-BTLS.
PROCTOR: The skin is wide open on the left side. Bleeding is difficult to control.
Student: I will continue to control the bleeding and call the receiving facility.
PROCTOR: Noted.

▸ **Assess for Jugular Vein Distention**

Student: Do I find any jugular vein distention (JVD)?
PROCTOR: No.

▸ **Assess for Tracheal Deviation**

Student: Do I see any tracheal deviation?
PROCTOR: No.

▾ Assess the Chest

Student: I am assessing the chest for DCAP-BTLS.
PROCTOR: Noted.

▸ **Inspect**
Student: What do I see when I look at the chest?
PROCTOR: There are no obvious injuries.
Student: Does the chest appear symmetric?
PROCTOR: Yes.

▸ **Palpate**
Student: When I touch the chest, do I feel crepitus or a flail segment?
PROCTOR: No.

▸ **Auscultate**
Student: Are lung sounds present in all fields?
PROCTOR: Yes.
Student: Do I hear any sucking sounds from the chest?
PROCTOR: No.

▾ Assess the Abdomen/Pelvis

▸ **Assess the Abdomen**
Student: I am assessing the abdomen for DCAP-BTLS. I am assessing all four quadrants. Do I find any problems?
PROCTOR: No.

▸ **Assess the Pelvis**
Student: I am assessing the pelvis for DCAP-BTLS. Is the pelvis stable?
PROCTOR: Yes.

▾ Assess the Genitalia/Perineum as Needed (Verbalize in Training)

Student: I am assessing the genitalia/perineum as necessary for DCAP-BTLS.
PROCTOR: The area is unremarkable.

▾ Assess the Extremities

▸ **Inspect**
Student: I am assessing the lower and upper extremities for DCAP-BTLS. Do I find anything?
PROCTOR: No.

▸ **Palpate**
Student: Do I feel anything unusual?
PROCTOR: No.

▸ **Assess Motor, Sensory, and Circulatory Function**
Student: I am checking for DCAP-BTLS, motor and sensory function, and pulses. Right leg?
PROCTOR: Negative DCAP-BTLS. Motor and sensory functions are present. Pulses are weak.
Student: Left leg?
PROCTOR: Negative DCAP-BTLS. Motor and sensory functions are present. Pulses are weak.
Student: Right arm?
PROCTOR: Negative DCAP-BTLS. Motor and sensory functions are present. Pulses are weak.
Student: Left arm?
PROCTOR: Negative DCAP-BTLS. Motor and sensory functions are present. Pulses are weak.

▾ Assess the Posterior

Note: This portion of the detailed physical exam would not be done if the patient were previously backboarded per local protocol.
Student: We will not check the back since it was previously checked and the patient is backboarded.
PROCTOR: Noted.

▾ Manage Secondary Injuries/Wounds

Student: I would direct my partner to continue direct pressure and bleeding control to the wound.
PROCTOR: Noted.

▾ Reassess Vital Signs

Student: I will reassess vital signs and mental status.
PROCTOR: Blood pressure, 94/70 mm Hg; pulse rate, 134 beats/min; respirations, 24 breaths/min; pulse oximetry reading, 95%; and the patient is dizzy/tired.
Student: The vital signs are deteriorating.
PROCTOR: Noted.

▾ Reassess Interventions

Student: I will reassess my interventions: airway, breathing, and oxygen; circulation and bleeding control; splints, immobilization, and straps; Trendelenburg position; and keep the patient warm.
PROCTOR: Noted.
ALS Student: I will reassess basic life support (BLS) interventions, plus the following: two large-bore IVs with fluid replacement to maintain a systolic blood pressure of 90 mm Hg and cardiac monitor.
ALS Proctor: Noted. The cardiac monitor shows sinus tachycardia.

> **Critical Criteria:**
> ❑ Did not find or manage problems associated with airway, breathing, hemorrhage or shock (hypoperfusion)

▼ Radio Report

(Provided by the student.)
PROCTOR: Noted.

▼ Ongoing Assessment

▾ Repeat Vital Signs

Student: I will reassess vital signs and mental status.
PROCTOR: Blood pressure, 90/66 mm Hg; pulse rate, 140 beats/min; respirations, 24 breaths/min; pulse oximetry reading, 95%; and the patient is responsive to verbal.
Student: The vital signs have deteriorated.
PROCTOR: Noted.

▾ Check Interventions

Student: I will check my interventions: airway, breathing, and oxygen; circulation and bleeding control; splints, immobilization, and straps; Trendelenburg position; and keep the patient warm.
PROCTOR: Noted.
ALS Student: I will check BLS interventions, plus the following: monitor IVs, maintain a systolic blood pressure of 90 mm Hg, and cardiac monitor.
ALS Proctor: Noted. The cardiac monitor shows sinus tachycardia.

> **Critical Criteria:**
> ❑ Did not find or manage problems associated with airway, breathing, hemorrhage or shock (hypoperfusion)

▼ Handoff Report to Emergency Department Staff

Student: The patient's condition deteriorated during transport.
PROCTOR: Noted.

> **Critical Criteria:**
> ❑ Did not transport patient within the (10) minute time limit

▼ Critical Criteria

(Inform the student of items missed, if any.)

❑ Pass ❑ Fail Date: ______________________

Proctor Comments: ______________________

Notes

Dispatch Information

PROCTOR: EMS 10, respond to a motor vehicle collision at the racetrack. The driver is pinned upside down in the car and the roll cage failed. No other information is available.

Pre-scene Action (BSI)

Student: I am wearing appropriate high-visibility personal protective equipment suitable for extrication, a helmet, extrication gloves, nonlatex gloves, safety glasses, mask, and gown.
PROCTOR: Noted.

Critical Criteria:
- ❑ Did not take, or verbalize, body substance isolation (BSI) precautions when necessary

Scene Size-up

Scene Safety

Student: Is the scene safe?
PROCTOR: Yes.

Mechanism of Injury

Student: What was the mechanism of injury?
PROCTOR: Motor vehicle collision. The patient is a 41-year-old male who was the driver in a rollover crash. He is pinned in the car.

Number of Patients

Student: How many patients are there?
PROCTOR: One.

Additional Resources

Student: I would call for advanced life support (ALS) assistance and additional resources: fire/rescue.
PROCTOR: Noted.
Student: I will let fire/rescue responders safely extricate the patient.
PROCTOR: Noted.

C-Spine Stabilization

Student: On the basis of the mechanism of injury, I would stabilize the cervical spine (c-spine) in a neutral in-line position.
PROCTOR: Noted.

Critical Criteria:
- ❑ Did not determine scene safety
- ❑ Did not assess for spinal protection
- ❑ Did not provide for spinal protection when indicated

Initial Assessment

Student: As I perform midline c-spine stabilization, I identify myself and ask the patient not to move.
PROCTOR: Noted.

General Impression

Student: My general impression is that the patient's condition is stable.
PROCTOR: Noted.

Responsiveness/Level of Consciousness

Student: What is the patient's level of consciousness?
PROCTOR: Alert.

Chief Complaint/Apparent Life Threats

Student: What is the patient's chief complaint?
PROCTOR: The patient is complaining of neck and back pain.
Student: There are no apparent life threats.
PROCTOR: Noted.

Assess the Airway and Breathing

Student: Is the airway open? Is the patient breathing?
PROCTOR: Yes, the airway is open and the patient is breathing.

Assessment

Student: What are the rate and the quality of breathing?
PROCTOR: Rate: Within normal limits. Quality: Normal.

Provide Oxygen

Student: I am applying oxygen at 15 L/min via nonrebreathing mask.
PROCTOR: Noted.

Ensure Adequate Ventilation

Student: The patient has adequate ventilations at this time.
PROCTOR: Noted.

Injury Management

Student: I will direct my partner to take over c-spine control as I continue assessment.
PROCTOR: Noted.

Assess Circulation

Student: I am assessing the patient's circulation.
PROCTOR: Noted.

Assess for and Control Major Bleeding

Student: Do I find any major bleeding?
PROCTOR: No.

Assess the Pulse

Student: What are the rate and the quality of pulses?
PROCTOR: Rate: Fast. Quality: Strong.

Assess the Skin

Student: I am assessing the skin. What are the color, temperature, and condition of the skin?
PROCTOR: Color: Flushed. Temperature: Hot. Condition: Moist.

Identify Priority Patients/Make Transport Decision

Student: The patient is a low priority and does not require immediate transport.
PROCTOR: Noted.

Critical Criteria:
- ❑ Did not provide high concentration of oxygen
- ❑ Did not find or manage problems associated with airway, breathing, hemorrhage or shock (hypoperfusion)
- ❑ Did not differentiate patient's need for transportation versus continued assessment at the scene
- ❑ Did other detailed examination before assessing the airway, breathing and circulation

Focused History and Physical Examination/Rapid Trauma Assessment

Select the Appropriate Assessment (Focused or Rapid)

Student: I am selecting the rapid physical exam to identify and treat life threats. I am checking for DCAP-BTLS. This acronym stands for deformities, contusions, abrasions, punctures, penetrations, and paradoxical motion in the chest, and burns, tenderness, lacerations, and swelling.
PROCTOR: Noted.

Head

Student: I am rapidly assessing the head.
PROCTOR: The patient was wearing a helmet that has deep gashes to its surface. The helmet protected the head from injury.

Neck

Student: I am rapidly assessing the neck.
PROCTOR: The patient complains of pain.
Student: I will follow local protocol for helmet removal and apply a cervical collar.
PROCTOR: Noted.

Chest

Student: I am rapidly assessing the chest. What are the lung sounds?
PROCTOR: There are no obvious injuries. Lung sounds are clear bilaterally.

▸ **Abdomen/Pelvis**

Student: I am rapidly assessing the abdomen.
PROCTOR: There are no obvious injuries.
Student: I am rapidly assessing the pelvis.
PROCTOR: There are no obvious injuries.

▸ **Extremities**

Student: I am rapidly assessing the extremities.
PROCTOR: There are no obvious injuries.

▸ **Assess Motor, Sensory, and Circulatory Function**

Student: I am checking for DCAP-BTLS. I am also checking motor and sensory function, and pulses. Right leg?
PROCTOR: Negative DCAP-BTLS. Motor and sensory functions are present. Pulses are present.
Student: Left leg?
PROCTOR: Negative DCAP-BTLS. Motor and sensory functions are present. Pulses are present.
Student: Right arm?
PROCTOR: Negative DCAP-BTLS. Motor and sensory functions are present. Pulses are present.
Student: Left arm?
PROCTOR: Negative DCAP-BTLS. Motor and sensory functions are present. Pulses are present.

▸ **Posterior**

Student: I will rapidly assess the back. We will now log roll the patient as a unit to check the back. The person at the head will count to three and we will roll the patient.
PROCTOR: Noted.

▸ **Assess the Thorax**

Student: I am assessing the thorax. Do I find injuries?
PROCTOR: No.

▸ **Assess the Lumbar Area**

Student: I am assessing the flanks and lumbar area. Do I find injuries?
PROCTOR: No.

▸ **Assess the Entire Backside**

Student: I am assessing the entire backside. Do I find injuries?
PROCTOR: No.

▸ **Manage Secondary Injuries/Wounds**

Student: We will apply a cervical collar and backboard with full immobilization per local protocol, if not yet done, at this time.
PROCTOR: Noted.
Student: Are there any changes in motor and sensory functions or pulses?
PROCTOR: No.
ALS Student: I will establish a large-bore IV en route to the hospital and maintain a systolic blood pressure of 90 mm Hg.
ALS Proctor: Noted.

▸ **Reevaluate Transport Decision**

Student: This patient does not require immediate transport.
PROCTOR: Noted.

▾ Baseline Vital Signs

Student: What are the patient's baseline vital signs, including blood pressure, pulse, respirations, pulse oximetry, and level of consciousness?
PROCTOR: Blood pressure, 148/84 mm Hg; pulse, 120 beats/min; respirations, 20 breaths/min; pulse oximetry reading, 98%; and the patient is alert.

▾ SAMPLE History

Student: At this time I will gather a SAMPLE history from the patient or family. What are the patient's signs and symptoms?
PROCTOR: He is only complaining of pain in the neck.
Student: Allergies?
PROCTOR: No allergies.
Student: Medications?
PROCTOR: No medications.
Student: Pertinent past medical history?
PROCTOR: No pertinent medical history.
Student: Last oral intake?
PROCTOR: 4 hours ago.
Student: Events leading up to the incident?
PROCTOR: The patient was driving in a race when he lost control and rolled the car. The roll cage failed and the helmet took the forces. There was no loss of consciousness.

Critical Criteria:
- ❑ Did not differentiate patient's need for transportation versus continued assessment at the scene
- ❑ Did not provide for spinal protection when indicated

▼ Detailed Physical Examination

Student: I am conducting the detailed physical exam. I am looking for DCAP-BTLS.
PROCTOR: Noted. The detailed physical exam will be performed during transport.

▾ Assess the Head

Student: I am assessing the head. Do I find any DCAP-BTLS? Do I find any evidence of Battle's sign or raccoon eyes?
PROCTOR: No, the patient was wearing a helmet that was damaged but is still intact.

▸ **Inspect and Palpate the Head and Ears**

Student: I am assessing the head and ears.
PROCTOR: There are no obvious injuries.

▸ **Assess the Eyes**

Student: I am assessing the eyes. Are the pupils equal, round, and regular in size, and react properly to light (PEARRL)?
PROCTOR: They are PEARRL.

▸ **Assess the Facial Area Including Oral and Nasal Areas**

Student: I am assessing the face, nose, and mouth. Do I see any discharge or hear any obstructions?
PROCTOR: No.

▾ Assess the Neck

▸ **Inspect and Palpate the Neck**

Student: I am assessing the neck for DCAP-BTLS.
PROCTOR: The patient complains of pain, but no deformity is felt.

▸ **Assess for Jugular Vein Distention**

Student: Do I find any jugular vein distention (JVD)?
PROCTOR: No.

▸ **Assess for Tracheal Deviation**

Student: Do I see any tracheal deviation?
PROCTOR: No.

▾ Assess the Chest

Student: I am assessing the chest for DCAP-BTLS.
PROCTOR: Noted.

▸ **Inspect**

Student: What do I see when I look at the chest?
PROCTOR: There are no obvious injuries.
Student: Does the chest appear symmetric?
PROCTOR: Yes.

▸ **Palpate**

Student: When I touch the chest, do I feel crepitus or a flail segment?
PROCTOR: No.

▸ **Auscultate**

Student: Are lung sounds present in all fields?
PROCTOR: Yes.
Student: Do I hear any sucking sounds from the chest?
PROCTOR: No.

▼ Assess the Abdomen/Pelvis

▸ **Assess the Abdomen**

Student: I am assessing the abdomen for DCAP-BTLS. I am assessing all four quadrants. Do I find any problems?

PROCTOR: No.

▸ **Assess the Pelvis**

Student: I am assessing the pelvis for DCAP-BTLS. Is the pelvis stable?

PROCTOR: Yes.

▼ Assess the Genitalia/Perineum as Needed (Verbalize in Training)

Student: I am assessing the genitalia/perineum as necessary for DCAP-BTLS.

PROCTOR: The area is unremarkable.

▼ Assess the Extremities

▸ **Inspect**

Student: I am assessing the lower and upper extremities for DCAP-BTLS. Do I find anything?

PROCTOR: No.

▸ **Palpate**

Student: Do I feel anything unusual?

PROCTOR: No.

▸ **Assess Motor, Sensory, and Circulatory Function**

Student: I am checking for DCAP-BTLS, motor and sensory function, and pulses. Right leg?

PROCTOR: Negative DCAP-BTLS. Motor and sensory functions are present. Pulses are present.

Student: Left leg?

PROCTOR: Negative DCAP-BTLS. Motor and sensory functions are present. Pulses are present.

Student: Right arm?

PROCTOR: Negative DCAP-BTLS. Motor and sensory functions are present. Pulses are present.

Student: Left arm?

PROCTOR: Negative DCAP-BTLS. Motor and sensory functions are present. Pulses are present.

▼ Assess the Posterior

Note: This portion of the detailed physical exam would not be done if the patient were previously backboarded per local protocol.

Student: We will not check the back since it was previously checked and the patient is backboarded.

PROCTOR: Noted.

▼ Manage Secondary Injuries/Wounds

Student: I would direct my partner to continue providing oxygen.

PROCTOR: Noted.

▼ Reassess Vital Signs

Student: I will reassess vital signs and mental status.

PROCTOR: Blood pressure, 140/78 mm Hg; pulse, 116 beats/min; respirations, 20 breaths/min; pulse oximetry reading, 99%; and the patient is alert.

Student: The vital signs have not changed significantly.

PROCTOR: Noted.

▼ Reassess Interventions

Student: I will reassess my interventions: oxygen, immobilization, and straps.

PROCTOR: Noted.

ALS Student: I will reassess basic life support (BLS) interventions, plus the following: IV access per local protocol.

ALS Proctor: Noted.

> **Critical Criteria:**
> ❑ Did not find or manage problems associated with airway, breathing, hemorrhage or shock (hypoperfusion)

Radio Report

(Provided by the student.)

PROCTOR: Noted.

Ongoing Assessment

▼ Repeat Vital Signs

Student: I will reassess vital signs and mental status.

PROCTOR: Blood pressure, 132/76 mm Hg; pulse, 108 beats/min; respirations, 20 breaths/min; pulse oximetry reading, 99%; and the patient is alert.

Student: The vital signs have not changed significantly.

PROCTOR: Noted.

▼ Check Interventions

Student: I will check my interventions: oxygen, immobilization, and straps.

PROCTOR: Noted.

ALS Student: I will check BLS interventions, plus the following: flow IV per local protocol.

ALS Proctor: Noted.

> **Critical Criteria:**
> ❑ Did not find or manage problems associated with airway, breathing, hemorrhage or shock (hypoperfusion)

Handoff Report to Emergency Department Staff

Student: There was no change during transport.

PROCTOR: Noted.

> **Critical Criteria:**
> ❑ Did not transport patient within the (10) minute time limit

Critical Criteria

(Inform the student of items missed, if any.)

❑ Pass ❑ Fail Date: ______________________________

Proctor Comments: ______________________________

____

____

Notes

CASE 26

Dispatch Information

PROCTOR: EMS 10, respond to a 23-year-old female who has been slashed across the face with a box cutter. She is conscious and breathing. The scene is said to be unsafe due to multiple fights. Police are not yet on the scene.

Pre-scene Action (BSI)

Student: I am wearing nonlatex gloves, safety glasses, mask, and gown.
PROCTOR: Noted.

Critical Criteria:
- ❑ Did not take, or verbalize, body substance isolation (BSI) precautions when necessary

Scene Size-up

Scene Safety

Student: Is the scene safe?
PROCTOR: Yes, police arrived, secured the scene, arrested the suspects, and have given you clearance to enter.

Mechanism of Injury

Student: What was the mechanism of injury?
PROCTOR: Penetrating trauma. The patient was standing in line to enter a club when a group of teens came up from behind; one of them slashed her face. She is standing up, crying, and holding a towel on her face.

Number of Patients

Student: How many patients are there?
PROCTOR: One.

Additional Resources

Student: I would call for advanced life support (ALS) assistance.
PROCTOR: Noted.

C-Spine Stabilization

Student: I would not stabilize the cervical spine (c-spine). I will immediately protect the airway and apply manual pressure and suction as necessary.
PROCTOR: Noted.

Critical Criteria:
- ❑ Did not determine scene safety
- ❑ Did not assess for spinal protection
- ❑ Did not provide for spinal protection when indicated

Initial Assessment

Student: As I approach the patient, I identify myself and ask the patient not to move.
PROCTOR: Noted.

General Impression

Student: My general impression is that the patient's condition is unstable.
PROCTOR: Noted.

Responsiveness/Level of Consciousness

Student: What is the patient's level of consciousness?
PROCTOR: Alert.

Chief Complaint/Apparent Life Threats

Student: What is the patient's chief complaint?
PROCTOR: The patient is complaining of her face being slashed from one cheek over the nose and to the other cheek.
Student: There are apparent life threats; the airway is compromised. I will immediately apply direct pressure to the wounds and suction the airway as needed.
PROCTOR: Noted.

Assess the Airway and Breathing

Student: Is the airway open? Is the patient breathing?
PROCTOR: Yes, the airway is open and the patient is breathing.

Assessment

Student: What are the rate and the quality of breathing?
PROCTOR: Rate: Rapid. Quality: Within normal limits.

Provide Oxygen

Student: I am applying oxygen at 15 L/min via nonrebreathing mask.
PROCTOR: Noted.

Ensure Adequate Ventilation

Student: The patient has adequate ventilations at this time.
PROCTOR: Noted.

Injury Management

Student: I will direct my partner to maintain the c-spine and direct pressure as I continue the assessment.
PROCTOR: Noted.

Assess Circulation

Student: I am assessing the patient's circulation.
PROCTOR: Noted.

Assess for and Control Major Bleeding

Student: Do I find any major bleeding?
PROCTOR: You have controlled the facial bleeding with direct pressure.
Student: I would suction the airway as needed. I would continue direct pressure and apply a dressing to control the bleeding.
PROCTOR: Noted.

Assess the Pulse

Student: What are the rate and the quality of pulses?
PROCTOR: Rate: Within normal limits. Quality: Strong.

Assess the Skin

Student: I am assessing the skin. What are the color, temperature, and condition of the skin?
PROCTOR: Color: Flushed. Temperature: Warm. Condition: Moist.

Identify Priority Patients/Make Transport Decision

Student: The patient is a high priority and is a load-and-go. I will begin packaging and transport.
PROCTOR: Noted.

Critical Criteria:
- ❑ Did not provide high concentration of oxygen
- ❑ Did not find or manage problems associated with airway, breathing, hemorrhage or shock (hypoperfusion)
- ❑ Did not differentiate patient's need for transportation versus continued assessment at the scene
- ❑ Did other detailed examination before assessing the airway, breathing and circulation

Focused History and Physical Examination/Rapid Trauma Assessment

Select the Appropriate Assessment (Focused or Rapid)

Student: I am selecting the rapid physical exam to identify and treat life threats. I am checking for DCAP-BTLS. This acronym stands for deformities, contusions, abrasions, punctures, penetrations, and paradoxical motion in the chest, and burns, tenderness, lacerations, and swelling.
PROCTOR: Noted.

Head

Student: I am rapidly assessing the head.
PROCTOR: You previously saw the incision gaping open into the face. You could see the teeth through the openings. Blood was flowing into the nasal passages.

Student: I would continue to control the bleeding with direct pressure and suction as necessary.
PROCTOR: Noted.

▸ **Neck**

Student: I am rapidly assessing the neck.
PROCTOR: There are no obvious injuries.

▸ **Chest**

Student: I am rapidly assessing the chest. What are the lung sounds?
PROCTOR: There are no obvious injuries. They are clear bilaterally.

▸ **Abdomen/Pelvis**

Student: I am rapidly assessing the abdomen.
PROCTOR: There are no obvious injuries.
Student: I am rapidly assessing the pelvis.
PROCTOR: There are no obvious injuries.

▸ **Extremities**

Student: I am rapidly assessing the extremities.
PROCTOR: There are no obvious injuries.

▸ **Assess Motor, Sensory, and Circulatory Function**

Student: I am checking for DCAP-BTLS. I am also checking motor and sensory function, and pulses. Right leg?
PROCTOR: Negative DCAP-BTLS. Motor and sensory functions are present. Pulses are present.
Student: Left leg?
PROCTOR: Negative DCAP-BTLS. Motor and sensory functions are present. Pulses are present.
Student: Right arm?
PROCTOR: Negative DCAP-BTLS. Motor and sensory functions are present. Pulses are present.
Student: Left arm?
PROCTOR: Negative DCAP-BTLS. Motor and sensory functions are present. Pulses are present.

▸ **Posterior**

Student: I will rapidly assess the back.
PROCTOR: Noted.

▸ **Assess the Thorax**

Student: I am assessing the thorax. Do I find injuries?
PROCTOR: No.

▸ **Assess the Lumbar Area**

Student: I am assessing the flanks and lumbar area. Do I find injuries?
PROCTOR: No.

▸ **Assess the Entire Backside**

Student: I am assessing the entire backside. Do I find injuries?
PROCTOR: No.

▸ **Manage Secondary Injuries/Wounds**

Student: We will transport her sitting up and leaning forward to prevent blood from flowing back into the airway while applying manual pressure on the wound. We will continue with 100% oxygen and suction as needed.
PROCTOR: Noted.
Student: Are there any changes in motor and sensory functions or pulses?
PROCTOR: No.
ALS Student: I will establish two large-bore IVs en route to the hospital and administer a bolus of 20 mL/kg in order to maintain a systolic blood pressure of 90 mm Hg.
ALS Proctor: Noted.

▸ **Reevaluate Transport Decision**

Student: This patient is a load-and-go due to airway compromise.
PROCTOR: Noted.

▾ Baseline Vital Signs

Student: What are the patient's baseline vital signs, including blood pressure, pulse, respirations, pulse oximetry, and level of consciousness?
PROCTOR: Blood pressure, 134/84 mm Hg; pulse rate, 100 beats/min; respirations, 24 breaths/min; pulse oximetry reading, 98%; and the patient is alert.

▾ SAMPLE History

Student: At this time I will gather a SAMPLE history from the patient or family. What are the patient's signs and symptoms?
PROCTOR: She is not speaking due to the direct pressure in the mouth. She will tap her hand yes or no; one tap for yes, two taps for no.
Student: Allergies?
PROCTOR: No allergies.
Student: Medications?
PROCTOR: No medications.
Student: Pertinent past medical history?
PROCTOR: No pertinent medical history.
Student: Last oral intake?
PROCTOR: Unknown.
Student: Events leading up to the incident?
PROCTOR: The patient was just standing in line when she was slashed.

Critical Criteria:
- ❑ Did not differentiate patient's need for transportation versus continued assessment at the scene
- ❑ Did not provide for spinal protection when indicated

Detailed Physical Examination

Student: I am conducting the detailed physical exam. I am looking for DCAP-BTLS.
PROCTOR: Noted. The detailed physical exam will be performed during transport.

▾ Assess the Head

Student: I am assessing the head. Do I find any DCAP-BTLS? Do I find any evidence of Battle's sign or raccoon eyes?
PROCTOR: You see only the facial incision.

▸ **Inspect and Palpate the Head and Ears**

Student: I am assessing the head and ears.
PROCTOR: You see only the facial incision.

▸ **Assess the Eyes**

Student: I am assessing the eyes. Are the pupils equal, round, and regular in size, and react properly to light (PEARRL)?
PROCTOR: They are PEARRL.

▸ **Assess the Facial Area Including Oral and Nasal Areas**

Student: I am assessing the face, nose, and mouth. Do I see any discharge or hear any obstructions?
PROCTOR: Yes, you occasionally hear gurgling.
Student: I would suction the airway as needed.
PROCTOR: Noted.

▾ Assess the Neck

▸ **Inspect and Palpate the Neck**

Student: I am assessing the neck for DCAP-BTLS.
PROCTOR: There are no obvious injuries.

▸ **Assess for Jugular Vein Distention**

Student: Do I find any jugular vein distention (JVD)?
PROCTOR: No.

▸ **Assess for Tracheal Deviation**

Student: Do I see any tracheal deviation?
PROCTOR: No.

▾ Assess the Chest

Student: I am assessing the chest for DCAP-BTLS.
PROCTOR: Noted.

▸ **Inspect**

Student: What do I see when I look at the chest?
PROCTOR: There are no obvious injuries.
Student: Does the chest appear symmetric?
PROCTOR: Yes.

▸ Palpate

Student: When I touch the chest, do I feel crepitus or a flail segment?

PROCTOR: No.

▸ Auscultate

Student: Are lung sounds present in all fields?

PROCTOR: Yes.

Student: Do I hear any sucking sounds from the chest?

PROCTOR: No.

▾ Assess the Abdomen/Pelvis

▸ Assess the Abdomen

Student: I am assessing the abdomen for DCAP-BTLS. I am assessing all four quadrants. Do I find any problems?

PROCTOR: No.

▸ Assess the Pelvis

Student: I am assessing the pelvis for DCAP-BTLS. Is the pelvis stable?

PROCTOR: Yes.

▾ Assess the Genitalia/Perineum as Needed (Verbalize in Training)

Student: I am assessing the genitalia/perineum as necessary for DCAP-BTLS.

PROCTOR: The area is unremarkable.

▾ Assess the Extremities

▸ Inspect

Student: I am assessing the lower and upper extremities for DCAP-BTLS. Do I find anything?

PROCTOR: No.

▸ Palpate

Student: Do I feel anything unusual?

PROCTOR: No.

▸ Assess Motor, Sensory, and Circulatory Function

Student: I am checking for DCAP-BTLS, motor and sensory function, and pulses. Right leg?

PROCTOR: Negative DCAP-BTLS. Motor and sensory functions are present. Pulses are present.

Student: Left leg?

PROCTOR: Negative DCAP-BTLS. Motor and sensory functions are present. Pulses are present.

Student: Right arm?

PROCTOR: Negative DCAP-BTLS. Motor and sensory functions are present. Pulses are present.

Student: Left arm?

PROCTOR: Negative DCAP-BTLS. Motor and sensory functions are present. Pulses are present.

▾ Assess the Posterior

Student: We will not check the back since it was previously checked.

PROCTOR: Noted.

▾ Manage Secondary Injuries/Wounds

Student: I would direct my partner to continue to maintain the airway and control bleeding.

PROCTOR: Noted.

▾ Reassess Vital Signs

Student: I will reassess vital signs and mental status.

PROCTOR: Blood pressure, 128/76 mm Hg; pulse rate, 82 beats/min; respirations, 20 breaths/min; pulse oximetry reading, 98%; and the patient is alert.

Student: The vital signs have not changed significantly.

PROCTOR: Noted.

▾ Reassess Interventions

Student: I will reassess my interventions: airway, breathing, oxygen, and suction; circulation and bleeding control; and treatment for shock.

PROCTOR: Noted.

ALS Student: I will reassess basic life support (BLS) interventions plus the following: two large-bore IVs.

ALS Proctor: Noted.

Critical Criteria:

❑ Did not find or manage problems associated with airway, breathing, hemorrhage or shock (hypoperfusion)

Radio Report

(Provided by the student.)

PROCTOR: Noted.

Ongoing Assessment

▾ Repeat Vital Signs

Student: I will reassess vital signs and mental status.

PROCTOR: Blood pressure, 130/78 mm Hg; pulse rate, 84 beats/min; respirations, 20 breaths/min; pulse oximetry reading, 97%; and the patient is alert.

Student: The vital signs have not changed significantly.

PROCTOR: Noted.

▾ Check Interventions

Student: I will check interventions: airway, breathing, oxygen, and suction; circulation and bleeding control; and treatment for shock.

PROCTOR: Noted.

ALS Student: I will check BLS interventions, plus the following: monitor the two large-bore IVs.

ALS Proctor: Noted.

Critical Criteria:

❑ Did not find or manage problems associated with airway, breathing, hemorrhage or shock (hypoperfusion)

Handoff Report to Emergency Department Staff

Student: There was no change during transport.

PROCTOR: Noted.

Critical Criteria:

❑ Did not transport patient within the (10) minute time limit

Critical Criteria

(Inform the student of items missed, if any.)

❑ Pass ❑ Fail Date: ____________________

Proctor Comments: ____________________

____

____

Notes

CASE 27

Dispatch Information

PROCTOR: EMS 10, respond to an 80-year-old female who has slipped and fallen on a throw rug. She thinks that her hip is broken. She is conscious and breathing. She says that her door is locked and she cannot get to the door. You will have to force entry.

Pre-scene Action (BSI)

Student: I am wearing nonlatex gloves and safety glasses.
PROCTOR: Noted.

Critical Criteria:
- ❑ Did not take, or verbalize, body substance isolation (BSI) precautions when necessary

Scene Size-up

Scene Safety
Student: Is the scene safe?
PROCTOR: Yes.

Mechanism of Injury
Student: What was the mechanism of injury?
PROCTOR: Fall. The patient was walking and slipped and fell on a throw rug.

Number of Patients
Student: How many patients are there?
PROCTOR: One.

Additional Resources
Student: I would call for advanced life support (ALS) and additional resources: fire/rescue and police to assist with forced entry.
PROCTOR: Noted. Law enforcement is able to gain entry for you.

C-Spine Stabilization
Student: On the basis of the mechanism of injury, I would stabilize the cervical spine (c-spine) in a neutral in-line position.
PROCTOR: Noted.

Critical Criteria:
- ❑ Did not determine scene safety
- ❑ Did not assess for spinal protection
- ❑ Did not provide for spinal protection when indicated

Initial Assessment

Student: As I perform midline c-spine stabilization, I identify myself and ask the patient not to move.
PROCTOR: Noted.

General Impression
Student: My general impression is that the patient's condition is stable.
PROCTOR: Noted.

Responsiveness/Level of Consciousness
Student: What is the patient's level of consciousness?
PROCTOR: Alert.

Chief Complaint/Apparent Life Threats
Student: What is the patient's chief complaint?
PROCTOR: The patient is complaining of right hip pain.
Student: There are no apparent life threats.
PROCTOR: Noted.

Assess the Airway and Breathing
Student: I am opening the airway. Is the patient breathing?
PROCTOR: Yes.

Assessment
Student: What are the rate and the quality of breathing?
PROCTOR: Rate: Within normal limits. Quality: Normal.

Provide Oxygen
Student: I am applying oxygen at 15 L/min via nonrebreathing mask.
PROCTOR: Noted.

Ensure Adequate Ventilation
Student: The patient has adequate ventilations at this time.
PROCTOR: Noted.

Injury Management
Student: I will direct my partner to take over c-spine control as I continue assessment.
PROCTOR: Noted.

Assess Circulation
Student: I am assessing the patient's circulation.
PROCTOR: Noted.

Assess for and Control Major Bleeding
Student: Do I find any major bleeding?
PROCTOR: No.

Assess the Pulse
Student: What are the rate and the quality of pulses?
PROCTOR: Rate: Within normal limits. Quality: Normal.

Assess the Skin
Student: I am assessing the skin. What are the color, temperature, and condition of the skin?
PROCTOR: Color: Flushed. Temperature: Warm. Condition: Dry.

Identify Priority Patients/Make Transport Decision
Student: The patient is a low priority and does not require immediate transport.
PROCTOR: Noted.

Critical Criteria:
- ❑ Did not provide high concentration of oxygen
- ❑ Did not find or manage problems associated with airway, breathing, hemorrhage or shock (hypoperfusion)
- ❑ Did not differentiate patient's need for transportation versus continued assessment at the scene
- ❑ Did other detailed examination before assessing the airway, breathing and circulation

Focused History and Physical Examination/Rapid Trauma Assessment

Select the Appropriate Assessment (Focused or Rapid)
Student: I am selecting the rapid physical exam to identify and treat life threats. I am checking for DCAP-BTLS. This acronym stands for deformities, contusions, abrasions, punctures, penetrations, and paradoxical motion in the chest, and burns, tenderness, lacerations, and swelling.
PROCTOR: Noted.

Head
Student: I am rapidly assessing the head.
PROCTOR: There are no obvious injuries.

Neck
Student: I am rapidly assessing the neck.
PROCTOR: There are no obvious injuries.
Student: I will apply a cervical collar.
PROCTOR: Noted.

Chest
Student: I am rapidly assessing the chest. What are the lung sounds?
PROCTOR: There are no obvious injuries. They are clear bilaterally.

Abdomen/Pelvis
Student: I am rapidly assessing the abdomen.
PROCTOR: There are no obvious injuries.
Student: I am rapidly assessing the pelvis.
PROCTOR: There are no obvious injuries.

▸ **Extremities**

Student: I am rapidly assessing the extremities.

PROCTOR: The right leg is shortened and externally rotated.

▸ **Assess Motor, Sensory, and Circulatory Function**

Student: I am checking for DCAP-BTLS. I am also checking motor and sensory function, and pulses. Right leg?

PROCTOR: It is shortened and externally rotated. Motor and sensory functions are present. Pulses are present.

Student: Left leg?

PROCTOR: Negative DCAP-BTLS. Motor and sensory functions are present. Pulses are present.

Student: Right arm?

PROCTOR: Negative DCAP-BTLS. Motor and sensory functions are present. Pulses are present.

Student: Left arm?

PROCTOR: Negative DCAP-BTLS. Motor and sensory functions are present. Pulses are present.

▸ **Posterior**

Student: I will rapidly assess the back. We will now log roll the patient as a unit to check the back. The person at the head will count to three and we will roll the patient.

PROCTOR: Noted.

▸ **Assess the Thorax**

Student: I am assessing the thorax. Do I find injuries?

PROCTOR: No.

▸ **Assess the Lumbar Area**

Student: I am assessing the flanks and lumbar area. Do I find injuries?

PROCTOR: No.

▸ **Assess the Entire Backside**

Student: I am assessing the entire backside. Do I find injuries?

PROCTOR: No.

▸ **Manage Secondary Injuries/Wounds**

Student: We will apply a cervical collar and backboard with full immobilization per local protocol, if not yet done, at this time. I will treat the hip per local protocol.

PROCTOR: Noted.

Student: Are there any changes in motor and sensory functions or pulses?

PROCTOR: No.

ALS Student: I will establish an IV en route to the hospital and administer pain management per local protocol.

ALS Proctor: Noted.

▸ **Reevaluate Transport Decision**

Student: This patient does not require immediate transport.

PROCTOR: Noted.

▼ Baseline Vital Signs

Student: What are the patient's baseline vital signs, including blood pressure, pulse, respirations, pulse oximetry, and level of consciousness?

PROCTOR: Blood pressure, 142/88 mm Hg; pulse rate, 92 beats/min; respirations, 20 breaths/min; pulse oximetry reading, 97%; and the patient is alert.

▼ SAMPLE History

Student: At this time I will gather a SAMPLE history from the patient or family. What are the patient's signs and symptoms?

PROCTOR: Pain in the right hip.

Student: Allergies?

PROCTOR: No allergies.

Student: Medications?

PROCTOR: Water pills and nitroglycerin.

Student: Pertinent past medical history?

PROCTOR: Congestive heart failure (CHF) and angina.

Student: Last oral intake?

PROCTOR: 2 hours ago.

Student: Events leading up to the incident?

PROCTOR: The patient was walking across the floor and slipped and fell on a throw rug.

Critical Criteria:

- ❑ Did not differentiate patient's need for transportation versus continued assessment at the scene
- ❑ Did not provide for spinal protection when indicated

▼ Detailed Physical Examination

Student: I am conducting the detailed physical exam. I am looking for DCAP-BTLS.

PROCTOR: Noted. The detailed physical exam will be performed during transport.

▼ Assess the Head

Student: I am assessing the head. Do I find any DCAP-BTLS? Do I find any evidence of Battle's sign or raccoon eyes?

PROCTOR: No.

▸ **Inspect and Palpate the Head and Ears**

Student: I am assessing the head and ears.

PROCTOR: There are no obvious injuries.

▸ **Assess the Eyes**

Student: I am assessing the eyes. Are the pupils equal, round, and regular in size, and react properly to light (PEARRL)?

PROCTOR: They are PEARRL.

▸ **Assess the Facial Area Including Oral and Nasal Areas**

Student: I am assessing the face, nose, and mouth. Do I see any discharge or hear any obstructions?

PROCTOR: No.

▼ Assess the Neck

▸ **Inspect and Palpate the Neck**

Student: I am assessing the neck for DCAP-BTLS.

PROCTOR: There are no obvious injuries.

▸ **Assess for Jugular Vein Distention**

Student: Do I find any jugular vein distention (JVD)?

PROCTOR: No.

▸ **Assess for Tracheal Deviation**

Student: Do I see any tracheal deviation?

PROCTOR: No.

▼ Assess the Chest

Student: I am assessing the chest for DCAP-BTLS.

PROCTOR: Noted.

▸ **Inspect**

Student: What do I see when I look at the chest?

PROCTOR: There are no obvious injuries.

Student: Does the chest appear symmetric?

PROCTOR: Yes.

▸ **Palpate**

Student: When I touch the chest, do I feel crepitus or a flail segment?

PROCTOR: No.

▸ **Auscultate**

Student: Are lung sounds present in all fields?

PROCTOR: Yes.

Student: Do I hear any sucking sounds from the chest?

PROCTOR: No.

▼ Assess the Abdomen/Pelvis

▸ **Assess the Abdomen**

Student: I am assessing the abdomen for DCAP-BTLS. I am assessing all four quadrants. Do I find any problems?

PROCTOR: No.

▸ **Assess the Pelvis**

Student: I am assessing the pelvis for DCAP-BTLS. Is the pelvis stable?

PROCTOR: Yes, but the patient complains of pain to the right hip area when you palpate the pelvis.

▼ **Assess the Genitalia/Perineum as Needed (Verbalize in Training)**

Student: I am assessing the genitalia/perineum as necessary for DCAP-BTLS.

PROCTOR: The area is unremarkable.

▼ **Assess the Extremities**

▸ **Inspect**

Student: I am assessing the lower and upper extremities for DCAP-BTLS. Do I find anything?

PROCTOR: Yes, the right leg is shortened and externally rotated.

▸ **Palpate**

Student: Do I feel anything unusual?

PROCTOR: No.

▸ **Assess Motor, Sensory, and Circulatory Function**

Student: I am checking for DCAP-BTLS, motor and sensory function, and pulses. Right leg?

PROCTOR: It is shortened and externally rotated. Motor and sensory functions are present. Pulses are present.

Student: Left leg?

PROCTOR: Negative DCAP-BTLS. Motor and sensory functions are present. Pulses are present.

Student: Right arm?

PROCTOR: Negative DCAP-BTLS. Motor and sensory functions are present. Pulses are present.

Student: Left arm?

PROCTOR: Negative DCAP-BTLS. Motor and sensory functions are present. Pulses are present.

▼ **Assess the Posterior**

Note: This portion of the detailed physical exam would not be done if the patient were previously backboarded per local protocol.

Student: We will not check the back since it was previously checked and the patient is backboarded.

PROCTOR: Noted.

▼ **Manage Secondary Injuries/Wounds**

Student: I would direct my partner to continue providing oxygen.

PROCTOR: Noted.

▼ **Reassess Vital Signs**

Student: I will reassess vital signs and mental status.

PROCTOR: Blood pressure, 136/82 mm Hg; pulse rate, 90 beats/min; respirations, 20 breaths/min; pulse oximetry reading, 97%; and the patient is alert.

Student: The vital signs have not changed significantly.

PROCTOR: Noted.

▼ **Reassess Interventions**

Student: I will reassess my interventions: oxygen, full immobilization, and splint the right leg and hip per local protocol.

PROCTOR: Noted.

ALS Student: I will reassess basic life support (BLS) interventions, plus the following: IV access and pain management per local protocol.

ALS Proctor: Noted.

Critical Criteria:

❑ Did not find or manage problems associated with airway, breathing, hemorrhage or shock (hypoperfusion)

Radio Report

(Provided by the student.)

PROCTOR: Noted.

Ongoing Assessment

▼ **Repeat Vital Signs**

Student: I will reassess vital signs and mental status.

PROCTOR: Blood pressure, 130/78 mm Hg; pulse rate, 84 beats/min; respirations, 20 breaths/min; pulse oximetry reading, 97%; and the patient is alert.

Student: The vital signs have not changed significantly.

PROCTOR: Noted.

▼ **Check Interventions**

Student: I will check my interventions: oxygen, full immobilization, and splinting.

PROCTOR: Noted.

ALS Student: I will check BLS interventions, plus the following: monitor IV and pain management.

ALS Proctor: Noted.

Critical Criteria:

❑ Did not find or manage problems associated with airway, breathing, hemorrhage or shock (hypoperfusion)

Handoff Report to Emergency Department Staff

Student: There was no change during transport.

PROCTOR: Noted.

Critical Criteria:

❑ Did not transport patient within the (10) minute time limit

Critical Criteria

(Inform the student of items missed, if any.)

❑ Pass ❑ Fail Date: ______________________________

Proctor Comments: ______________________________

____

____

Notes

Dispatch Information

PROCTOR: EMS 10, respond to a 60-year-old male patient who has been shot in the chest. He is breathing and conscious. Police are en route to the scene.

Pre-scene Action (BSI)

Student: I am wearing nonlatex gloves, safety glasses, mask, and gown.
PROCTOR: Noted.

Critical Criteria:
- ❑ Did not take, or verbalize, body substance isolation (BSI) precautions when necessary

Scene Size-up

Scene Safety

Student: Is the scene safe?
PROCTOR: Yes, police are on scene and you are given clearance to enter.

Mechanism of Injury

Student: What was the mechanism of injury?
PROCTOR: Gunshot wound. The patient was shot by his girlfriend's ex-husband.

Number of Patients

Student: How many patients are there?
PROCTOR: One.

Additional Resources

Student: I would call for advanced life support (ALS) assistance.
PROCTOR: Noted.

C-Spine Stabilization

Student: On the basis of the mechanism of injury, I would stabilize the cervical spine (c-spine) in a neutral in-line position.
PROCTOR: Noted.

Critical Criteria:
- ❑ Did not determine scene safety
- ❑ Did not assess for spinal protection
- ❑ Did not provide for spinal protection when indicated

Initial Assessment

Student: As I perform midline c-spine stabilization, I identify myself and ask the patient not to move.
PROCTOR: Noted.

General Impression

Student: My general impression is that the patient's condition is unstable.
PROCTOR: Noted.

Responsiveness/Level of Consciousness

Student: What is the patient's level of consciousness?
PROCTOR: Alert.

Chief Complaint/Apparent Life Threats

Student: What is the patient's chief complaint?
PROCTOR: The patient is complaining of chest pain.
Student: There is an apparent life threat; the life threat is a chest wound.
PROCTOR: Noted.

Assess the Airway and Breathing

Student: Is the airway open? Is the patient breathing?
PROCTOR: Yes, the airway is open and the patient is breathing.

Assessment

Student: What are the rate and the quality of breathing?
PROCTOR: Rate: Within normal limits. Quality: Normal.

Provide Oxygen

Student: I am applying oxygen at 15 L/min via nonrebreathing mask.
PROCTOR: Noted.

Ensure Adequate Ventilation

Student: The patient has adequate ventilations at this time. I will apply an occlusive dressing.
PROCTOR: Noted.

Injury Management

Student: I will direct my partner to take over c-spine control as I continue assessment.
PROCTOR: Noted.

Assess Circulation

Student: I am assessing the patient's circulation.
PROCTOR: Noted.

Assess for and Control Major Bleeding

Student: Do I find any major bleeding?
PROCTOR: No.

Assess the Pulse

Student: What are the rate and the quality of pulses?
PROCTOR: Rate: Tachycardic. Quality: Bounding.

Assess the Skin

Student: I am assessing the skin. What are the color, temperature, and condition of the skin?
PROCTOR: Color: Flushed. Temperature: Normal. Condition: Normal.

Identify Priority Patients/Make Transport Decision

Student: The patient is a high priority and is a load-and-go. I will begin packaging and transport.
PROCTOR: Noted.

Critical Criteria:
- ❑ Did not provide high concentration of oxygen
- ❑ Did not find or manage problems associated with airway, breathing, hemorrhage or shock (hypoperfusion)
- ❑ Did not differentiate patient's need for transportation versus continued assessment at the scene
- ❑ Did other detailed examination before assessing the airway, breathing and circulation

Focused History and Physical Examination/Rapid Trauma Assessment

Select the Appropriate Assessment (Focused or Rapid)

Student: I am selecting the rapid physical exam to identify and treat life threats. I am checking for DCAP-BTLS. This acronym stands for deformities, contusions, abrasions, punctures, penetrations, and paradoxical motion in the chest, and burns, tenderness, lacerations, and swelling.
PROCTOR: Noted.

Head

Student: I am rapidly assessing the head.
PROCTOR: There are no obvious injuries.

▸ Neck

Student: I am rapidly assessing the neck.
PROCTOR: There are no obvious injuries.
Student: I will apply a cervical collar.
PROCTOR: Noted.

▸ Chest

Student: I am rapidly assessing the chest.
PROCTOR: You note that the bullet entered the chest at the sternum and followed a rib around to the side without entering the chest cavity. The bullet exited from the left chest.
Student: I will apply occlusive dressings to the chest at the entrance and exit wound.
PROCTOR: Noted.
Student: What are lung sounds?
PROCTOR: They are clear bilaterally.
Student: I will assess the chest for tension pneumothorax by auscultation, and assessment (jugular vein distention [JVD], tracheal deviation, and decreased lung sounds).
PROCTOR: The lung sounds appear clear bilaterally, jugular vein distention is not present, and the trachea is midline.
ALS Student: I will assess the chest for hyperresonance to percussion.
ALS Proctor: Noted. There is no tension pneumothorax.
ALS Student: I will continuously reassess the chest.
ALS Proctor: Noted.

▸ Abdomen/Pelvis

Student: I am rapidly assessing the abdomen.
PROCTOR: There are no obvious injuries.
Student: I am rapidly assessing the pelvis.
PROCTOR: There are no obvious injuries.

▸ Extremities

Student: I am rapidly assessing the extremities.
PROCTOR: There are no obvious injuries.

▸ Assess Motor, Sensory, and Circulatory Function

Student: I am checking for DCAP-BTLS. I am also checking motor and sensory function, and pulses. Right leg?
PROCTOR: Negative DCAP-BTLS. Motor and sensory functions are present. Pulses are present.
Student: Left leg?
PROCTOR: Negative DCAP-BTLS. Motor and sensory functions are present. Pulses are present.
Student: Right arm?
PROCTOR: Negative DCAP-BTLS. Motor and sensory functions are present. Pulses are present.
Student: Left arm?
PROCTOR: Negative DCAP-BTLS. Motor and sensory functions are present. Pulses are present.

▸ Posterior

Student: I am rapidly assessing the back. We will now log roll the patient as a unit to check the back. The person at the head will count to three and we will roll the patient.
PROCTOR: Noted.

▸ Assess the Thorax

Student: I am assessing the thorax. Do I find injuries?
PROCTOR: No.

▸ Assess the Lumbar Area

Student: I am assessing the flanks and lumbar area. Do I find injuries?
PROCTOR: No.

▸ Assess the Entire Backside

Student: I am assessing the entire backside. Do I find injuries?
PROCTOR: No.

▸ Manage Secondary Injuries/Wounds

Student: We will apply a cervical collar and backboard with full immobilization per local protocol, if not yet done, at this time.
PROCTOR: Noted.
Student: Are there any changes in motor and sensory functions and pulses?
PROCTOR: No.
ALS Student: I will establish a large-bore IV en route to the hospital and maintain a systolic blood pressure of 90 mm Hg.
ALS Proctor: Noted.

▸ Reevaluate Transport Decision

Student: This patient needs immediate transport due to the mechanism of injury.
PROCTOR: Noted.

▾ Baseline Vital Signs

Student: What are the patient's baseline vital signs, including blood pressure, pulse, respirations, pulse oximetry, and level of consciousness?
PROCTOR: Blood pressure, 160/90 mm Hg; pulse rate, 134 beats/min; respirations, 24 breaths/min; pulse oximetry reading, 98%; and the patient is alert.

▾ SAMPLE History

Student: At this time I will gather a SAMPLE history from the patient or family. What are the patient's signs and symptoms?
PROCTOR: Pain in the chest.
Student: Allergies?
PROCTOR: Sulfa medications.
Student: Medications?
PROCTOR: Blood pressure medications (he did not take them today).
Student: Pertinent past medical history?
PROCTOR: High blood pressure.
Student: Last oral intake?
PROCTOR: 3 hours ago.
Student: Events leading up to the incident?
PROCTOR: He was on a date when he was shot by his girlfriend's ex-husband.

Critical Criteria:
- ❑ Did not differentiate patient's need for transportation versus continued assessment at the scene
- ❑ Did not provide for spinal protection when indicated

▾ Detailed Physical Examination

Student: I am conducting the detailed physical exam. I am looking for DCAP-BTLS.
PROCTOR: Noted. The detailed physical exam will be performed during transport.

▾ Assess the Head

Student: I am assessing the head. Do I find any DCAP-BTLS? Do I find any evidence of Battle's sign or raccoon eyes?
PROCTOR: No.

▸ Inspect and Palpate the Head and Ears

Student: I am assessing the head and ears.
PROCTOR: There are no obvious injuries.

▸ Assess the Eyes

Student: I am assessing the eyes. Are the pupils equal, round, and regular in size, and react properly to light (PEARRL)?
PROCTOR: They are PEARRL.

▸ Assess the Facial Area Including Oral and Nasal Areas

Student: I am assessing the face, nose, and mouth. Do I see any discharge or hear any obstructions?
PROCTOR: No.

▼ Assess the Neck

▸ **Inspect and Palpate the Neck**

Student: I am assessing the neck for DCAP-BTLS.

PROCTOR: There are no obvious injuries.

▸ **Assess for Jugular Vein Distention**

Student: Do I find any jugular vein distention (JVD)?

PROCTOR: No.

▸ **Assess for Tracheal Deviation**

Student: Do I see any tracheal deviation?

PROCTOR: No.

▼ Assess the Chest

Student: I am assessing the chest for DCAP-BTLS.

PROCTOR: Noted.

▸ **Inspect**

Student: What do I see when I look at the chest?

PROCTOR: A bullet entered the skin but appears to have deflected off the sternum and followed a rib around to exit the left chest.

Student: Does the chest appear symmetric?

PROCTOR: Yes.

▸ **Palpate**

Student: When I touch the chest, do I feel crepitus or a flail segment?

PROCTOR: No.

▸ **Auscultate**

Student: Are lung sounds present in all fields?

PROCTOR: Yes.

Student: Do I hear any sucking sounds from the chest?

PROCTOR: No.

Student: I would control any bleeding with an occlusive dressing.

PROCTOR: Noted.

▼ Assess the Abdomen/Pelvis

▸ **Assess the Abdomen**

Student: I am assessing the abdomen for DCAP-BTLS. I am assessing all four quadrants. Do I find any problems?

PROCTOR: No.

▸ **Assess the Pelvis**

Student: I am assessing the pelvis for DCAP-BTLS. Is the pelvis stable?

PROCTOR: Yes.

▼ Assess the Genitalia/Perineum as Needed (Verbalize in Training)

Student: I am assessing the genitalia/perineum as necessary for DCAP-BTLS.

PROCTOR: The area is unremarkable.

▼ Assess the Extremities

▸ **Inspect**

Student: I am assessing the lower and upper extremities for DCAP-BTLS. Do I find anything?

PROCTOR: No.

▸ **Palpate**

Student: Do I feel anything unusual?

PROCTOR: No.

▸ **Assess Motor, Sensory, and Circulatory Function**

Student: I am checking for DCAP-BTLS, motor and sensory function, and pulses. Right leg?

PROCTOR: Negative DCAP-BTLS. Motor and sensory functions are present. Pulses are present.

Student: Left leg?

PROCTOR: Negative DCAP-BTLS. Motor and sensory functions are present. Pulses are present.

Student: Right arm?

PROCTOR: Negative DCAP-BTLS. Motor and sensory functions are present. Pulses are present.

Student: Left arm?

PROCTOR: Negative DCAP-BTLS. Motor and sensory functions are present. Pulses are present.

▼ Assess the Posterior

Note: This portion of the detailed physical exam would not be done if the patient were previously backboarded per local protocol.

Student: We will not check the back because it was previously checked and the patient is backboarded.

PROCTOR: Noted.

▼ Manage Secondary Injuries/Wounds

Student: I will direct my partner to monitor the patient's airway, breathing, occlusive dressings, and for the possibility of pneumothorax.

PROCTOR: Noted.

▼ Reassess Vital Signs

Student: I will reassess vital signs and mental status.

PROCTOR: Blood pressure, 150/88 mm Hg; pulse rate, 120 beats/min; respirations, 24 breaths/min; pulse oximetry reading, 98%; and the patient is alert.

Student: The vital signs are improving.

PROCTOR: Noted.

▼ Reassess Interventions

Student: I will reassess my interventions: airway, breathing, and oxygen; circulation and bleeding control; and immobilization and straps.

PROCTOR: Noted.

ALS Student: I will reassess basic life support (BLS) interventions, plus the following: establish two large-bore IVs and perform cardiac monitoring.

ALS Proctor: Noted. The cardiac monitor shows sinus tachycardia.

Critical Criteria:

- ❑ Did not find or manage problems associated with airway, breathing, hemorrhage or shock (hypoperfusion)

▼ Radio Report

(Provided by the student.)

PROCTOR: Noted.

▼ Ongoing Assessment

▼ Repeat Vital Signs

Student: I will reassess vital signs and mental status.

PROCTOR: Blood pressure, 144/86 mm Hg; pulse rate, 110 beats/min; respirations, 18 breaths/min; pulse oximetry reading, 98%; and the patient is alert.

Student: The vital signs have improved.

PROCTOR: Noted.

Check Interventions

Student: I will check my interventions: airway, breathing, and oxygen; circulation and bleeding control; and immobilization and straps.

PROCTOR: Noted.

ALS Student: I will check BLS interventions, plus the following: monitor IVs and cardiac monitor.

ALS Proctor: Noted. The cardiac monitor shows sinus tachycardia.

Critical Criteria:

- ❑ Did not find or manage problems associated with airway, breathing, hemorrhage or shock (hypoperfusion)

Handoff Report to Emergency Department Staff

Student: The patient's condition improved during transport.

PROCTOR: Noted.

Critical Criteria:

- ❑ Did not transport patient within the (10) minute time limit

Critical Criteria

(Inform the student of items missed, if any.)

❑ Pass ❑ Fail Date: ____________________

Proctor Comments: ____________________

____

____

Dispatch Information

PROCTOR: EMS 10, respond to a motor vehicle collision. An SUV went off a cliff. Police are protecting the scene from traffic.

Pre-scene Action (BSI)

Student: I am wearing appropriate high-visibility personal protective equipment suitable for extrication, a helmet, extrication gloves, nonlatex gloves, safety glasses, mask, and gown.
PROCTOR: Noted.

Critical Criteria:
- ❑ Did not take, or verbalize, body substance isolation (BSI) precautions when necessary

Scene Size-up

Scene Safety

Student: Is the scene safe?
PROCTOR: Yes, police are on scene and you are given clearance to enter.

Mechanism of Injury

Student: What was the mechanism of injury?
PROCTOR: Motor vehicle collision. The patient is a 17-year-old male unrestrained driver who lost control on a curve and rolled over several times down a cliff. The teenage driver cannot feel his legs.

Number of Patients

Student: How many patients are there?
PROCTOR: One.

Additional Resources

Student: I would call for advanced life support (ALS) assistance and additional resources: fire/rescue.
PROCTOR: Noted.

C-Spine Stabilization

Student: On the basis of the mechanism of injury, I would stabilize the cervical spine (c-spine) in a neutral in-line position.
PROCTOR: Noted.

Critical Criteria:
- ❑ Did not determine scene safety
- ❑ Did not assess for spinal protection
- ❑ Did not provide for spinal protection when indicated

Initial Assessment

Student: As I perform midline c-spine stabilization, I identify myself and ask the patient not to move.
PROCTOR: Noted.

General Impression

Student: My general impression is that the patient's condition is unstable.
PROCTOR: Noted.

Responsiveness/Level of Consciousness

Student: What is the patient's level of consciousness?
PROCTOR: Alert but suicidal.

Chief Complaint/Apparent Life Threats

Student: What is the patient's chief complaint?
PROCTOR: The patient is complaining of not being able to feel his legs. He says that if he is paralyzed, he will kill himself.
Student: There are apparent life threats; the life threats are the mechanism of injury and shock.
PROCTOR: Noted.

Assess the Airway and Breathing

Student: Is the airway open? Is the patient breathing?
PROCTOR: Yes, the airway is open and the patient is breathing.

Assessment

Student: What are the rate and the quality of breathing?
PROCTOR: Rate: Tachypneic. Quality: Crying.

Provide Oxygen

Student: I am applying oxygen at 15 L/min via nonrebreathing mask.
PROCTOR: Noted.

Ensure Adequate Ventilation

Student: The patient has adequate ventilations at this time.
PROCTOR: Noted.

Injury Management

Student: I will direct my partner to take over c-spine control as I continue assessment.
PROCTOR: Noted.

Assess Circulation

Student: I am assessing the patient's circulation.
PROCTOR: Noted.

Assess for and Control Major Bleeding

Student: Do I find any major bleeding?
PROCTOR: No.

Assess the Pulse

Student: What are the rate and the quality of pulses?
PROCTOR: Rate: Tachycardic. Quality: Thready.

Assess the Skin

Student: I am assessing the skin. What are the color, temperature, and condition of the skin?
PROCTOR: Color: Pale. Temperature: Cool. Condition: Moist.

Identify Priority Patients/Make Transport Decision

Student: The patient is a high priority and is a load-and-go. I will begin packaging and transport.
PROCTOR: Noted.

Critical Criteria:
- ❑ Did not provide high concentration of oxygen
- ❑ Did not find or manage problems associated with airway, breathing, hemorrhage or shock (hypoperfusion)
- ❑ Did not differentiate patient's need for transportation versus continued assessment at the scene
- ❑ Did other detailed examination before assessing the airway, breathing and circulation

Focused History and Physical Examination/Rapid Trauma Assessment

Select the Appropriate Assessment (Focused or Rapid)

Student: I am selecting the rapid physical exam to identify and treat life threats. I am checking for DCAP-BTLS. This acronym stands for deformities, contusions, abrasions, punctures, penetrations, and paradoxical motion in the chest, and burns, tenderness, lacerations, and swelling.
PROCTOR: Noted.

Head

Student: I am rapidly assessing the head.
PROCTOR: Some bruising is noted to the forehead.

Neck

Student: I am rapidly assessing the neck.
PROCTOR: There are no obvious injuries.
Student: I will apply a cervical collar.
PROCTOR: Noted.

▸ Chest

Student: I am rapidly assessing the chest. What are the lung sounds?

PROCTOR: Some bruising is noted across the upper chest, but the chest appears stable. The lung sounds are clear bilaterally.

Student: I will assess the chest for tension pneumothorax by auscultation, and assessment (jugular vein distention [JVD], tracheal deviation, and decreased lung sounds).

PROCTOR: The lung sounds appear clear bilaterally, jugular vein distention is not present, and the trachea is midline.

ALS Student: I will assess the chest for hyperresonance to percussion.

ALS Proctor: Noted. There is no tension pneumothorax.

ALS Student: I will continuously reassess the chest.

ALS Proctor: Noted.

▸ Abdomen/Pelvis

Student: I am rapidly assessing the abdomen.

PROCTOR: There are no obvious injuries.

Student: I am rapidly assessing the pelvis.

PROCTOR: Some bruising is noted to the crests, but the pelvis is stable.

▸ Extremities

Student: I am rapidly assessing the extremities.

PROCTOR: There are no obvious injuries.

▸ Assess Motor, Sensory, and Circulatory Function

Student: I am checking for DCAP-BTLS. I am also checking motor and sensory function, and pulses. Right leg?

PROCTOR: Negative DCAP-BTLS. Motor and sensory functions are absent. Pulses are weak.

Student: Left leg?

PROCTOR: Negative DCAP-BTLS. Motor and sensory functions are absent. Pulses are weak.

Student: Right arm?

PROCTOR: Negative DCAP-BTLS. Motor and sensory functions are present. Pulses are weak.

Student: Left arm?

PROCTOR: Negative DCAP-BTLS. Motor and sensory functions are present. Pulses are weak.

▸ Posterior

Student: I will rapidly assess the back. We will now log roll the patient as a unit to check the back. The person at the head will count to three and we will roll the patient.

PROCTOR: Noted.

▸ Assess the Thorax

Student: I am assessing the thorax. Do I find injuries?

PROCTOR: No.

▸ Assess the Lumbar Area

Student: I am assessing the flanks and lumbar area. Do I find injuries?

PROCTOR: He has a bruise across his lumbar spine and is complaining of pain to that area of his back. He says that he cannot feel anything below that point.

▸ Assess the Entire Backside

Student: I am assessing the entire backside. Do I find injuries?

PROCTOR: Just the bruised area of the lower back.

▸ Manage Secondary Injuries/Wounds

Student: We will apply a cervical collar and backboard with full immobilization per local protocol, if not yet done, at this time.

PROCTOR: Noted.

ALS Student: I will apply basic life support (BLS) interventions, plus the following: establish two large-bore IVs, administer 20 mL/kg of normal saline, and maintain a systolic blood pressure of 90 mm Hg.

ALS Proctor: Noted.

Student: Are there any changes in motor and sensory functions or pulses?

PROCTOR: No.

▸ Reevaluate Transport Decision

Student: This patient is a load-and-go due to shock.

PROCTOR: Noted.

▾ Baseline Vital Signs

Student: What are the patient's baseline vital signs, including blood pressure, pulse, respirations, pulse oximetry, and level of consciousness?

PROCTOR: Blood pressure, 110/68 mm Hg; pulse rate, 132 beats/min; respirations, 24 breaths/min; pulse oximetry reading, 96%; and the patient is alert.

▾ SAMPLE History

Student: At this time I will gather a SAMPLE history from the patient or family. What are the patient's signs and symptoms?

PROCTOR: Pain in the lower back and he cannot move or feel his legs.

Student: Allergies?

PROCTOR: No allergies.

Student: Medications?

PROCTOR: No medications.

Student: Pertinent past medical history?

PROCTOR: No pertinent medical history.

Student: Last oral intake?

PROCTOR: 2 hours ago.

Student: Events leading up to the incident?

PROCTOR: He lost control of the car and rolled several times down a cliff.

Critical Criteria:
- ❑ Did not differentiate patient's need for transportation versus continued assessment at the scene
- ❑ Did not provide for spinal protection when indicated

Detailed Physical Examination

Student: I am conducting the detailed physical exam. I am looking for DCAP-BTLS.

PROCTOR: Noted. The detailed physical exam will be performed during transport.

▾ Assess the Head

Student: I am assessing the head. Do I find any DCAP-BTLS? Do I find any evidence of Battle's sign or raccoon eyes?

PROCTOR: No.

▸ Inspect and Palpate the Head and Ears

Student: I am assessing the head and ears.

PROCTOR: Some bruising is noted to the forehead.

▸ Assess the Eyes

Student: I am assessing the eyes. Are the pupils equal, round, and regular in size, and react properly to light (PEARRL)?

PROCTOR: They are PEARRL.

▸ Assess the Facial Area Including Oral and Nasal Areas

Student: I am assessing the face, nose, and mouth. Do I see any discharge or hear any obstructions?

PROCTOR: No.

▾ Assess the Neck

▸ Inspect and Palpate the Neck

Student: I am assessing the neck for DCAP-BTLS.

PROCTOR: There are no obvious injuries.

▸ Assess for Jugular Vein Distention

Student: Do I find any jugular vein distention (JVD)?

PROCTOR: No.

▸ Assess for Tracheal Deviation

Student: Do I see any tracheal deviation?

PROCTOR: No.

▾ Assess the Chest

Student: I am assessing the chest for DCAP-BTLS.

PROCTOR: Noted.

▸ Inspect

Student: What do I see when I look at the chest?

PROCTOR: Some bruising is noted across the upper chest.

Student: Does the chest appear symmetric?

PROCTOR: Yes.

▸ Palpate

Student: When I touch the chest, do I feel crepitus or a flail segment?

PROCTOR: No.

▸ Auscultate

Student: Are lung sounds present in all fields?

PROCTOR: Yes.

Student: Do I hear any sucking sounds from the chest?

PROCTOR: No.

▾ Assess the Abdomen/Pelvis

▸ Assess the Abdomen

Student: I am assessing the abdomen for DCAP-BTLS. I am assessing all four quadrants. Do I find any problems?

PROCTOR: No.

▸ Assess the Pelvis

Student: I am assessing the pelvis for DCAP-BTLS. Is the pelvis stable?

PROCTOR: Yes, with some bruising noted to the crests.

▾ Assess the Genitalia/Perineum as Needed (Verbalize in Training)

Student: I am assessing the genitalia/perineum as necessary for DCAP-BTLS.

PROCTOR: The area is unremarkable.

▾ Assess the Extremities

▸ Inspect

Student: I am assessing the lower and upper extremities for DCAP-BTLS. Do I find anything?

PROCTOR: No.

▸ Palpate

Student: Do I feel anything unusual?

PROCTOR: No.

▸ Assess Motor, Sensory, and Circulatory Function

Student: I am checking for DCAP-BTLS, motor and sensory function, and pulses. Right leg?

PROCTOR: Negative DCAP-BTLS. Motor and sensory functions are absent. Pulses are weak.

Student: Left leg?

PROCTOR: Negative DCAP-BTLS. Motor and sensory functions are absent. Pulses are weak.

Student: Right arm?

PROCTOR: Negative DCAP-BTLS. Motor and sensory functions are present. Pulses are weak.

Student: Left arm?

PROCTOR: Negative DCAP-BTLS. Motor and sensory functions are present. Pulses are weak.

▾ Assess the Posterior

Note: This portion of the detailed physical exam would not be done if the patient were previously backboarded per local protocol.

Student: We will not check the back since it was previously checked and the patient is backboarded.

PROCTOR: Noted.

▾ Manage Secondary Injuries/Wounds

Student: I would direct my partner to continue monitoring the patient.

PROCTOR: Noted.

▾ Reassess Vital Signs

Student: I will reassess vital signs and mental status.

PROCTOR: Blood pressure, 110/66 mm Hg; pulse rate, 134 beats/min; respirations, 24 breaths/min; pulse oximetry reading, 97%; and the patient is alert.

Student: The vital signs have not changed significantly.

PROCTOR: Noted.

▾ Reassess Interventions

Student: I will reassess my interventions: oxygen, full immobilization, and treatment for shock.

PROCTOR: Noted.

ALS Student: I will reassess BLS interventions, plus the following: two large-bore IVs, maintain a systolic blood pressure of 90 mm Hg, and cardiac monitoring.

ALS Proctor: Noted. The cardiac monitor shows sinus tachycardia.

Critical Criteria:

❑ Did not find or manage problems associated with airway, breathing, hemorrhage or shock (hypoperfusion)

Radio Report

(Provided by the student.)

PROCTOR: Noted.

Ongoing Assessment

▾ Repeat Vital Signs

Student: I will reassess vital signs and mental status.

PROCTOR: Blood pressure, 108/68 mm Hg; pulse rate, 132 beats/min; respirations, 24 breaths/min; pulse oximetry reading, 98%; and the patient is alert.

Student: The vital signs have not changed significantly.

PROCTOR: Noted.

▾ Check Interventions

Student: I will check my interventions: oxygen, full immobilization, and treatment for shock.

PROCTOR: Noted.

ALS Student: I will check BLS interventions, plus the following: flow of the two large-bore IVs to maintain a systolic blood pressure of 90 mm Hg and cardiac monitoring.

ALS Proctor: Noted. The cardiac monitor shows sinus tachycardia.

Critical Criteria:

❑ Did not find or manage problems associated with airway, breathing, hemorrhage or shock (hypoperfusion)

Handoff Report to Emergency Department Staff

Student: There was no change during transport.

PROCTOR: Noted.

Critical Criteria:

❑ Did not transport patient within the (10) minute time limit

Critical Criteria

(Inform the student of items missed, if any.)

❑ Pass ❑ Fail Date: ______________________________

Proctor Comments: ______________________________

____

____

Notes

Dispatch Information

PROCTOR: EMS 10, respond to a 52-year-old male patient who was held and struck several times in the chest with a baseball bat. He is conscious and breathing. Police officers are on the scene.

Pre-scene Action (BSI)

Student: I am wearing nonlatex gloves, safety glasses, mask, and gown.
PROCTOR: Noted.

Critical Criteria:
- ❑ Did not take, or verbalize, body substance isolation (BSI) precautions when necessary

Scene Size-up

Scene Safety

Student: Is the scene safe?
PROCTOR: Yes, police are on scene and you are given clearance to enter.

Mechanism of Injury

Student: What was the mechanism of injury?
PROCTOR: Blunt trauma. The patient was held by two men while he was hit in the chest with a baseball bat by a third man.

Number of Patients

Student: How many patients are there?
PROCTOR: One.

Additional Resources

Student: I would call for advanced life support (ALS) assistance.
PROCTOR: Noted.

C-Spine Stabilization

Student: On the basis of the mechanism of injury, I would stabilize the cervical spine (c-spine) in a neutral in-line position.
PROCTOR: Noted.

Critical Criteria:
- ❑ Did not determine scene safety
- ❑ Did not assess for spinal protection
- ❑ Did not provide for spinal protection when indicated

Initial Assessment

Student: As I perform midline c-spine stabilization, I identify myself and ask the patient not to move.
PROCTOR: Noted.

General Impression

Student: My general impression is that the patient's condition is unstable.
PROCTOR: Noted.

Responsiveness/Level of Consciousness

Student: What is the patient's level of consciousness?
PROCTOR: Alert.

Chief Complaint/Apparent Life Threats

Student: What is the patient's chief complaint?
PROCTOR: The patient is complaining of chest pain.
Student: There is an apparent life threat; the life threat is chest trauma.
PROCTOR: Noted.

Assess the Airway and Breathing

Student: Is the airway open? Is the patient breathing?
PROCTOR: Yes, the airway is open and the patient is breathing.

Assessment

Student: What are the rate and the quality of breathing?
PROCTOR: Rate: Tachypneic. Quality: Guarded.

Provide Oxygen

Student: I am applying oxygen at 15 L/min via nonrebreathing mask.
PROCTOR: Noted.

Ensure Adequate Ventilation

Student: The patient has adequate ventilations at this time.
PROCTOR: Noted.

Injury Management

Student: I will direct my partner to take over c-spine control as I continue assessment.
PROCTOR: Noted.

Assess Circulation

Student: I am assessing the patient's circulation.
PROCTOR: Noted.

Assess for and Control Major Bleeding

Student: Do I find any major bleeding?
PROCTOR: No.

Assess the Pulse

Student: What are the rate and the quality of pulses?
PROCTOR: Rate: Tachycardic. Quality: Thready.

Assess the Skin

Student: I am assessing the skin. What are the color, temperature, and condition of the skin?
PROCTOR: Color: Cyanotic. Temperature: Cool. Condition: Diaphoretic.

Identify Priority Patients/Make Transport Decision

Student: The patient is a high priority and is a load-and-go. I will begin packaging and transport.
PROCTOR: Noted.

Critical Criteria:
- ❑ Did not provide high concentration of oxygen
- ❑ Did not find or manage problems associated with airway, breathing, hemorrhage or shock (hypoperfusion)
- ❑ Did not differentiate patient's need for transportation versus continued assessment at the scene
- ❑ Did other detailed examination before assessing the airway, breathing and circulation

Focused History and Physical Examination/Rapid Trauma Assessment

Select the Appropriate Assessment (Focused or Rapid)

Student: I am selecting the rapid physical exam to identify and treat life threats. I am checking for DCAP-BTLS. This acronym stands for deformities, contusions, abrasions, punctures, penetrations, and paradoxical motion in the chest, and burns, tenderness, lacerations, and swelling.
PROCTOR: Noted.

Head

Student: I am rapidly assessing the head.
PROCTOR: There are no obvious injuries.

Neck

Student: I am rapidly assessing the neck.
PROCTOR: There is deviation of the trachea to the right.
Student: I will quickly assess the chest and apply a cervical collar.
PROCTOR: Noted.

Chest

Student: I am rapidly assessing the chest.
PROCTOR: You see paradoxical motion on the left side of the chest.
Student: I will treat the flail segment with a bulky dressing per local protocol and ensure adequate breathing.
PROCTOR: Noted.
Student: I will listen to the lung sounds.
PROCTOR: Lung sounds are diminished on the left.

Student: I will ensure ALS assistance.
PROCTOR: Noted.
Student: I will assess the chest for tension pneumothorax by auscultation, and assessment (jugular vein distention [JVD], tracheal deviation, and decreased lung sounds).
PROCTOR: The lung sounds appear diminished on the left, jugular vein distention is present, and the trachea is deviated to the right.
ALS Student: I will assess the chest for hyperresonance to percussion.
ALS Proctor: Noted. There is a tension pneumothorax on the left side.
ALS Student: I will decompress the left chest.
ALS Proctor: Noted. The treatment was effective.
ALS Student: I will continuously reassess the chest.
ALS Proctor: Noted.
ALS Student: I will apply basic life support (BLS) interventions, plus the following: I will decompress the left chest.
ALS Proctor: Noted. There is an improvement in lung sounds and chest rise.

▸ **Abdomen/Pelvis**
Student: I am rapidly assessing the abdomen.
PROCTOR: There are no obvious injuries.
Student: I am rapidly assessing the pelvis.
PROCTOR: There are no obvious injuries.

▸ **Extremities**
Student: I am rapidly assessing the extremities.
PROCTOR: There are no obvious injuries.

▸ **Assess Motor, Sensory, and Circulatory Function**
Student: I am checking for DCAP-BTLS. I am also checking motor and sensory function, and pulses. Right leg?
PROCTOR: Negative DCAP-BTLS. Motor and sensory functions are present. Pulses are weak.
Student: Left leg?
PROCTOR: Negative DCAP-BTLS. Motor and sensory functions are present. Pulses are weak.
Student: Right arm?
PROCTOR: Negative DCAP-BTLS. Motor and sensory functions are present. Pulses are weak.
Student: Left arm?
PROCTOR: Negative DCAP-BTLS. Motor and sensory functions are present. Pulses are weak.

▸ **Posterior**
Student: I will rapidly assess the back. We will now log roll the patient as a unit to check the back. The person at the head will count to three and we will roll the patient.
PROCTOR: Noted.

▸ **Assess the Thorax**
Student: I am assessing the thorax. Do I find injuries?
PROCTOR: No.

▸ **Assess the Lumbar Area**
Student: I am assessing the flanks and lumbar area. Do I find injuries?
PROCTOR: No.

▸ **Assess the Entire Backside**
Student: I am assessing the entire backside. Do I find injuries?
PROCTOR: No.

▸ **Manage Secondary Injuries/Wounds**
Student: We will apply a cervical collar and backboard with full immobilization per local protocol, if not yet done, at this time.
PROCTOR: Noted.
Student: Are there any changes in motor and sensory functions or pulses?
PROCTOR: No.

ALS Student: I will establish two large-bore IVs en route to the hospital and administer a bolus of 20 mL/kg in order to maintain a systolic blood pressure of 90 mm Hg.
ALS Proctor: Noted.

▸ **Reevaluate Transport Decision**
Student: This patient is a load-and-go due to the mechanism of injury.
PROCTOR: Noted.

▾ Baseline Vital Signs
Student: What are the patient's baseline vital signs, including blood pressure, pulse, respirations, pulse oximetry, and level of consciousness?
PROCTOR: Blood pressure, 110/74 mm Hg; pulse rate, 130 beats/min; respirations, 28 breaths/min; pulse oximetry reading, 92%; and the patient is alert.

▾ SAMPLE History
Student: At this time I will gather a SAMPLE history from the patient or family. What are the patient's signs and symptoms?
PROCTOR: Pain in the chest.
Student: Allergies?
PROCTOR: No allergies.
Student: Medications?
PROCTOR: No medications.
Student: Pertinent past medical history?
PROCTOR: Heart problems.
Student: Last oral intake?
PROCTOR: 4 hours ago.
Student: Events leading up to the incident?
PROCTOR: The patient was assaulted for not paying a gambling debt.

Critical Criteria:
- ❑ Did not differentiate patient's need for transportation versus continued assessment at the scene
- ❑ Did not provide for spinal protection when indicated

Detailed Physical Examination
Student: I am conducting the detailed physical exam. I am looking for DCAP-BTLS.
PROCTOR: Noted. The detailed physical exam will be performed during transport.

▾ Assess the Head
Student: I am assessing the head. Do I find any DCAP-BTLS? Do I find any evidence of Battle's sign or raccoon eyes?
PROCTOR: No.

▸ **Inspect and Palpate the Head and Ears**
Student: I am assessing the head and ears.
PROCTOR: There are no obvious injuries.

▸ **Assess the Eyes**
Student: I am assessing the eyes. Are the pupils equal, round, and regular in size, and react properly to light (PEARRL)?
PROCTOR: They are PEARRL.

▸ **Assess the Facial Area Including Oral and Nasal Areas**
Student: I am assessing the face, nose, and mouth. Do I see any discharge or hear any obstructions?
PROCTOR: Yes, you hear gurgling.
Student: I would suction as necessary.
PROCTOR: Noted.

▾ Assess the Neck
▸ **Inspect and Palpate the Neck**
Student: I am assessing the neck for DCAP-BTLS.
PROCTOR: There are no obvious injuries.

▸ **Assess for Jugular Vein Distention**

Student: Do I find any jugular vein distention (JVD)?

PROCTOR: Yes.

▸ **Assess for Tracheal Deviation**

Student: Do I see any tracheal deviation?

PROCTOR: Yes, to the right side (if ALS is not on scene). No, if the chest has been decompressed.

▾ Assess the Chest

Student: I am assessing the chest for DCAP-BTLS.

PROCTOR: Noted.

▸ **Inspect**

Student: What do I see when I look at the chest?

PROCTOR: You saw abrasions and contusions across the left side of the chest before the placement of a bulky dressing.

Student: Does the chest appear symmetric?

PROCTOR: No, but it has been stabilized with a bulky dressing.

▸ **Palpate**

Student: When I touch the chest, do I feel crepitus or a flail segment?

PROCTOR: Yes, there was crepitus on the left side of the chest that has been stabilized with a bulky dressing.

▸ **Auscultate**

Student: Are lung sounds present in all fields?

PROCTOR: Yes, they were diminished on the left side of the chest, but are equal after decompression by an ALS provider.

Student: Do I hear any sucking sounds from the chest?

PROCTOR: No.

▾ Assess the Abdomen/Pelvis

▸ **Assess the Abdomen**

Student: I am assessing the abdomen for DCAP-BTLS. I am assessing all four quadrants. Do I find any problems?

PROCTOR: No.

▸ **Assess the Pelvis**

Student: I am assessing the pelvis for DCAP-BTLS. Is the pelvis stable?

PROCTOR: Yes.

▾ Assess the Genitalia/Perineum as Needed (Verbalize in Training)

Student: I am assessing the genitalia/perineum as necessary for DCAP-BTLS.

PROCTOR: The area is unremarkable.

▾ Assess the Extremities

▸ **Inspect**

Student: I am assessing the lower and upper extremities for DCAP-BTLS. Do I find anything?

PROCTOR: No.

▸ **Palpate**

Student: Do I feel anything unusual?

PROCTOR: No.

▸ **Assess Motor, Sensory, and Circulatory Function**

Student: I am checking for DCAP-BTLS, motor and sensory function, and pulses. Right leg?

PROCTOR: Negative DCAP-BTLS. Motor and sensory functions are present. Pulses are weak.

Student: Left leg?

PROCTOR: Negative DCAP-BTLS. Motor and sensory functions are present. Pulses are weak.

Student: Right arm?

PROCTOR: Negative DCAP-BTLS. Motor and sensory functions are present. Pulses are weak.

Student: Left arm?

PROCTOR: Negative DCAP-BTLS. Motor and sensory functions are present. Pulses are weak.

▾ Assess the Posterior

Note: This portion of the detailed physical exam would not be done if the patient were previously backboarded per local protocol.

Student: We will not check the back since it was previously checked and the patient is backboarded.

PROCTOR: Noted.

▾ Manage Secondary Injuries/Wounds

Student: I would direct my partner to monitor the patient.

PROCTOR: Noted.

▾ Reassess Vital Signs

Student: I will reassess vital signs and mental status.

PROCTOR: Blood pressure, 100/68 mm Hg; pulse rate, 134 beats/min; respirations, 28 breaths/min; pulse oximetry reading, 91%; and the patient is tired.

Student: The vital signs are deteriorating.

PROCTOR: Noted.

▾ Reassess Interventions

Student: I will reassess my interventions: airway, breathing, and oxygen; suction as needed; circulation and bleeding control; chest stabilization; immobilization and straps; and treatment for shock.

PROCTOR: Noted.

ALS Student: I will reassess BLS interventions, plus the following: assess the chest decompression, monitor the two large-bore IVs, and cardiac monitoring.

ALS Proctor: Noted. The cardiac monitor shows sinus tachycardia.

Critical Criteria:

❑ Did not find or manage problems associated with airway, breathing, hemorrhage or shock (hypoperfusion)

Radio Report

(Provided by the student.)

PROCTOR: Noted.

Ongoing Assessment

▾ Repeat Vital Signs

Student: I will reassess vital signs and mental status.

PROCTOR: Blood pressure, 90/50 mm Hg; pulse rate, 140 beats/min; respirations, 28 breaths/min; pulse oximetry reading, 91%; and the patient is responsive to pain.

Student: The vital signs have deteriorated.

PROCTOR: Noted.

Check Interventions

Student: I will check my interventions: airway, breathing, and oxygen; suction as needed; circulation and bleeding control; chest stabilization; immobilization and straps; and treatment for shock.
PROCTOR: Noted.
ALS Student: I will check BLS interventions, plus the following: assess the chest decompression, flow of the two large-bore IVs per local protocol, and cardiac monitoring.
ALS Proctor: Noted. The cardiac monitor shows sinus tachycardia.

Critical Criteria:
- ❑ Did not find or manage problems associated with airway, breathing, hemorrhage or shock (hypoperfusion)

Handoff Report to Emergency Department Staff

Student: The patient's condition deteriorated during transport.
PROCTOR: Noted.

Critical Criteria:
- ❑ Did not transport patient within the (10) minute time limit

Critical Criteria

(Inform the student of items missed, if any.)

❑ Pass ❑ Fail Date: ______________________

Proctor Comments: ______________________

____

____

Dispatch Information

PROCTOR: EMS 10, respond to a 30-year-old male who was shot in the neck. It is unknown if the patient is conscious or breathing. Police have been dispatched.

Pre-scene Action (BSI)

Student: I am wearing nonlatex gloves, safety glasses, mask, and gown.
PROCTOR: Noted.

Critical Criteria:
- ❑ Did not take, or verbalize, body substance isolation (BSI) precautions when necessary

Scene Size-up

Scene Safety

Student: Is the scene safe?
PROCTOR: Yes, police are on scene and you are given clearance to enter.

Mechanism of Injury

Student: What was the mechanism of injury?
PROCTOR: Gunshot wound. The patient opened the front door and was shot in the throat. He is lying in the entryway of the home.

Number of Patients

Student: How many patients are there?
PROCTOR: One.

Additional Resources

Student: I would call for advanced life support (ALS) assistance.
PROCTOR: Noted.

C-Spine Stabilization

Student: On the basis of the mechanism of injury, I would stabilize the cervical spine (c-spine) in a neutral in-line position.
PROCTOR: Noted.

Critical Criteria:
- ❑ Did not determine scene safety
- ❑ Did not assess for spinal protection
- ❑ Did not provide for spinal protection when indicated

Initial Assessment

Student: As I perform midline c-spine stabilization, I identify myself and ask the patient not to move.
PROCTOR: Noted.

General Impression

Student: My general impression is that the patient's condition is unstable.
PROCTOR: Noted.

Responsiveness/Level of Consciousness

Student: What is the patient's level of consciousness?
PROCTOR: Unresponsive.

Chief Complaint/Apparent Life Threats

Student: What is the patient's chief complaint?
PROCTOR: The patient is unresponsive.
Student: There are apparent life threats; the life threats are a gunshot wound to the neck and unconsciousness.
PROCTOR: Noted.

Assess the Airway and Breathing

Student: I am opening the airway using the jaw-thrust maneuver.
PROCTOR: Noted. There is blood in the mouth.
Student: I will suction the airway as needed.
PROCTOR: Noted.

▸ Assessment

Student: What are the rate and the quality of breathing?
PROCTOR: Rate: Absent. Quality: Absent.

▸ Provide Oxygen

Student: I am assisting ventilations with a bag-valve device with 100% oxygen and an oral/advanced airway.
PROCTOR: Noted.
ALS Student: I will perform midline intubation and confirm tube placement with lung sounds and end tidal CO_2.
ALS Proctor: Noted. Lung sounds and end tidal CO_2 confirm tube placement.

▸ Ensure Adequate Ventilation

Student: I will protect the airway and dress the wound.
PROCTOR: Noted.

▸ Injury Management

Student: I will direct my partner to take over c-spine control and ventilation as I continue the assessment.
PROCTOR: Noted.

Assess Circulation

Student: I am assessing the patient's circulation.
PROCTOR: Noted.

▸ Assess for and Control Major Bleeding

Student: Do I find any major bleeding?
PROCTOR: Yes, from the neck.
Student: I would apply direct pressure and a dressing.
PROCTOR: Noted.

▸ Assess the Pulse

Student: What are the rate and the quality of pulses?
PROCTOR: Rate: Tachycardic. Quality: Thready.

▸ Assess the Skin

Student: I am assessing the skin. What are the color, temperature, and condition of the skin?
PROCTOR: Color: Pale. Temperature: Cool. Condition: Diaphoretic.

Identify Priority Patients/Make Transport Decision

Student: The patient is a high priority and is a load-and-go. I will begin packaging and transport.
PROCTOR: Noted.

Critical Criteria:
- ❑ Did not provide high concentration of oxygen
- ❑ Did not find or manage problems associated with airway, breathing, hemorrhage or shock (hypoperfusion)
- ❑ Did not differentiate patient's need for transportation versus continued assessment at the scene
- ❑ Did other detailed examination before assessing the airway, breathing and circulation

Focused History and Physical Examination/Rapid Trauma Assessment

Select the Appropriate Assessment (Focused or Rapid)

Student: I am selecting the rapid physical exam to identify and treat life threats.
PROCTOR: Noted.
Student: I am checking for DCAP-BTLS. This acronym stands for deformities, contusions, abrasions, punctures, penetrations, paradoxical motion in the chest, and burns, tenderness, lacerations, and swelling. I am also checking for motor and sensory function and pulses.
PROCTOR: Noted.

▸ Head

Student: I am rapidly assessing the head.
PROCTOR: There are no obvious injuries.

▸ Neck

Student: I am rapidly assessing the neck.

PROCTOR: There is an open wound to the neck.

Student: I will check the dressing and will apply a cervical collar if it does not interfere with the airway. If the cervical collar interferes with the airway and bleeding control, we will manually stabilize the c-spine, maintain the airway, ventilate, and control bleeding.

PROCTOR: Noted.

▸ Chest

Student: I am rapidly inspecting and palpating the chest.

PROCTOR: There are no obvious injuries.

Student: Are there lung sounds present?

PROCTOR: They are clear bilaterally.

▸ Abdomen/Pelvis

Student: I am rapidly assessing the abdomen.

PROCTOR: There are no obvious injuries.

Student: I am rapidly assessing the pelvis.

PROCTOR: There are no obvious injuries.

▸ Extremities

Student: I am rapidly assessing the extremities.

PROCTOR: There are no obvious injuries.

▸ Assess Motor, Sensory, and Circulatory Function

Student: I am checking for DCAP-BTLS, motor and sensory function, and pulses. Right leg?

PROCTOR: Negative DCAP-BTLS. Motor and sensory functions are absent. Pulses are weak.

Student: Left leg?

PROCTOR: Negative DCAP-BTLS. Motor and sensory functions are absent. Pulses are weak.

Student: Right arm?

PROCTOR: Negative DCAP-BTLS. Motor and sensory functions are absent. Pulses are weak.

Student: Left arm?

PROCTOR: Negative DCAP-BTLS. Motor and sensory functions are absent. Pulses are weak.

▸ Posterior

Student: I am rapidly assessing the back. We will now log roll the patient as a unit to check the back. The person at the head will count to three and we will roll the patient.

PROCTOR: Noted.

▸ Assess the Thorax

Student: I am assessing the thorax. Do I find injuries?

PROCTOR: No.

▸ Assess the Lumbar Area

Student: I am assessing the flanks and lumbar area. Do I find injuries?

PROCTOR: No.

▸ Assess the Entire Backside

Student: I am assessing the entire backside. Do I find injuries?

PROCTOR: No.

▸ Manage Secondary Injuries/Wounds

Student: We will maintain the airway, control bleeding, and manually stabilize the c-spine. We will apply a cervical collar if it does not compromise ventilations and backboard with full immobilization, if not yet done, at this time.

PROCTOR: Noted.

Student: Are there any changes in motor and sensory functions and pulses?

PROCTOR: No.

ALS Student: I will establish two large-bore IVs en route to the hospital and administer a bolus of 20 mL/kg to maintain a systolic blood pressure of 90 mm Hg.

ALS Proctor: Noted.

▸ Reevaluate Transport Decision

Student: This patient is a high priority and is a load-and-go to a trauma center due to an open neck wound, respiratory compromise, critical trauma, and unconsciousness.

PROCTOR: Noted.

▾ Baseline Vital Signs

Student: What are the patient's baseline vital signs, including blood pressure, pulse, respirations, pulse oximetry, and level of consciousness?

PROCTOR: Blood pressure, 110/74 mm Hg; pulse, 114 beats/min; respirations per bag-valve device; pulse oximetry reading, 94%; and the patient is unresponsive.

▾ SAMPLE History

Student: At this time I will gather a SAMPLE history from the patient or family. What are the patient's signs and symptoms?

PROCTOR: Open neck wound.

Student: Allergies?

PROCTOR: Unknown.

Student: Medications?

PROCTOR: Unknown.

Student: Pertinent past medical history?

PROCTOR: Unknown.

Student: Last oral intake?

PROCTOR: Unknown.

Student: Events leading up to the injury or illness?

PROCTOR: The patient opened his front door and he was shot.

Critical Criteria:

- ❑ Did not differentiate patient's need for transportation versus continued assessment at the scene
- ❑ Did not provide for spinal protection when indicated

Detailed Physical Exam

Student: I am conducting the detailed physical exam.

PROCTOR: Noted. The detailed physical exam will be performed during transport.

▾ Assess the Head

Student: I am assessing the head. Do I find any DCAP-BTLS?

PROCTOR: No.

Student: Do I find any evidence of Battle's sign or raccoon eyes?

PROCTOR: No.

▸ Inspect and Palpate the Head and Ears

Student: I am assessing the head and ears.

PROCTOR: There are no obvious injuries.

▸ Assess the Eyes

Student: I am assessing the eyes. Are the pupils equal, round, and regular in size, and react properly to light (PEARRL)?

PROCTOR: They are sluggish.

▸ Assess the Facial Area Including Oral and Nasal Areas

Student: I am assessing the face, nose, and mouth. Do I see any discharge or hear any obstructions?

PROCTOR: Yes, you hear occasional gurgling.

Student: I will suction the airway as needed and reassess.

PROCTOR: Noted.

Assess the Neck

Inspect and Palpate the Neck

Student: I am assessing the neck for DCAP-BTLS.

PROCTOR: There is an open wound to the neck, crepitus is noted, and there is heavy damage to the soft tissue.

Student: I will reassess my interventions.

PROCTOR: Noted. Bleeding is controlled.

Assess for Jugular Vein Distention

Student: Do I find any jugular vein distention (JVD)?

PROCTOR: No.

Assess for Tracheal Deviation

Student: Do I see any tracheal deviation?

PROCTOR: No.

Assess the Chest

Student: I am assessing the chest for DCAP-BTLS.

PROCTOR: Noted.

Inspect

Student: What do I see when I look at the chest?

PROCTOR: There are no obvious injuries.

Student: Does the chest appear symmetric?

PROCTOR: Yes.

Palpate

Student: When I touch the chest, do I feel crepitus or a flail segment?

PROCTOR: No.

Auscultate

Student: I will reassess the patient's lung sounds. Are they present in all fields?

PROCTOR: Yes.

Student: Do I hear any sucking sounds coming from the chest?

PROCTOR: No.

Assess the Abdomen/Pelvis

Assess the Abdomen

Student: I am assessing the abdomen for DCAP-BTLS. I am assessing all four quadrants. Do I find any problems?

PROCTOR: No.

Assess the Pelvis

Student: I am assessing the pelvis for DCAP-BTLS. Is the pelvis stable?

PROCTOR: Yes.

Assess the Genitalia/Perineum as Needed (Verbalize in Training)

Student: I am assessing the genitalia/perineum as needed for DCAP-BTLS.

PROCTOR: The area is unremarkable.

Assess the Extremities

Inspect

Student: I am assessing the lower and upper extremities for DCAP-BTLS. Do I find anything?

PROCTOR: No.

Palpate

Student: Do I feel anything unusual?

PROCTOR: No.

Assess Motor, Sensory, and Circulatory Function

Student: I am checking for DCAP-BTLS, motor and sensory function, and pulses. Right leg?

PROCTOR: Negative DCAP-BTLS. Motor and sensory functions are absent. Pulses are weak.

Student: Left leg?

PROCTOR: Negative DCAP-BTLS. Motor and sensory functions are absent. Pulses are weak.

Student: Right arm?

PROCTOR: Negative DCAP-BTLS. Motor and sensory functions are absent. Pulses are weak.

Student: Left arm?

PROCTOR: Negative DCAP-BTLS. Motor and sensory functions are absent. Pulses are weak.

Assess the Posterior

Note: This portion of the detailed physical exam would not be done if the patient were previously backboarded per local protocol.

Student: We will not check the back since it was previously checked and the patient is backboarded.

PROCTOR: Noted.

Manage Secondary Injuries/Wounds

Student: I would direct my partner to reassess the neck.

PROCTOR: Noted.

Reassess Vital Signs

Student: At this time I will reassess vital signs and mental status.

PROCTOR: Blood pressure, 100/66 mm Hg; pulse, 128 beats/min; respirations per bag-valve device; pulse oximetry reading, 92%; and the patient is unresponsive.

Student: The vital signs are deteriorating.

PROCTOR: Noted.

Reassess Interventions

Student: I will reassess my interventions: oral/advanced airway, bag-valve device and oxygen; suction as needed; circulation and bleeding control; immobilization and straps; and treatment for shock.

PROCTOR: Noted.

ALS Student: I will reassess basic life support (BLS) interventions, plus the following: intubation, two large-bore IVs, maintain a systolic blood pressure of 90 mm Hg, and cardiac monitoring.

ALS Proctor: Noted. The cardiac monitor shows normal sinus rhythm.

Critical Criteria:

- ❑ Did not find or manage problems associated with airway, breathing, hemorrhage or shock (hypoperfusion)

Radio Report

(Provided by the student.)

PROCTOR: Noted.

Ongoing Assessment

Reassess and Record Vital Signs

Student: I will reassess vital signs and mental status.

PROCTOR: Blood pressure, 92/60 mm Hg; pulse, 128 beats/min; respirations per bag-valve device; pulse oximetry reading, 90%; and the patient is unresponsive.

Student: The vital signs have deteriorated.

PROCTOR: Noted.

Check Interventions

Student: I will check my interventions: oral/advanced airway, bag-valve device, and oxygen; suction as needed; circulation and bleeding control; immobilization and straps; and treatment for shock.

PROCTOR: Noted.

ALS Student: I will check BLS interventions, plus the following: intubation, two large-bore IVs, maintain a systolic blood pressure of 90 mm Hg, and cardiac monitoring.

ALS Proctor: Noted. The cardiac monitor shows normal sinus rhythm.

Critical Criteria:

❑ Did not find or manage problems associated with airway, breathing, hemorrhage or shock (hypoperfusion)

Handoff Report to Emergency Department Staff

Student: The patient's condition deteriorated during transport.

PROCTOR: Noted.

Critical Criteria:

❑ Did not transport patient within the (10) minute time limit

Critical Criteria

(Inform the student of items missed, if any.)

❑ Pass ❑ Fail Date: ______________________

Proctor Comments: ______________________

____

____

Dispatch Information

PROCTOR: EMS 10, respond to a 16-year-old female who has fallen from a trampoline onto a concrete sidewalk. She is conscious and breathing.

Pre-scene Action (BSI)

Student: I am wearing nonlatex gloves, safety glasses, mask, and gown.
PROCTOR: Noted.

Critical Criteria:
- ❑ Did not take, or verbalize, body substance isolation (BSI) precautions when necessary

Scene Size-up

Scene Safety

Student: Is the scene safe?
PROCTOR: Yes.

Mechanism of Injury

Student: What was the mechanism of injury?
PROCTOR: Fall. The patient was playing on a trampoline when she fell onto the sidewalk. She got up, walked around, and then collapsed to the ground.

Number of Patients

Student: How many patients are there?
PROCTOR: One.

Additional Resources

Student: I would call for advanced life support (ALS) assistance.
PROCTOR: Noted.

C-Spine Stabilization

Student: On the basis of the mechanism of injury, I would stabilize the cervical spine (c-spine) in a neutral in-line position.
PROCTOR: Noted.

Critical Criteria:
- ❑ Did not determine scene safety
- ❑ Did not assess for spinal protection
- ❑ Did not provide for spinal protection when indicated

Initial Assessment

Student: As I perform midline c-spine stabilization, I identify myself and ask the patient not to move.
PROCTOR: Noted.

General Impression

Student: My general impression is that the patient's condition is unstable.
PROCTOR: Noted.

Responsiveness/Level of Consciousness

Student: What is the patient's level of consciousness?
PROCTOR: Alert and very upset.

Chief Complaint/Apparent Life Threats

Student: What is the patient's chief complaint?
PROCTOR: The patient is complaining of being unable to move her legs.
Student: There are apparent life threats; the life threats are spinal shock and the mechanism of injury.
PROCTOR: Noted.

Assess the Airway and Breathing

Student: Is the airway open? Is the patient breathing?
PROCTOR: Yes, the airway is open and the patient is breathing.

Assessment

Student: What are the rate and the quality of breathing?
PROCTOR: Rate: Rapid. Quality: Diaphragmatic.

Provide Oxygen

Student: I am assisting ventilations with a bag-valve device with 100% oxygen.
PROCTOR: Noted.

Ensure Adequate Ventilation

Student: I am assisting ventilations with a bag-valve device.
PROCTOR: Noted.

Injury Management

Student: I will direct my partner to take over c-spine control and bag-valve ventilations as I continue the assessment.
PROCTOR: Noted.

Assess Circulation

Student: I am assessing the patient's circulation.
PROCTOR: Noted.

Assess for and Control Major Bleeding

Student: Do I find any major bleeding?
PROCTOR: No.

Assess the Pulse

Student: What are the rate and the quality of pulses?
PROCTOR: Rate: Within normal limits. Quality: Normal.

Assess the Skin

Student: I am assessing the skin. What are the color, temperature, and condition of the skin?
PROCTOR: Color: Normal. Temperature: Normal. Condition: Dry.

Identify Priority Patients/Make Transport Decision

Student: The patient is a high priority and is a load-and-go. I will begin packaging and transport to a trauma center.
PROCTOR: Noted.

Critical Criteria:
- ❑ Did not provide high concentration of oxygen
- ❑ Did not find or manage problems associated with airway, breathing, hemorrhage, or shock (hypoperfusion)
- ❑ Did not differentiate patient's need for transportation versus continued assessment at the scene
- ❑ Did other detailed examination before assessing the airway, breathing and circulation

Focused History and Physical Examination/Rapid Trauma Assessment

Select the Appropriate Assessment (Focused or Rapid)

Student: I am selecting the rapid physical exam to identify and treat life threats. I am checking for DCAP-BTLS. This acronym stands for deformities, contusions, abrasions, punctures, penetrations, and paradoxical motion in the chest, and burns, tenderness, lacerations, and swelling.
PROCTOR: Noted.

Head

Student: I am rapidly assessing the head.
PROCTOR: There is a hematoma or a deformity felt on the back of the head.

Neck

Student: I am rapidly assessing the neck.
PROCTOR: There is deformity noted to the cervical spine.
Student: I will apply a cervical collar as soon as possible.
PROCTOR: Noted.

Chest

Student: I am rapidly assessing the chest.
PROCTOR: The patient appears to be breathing only with her diaphragm.

▸ **Abdomen/Pelvis**

Student: I am rapidly assessing the abdomen.
PROCTOR: There are no obvious injuries.
Student: I am rapidly assessing the pelvis.
PROCTOR: There are no obvious injuries.

▸ **Extremities**

Student: I am rapidly assessing the extremities.
PROCTOR: The patient is unable to move her extremities.

▸ **Assess Motor, Sensory, and Circulatory Function**

Student: I am checking for DCAP-BTLS. I am also checking motor and sensory function, and pulses. Right leg?
PROCTOR: There is no purposeful motion. Motor and sensory functions are absent. Pulses are present.
Student: Left leg?
PROCTOR: There is no purposeful motion. Motor and sensory functions are absent. Pulses are present.
Student: Right arm?
PROCTOR: There is no purposeful motion. Motor and sensory functions are absent. Pulses are present.
Student: Left arm?
PROCTOR: There is no purposeful motion. Motor and sensory functions are absent. Pulses are present.

▸ **Posterior**

Student: I will rapidly assess the back. We will now log roll the patient as a unit to check the back. The person at the head will count to three and we will roll the patient.
PROCTOR: Noted.

▸ **Assess the Thorax**

Student: I am assessing the thorax. Do I find injuries?
PROCTOR: No.

▸ **Assess the Lumbar Area**

Student: I am assessing the flanks and lumbar area. Do I find injuries?
PROCTOR: No.

▸ **Assess the Entire Backside**

Student: I am assessing the entire backside. Do I find injuries?
PROCTOR: No.

▸ **Manage Secondary Injuries/Wounds**

Student: We will apply a cervical collar and backboard with full immobilization per local protocol, if not yet done, at this time.
PROCTOR: Noted.
Student: Are there any changes in motor and sensory functions or pulses?
PROCTOR: No.
ALS Student: I will establish two large-bore IVs while en route to the hospital and administer a bolus of 20 mL/kg to maintain a systolic blood pressure of 90 mm Hg. I will be prepared to intubate using rapid sequence intubation (RSI) per local protocol.
ALS Proctor: Noted.

▸ **Reevaluate Transport Decision**

Student: This patient is a load-and-go due to dry or neurologic shock.
PROCTOR: Noted.

▾ Baseline Vital Signs

Student: What are the patient's baseline vital signs, including blood pressure, pulse, respirations, pulse oximetry, and level of consciousness?
PROCTOR: Blood pressure, 122/72 mm Hg; pulse rate, 90 beats/min; respirations, 24 breaths/min; pulse oximetry reading, 96%; and the patient is alert.

▾ SAMPLE History

Student: At this time I will gather a SAMPLE history from the patient or family. What are the patient's signs and symptoms?
PROCTOR: Pain in the neck.
Student: Allergies?
PROCTOR: No allergies.
Student: Medications?
PROCTOR: Asthma medications and inhaler.
Student: Pertinent past medical history?
PROCTOR: Asthma.
Student: Last oral intake?
PROCTOR: 3 hours ago.
Student: Events leading up to the incident?
PROCTOR: The patient was jumping up and down on a trampoline when she fell to the sidewalk, landing on the back of her head and neck. She then stood up, walked around, and suddenly collapsed.

Critical Criteria:
- ❑ Did not differentiate patient's need for transportation versus continued assessment at the scene
- ❑ Did not provide for spinal protection when indicated

▾ Detailed Physical Examination

Student: I am conducting the detailed physical exam. I am looking for DCAP-BTLS.
PROCTOR: Noted. The detailed physical exam will be performed during transport.

▾ Assess the Head

Student: I am assessing the head. Do I find any DCAP-BTLS? Do I find any evidence of Battle's sign or raccoon eyes?
PROCTOR: There is a large bump on the back of the head.

▸ **Inspect and Palpate the Head and Ears**

Student: I am assessing the head and ears.
PROCTOR: There is a large bump on the back of the head.

▸ **Assess the Eyes**

Student: I am assessing the eyes. Are the pupils equal, round, and regular in size, and react properly to light (PEARRL)?
PROCTOR: They are PEARRL.

▸ **Assess the Facial Area Including Oral and Nasal Areas**

Student: I am assessing the face, nose, and mouth. Do I see any discharge or hear any obstructions?
PROCTOR: No.

▾ Assess the Neck

▸ **Inspect and Palpate the Neck**

Student: I am assessing the neck for DCAP-BTLS.
PROCTOR: The neck was previously assessed and now there is a cervical collar in place.

▸ **Assess for Jugular Vein Distention**

Student: Do I find any jugular vein distention (JVD)?
PROCTOR: No.

▸ **Assess for Tracheal Deviation**

Student: Do I see any tracheal deviation?
PROCTOR: No.

▾ Assess the Chest

Student: I am assessing the chest for DCAP-BTLS.
PROCTOR: Noted.

▸ **Inspect**

Student: What do I see when I look at the chest?
PROCTOR: The patient is breathing with her diaphragm.
Student: Does the chest appear symmetric?
PROCTOR: Yes.

▸ **Palpate**

Student: When I touch the chest, do I feel crepitus or a flail segment?
PROCTOR: No.

▸ **Auscultate**

Student: Are lung sounds present in all fields?
PROCTOR: Yes.
Student: Do I hear any sucking sounds from the chest?
PROCTOR: No.

▼ Assess the Abdomen/Pelvis

▸ **Assess the Abdomen**

Student: I am assessing the abdomen for DCAP-BTLS. I am assessing all four quadrants. Do I find any problems?

PROCTOR: No.

▸ **Assess the Pelvis**

Student: I am assessing the pelvis for DCAP-BTLS. Is the pelvis stable?

PROCTOR: Yes.

▼ Assess the Genitalia/Perineum as Needed (Verbalize in Training)

Student: I am assessing the genitalia/perineum as necessary for DCAP-BTLS.

PROCTOR: The patient is incontinent of urine.

▼ Assess the Extremities

▸ **Inspect**

Student: I am assessing the lower and upper extremities for DCAP-BTLS. Do I find anything?

PROCTOR: No.

▸ **Palpate**

Student: Do I feel anything unusual?

PROCTOR: No.

▸ **Assess Motor, Sensory, and Circulatory Function**

Student: I am checking for DCAP-BTLS, motor and sensory function, and pulses. Right leg?

PROCTOR: There is no purposeful motion. Motor and sensory functions are absent. Pulses are present.

Student: Left leg?

PROCTOR: There is no purposeful motion. Motor and sensory functions are absent. Pulses are present.

Student: Right arm?

PROCTOR: There is no purposeful motion. Motor and sensory functions are absent. Pulses are present.

Student: Left arm?

PROCTOR: There is no purposeful motion. Motor and sensory functions are absent. Pulses are present.

▼ Assess the Posterior

Note: This portion of the detailed physical exam would not be done if the patient were previously backboarded per local protocol.

Student: We will not check the back since it was previously checked and the patient is backboarded.

PROCTOR: Noted.

▼ Manage Secondary Injuries/Wounds

Student: I would direct my partner to maintain the airway and ventilations.

PROCTOR: Noted.

▼ Reassess Vital Signs

Student: I will reassess vital signs and mental status.

PROCTOR: Blood pressure, 100/60 mm Hg; pulse rate, 80 beats/min; respirations, per bag-valve device; pulse oximetry reading, 96%; and the patient is alert.

Student: The vital signs are deteriorating.

PROCTOR: Noted.

▼ Reassess Interventions

Student: I will reassess my interventions: airway, breathing, bag-valve device, and oxygen; immobilization and straps; and treatment for shock.

PROCTOR: Noted.

ALS Student: I will reassess basic life support (BLS) interventions, plus the following: two large-bore IVs, and consider rapid sequence intubation (RSI) per local protocol.

ALS Proctor: Noted.

Critical Criteria:
- ☐ Did not find or manage problems associated with airway, breathing, hemorrhage or shock (hypoperfusion)

▼ Radio Report

(Provided by the student.)

PROCTOR: Noted.

▼ Ongoing Assessment

▼ Repeat Vital Signs

Student: I will reassess vital signs and mental status.

PROCTOR: Blood pressure, 90/50 mm Hg; pulse rate, 80 beats/min; respirations, per bag-valve device; pulse oximetry reading, 96%; and the patient is alert.

Student: The vital signs have deteriorated.

PROCTOR: Noted.

▼ Check Interventions

Student: I will check my interventions: airway, breathing, bag-valve device, and oxygen; immobilization and straps; and treatment for shock.

PROCTOR: Noted.

ALS Student: I will check BLS interventions, plus the following: maintain the blood pressure via two large-bore IVs.

ALS Proctor: Noted.

Critical Criteria:
- ☐ Did not find or manage problems associated with airway, breathing, hemorrhage or shock (hypoperfusion)

▼ Handoff Report to Emergency Department Staff

Student: The patient's condition deteriorated during transport.

PROCTOR: Noted.

Critical Criteria:
- ☐ Did not transport patient within the (10) minute time limit

▼ Critical Criteria

(Inform the student of items missed, if any.)

☐ Pass ☐ Fail Date: ____________________

Proctor Comments: ____________________

Notes

Dispatch Information

PROCTOR: EMS 10, respond to an 82-year-old female who has cut her hand on a metal can. She is conscious and breathing.

Pre-scene Action (BSI)

Student: I am wearing nonlatex gloves, safety glasses, mask, and gown.
PROCTOR: Noted.

Critical Criteria:
- ❑ Did not take, or verbalize, body substance isolation (BSI) precautions when necessary

Scene Size-up

Scene Safety

Student: Is the scene safe?
PROCTOR: Yes.

Mechanism of Injury

Student: What was the mechanism of injury?
PROCTOR: Penetrating trauma. The patient was opening a can with a can opener when she cut her thumb.

Number of Patients

Student: How many patients are there?
PROCTOR: One.

Additional Resources

Student: No additional resources are needed.
PROCTOR: Noted.

C-Spine Stabilization

Student: I would not stabilize the cervical spine (c-spine).
PROCTOR: Noted.

Critical Criteria:
- ❑ Did not determine scene safety
- ❑ Did not assess for spinal protection
- ❑ Did not provide for spinal protection when indicated

Initial Assessment

Student: I identify myself and ask the patient not to move.
PROCTOR: Noted.

General Impression

Student: My general impression is that the patient's condition is stable.
PROCTOR: Noted.

Responsiveness/Level of Consciousness

Student: What is the patient's level of consciousness?
PROCTOR: Alert.

Chief Complaint/Apparent Life Threats

Student: What is the patient's chief complaint?
PROCTOR: The patient is complaining of a cut thumb that will not stop bleeding.
Student: There are no apparent life threats.
PROCTOR: Noted.

Assess the Airway and Breathing

Student: Is the airway open? Is the patient breathing?
PROCTOR: Yes, the airway is open and the patient is breathing.

▸ Assessment

Student: What are the rate and the quality of breathing?
PROCTOR: Rate: Within normal limits. Quality: Normal.

▸ Provide Oxygen

Student: I am applying oxygen at 15 L/min via nonrebreathing mask.
PROCTOR: Noted.

▸ Ensure Adequate Ventilation

Student: The patient has adequate ventilations at this time.
PROCTOR: Noted.

Injury Management

Student: I will direct my partner to control bleeding with a dressing and direct pressure as I continue the assessment.
PROCTOR: Noted.

Assess Circulation

Student: I am assessing the patient's circulation.
PROCTOR: Noted.

▸ Assess for and Control Major Bleeding

Student: Do I find any major bleeding?
PROCTOR: Yes, the thumb is still bleeding.
Student: I would continue with direct pressure and apply a pressure dressing.
PROCTOR: Noted. Bleeding is now being controlled.

▸ Assess the Pulse

Student: What are the rate and the quality of pulses?
PROCTOR: Rate: Within normal limits. Quality: Bounding.

▸ Assess the Skin

Student: I am assessing the skin. What are the color, temperature, and condition of the skin?
PROCTOR: Color: Pale. Temperature: Cool. Condition: Moist.

Identify Priority Patients/Make Transport Decision

Student: The patient is a low priority and does not require immediate transport.
PROCTOR: Noted.

Critical Criteria:
- ❑ Did not provide high concentration of oxygen
- ❑ Did not find or manage problems associated with airway, breathing, hemorrhage or shock (hypoperfusion)
- ❑ Did not differentiate patient's need for transportation versus continued assessment at the scene
- ❑ Did other detailed examination before assessing the airway, breathing and circulation

Focused History and Physical Examination/Rapid Trauma Assessment

Select the Appropriate Assessment (Focused or Rapid)

Student: I am selecting the focused assessment.
PROCTOR: Noted.
Student: I would assess whether the cut on the thumb is the only injury.
PROCTOR: It is the only injury.
Student: I would estimate blood loss based on the time of the injury and the evidence of blood.
PROCTOR: Noted. She has lost about 100 mL of blood.
Student: I will apply direct pressure and a dressing.
PROCTOR: Noted.

Baseline Vital Signs

Student: What are the patient's baseline vital signs, including blood pressure, pulse, respirations, pulse oximetry, and level of consciousness?
PROCTOR: Blood pressure, 138/86 mm Hg; pulse rate, 96 beats/min; respirations, 20 breaths/min; pulse oximetry reading, 96%; and the patient is alert.

▼ **SAMPLE History**

Student: At this time I will gather a SAMPLE history from the patient or family. What are the patient's signs and symptoms?
PROCTOR: Pain in the thumb.
Student: Allergies?
PROCTOR: Sulfa medications.
Student: Medications?
PROCTOR: Blood thinners and nitroglycerin.
Student: Pertinent past medical history?
PROCTOR: Heart problems.
Student: Last oral intake?
PROCTOR: 4 hours ago.
Student: Events leading up to the incident?
PROCTOR: The patient was opening a can with a can opener and cut her thumb.
Student: Interventions?
PROCTOR: She attempted to control the bleeding with a rag.

Critical Criteria:
- ❑ Did not differentiate patient's need for transportation versus continued assessment at the scene
- ❑ Did not provide for spinal protection when indicated

Detailed Physical Examination

Student: I would not conduct a detailed physical exam.
PROCTOR: Noted.

▼ **Manage Secondary Injuries/Wounds**

Student: I would direct my partner to control bleeding.
PROCTOR: Noted.

▼ **Reassess Vital Signs**

Student: I will reassess vital signs and mental status.
PROCTOR: Blood pressure, 142/82 mm Hg; pulse rate, 88 beats/min; respirations, 20 breaths/min; pulse oximetry reading, 97%; and the patient is alert.
Student: The vital signs have not changed significantly.
PROCTOR: Noted.

▼ **Reassess Interventions**

Student: I will reassess my interventions: oxygen and bleeding control.
PROCTOR: Noted.

Critical Criteria:
- ❑ Did not find or manage problems associated with airway, breathing, hemorrhage or shock (hypoperfusion)

Radio Report

(Provided by the student.)
PROCTOR: Noted.

Ongoing Assessment

▼ **Repeat Vital Signs**

Student: I will reassess vital signs and mental status.
PROCTOR: Blood pressure, 136/78 mm Hg; pulse rate, 82 beats/min; respirations, 20 breaths/min; pulse oximetry reading, 97%; and the patient is alert.
Student: The vital signs have not changed significantly.
PROCTOR: Noted.

▼ **Check Interventions**

Student: I will check my interventions: oxygen and bleeding control.
PROCTOR: Noted.

Critical Criteria:
- ❑ Did not find or manage problems associated with airway, breathing, hemorrhage or shock (hypoperfusion)

Handoff Report to Emergency Department Staff

Student: There was no change in the patient's condition during transport.
PROCTOR: Noted.

Critical Criteria:
- ❑ Did not transport patient within the (10) minute time limit

Critical Criteria

(Inform the student of items missed, if any.)

❑ Pass ❑ Fail Date: ______________________

Proctor Comments: ______________________

____

____

CASE 34

Dispatch Information

PROCTOR: EMS 10, respond to a one-car motor vehicle collision. A 53-year-old female has been ejected and thrown down a cliff. She is alert and breathing. Police are on scene.

Pre-scene Action (BSI)

Student: I am wearing appropriate high-visibility personal protective equipment suitable for extrication, a helmet, extrication gloves, nonlatex gloves, and safety glasses.
PROCTOR: Noted.

Critical Criteria:
- ❑ Did not take, or verbalize, body substance isolation (BSI) precautions when necessary

Scene Size-up

Scene Safety

Student: Is the scene safe?
PROCTOR: Yes. You will enter the scene through a lower road.

Mechanism of Injury

Student: What was the mechanism of injury?
PROCTOR: Motor vehicle collision. The patient was driving without a seat belt; she was ejected from the car and caught in a barbed-wire fence that removed the skin from her back, buttocks, and legs. She is at the bottom of a cliff.

Number of Patients

Student: How many patients are there?
PROCTOR: One.

Additional Resources

Student: I would call for advanced life support (ALS) assistance and additional resources: fire/rescue.
PROCTOR: Noted.

C-Spine Stabilization

Student: On the basis of the mechanism of injury, I would stabilize the cervical spine (c-spine) in a neutral in-line position.
PROCTOR: Noted.

Critical Criteria:
- ❑ Did not determine scene safety
- ❑ Did not assess for spinal protection
- ❑ Did not provide for spinal protection when indicated

Initial Assessment

Student: As I perform midline c-spine stabilization, I identify myself and ask the patient not to move.
PROCTOR: Noted.

General Impression

Student: My general impression is that the patient's condition is unstable.
PROCTOR: Noted.

Responsiveness/Level of Consciousness

Student: What is the patient's level of consciousness?
PROCTOR: Alert.

Chief Complaint/Apparent Life Threats

Student: What is the patient's chief complaint?
PROCTOR: The patient is complaining of the skin of her backside being removed by the barbed-wire fence.
Student: There is an apparent life threat; the life threat is the mechanism of injury.
PROCTOR: Noted.

Assess the Airway and Breathing

Student: Is the airway open? Is the patient breathing?
PROCTOR: Yes, the airway is open and the patient is breathing.

Assessment

Student: What are the rate and the quality of breathing?
PROCTOR: Rate: A little fast. Quality: Normal.

Provide Oxygen

Student: I am applying oxygen at 15 L/min via nonrebreathing mask.
PROCTOR: Noted.

Ensure Adequate Ventilation

Student: The patient has adequate ventilations at this time.
PROCTOR: Noted.

Injury Management

Student: I will direct my partner to maintain c-spine control as I continue the assessment.
PROCTOR: Noted.

Assess Circulation

Student: I am assessing the patient's circulation.
PROCTOR: Noted.

Assess for and Control Major Bleeding

Student: Do I find any major bleeding?
PROCTOR: Yes, the patient has bleeding noted throughout her backside where skin has been removed by the barbed-wire fence.
Student: We will log roll the patient and control bleeding with trauma dressings and direct pressure.
PROCTOR: Noted.

Assess the Pulse

Student: What are the rate and the quality of pulses?
PROCTOR: Rate: Tachycardic. Quality: Bounding.

Assess the Skin

Student: I am assessing the skin. What are the color, temperature, and condition of the skin?
PROCTOR: Color: Flushed. Temperature: Warm. Condition: Moist.

Identify Priority Patients/Make Transport Decision

Student: The patient is a high priority and is a load-and-go. I will begin packaging and transport.
PROCTOR: Noted.

Critical Criteria:
- ❑ Did not provide high concentration of oxygen
- ❑ Did not find or manage problems associated with airway, breathing, hemorrhage or shock (hypoperfusion)
- ❑ Did not differentiate patient's need for transportation versus continued assessment at the scene
- ❑ Did other detailed examination before assessing the airway, breathing and circulation

Focused History and Physical Examination/Rapid Trauma Assessment

Select the Appropriate Assessment (Focused or Rapid)

Student: I am selecting the rapid physical exam to identify and treat life threats. I am checking for DCAP-BTLS. This acronym stands for deformities, contusions, abrasions, punctures, penetrations, and paradoxical motion in the chest, and burns, tenderness, lacerations, and swelling.
PROCTOR: Noted.

Head

Student: I am rapidly assessing the head.
PROCTOR: There are no obvious injuries.

Neck

Student: I am rapidly assessing the neck.
PROCTOR: There are no obvious injuries.

Student: I will apply a cervical collar.
PROCTOR: Noted.

▸ **Chest**

Student: I am rapidly assessing the chest. What are the lung sounds?
PROCTOR: There are no obvious injuries. Lung sounds are clear bilaterally.

▸ **Abdomen/Pelvis**

Student: I am rapidly assessing the abdomen.
PROCTOR: There are no obvious injuries.
Student: I am rapidly assessing the pelvis.
PROCTOR: There are no obvious injuries.

▸ **Extremities**

Student: I am rapidly assessing the extremities.
PROCTOR: The patient has an obvious deformity to her right humerus.
Student: I will splint the injury per local protocol.
PROCTOR: Noted.

▸ **Assess Motor, Sensory, and Circulatory Function**

Student: I am checking for DCAP-BTLS. I am also checking motor and sensory function, and pulses. Right leg?
PROCTOR: Bleeding from the backside is controlled. Motor and sensory functions are present. Pulses are present.
Student: Left leg?
PROCTOR: Bleeding from the backside is controlled. Motor and sensory functions are present. Pulses are present.
Student: Right arm?
PROCTOR: The right arm is fractured at the humerus. Motor and sensory functions are present. Pulses are present.
Student: I will splint the arm en route to the hospital.
PROCTOR: Noted.
Student: Left arm?
PROCTOR: Negative DCAP-BTLS. Motor and sensory functions are present. Pulses are present.

▸ **Posterior**

Student: I will rapidly assess the back. We will now log roll the patient as a unit to check the back. The person at the head will count to three and we will roll the patient.
PROCTOR: The skin from the patient's back, buttocks, and upper legs is missing. This was treated during the initial assessment.
Student: I will assess trauma dressings and bleeding control.
PROCTOR: Noted. Bleeding is controlled.

▸ **Assess the Thorax**

Student: I am assessing the thorax. Do I find injuries?
PROCTOR: She has multiple large abrasions and skin avulsions that have been dressed.

▸ **Assess the Lumbar Area**

Student: I am assessing the flanks and lumbar area. Do I find injuries?
PROCTOR: She has multiple large abrasions and skin avulsions.
Student: I will apply dressings and control bleeding.
PROCTOR: Noted.

▸ **Assess the Entire Backside**

Student: I am assessing the entire backside. Do I find injuries?
PROCTOR: She has multiple large abrasions and skin avulsions.
Student: I will apply dressings and control bleeding.
PROCTOR: Noted.

▸ **Manage Secondary Injuries/Wounds**

Student: We will apply a cervical collar and backboard with full immobilization per local protocol, if not yet done, at this time.
PROCTOR: Noted.
Student: Are there any changes in motor and sensory functions or pulses?
PROCTOR: No.

ALS Student: I will establish two large-bore IVs while en route to the hospital and maintain a systolic blood pressure of 90 mm Hg.
ALS Proctor: Noted.

▸ **Reevaluate Transport Decision**

Student: This patient is a load-and-go due to the mechanism of injury.
PROCTOR: Noted.

▾ Baseline Vital Signs

Student: What are the patient's baseline vital signs, including blood pressure, pulse, respirations, pulse oximetry, and level of consciousness?
PROCTOR: Blood pressure, 156/90 mm Hg; pulse rate, 134 beats/min; respirations, 24 breaths/min; pulse oximetry reading, 97%; and the patient is alert.

▾ SAMPLE History

Student: At this time I will gather a SAMPLE history from the patient or family. What are the patient's signs and symptoms?
PROCTOR: Pain to her backside.
Student: Allergies?
PROCTOR: Penicillin (PCN).
Student: Medications?
PROCTOR: No medications.
Student: Pertinent past medical history?
PROCTOR: No pertinent medical history.
Student: Last oral intake?
PROCTOR: 2 hours ago.
Student: Events leading up to the incident?
PROCTOR: The patient was driving at high speed in rainy conditions when her car ran off the road. She was not wearing a seat belt and was ejected from the vehicle. The skin on her backside was removed by a barbed-wire fence as she fell down the cliff. The patient weighs more than 300 pounds.
Student: I would enlist the fire and rescue personnel for packaging and moving assistance.
PROCTOR: Noted.

Critical Criteria:
- ❑ Did not differentiate patient's need for transportation versus continued assessment at the scene
- ❑ Did not provide for spinal protection when indicated

▼ Detailed Physical Examination

Student: I am conducting the detailed physical exam. I am looking for DCAP-BTLS.
PROCTOR: Noted. The detailed physical exam will be performed during transport.

▾ Assess the Head

Student: I am assessing the head. Do I find any DCAP-BTLS? Do I find any evidence of Battle's sign or raccoon eyes?
PROCTOR: No.

▸ **Inspect and Palpate the Head and Ears**

Student: I am assessing the head and ears.
PROCTOR: There are no obvious injuries.

▸ **Assess the Eyes**

Student: I am assessing the eyes. Are the pupils equal, round, and regular in size, and react properly to light (PEARRL)?
PROCTOR: They are PEARRL.

▸ **Assess the Facial Area Including Oral and Nasal Areas**

Student: I am assessing the face, nose, and mouth. Do I see any discharge or hear any obstructions?
PROCTOR: No.

Assess the Neck

Inspect and Palpate the Neck

Student: I am assessing the neck for DCAP-BTLS.
PROCTOR: There are no obvious injuries.

Assess for Jugular Vein Distention

Student: Do I find any jugular vein distention (JVD)?
PROCTOR: No.

Assess for Tracheal Deviation

Student: Do I see any tracheal deviation?
PROCTOR: No.

Assess the Chest

Student: I am assessing the chest for DCAP-BTLS.
PROCTOR: Noted.

Inspect

Student: What do I see when I look at the chest?
PROCTOR: There are no obvious injuries.
Student: Does the chest appear symmetric?
PROCTOR: Yes.

Palpate

Student: When I touch the chest, do I feel crepitus or a flail segment?
PROCTOR: No.

Auscultate

Student: Are lung sounds present in all fields?
PROCTOR: Yes.
Student: Do I hear any sucking sounds from the chest?
PROCTOR: No.

Assess the Abdomen/Pelvis

Assess the Abdomen

Student: I am assessing the abdomen for DCAP-BTLS. I am assessing all four quadrants. Do I find any problems?
PROCTOR: No.

Assess the Pelvis

Student: I am assessing the pelvis for DCAP-BTLS. Is the pelvis stable?
PROCTOR: Yes.

Assess the Genitalia/Perineum as Needed (Verbalize in Training)

Student: I am assessing the genitalia/perineum as necessary for DCAP-BTLS.
PROCTOR: The area is unremarkable.

Assess the Extremities

Inspect

Student: I am assessing the lower and upper extremities for DCAP-BTLS. Do I find anything?
PROCTOR: Yes, the lacerations and avulsions.

Palpate

Student: Do I feel anything unusual?
PROCTOR: Yes, the fracture to the right arm.
Student: I will splint the right arm.
PROCTOR: Noted.

Assess Motor, Sensory, and Circulatory Function

Student: I am checking for DCAP-BTLS, motor and sensory function, and pulses. Right leg?
PROCTOR: Bleeding from the backside is dressed per local protocol. Motor and sensory functions are present. Pulses are present.
Student: Left leg?
PROCTOR: Bleeding from the backside is dressed per local protocol. Motor and sensory functions are present. Pulses are present.
Student: Right arm?
PROCTOR: The right arm is splinted. Motor and sensory functions are present. Pulses are present.
Student: Left arm?
PROCTOR: Negative DCAP-BTLS. Motor and sensory functions are present. Pulses are present.

Assess the Posterior

Note: This portion of the detailed physical exam would not be done if the patient were previously backboarded per local protocol.
Student: We will not check the back since it was previously checked and the patient is backboarded.
PROCTOR: Noted.

Manage Secondary Injuries/Wounds

Student: I would direct my partner to monitor the patient.
PROCTOR: Noted.

Reassess Vital Signs

Student: I will reassess vital signs and mental status.
PROCTOR: Blood pressure, 148/88 mm Hg; pulse rate, 136 beats/min; respirations, 24 breaths/min; pulse oximetry reading, 98%; and the patient is alert.
Student: The vital signs have not changed significantly.
PROCTOR: Noted.

Reassess Interventions

Student: I will reassess my interventions: oxygen, bleeding control, full immobilization, and a splint to the right arm, and treatment for possible shock. I will ensure that the patient is secure on the backboard prior to being placed in the Stokes or rescue basket and transported. I will work with the haul team to ensure safe patient movement.
PROCTOR: Noted.
ALS Student: I will reassess basic life support (BLS) interventions, plus the following: establish two large-bore IVs and perform cardiac monitoring.
ALS Proctor: Noted. The cardiac monitor shows sinus tachycardia.

Critical Criteria:
- ❑ Did not find or manage problems associated with airway, breathing, hemorrhage or shock (hypoperfusion)

Radio Report

(Provided by the student.)
PROCTOR: Noted.

Ongoing Assessment

Repeat Vital Signs

Student: I will reassess vital signs and mental status.
PROCTOR: Blood pressure, 142/82 mm Hg; pulse rate, 128 beats/min; respirations, 24 breaths/min; pulse oximetry reading, 98%; and the patient is alert.
Student: The vital signs have not changed significantly.
PROCTOR: Noted.

Check Interventions

Student: I will check my interventions: oxygen, bleeding control, full immobilization, and a splint to the right arm, and treatment for possible shock. I will continuously monitor the patient during the raise operation.

PROCTOR: Noted.

ALS Student: I will check BLS interventions, plus the following: two large-bore IVs and cardiac monitor.

ALS Proctor: Noted. The cardiac monitor shows sinus tachycardia.

Critical Criteria:
- ❑ Did not find or manage problems associated with airway, breathing, hemorrhage or shock (hypoperfusion)

Handoff Report to Emergency Department Staff

Student: There was no change in the patient's condition during transport.

PROCTOR: Noted.

Critical Criteria:
- ❑ Did not transport patient within the (10) minute time limit

Critical Criteria

(Inform the student of items missed, if any.)

❑ Pass ❑ Fail Date: ____________________

Proctor Comments: ____________________

____

____

CASE 35

Dispatch Information

PROCTOR: EMS 10, respond to an assault of a 36-year-old male trying to buy drugs. The dealers tied his hands with an extension cord, and then beat his hands and head with an axe handle. The patient is conscious and breathing. Police are on the scene.

Pre-scene Action (BSI)

Student: I am wearing nonlatex gloves, safety glasses, mask, and gown.
PROCTOR: Noted.

> **Critical Criteria:**
> ❑ Did not take, or verbalize, body substance isolation (BSI) precautions when necessary

Scene Size-up

Scene Safety

Student: Is the scene safe?
PROCTOR: Yes, police are on scene and you are given clearance to enter.

Mechanism of Injury

Student: What was the mechanism of injury?
PROCTOR: Blunt trauma. The patient was assaulted with an axe handle to his head and hands.

Number of Patients

Student: How many patients are there?
PROCTOR: One.

Additional Resources

Student: I would call for advanced life support (ALS) assistance.
PROCTOR: Noted.

C-Spine Stabilization

Student: On the basis of the mechanism of injury, I would stabilize the cervical spine (c-spine) in a neutral in-line position.
PROCTOR: Noted.

> **Critical Criteria:**
> ❑ Did not determine scene safety
> ❑ Did not assess for spinal protection
> ❑ Did not provide for spinal protection when indicated

Initial Assessment

Student: As I perform midline c-spine stabilization, I identify myself and ask the patient not to move.
PROCTOR: Noted.

General Impression

Student: My general impression is that the patient's condition is unstable.
PROCTOR: Noted.

Responsiveness/Level of Consciousness

Student: What is the patient's level of consciousness?
PROCTOR: He is very anxious.

Chief Complaint/Apparent Life Threats

Student: What is the patient's chief complaint?
PROCTOR: The patient is complaining of pain in his hands and his head.
Student: There is an apparent life threat; the life threat is the head injury.
PROCTOR: Noted.

Assess the Airway and Breathing

Student: Is the airway open? Is the patient breathing?
PROCTOR: Yes, the airway is open and the patient is breathing.

Assessment

Student: What are the rate and the quality of breathing?
PROCTOR: Rate: Within normal limits. Quality: Normal.

Provide Oxygen

Student: I am applying oxygen at 15 L/min via nonrebreathing mask.
PROCTOR: Noted.

Ensure Adequate Ventilation

Student: The patient has adequate ventilations at this time.
PROCTOR: Noted.

Injury Management

Student: I will direct my partner to take over c-spine control as I continue the assessment.
PROCTOR: Noted.

Assess Circulation

Student: I am assessing the patient's circulation.
PROCTOR: Noted.

Assess for and Control Major Bleeding

Student: Do I find any major bleeding?
PROCTOR: You see large open lacerations on top of the patient's head with severe bleeding.
Student: I would apply direct pressure and a dressing. I would also do a halo test.
PROCTOR: Noted. The halo test is positive for cerebrospinal fluid (CSF).

Assess the Pulse

Student: What are the rate and the quality of pulses?
PROCTOR: Rate: Tachycardic. Quality: Bounding.

Assess the Skin

Student: I am assessing the skin. What are the color, temperature, and condition of the skin?
PROCTOR: Color: Flushed. Temperature: Cool. Condition: Moist.

Identify Priority Patients/Make Transport Decision

Student: The patient is a high priority and is a load-and-go. I will begin packaging and transport to a trauma center.
PROCTOR: Noted.

> **Critical Criteria:**
> ❑ Did not provide high concentration of oxygen
> ❑ Did not find or manage problems associated with airway, breathing, hemorrhage or shock (hypoperfusion)
> ❑ Did not differentiate patient's need for transportation versus continued assessment at the scene
> ❑ Did other detailed examination before assessing the airway, breathing and circulation

Focused History and Physical Examination/Rapid Trauma Assessment

Select the Appropriate Assessment (Focused or Rapid)

Student: I am selecting the rapid physical exam to identify and treat life threats. I am checking for DCAP-BTLS. This acronym stands for deformities, contusions, abrasions, punctures, penetrations, and paradoxical motion in the chest, and burns, tenderness, lacerations, and swelling.
PROCTOR: Noted.

Head

Student: I am rapidly assessing the head.
PROCTOR: You notice a large laceration to the top of the head and feel a deformity in the head.
Student: I would continue to control bleeding and dress the head.
PROCTOR: Noted.

▶ **Neck**

Student: I am rapidly assessing the neck.

PROCTOR: Nothing is noted.

Student: I will apply a cervical collar if dictated by local protocol.

PROCTOR: Noted.

▶ **Chest**

Student: I am rapidly assessing the chest. What are the lung sounds?

PROCTOR: There are no obvious injuries. Lung sounds are clear bilaterally.

▶ **Abdomen/Pelvis**

Student: I am rapidly assessing the abdomen.

PROCTOR: There are no obvious injuries.

Student: I am rapidly assessing the pelvis.

PROCTOR: There are no obvious injuries.

▶ **Extremities**

Student: I am rapidly assessing the extremities.

PROCTOR: You see that the patient's hands have been bound and are covered with blood.

Student: I will remove any binding material, assess the hands, and dress the patient's hands en route to the hospital. I will save binding material as evidence.

PROCTOR: Noted.

▶ **Assess Motor, Sensory, and Circulatory Function**

Student: I am checking for DCAP-BTLS. I am also checking motor and sensory function, and pulses. Right leg?

PROCTOR: Negative DCAP-BTLS. Motor and sensory functions are present. Pulses are present.

Student: Left leg?

PROCTOR: Negative DCAP-BTLS. Motor and sensory functions are present. Pulses are present.

Student: Right arm?

PROCTOR: The right arm is swollen and heavily bruised with lacerations and evidence of being bound. Motor and sensory functions are present. Pulses are present.

Student: Left arm?

PROCTOR: The left arm is swollen and heavily bruised with lacerations and evidence of being bound. Motor and sensory functions are present. Pulses are present.

▶ **Posterior**

Student: I will rapidly assess the back. We will now log roll the patient as a unit to check the back. The person at the head will count to three and we will roll the patient.

PROCTOR: Noted.

▶ **Assess the Thorax**

Student: I am assessing the thorax. Do I find injuries?

PROCTOR: No.

▶ **Assess the Lumbar Area**

Student: I am assessing the flanks and lumbar area. Do I find injuries?

PROCTOR: No.

▶ **Assess the Entire Backside**

Student: I am assessing the entire backside. Do I find injuries?

PROCTOR: No.

▶ **Manage Secondary Injuries/Wounds**

Student: We will apply a cervical collar and backboard with full immobilization per local protocol, if not yet done, at this time.

PROCTOR: Noted.

Student: Are there any changes in motor and sensory functions or pulses?

PROCTOR: No.

ALS Student: I will establish two large-bore IVs while en route to the hospital and maintain a systolic blood pressure of 90 mm Hg.

ALS Proctor: Noted.

▶ **Reevaluate Transport Decision**

Student: This patient is a load-and-go due to the head injury.

PROCTOR: Noted.

▼ **Baseline Vital Signs**

Student: What are the patient's baseline vital signs, including blood pressure, pulse, respirations, pulse oximetry, and level of consciousness?

PROCTOR: Blood pressure, 136/88 mm Hg; pulse rate, 114 beats/min; respirations, 16 breaths/min; pulse oximetry reading, 97%; and the patient is tired.

▼ **SAMPLE History**

Student: At this time I will gather a SAMPLE history from the patient or family. What are the patient's signs and symptoms?

PROCTOR: Pain in the hands and head.

Student: Allergies?

PROCTOR: No allergies.

Student: Medications?

PROCTOR: Cocaine.

Student: Pertinent past medical history?

PROCTOR: Drug problems.

Student: Last oral intake?

PROCTOR: 12 hours ago.

Student: Events leading up to the incident?

PROCTOR: The patient was buying drugs when he was beaten.

Critical Criteria:

- ❑ Did not differentiate patient's need for transportation versus continued assessment at the scene
- ❑ Did not provide for spinal protection when indicated

Detailed Physical Examination

Student: I am conducting the detailed physical exam. I am looking for DCAP-BTLS.

PROCTOR: Noted. The detailed physical exam will be performed during transport.

▼ **Assess the Head**

Student: I am assessing the head. Do I find any DCAP-BTLS? Do I find any evidence of Battle's sign or raccoon eyes?

PROCTOR: Yes, there is a deformity to the top of the head consistent with an axe handle. It has been dressed.

▶ **Inspect and Palpate the Head and Ears**

Student: I am assessing the head and ears.

PROCTOR: Cerebrospinal fluid is obvious in the blood.

▶ **Assess the Eyes**

Student: I am assessing the eyes. Are the pupils equal, round, and regular in size, and react properly to light (PEARRL)?

PROCTOR: The left pupil is larger than the right pupil.

▶ **Assess the Facial Area Including Oral and Nasal Areas**

Student: I am assessing the face, nose, and mouth. Do I see any discharge or hear any obstructions?

PROCTOR: No.

▼ **Assess the Neck**

▶ **Inspect and Palpate the Neck**

Student: I am assessing the neck for DCAP-BTLS.

PROCTOR: There are no obvious injuries.

▶ **Assess for Jugular Vein Distention**

Student: Do I find any jugular vein distention (JVD)?

PROCTOR: No.

▶ **Assess for Tracheal Deviation**

Student: Do I see any tracheal deviation?

PROCTOR: No.

▼ **Assess the Chest**

Student: I am assessing the chest for DCAP-BTLS.

PROCTOR: Noted.

▸ **Inspect**

Student: What do I see when I look at the chest?
PROCTOR: There are no obvious injuries.
Student: Does the chest appear symmetric?
PROCTOR: Yes.

▸ **Palpate**

Student: When I touch the chest, do I feel crepitus or a flail segment?
PROCTOR: No.

▸ **Auscultate**

Student: Are lung sounds present in all fields?
PROCTOR: Yes.
Student: Do I hear any sucking sounds from the chest?
PROCTOR: No.

▼ Assess the Abdomen/Pelvis

▸ **Assess the Abdomen**

Student: I am assessing the abdomen for DCAP-BTLS. I am assessing all four quadrants. Do I find any problems?
PROCTOR: No.

▸ **Assess the Pelvis**

Student: I am assessing the pelvis for DCAP-BTLS. Is the pelvis stable?
PROCTOR: Yes.

▼ Assess the Genitalia/Perineum as Needed (Verbalize in Training)

Student: I am assessing the genitalia/perineum as necessary for DCAP-BTLS.
PROCTOR: The area is unremarkable.

▼ Assess the Extremities

▸ **Inspect**

Student: I am assessing the lower and upper extremities for DCAP-BTLS. Do I find anything?
PROCTOR: Yes, the wrists were bound and beaten. They are bruised and swollen.

▸ **Palpate**

Student: Do I feel anything unusual?
PROCTOR: Yes, the hands are swollen and have crepitus.

▸ **Assess Motor, Sensory, and Circulatory Function**

Student: I am checking for DCAP-BTLS, motor and sensory function, and pulses. Right leg?
PROCTOR: Negative DCAP-BTLS. Motor and sensory functions are present. Pulses are present.
Student: Left leg?
PROCTOR: Negative DCAP-BTLS. Motor and sensory functions are present. Pulses are present.
Student: Right arm?
PROCTOR: The right arm is swollen and heavily bruised with lacerations and evidence of being bound. Motor and sensory functions are present. Pulses are present.
Student: Left arm?
PROCTOR: The left arm is swollen and heavily bruised with lacerations and evidence of being bound. Motor and sensory functions are present. Pulses are present.
Student: I will dress and splint the hands and wrists.
PROCTOR: Noted.

▼ Assess the Posterior

Note: This portion of the detailed physical exam would not be done if the patient were previously backboarded per local protocol.
Student: We will not check the back since it was previously checked and the patient is backboarded.
PROCTOR: Noted.

▼ Manage Secondary Injuries/Wounds

Student: I would direct my partner to continuously assess the level of consciousness, bleeding control, and dressings to the head and hands.
PROCTOR: Noted.

▼ Reassess Vital Signs

Student: I will reassess vital signs and mental status.
PROCTOR: Blood pressure, 130/80 mm Hg; pulse rate, 94 beats/min; respirations, 16 breaths/min; pulse oximetry reading, 98%; and the patient is tired.
Student: The vital signs have not changed significantly.
PROCTOR: Noted.

▼ Reassess Interventions

Student: I will reassess my interventions: airway, breathing, and oxygen; circulation and bleeding control; and immobilization, splints, and straps.
PROCTOR: Noted.
ALS Student: I will reassess basic life support (BLS) interventions, plus the following: establish two large-bore IVs, consider rapid sequence intubation (RSI) per local protocol, and perform cardiac monitoring.
ALS Proctor: Noted. The cardiac monitor shows normal sinus rhythm.

Critical Criteria:
- ☐ Did not find or manage problems associated with airway, breathing, hemorrhage or shock (hypoperfusion)

▼ Radio Report

(Provided by the student.)
PROCTOR: Noted.

▼ Ongoing Assessment

▼ Repeat Vital Signs

Student: I will reassess vital signs and mental status.
PROCTOR: Blood pressure, 132/78; pulse rate, 88 beats/min; respirations, 16 breaths/min; pulse oximetry reading, 98%; and the patient is tired.
Student: The vital signs have not changed significantly.
PROCTOR: Noted.

▼ Check Interventions

Student: I will check my interventions: airway, breathing, and oxygen; circulation and bleeding control; and immobilization, splints, and straps.
PROCTOR: Noted.

ALS Student: I will check BLS interventions, plus the following: check IVs, consider RSI per local protocol, and cardiac monitor.

ALS Proctor: Noted. The cardiac monitor shows normal sinus rhythm.

Critical Criteria:

- ❑ Did not find or manage problems associated with airway, breathing, hemorrhage or shock (hypoperfusion)

Handoff Report to Emergency Department Staff

Student: There was no change to the patient's condition during transport.

PROCTOR: Noted.

Critical Criteria:

- ❑ Did not transport patient within the (10) minute time limit

Critical Criteria

(Inform the student of items missed, if any.)

❑ Pass ❑ Fail Date: ____________________

Proctor Comments: ____________________

Dispatch Information

PROCTOR: EMS 10, respond to a one-car motor vehicle collision. The 60-year-old female driver has impaled herself on the gear shifter after striking a concrete culvert. She weighs more than 350 pounds. Police are on the scene.

Pre-scene Action (BSI)

Student: I am wearing nonlatex gloves and safety glasses.
PROCTOR: Noted.

> **Critical Criteria:**
> ❑ Did not take, or verbalize, body substance isolation (BSI) precautions when necessary

Scene Size-up

Scene Safety

Student: Is the scene safe?
PROCTOR: Yes, police are on scene and you are given clearance to enter.

Mechanism of Injury

Student: What was the mechanism of injury?
PROCTOR: Motor vehicle collision. The patient impaled herself on the gear shifter. She has removed herself from the gear shifter prior to your arrival.

Number of Patients

Student: How many patients are there?
PROCTOR: One.

Additional Resources

Student: I would call for advanced life support (ALS) assistance and additional resources: fire/rescue.
PROCTOR: Noted.

C-Spine Stabilization

Student: On the basis of the mechanism of injury, I would stabilize the cervical spine (c-spine) in a neutral in-line position.
PROCTOR: Noted.

> **Critical Criteria:**
> ❑ Did not determine scene safety
> ❑ Did not assess for spinal protection
> ❑ Did not provide for spinal protection when indicated

Initial Assessment

Student: As I perform midline c-spine stabilization, I identify myself and ask the patient not to move.
PROCTOR: Noted.

General Impression

Student: My general impression is that the patient's condition is unstable.
PROCTOR: Noted.

Responsiveness/Level of Consciousness

Student: What is the patient's level of consciousness?
PROCTOR: Alert.

Chief Complaint/Apparent Life Threats

Student: What is the patient's chief complaint?
PROCTOR: The patient is complaining of vaginal, back, and neck pain.
Student: The life threats are the mechanism of injury and impalement.
PROCTOR: Noted.

Assess the Airway and Breathing

Student: Is the airway open? Is the patient breathing?
PROCTOR: Yes, the airway is open and the patient is breathing.

Assessment

Student: What are the rate and the quality of breathing?
PROCTOR: Rate: Tachypneic. Quality: Normal.

Provide Oxygen

Student: I am applying oxygen at 15 L/min via nonrebreathing mask.
PROCTOR: Noted.

Ensure Adequate Ventilation

Student: The patient has adequate ventilations at this time.
PROCTOR: Noted.

Injury Management

Student: I will direct my partner to take over c-spine control as I continue the assessment.
PROCTOR: Noted.

Assess Circulation

Student: I am assessing the patient's circulation.
PROCTOR: Noted.

Assess for and Control Major Bleeding

Student: Do I find any major bleeding?
PROCTOR: No.

Assess the Pulse

Student: What are the rate and the quality of pulses?
PROCTOR: Rate: Tachycardic. Quality: Bounding.

Assess the Skin

Student: I am assessing the skin. What are the color, temperature, and condition of the skin?
PROCTOR: Color: Flushed. Temperature: Normal. Condition: Moist.

Identify Priority Patients/Make Transport Decision

Student: The patient is a high priority and a load-and-go. We will rapidly package and transport to a trauma center.
PROCTOR: Noted.

> **Critical Criteria:**
> ❑ Did not provide high concentration of oxygen
> ❑ Did not find or manage problems associated with airway, breathing, hemorrhage or shock (hypoperfusion)
> ❑ Did not differentiate patient's need for transportation versus continued assessment at the scene
> ❑ Did other detailed examination before assessing the airway, breathing and circulation

Focused History and Physical Examination/Rapid Trauma Assessment

Select the Appropriate Assessment (Focused or Rapid)

Student: I am selecting the rapid physical exam to identify and treat life threats. I am checking for DCAP-BTLS. This acronym stands for deformities, contusions, abrasions, punctures, penetrations, and paradoxical motion in the chest, and burns, tenderness, lacerations, and swelling.
PROCTOR: Noted.

Head

Student: I am rapidly assessing the head.
PROCTOR: There is a large laceration to the top of the head.
Student: I will control bleeding with direct pressure.
PROCTOR: Noted.

Neck

Student: I am rapidly assessing the neck.
PROCTOR: The patient is complaining of pain to the neck.
Student: I will apply a cervical collar.
PROCTOR: Noted.

Chest

Student: I am rapidly assessing the chest. What are the lung sounds?
PROCTOR: There are no obvious injuries. Lung sounds are clear bilaterally.

▸ **Abdomen/Pelvis**

Student: I am rapidly assessing the abdomen.
PROCTOR: There are no obvious injuries.
Student: I am rapidly assessing the pelvis.
PROCTOR: The patient has some vaginal bleeding noted.
Student: I will treat with dressings and local protocol at this time.
PROCTOR: Noted.

▸ **Extremities**

Student: I am rapidly assessing the extremities.
PROCTOR: There are no obvious injuries.

▸ **Assess Motor, Sensory, and Circulatory Function**

Student: I am checking for DCAP-BTLS. I am also checking motor and sensory function, and pulses. Right leg?
PROCTOR: Negative DCAP-BTLS. Motor and sensory functions are present. Pulses are present.
Student: Left leg?
PROCTOR: Negative DCAP-BTLS. Motor and sensory functions are present. Pulses are present.
Student: Right arm?
PROCTOR: Negative DCAP-BTLS. Motor and sensory functions are present. Pulses are present.
Student: Left arm?
PROCTOR: Negative DCAP-BTLS. Motor and sensory functions are present. Pulses are present.

▸ **Posterior**

Student: I will rapidly assess the back. We will now log roll the patient as a unit to check the back. The person at the head will count to three and we will roll the patient.
PROCTOR: Noted.

▸ **Assess the Thorax**

Student: I am assessing the thorax. Do I find injuries?
PROCTOR: No, but the patient complains of neck and back pain.

▸ **Assess the Lumbar Area**

Student: I am assessing the flanks and lumbar area. Do I find injuries?
PROCTOR: No.

▸ **Assess the Entire Backside**

Student: I am assessing the entire backside. Do I find injuries?
PROCTOR: No.

▸ **Manage Secondary Injuries/Wounds**

Student: We will apply a cervical collar and backboard with full immobilization per local protocol, if not yet done, at this time. We will dress the wounds and control bleeding.
PROCTOR: Noted.
Student: Are there any changes in motor and sensory functions or pulses?
PROCTOR: No.
ALS Student: I will establish two large-bore IVs while en route to the hospital and maintain a systolic blood pressure of 90 mm Hg.
ALS Proctor: Noted.

▸ **Reevaluate Transport Decision**

Student: This patient is a high priority and requires immediate transport.
PROCTOR: Noted.

▾ Baseline Vital Signs

Student: What are the patient's baseline vital signs, including blood pressure, pulse, respirations, pulse oximetry, and level of consciousness?
PROCTOR: Blood pressure, 160/90 mm Hg; pulse rate, 128 beats/min; respirations, 28 breaths/min; pulse oximetry reading, 98%; and the patient is alert.

▾ SAMPLE History

Student: At this time I will gather a SAMPLE history from the patient or family. What are the patient's signs and symptoms?
PROCTOR: Pain in the vagina, back, and neck.
Student: Allergies?
PROCTOR: Penicillin (PCN).
Student: Medications?
PROCTOR: Insulin.
Student: Pertinent past medical history?
PROCTOR: Diabetes.
Student: I will check her blood glucose level.
PROCTOR: Noted. It is 124 mg/dL.
Student: Last oral intake?
PROCTOR: 2 hours ago.
Student: Events leading up to the incident?
PROCTOR: The patient was driving in heavy rain and slid off of the road; her car struck and bounced over a concrete culvert. The patient weighs more than 350 pounds.

Critical Criteria:
- ❑ Did not differentiate patient's need for transportation versus continued assessment at the scene
- ❑ Did not provide for spinal protection when indicated

▼ Detailed Physical Examination

Student: I am conducting the detailed physical exam. I am looking for DCAP-BTLS.
PROCTOR: Noted. The detailed physical exam will be performed during transport.

▾ Assess the Head

Student: I am assessing the head. Do I find any DCAP-BTLS? Do I find any evidence of Battle's sign or raccoon eyes?
PROCTOR: There is a large laceration to the top of the head.

▸ **Inspect and Palpate the Head and Ears**

Student: I am assessing the head and ears.
PROCTOR: There is a large laceration to the top of the head, treated earlier.
Student: I will apply a dressing per local protocol.
PROCTOR: Noted. Bleeding is controlled.

▸ **Assess the Eyes**

Student: I am assessing the eyes. Are the pupils equal, round, and regular in size, and react properly to light (PEARRL)?
PROCTOR: They are PEARRL.

▸ **Assess the Facial Area Including Oral and Nasal Areas**

Student: I am assessing the face, nose, and mouth. Do I see any discharge or hear any obstructions?
PROCTOR: No.

▾ Assess the Neck

▸ **Inspect and Palpate the Neck**

Student: I am assessing the neck for DCAP-BTLS.
PROCTOR: There are no obvious injuries.

▸ **Assess for Jugular Vein Distention**

Student: Do I find any jugular vein distention (JVD)?
PROCTOR: No.

▸ **Assess for Tracheal Deviation**

Student: Do I see any tracheal deviation?
PROCTOR: No.

▾ Assess the Chest

Student: I am assessing the chest for DCAP-BTLS.
PROCTOR: Noted.

▸ **Inspect**

Student: What do I see when I look at the chest?
PROCTOR: There are no obvious injuries.
Student: Does the chest appear symmetric?
PROCTOR: Yes.

▸ **Palpate**

Student: When I touch the chest, do I feel crepitus or a flail segment?
PROCTOR: No.

▸ **Auscultate**

Student: Are lung sounds present in all fields?
PROCTOR: Yes.

Student: Do I hear any sucking sounds from the chest?
PROCTOR: No.

Assess the Abdomen/Pelvis

Assess the Abdomen

Student: I am assessing the abdomen for DCAP-BTLS. I am assessing all four quadrants. Do I find any problems?
PROCTOR: No.

Assess the Pelvis

Student: I am assessing the pelvis for DCAP-BTLS. Is the pelvis stable?
PROCTOR: Yes.

Assess the Genitalia/Perineum as Needed (Verbalize in Training)

Student: I am assessing the genitalia/perineum as necessary for DCAP-BTLS.
PROCTOR: The patient's minimal vaginal bleeding was treated with dressings and per local protocol earlier in the assessment; now she is backboarded.
Student: I will reassess the dressing.
PROCTOR: Noted. Blood is minimally visible on the dressing.

Assess the Extremities

Inspect

Student: I am assessing the lower and upper extremities for DCAP-BTLS. Do I find anything?
PROCTOR: No.

Palpate

Student: Do I feel anything unusual?
PROCTOR: No.

Assess Motor, Sensory, and Circulatory Function

Student: I am checking for DCAP-BTLS, motor and sensory function, and pulses. Right leg?
PROCTOR: Negative DCAP-BTLS. Motor and sensory functions are present. Pulses are present.
Student: Left leg?
PROCTOR: Negative DCAP-BTLS. Motor and sensory functions are present. Pulses are present.
Student: Right arm?
PROCTOR: Negative DCAP-BTLS. Motor and sensory functions are present. Pulses are present.
Student: Left arm?
PROCTOR: Negative DCAP-BTLS. Motor and sensory functions are present. Pulses are present.

Assess the Posterior

Note: This portion of the detailed physical exam would not be done if the patient were previously backboarded per local protocol.
Student: We will not check the back since it was previously checked and the patient is backboarded.
PROCTOR: Noted.

Manage Secondary Injuries/Wounds

Student: I would direct my partner to continue providing oxygen and bleeding control to the head laceration.
PROCTOR: Noted.

Reassess Vital Signs

Student: I will reassess vital signs and mental status.
PROCTOR: Blood pressure, 152/84 mm Hg; pulse rate, 118 beats/min; respirations, 24 breaths/min; pulse oximetry reading, 98%; and the patient is alert.
Student: The vital signs have not changed significantly.
PROCTOR: Noted.

Reassess Interventions

Student: I will reassess my interventions: oxygen, bleeding control, full immobilization, and treatment for possible shock.
PROCTOR: Noted.
ALS Student: I will reassess basic life support (BLS) interventions, plus the following: establish two large-bore IVs and perform cardiac monitoring.
ALS Proctor: Noted. The cardiac monitor shows sinus tachycardia.

Critical Criteria:
- ❑ Did not find or manage problems associated with airway, breathing, hemorrhage or shock (hypoperfusion)

Radio Report

(Provided by the student.)
PROCTOR: Noted.

Ongoing Assessment

Repeat Vital Signs

Student: I will reassess vital signs and mental status.
PROCTOR: Blood pressure, 144/86 mm Hg; pulse rate, 122 beats/min; respirations 20 breaths/min; pulse oximetry reading, 98%; and the patient is alert.
Student: The vital signs have not changed significantly.
PROCTOR: Noted.

Check Interventions

Student: I will check my interventions: oxygen, bleeding control, and full immobilization.
PROCTOR: Noted.
ALS Student: I will check BLS interventions, plus the following: maintain two large-bore IVs and cardiac monitor.
ALS Proctor: Noted. The cardiac monitor shows sinus tachycardia.

Critical Criteria:
- ❑ Did not find or manage problems associated with airway, breathing, hemorrhage or shock (hypoperfusion)

Handoff Report to Emergency Department Staff

Student: There was no change in the patient's condition during transport.
PROCTOR: Noted.

Critical Criteria:
- ❑ Did not transport patient within the (10) minute time limit

Critical Criteria

(Inform the student of items missed, if any.)

❑ Pass ❑ Fail Date: ____________________

Proctor Comments: ____________________

Notes

CASE 37

Dispatch Information

PROCTOR: EMS 10, respond to a 24-year-old driver who has reportedly been shot multiple times. He is conscious and breathing. Police are on scene.

Pre-scene Action (BSI)

Student: I am wearing nonlatex gloves, safety glasses, mask, and gown.
PROCTOR: Noted.

Critical Criteria:
- ❑ Did not take, or verbalize, body substance isolation (BSI) precautions when necessary

Scene Size-up

Scene Safety

Student: Is the scene safe?
PROCTOR: Yes, police are on scene and you are given clearance to enter. The patient is sitting in the driver's seat of his car.

Mechanism of Injury

Student: What was the mechanism of injury?
PROCTOR: Gunshot wound. The patient was shot while stopped at a stop sign.

Number of Patients

Student: How many patients are there?
PROCTOR: One.

Additional Resources

Student: I would call for advanced life support (ALS) assistance.
PROCTOR: Noted.

C-Spine Stabilization

Student: On the basis of the mechanism of injury, I would stabilize the cervical spine (c-spine) in a neutral in-line position.
PROCTOR: Noted.

Critical Criteria:
- ❑ Did not determine scene safety
- ❑ Did not assess for spinal protection
- ❑ Did not provide for spinal protection when indicated

Initial Assessment

Student: As I perform midline c-spine stabilization, I identify myself and ask the patient not to move.
PROCTOR: Noted.

General Impression

Student: My general impression is that the patient's condition is unstable.
PROCTOR: Noted.

Responsiveness/Level of Consciousness

Student: What is the patient's level of consciousness?
PROCTOR: Alert.

Chief Complaint/Apparent Life Threats

Student: What is the patient's chief complaint?
PROCTOR: The patient is complaining of chest, left arm, left hip, and left leg pain.
Student: There are apparent life threats; the life threats are chest pain and multi-trauma.
PROCTOR: Noted.

Assess the Airway and Breathing

Student: Is the airway open? Is the patient breathing?
PROCTOR: Yes, the airway is open and the patient is breathing.

► Assessment

Student: What are the rate and the quality of breathing?
PROCTOR: Rate: Within normal limits. Quality: Deep.

► Provide Oxygen

Student: I am applying oxygen at 15 L/min via nonrebreathing mask.
PROCTOR: Noted.

► Ensure Adequate Ventilation

Student: The patient has adequate ventilations at this time.
PROCTOR: Noted.

Injury Management

Student: I will direct my partner to take over c-spine control as I continue the assessment.
PROCTOR: Noted.

Assess Circulation

Student: I am assessing the patient's circulation.
PROCTOR: Noted.

► Assess for and Control Major Bleeding

Student: Do I find any major bleeding?
PROCTOR: No.

► Assess the Pulse

Student: What are the rate and the quality of pulses?
PROCTOR: Rate: Tachycardic. Quality: Normal.

► Assess the Skin

Student: I am assessing the skin. What are the color, temperature, and condition of the skin?
PROCTOR: Color: Normal. Temperature: Normal. Condition: Moist.

Identify Priority Patients/Make Transport Decision

Student: The patient is a high priority and is a load-and-go. I will begin packaging and transport.
PROCTOR: Noted.

Critical Criteria:
- ❑ Did not provide high concentration of oxygen
- ❑ Did not find or manage problems associated with airway, breathing, hemorrhage or shock (hypoperfusion)
- ❑ Did not differentiate patient's need for transportation versus continued assessment at the scene
- ❑ Did other detailed examination before assessing the airway, breathing and circulation

Focused History and Physical Examination/Rapid Trauma Assessment

Select the Appropriate Assessment (Focused or Rapid)

Student: I am selecting the rapid physical exam to identify and treat life threats. I am checking for DCAP-BTLS. This acronym stands for deformities, contusions, abrasions, punctures, penetrations, and paradoxical motion in the chest, and burns, tenderness, lacerations, and swelling.
PROCTOR: Noted.

► Head

Student: I am rapidly assessing the head.
PROCTOR: There are no obvious injuries.

► Neck

Student: I am rapidly assessing the neck.
PROCTOR: There are no obvious injuries.
Student: I will apply a cervical collar.
PROCTOR: Noted.

► Chest

Student: I am rapidly assessing the chest. What are the lung sounds?
PROCTOR: You see an apparent gunshot wound through the left clavicle. Lung sounds are clear bilaterally.
Student: I would apply an occlusive dressing.
PROCTOR: Noted.
Student: I will assess the chest for tension pneumothorax by auscultation, and assessment (jugular vein distention [JVD], tracheal deviation, and decreased lung sounds).
PROCTOR: The lung sounds appear clear bilaterally, jugular vein distention is not present, and the trachea is midline.

ALS Student: I will assess the chest for hyperresonance to percussion.
ALS Proctor: Noted. There is no tension pneumothorax.
ALS Student: I will continuously reassess the chest.
ALS Proctor: Noted.

▸ **Abdomen/Pelvis**

Student: I am rapidly assessing the abdomen.
PROCTOR: There are no obvious injuries.
Student: I am rapidly assessing the pelvis.
PROCTOR: There are no obvious injuries.

▸ **Extremities**

Student: I am rapidly assessing the extremities.
PROCTOR: There are possible gunshot wounds to the left forearm, left hip, and left leg.
Student: I would apply dressings to all of these wounds.
PROCTOR: Noted.

▸ **Assess Motor, Sensory, and Circulatory Function**

Student: I am checking for DCAP-BTLS. I am also checking motor and sensory function, and pulses. Right leg?
PROCTOR: Negative DCAP-BTLS. Motor and sensory functions are present. Pulses are present.
Student: Left leg?
PROCTOR: Puncture wound in the lateral leg. Motor and sensory functions are present. Pulses are present.
Student: I would assess the dressing.
PROCTOR: Noted. Bleeding is controlled.
Student: Right arm?
PROCTOR: Negative DCAP-BTLS. Motor and sensory functions are present. Pulses are present.
Student: Left arm?
PROCTOR: Puncture wound in the lateral arm. Motor and sensory functions are present. Pulses are present.
Student: I would assess the dressing.
PROCTOR: Noted. Bleeding is controlled.

▸ **Posterior**

Student: I will rapidly assess the back. We will now log roll the patient as a unit to check the back. The person at the head will count to three and we will roll the patient.
PROCTOR: Noted.

▸ **Assess the Thorax**

Student: I am assessing the thorax. Do I find injuries?
PROCTOR: No.

▸ **Assess the Lumbar Area**

Student: I am assessing the flanks and lumbar area. Do I find injuries?
PROCTOR: No.

▸ **Assess the Entire Backside**

Student: I am assessing the entire backside. Do I find injuries?
PROCTOR: No.

▸ **Manage Secondary Injuries/Wounds**

Student: We will apply a cervical collar and backboard with full immobilization per local protocol, if not yet done, at this time.
PROCTOR: Noted.
Student: Are there any changes in motor and sensory functions or pulses?
PROCTOR: No.
Student: I will reevaluate the dressings and monitor the patient.
PROCTOR: Noted.
ALS Student: I will establish two large-bore IVs while en route to the hospital and maintain a systolic blood pressure of 90 mm Hg.
ALS Proctor: Noted.

▸ **Reevaluate Transport Decision**

Student: This patient is a high priority and a load-and-go due to the puncture wound to the chest and multiple trauma.
PROCTOR: Noted.

▾ Baseline Vital Signs

Student: What are the patient's baseline vital signs, including blood pressure, pulse, respirations, pulse oximetry, and level of consciousness?
PROCTOR: Blood pressure, 130/90 mm Hg; pulse rate, 130 beats/min; respirations, 18 breaths/min; pulse oximetry reading, 98%; and the patient is alert.

▾ SAMPLE History

Student: At this time I will gather a SAMPLE history from the patient or family. What are the patient's signs and symptoms?
PROCTOR: He has pain to the left chest, left arm, left hip, and left leg.
Student: Allergies?
PROCTOR: No allergies.
Student: Medications?
PROCTOR: No medications.
Student: Pertinent past medical history?
PROCTOR: No pertinent medical history.
Student: Last oral intake?
PROCTOR: 2 hours ago.
Student: Events leading up to the incident?
PROCTOR: The patient was driving his car when he stopped at a stop sign and was shot. His window was rolled down and his arm was out the window. The other shots came through the door.

Critical Criteria:
- ❑ Did not differentiate patient's need for transportation versus continued assessment at the scene
- ❑ Did not provide for spinal protection when indicated

Detailed Physical Examination

Student: I am conducting the detailed physical exam. I am looking for DCAP-BTLS.
PROCTOR: Noted. The detailed physical exam will be performed during transport.

▾ Assess the Head

Student: I am assessing the head. Do I find any DCAP-BTLS? Do I find any evidence of Battle's sign or raccoon eyes?
PROCTOR: No.

▸ **Inspect and Palpate the Head and Ears**

Student: I am assessing the head and ears.
PROCTOR: There are no obvious injuries.

▸ **Assess the Eyes**

Student: I am assessing the eyes. Are the pupils equal, round, and regular in size, and react properly to light (PEARRL)?
PROCTOR: They are PEARRL.

▸ **Assess the Facial Area Including Oral and Nasal Areas**

Student: I am assessing the face, nose, and mouth. Do I see any discharge or hear any obstructions?
PROCTOR: No.

▾ Assess the Neck

▸ **Inspect and Palpate the Neck**

Student: I am assessing the neck for DCAP-BTLS.
PROCTOR: There are no obvious injuries.

▸ **Assess for Jugular Vein Distention**

Student: Do I find any jugular vein distention (JVD)?
PROCTOR: No.

Assess for Tracheal Deviation

Student: Do I see any tracheal deviation?
PROCTOR: No.

Assess the Chest

Student: I am assessing the chest for DCAP-BTLS.
PROCTOR: Noted.

Inspect

Student: What do I see when I look at the chest?
PROCTOR: The occlusive dressing is in place, covering the small puncture wound through the left clavicle. Bleeding is controlled.
Student: Does the chest appear symmetric?
PROCTOR: Yes.

Palpate

Student: When I touch the chest, do I feel crepitus or a flail segment?
PROCTOR: No.

Auscultate

Student: Are lung sounds present in all fields?
PROCTOR: Yes.
Student: Do I hear any sucking sounds from the chest?
PROCTOR: No.

Assess the Abdomen/Pelvis

Assess the Abdomen

Student: I am assessing the abdomen for DCAP-BTLS. I am assessing all four quadrants. Do I find any problems?
PROCTOR: No.

Assess the Pelvis

Student: I am assessing the pelvis for DCAP-BTLS. Is the pelvis stable?
PROCTOR: Yes, there is a puncture wound to the left hip.
Student: I would assess the dressing.
PROCTOR: Noted. Bleeding is controlled.

Assess the Genitalia/Perineum as Needed (Verbalize in Training)

Student: I am assessing the genitalia/perineum as necessary for DCAP-BTLS.
PROCTOR: The area is unremarkable.

Assess the Extremities

Inspect

Student: I am assessing the lower and upper extremities for DCAP-BTLS. Do I find anything?
PROCTOR: Yes.

Palpate

Student: Do I feel anything unusual?
PROCTOR: No.

Assess Motor, Sensory, and Circulatory Function

Student: I am checking for DCAP-BTLS, motor and sensory function, and pulses. Right leg?
PROCTOR: Negative DCAP-BTLS. Motor and sensory functions are present. Pulses are present.
Student: Left leg?
PROCTOR: Puncture wound in the lateral leg. Motor and sensory functions are present. Pulses are present.
Student: I would assess the dressing.
PROCTOR: Noted. Bleeding is controlled.
Student: Right arm?
PROCTOR: Negative DCAP-BTLS. Motor and sensory functions are present. Pulses are present.
Student: Left arm?
PROCTOR: Puncture wound in the lateral arm. Motor and sensory functions are present. Pulses are present.
Student: I would assess the dressing.
PROCTOR: Noted. Bleeding is controlled.

Assess the Posterior

Note: This portion of the detailed physical exam would not be done if the patient were previously backboarded per local protocol.
Student: We will not check the back since it was previously checked and the patient is backboarded.
PROCTOR: Noted.

Manage Secondary Injuries/Wounds

Student: I would direct my partner to splint the extremities.
PROCTOR: Noted.

Reassess Vital Signs

Student: I will reassess vital signs and mental status.
PROCTOR: Blood pressure, 124/88 mm Hg; pulse rate, 120 beats/min; respirations, 18 breaths/min; pulse oximetry reading, 98%; and the patient is alert.
Student: The vital signs are improving.
PROCTOR: Noted.

Reassess Interventions

Student: I will reassess my interventions: airway, breathing, and oxygen; circulation and bleeding control; occlusive dressing to the left chest; bleeding control to the left arm, left hip, and left leg; and full immobilization and splints.
PROCTOR: Noted.
ALS Student: I will reassess basic life support (BLS) interventions, plus the following: two large-bore IVs and cardiac monitor.
ALS Proctor: Noted. The cardiac monitor shows sinus tachycardia.

Critical Criteria:
- ❑ Did not find or manage problems associated with airway, breathing, hemorrhage or shock (hypoperfusion)

Radio Report

(Provided by the student.)
PROCTOR: Noted.

Ongoing Assessment

Repeat Vital Signs

Student: I will reassess vital signs and mental status.
PROCTOR: Blood pressure, 122/80 mm Hg; pulse rate, 108 beats/min; respirations, 18 breaths/min; pulse oximetry reading, 98%; and the patient is alert.
Student: The vital signs have improved.
PROCTOR: Noted.

▼ **Check Interventions**

Student: I will check interventions: airway, breathing, and oxygen; circulation and bleeding control; occlusive dressing to the left chest; bleeding control to the left arm, left hip, and left leg; and full immobilization and splints.

PROCTOR: Noted.

ALS Student: I will check BLS interventions, plus the following: two large-bore IVs and cardiac monitor.

ALS Proctor: Noted. The cardiac monitor shows sinus tachycardia.

Critical Criteria:

- ❑ Did not find or manage problems associated with airway, breathing, hemorrhage or shock (hypoperfusion)

Handoff Report to Emergency Department Staff

Student: The patient's condition improved during transport.

PROCTOR: Noted.

Critical Criteria:

- ❑ Did not transport patient within the (10) minute time limit

Critical Criteria

(Inform the student of items missed, if any.)

❑ Pass ❑ Fail Date: ______________________________

Proctor Comments: ______________________________

____

____

CASE 38

Dispatch Information

PROCTOR: EMS 10, respond to a 38-year-old male who has been stabbed in the abdomen. He is conscious and breathing. Police officers are en route.

Pre-scene Action (BSI)

Student: I am wearing nonlatex gloves and safety glasses.
PROCTOR: Noted.

Critical Criteria:
- ❑ Did not take, or verbalize, body substance isolation (BSI) precautions when necessary

Scene Size-up

Scene Safety

Student: Is the scene safe?
PROCTOR: Yes, police are on scene and you are given clearance to enter.

Mechanism of Injury

Student: What was the mechanism of injury?
PROCTOR: Penetrating trauma. The patient was stabbed during a robbery, and his intestines are protruding from his abdomen.

Number of Patients

Student: How many patients are there?
PROCTOR: One.

Additional Resources

Student: I would call for advanced life support (ALS) assistance.
PROCTOR: Noted.

C-Spine Stabilization

Student: On the basis of the mechanism of injury, I would stabilize the cervical spine (c-spine) in a neutral in-line position.
PROCTOR: Noted.

Critical Criteria:
- ❑ Did not determine scene safety
- ❑ Did not assess for spinal protection
- ❑ Did not provide for spinal protection when indicated

Initial Assessment

Student: As I perform midline c-spine stabilization, I identify myself and ask the patient not to move.
PROCTOR: Noted.

General Impression

Student: My general impression is that the patient's condition is unstable.
PROCTOR: Noted.

Responsiveness/Level of Consciousness

Student: What is the patient's level of consciousness?
PROCTOR: Alert.

Chief Complaint/Apparent Life Threats

Student: What is the patient's chief complaint?
PROCTOR: The patient is complaining of his guts hanging out.
Student: There are no apparent life threats.
PROCTOR: Noted.

Assess the Airway and Breathing

Student: Is the airway open? Is the patient breathing?
PROCTOR: Yes, the airway is open and the patient is breathing.

Assessment

Student: What are the rate and the quality of breathing?
PROCTOR: Rate: Within normal limits. Quality: Normal.

Provide Oxygen

Student: I am applying oxygen at 15 L/min via nonrebreathing mask.
PROCTOR: Noted.

Ensure Adequate Ventilation

Student: The patient has adequate ventilations at this time.
PROCTOR: Noted.

Injury Management

Student: I will direct my partner to maintain c-spine control while I continue the assessment.
PROCTOR: Noted.

Assess Circulation

Student: I am assessing the patient's circulation.
PROCTOR: Noted.

Assess for and Control Major Bleeding

Student: Do I find any major bleeding?
PROCTOR: Yes, you see a large laceration with an evisceration of intestines.
Student: I will apply a moist dressing covered by an occlusive and a dry dressing to the evisceration.
PROCTOR: Noted.

Assess the Pulse

Student: What are the rate and the quality of pulses?
PROCTOR: Rate: Tachycardic. Quality: Bounding.

Assess the Skin

Student: I am assessing the skin. What are the color, temperature, and condition of the skin?
PROCTOR: Color: Pale. Temperature: Normal. Condition: Moist.

Identify Priority Patients/Make Transport Decision

Student: The patient is a high priority and is a load-and-go. I will begin packaging and transport to a trauma center.
PROCTOR: Noted.

Critical Criteria:
- ❑ Did not provide high concentration of oxygen
- ❑ Did not find or manage problems associated with airway, breathing, hemorrhage or shock (hypoperfusion)
- ❑ Did not differentiate patient's need for transportation versus continued assessment at the scene
- ❑ Did other detailed examination before assessing the airway, breathing and circulation

Focused History and Physical Examination/Rapid Trauma Assessment

Select the Appropriate Assessment (Focused or Rapid)

Student: I am selecting the rapid physical exam to identify and treat life threats. I am checking for DCAP-BTLS. This acronym stands for deformities, contusions, abrasions, punctures, penetrations, and paradoxical motion in the chest, and burns, tenderness, lacerations, and swelling.
PROCTOR: Noted.

Head

Student: I am rapidly assessing the head.
PROCTOR: There are no obvious injuries.

Neck

Student: I am rapidly assessing the neck.
PROCTOR: There are no obvious injuries.
Student: I will apply a cervical collar.
PROCTOR: Noted.

Chest

Student: I am rapidly assessing the chest. What are the lung sounds?
PROCTOR: There are no obvious injuries. Lung sounds are clear bilaterally.

Abdomen/Pelvis

Student: I am rapidly assessing the abdomen.
PROCTOR: The patient has an evisceration covered by a moist dressing and an occlusive dressing.

Student: I will check the occlusive dressing.
PROCTOR: Noted. Bleeding is controlled.

▸ **Extremities**

Student: I am rapidly assessing the extremities.
PROCTOR: There are no obvious injuries.

▸ **Assess Motor, Sensory, and Circulatory Function**

Student: I am checking for DCAP-BTLS. I am also checking motor and sensory function, and pulses. Right leg?
PROCTOR: Negative DCAP-BTLS. Motor and sensory functions are present. Pulses are present.
Student: Left leg?
PROCTOR: Negative DCAP-BTLS. Motor and sensory functions are present. Pulses are present.
Student: Right arm?
PROCTOR: Negative DCAP-BTLS. Motor and sensory functions are present. Pulses are present.
Student: Left arm?
PROCTOR: Negative DCAP-BTLS. Motor and sensory functions are present. Pulses are present.

▸ **Posterior**

Student: I will rapidly assess the back. We will now log roll the patient as a unit to check the back. The person at the head will count to three and we will roll the patient.
PROCTOR: Noted.

▸ **Assess the Thorax**

Student: I am assessing the thorax. Do I find injuries?
PROCTOR: No.

▸ **Assess the Lumbar Area**

Student: I am assessing the flanks and lumbar area. Do I find injuries?
PROCTOR: No.

▸ **Assess the Entire Backside**

Student: I am assessing the entire backside. Do I find injuries?
PROCTOR: No.

▸ **Manage Secondary Injuries/Wounds**

Student: We will apply a cervical collar and backboard with full immobilization per local protocol, if not yet done, at this time.
PROCTOR: Noted.
Student: Are there any changes in motor and sensory functions or pulses?
PROCTOR: No.
ALS Student: I will establish two large-bore IVs while en route to the hospital and maintain a systolic blood pressure of 90 mm Hg.
ALS Proctor: Noted.

▸ **Reevaluate Transport Decision**

Student: This patient is a high priority and is a load-and-go.
PROCTOR: Noted.

▾ Baseline Vital Signs

Student: What are the patient's baseline vital signs, including blood pressure, pulse, respirations, pulse oximetry, and level of consciousness?
PROCTOR: Blood pressure, 134/82 mm Hg; pulse rate, 120 beats/min; respirations, 16 breaths/min; pulse oximetry reading, 98%; and the patient is alert.

▾ SAMPLE History

Student: At this time I will gather a SAMPLE history from the patient or family. What are the patient's signs and symptoms?
PROCTOR: Pain in the abdomen.
Student: Allergies?
PROCTOR: Penicillin (PCN).
Student: Medications?
PROCTOR: Asthma medications.
Student: Pertinent past medical history?
PROCTOR: Asthma.
Student: Last oral intake?
PROCTOR: 4 hours ago.
Student: Events leading up to the incident?
PROCTOR: The patient was walking to a restaurant when he was stabbed and robbed.
Student: Interventions?
PROCTOR: The patient held pressure on the wound.

Critical Criteria:
- ❑ Did not differentiate patient's need for transportation versus continued assessment at the scene
- ❑ Did not provide for spinal protection when indicated

▼ Detailed Physical Examination

Student: I am conducting the detailed physical exam. I am looking for DCAP-BTLS.
PROCTOR: Noted. The detailed physical exam will be performed during transport.

▾ Assess the Head

Student: I am assessing the head. Do I find any DCAP-BTLS? Do I find any evidence of Battle's sign or raccoon eyes?
PROCTOR: No.

▸ **Inspect and Palpate the Head and Ears**

Student: I am assessing the head and ears.
PROCTOR: There are no obvious injuries.

▸ **Assess the Eyes**

Student: I am assessing the eyes. Are the pupils equal, round, and regular in size, and react properly to light (PEARRL)?
PROCTOR: They are PEARRL.

▸ **Assess the Facial Area Including Oral and Nasal Areas**

Student: I am assessing the face, nose, and mouth. Do I see any discharge or hear any obstructions?
PROCTOR: No.

▾ Assess the Neck

▸ **Inspect and Palpate the Neck**

Student: I am assessing the neck for DCAP-BTLS.
PROCTOR: There are no obvious injuries.

▸ **Assess for Jugular Vein Distention**

Student: Do I find any jugular vein distention (JVD)?
PROCTOR: No.

▸ **Assess for Tracheal Deviation**

Student: Do I see any tracheal deviation?
PROCTOR: No.

▾ Assess the Chest

Student: I am assessing the chest for DCAP-BTLS.
PROCTOR: Noted.

▸ **Inspect**

Student: What do I see when I look at the chest?
PROCTOR: There are no obvious injuries.
Student: Does the chest appear symmetric?
PROCTOR: Yes.

▸ **Palpate**

Student: When I touch the chest, do I feel crepitus or a flail segment?
PROCTOR: No.

▸ **Auscultate**

Student: Are lung sounds present in all fields?
PROCTOR: Yes.
Student: Do I hear any sucking sounds from the chest?
PROCTOR: No.

▼ Assess the Abdomen/Pelvis

▸ Assess the Abdomen

Student: I am assessing the abdomen for DCAP-BTLS. I am assessing all four quadrants. Do I find any problems?

PROCTOR: The patient has an evisceration with minimal bleeding.

Student: I would assess the dressings.

PROCTOR: Noted.

▸ Assess the Pelvis

Student: I am assessing the pelvis for DCAP-BTLS. Is the pelvis stable?

PROCTOR: Yes.

▼ Assess the Genitalia/Perineum as Needed (Verbalize in Training)

Student: I am assessing the genitalia/perineum as necessary for DCAP-BTLS.

PROCTOR: The area is unremarkable.

▼ Assess the Extremities

▸ Inspect

Student: I am assessing the lower and upper extremities for DCAP-BTLS. Do I find anything?

PROCTOR: No.

▸ Palpate

Student: Do I feel anything unusual?

PROCTOR: No.

▸ Assess Motor, Sensory, and Circulatory Function

Student: I am checking for DCAP-BTLS, motor and sensory function, and pulses. Right leg?

PROCTOR: Negative DCAP-BTLS. Motor and sensory functions are present. Pulses are present.

Student: Left leg?

PROCTOR: Negative DCAP-BTLS. Motor and sensory functions are present. Pulses are present.

Student: Right arm?

PROCTOR: Negative DCAP-BTLS. Motor and sensory functions are present. Pulses are present.

Student: Left arm?

PROCTOR: Negative DCAP-BTLS. Motor and sensory functions are present. Pulses are present.

▼ Assess the Posterior

Note: This portion of the detailed physical exam would not be done if the patient were previously backboarded per local protocol.

Student: We will not check the back since it was previously checked and the patient is backboarded.

PROCTOR: Noted.

▼ Manage Secondary Injuries/Wounds

Student: I would direct my partner to recheck the abdomen and maintain the airway.

PROCTOR: Noted.

▼ Reassess Vital Signs

Student: I will reassess vital signs and mental status.

PROCTOR: Blood pressure, 136/80 mm Hg; pulse rate, 96 beats/min; respirations, 16 breaths/min; pulse oximetry reading, 98%; and the patient is alert.

Student: The vital signs have not changed significantly.

PROCTOR: Noted.

▼ Reassess Interventions

Student: I will reassess my interventions: airway, breathing, and oxygen; occlusive dressing; immobilization and straps; and treatment for shock.

PROCTOR: Noted.

ALS Student: I will reassess basic life support (BLS) interventions, plus the following: two large-bore IVs and cardiac monitor.

ALS Proctor: Noted. The cardiac monitor shows normal sinus rhythm.

Critical Criteria:

❑ Did not find or manage problems associated with airway, breathing, hemorrhage or shock (hypoperfusion)

Radio Report

(Provided by the student.)

PROCTOR: Noted.

Ongoing Assessment

▼ Repeat Vital Signs

Student: I will reassess vital signs and mental status.

PROCTOR: Blood pressure, 132/78 mm Hg; pulse rate, 90 beats/min; respirations, 16 breaths/min; pulse oximetry reading, 98%; and the patient is alert.

Student: The vital signs have not changed significantly.

PROCTOR: Noted.

▼ Check Interventions

Student: I will check interventions: airway, breathing, and oxygen; occlusive dressing; immobilization and straps; and treatment for shock.

PROCTOR: Noted.

ALS Student: I will check BLS interventions, plus the following: maintain two large-bore IVs and cardiac monitor.

ALS Proctor: Noted. The cardiac monitor shows normal sinus rhythm.

Critical Criteria:

❑ Did not find or manage problems associated with airway, breathing, hemorrhage or shock (hypoperfusion)

Handoff Report to Emergency Department Staff

Student: There was no change during transport.

PROCTOR: Noted.

Critical Criteria:

❑ Did not transport patient within the (10) minute time limit

Critical Criteria

(Inform the student of items missed, if any.)

❑ Pass ❑ Fail Date: ____________________

Proctor Comments: ____________________

____

____

Notes

CASE 39

Dispatch Information

PROCTOR: EMS 10, respond to a motor vehicle collision for a 55-year-old obese female with a large abdominal laceration. She is conscious and breathing.

Pre-scene Action (BSI)

Student: I am wearing appropriate high-visibility personal protective equipment suitable for extrication, a helmet, extrication gloves, nonlatex gloves, and safety glasses.
PROCTOR: Noted.

Critical Criteria:
- ❑ Did not take, or verbalize, body substance isolation (BSI) precautions when necessary

Scene Size-up

Scene Safety

Student: Is the scene safe?
PROCTOR: Yes.

Mechanism of Injury

Student: What was the mechanism of injury?
PROCTOR: Motor vehicle collision. The obese patient was the front-seat passenger and was not wearing a seat belt. When she flew forward, her right side was lacerated by the window crank and there is an organ protruding.

Number of Patients

Student: How many patients are there?
PROCTOR: One, with two refusals of service. You have only this patient.

Additional Resources

Student: I would call for advanced life support (ALS) assistance and additional resources: fire/rescue and police.
PROCTOR: Noted.

C-Spine Stabilization

Student: On the basis of the mechanism of injury, I would stabilize the cervical spine (c-spine) in a neutral in-line position.
PROCTOR: Noted.

Critical Criteria:
- ❑ Did not determine scene safety
- ❑ Did not assess for spinal protection
- ❑ Did not provide for spinal protection when indicated

Initial Assessment

Student: As I perform midline c-spine stabilization, I identify myself and ask the patient not to move.
PROCTOR: Noted.

General Impression

Student: My general impression is that the patient's condition is unstable.
PROCTOR: Noted.

Responsiveness/Level of Consciousness

Student: What is the patient's level of consciousness?
PROCTOR: Alert.

Chief Complaint/Apparent Life Threats

Student: What is the patient's chief complaint?
PROCTOR: The patient is complaining of pain to the right upper abdomen. The liver appears to be hanging out.
Student: I will apply a moist dressing and cover with an occlusive dressing (if possible) and a dry dressing on top to prevent heat loss.
PROCTOR: Noted.
Student: There is an apparent life threat; the life threat is the possibility of internal bleeding.
PROCTOR: Noted.

Assess the Airway and Breathing

Student: Is the airway open? Is the patient breathing?
PROCTOR: Yes, the airway is open and the patient is breathing.

Assessment

Student: What are the rate and the quality of breathing?
PROCTOR: Rate: Tachypneic. Quality: Normal.

Provide Oxygen

Student: I am applying oxygen at 15 L/min via nonrebreathing mask.
PROCTOR: Noted.

Ensure Adequate Ventilation

Student: The patient has adequate ventilations at this time.
PROCTOR: Noted.

Injury Management

Student: I will direct my partner to take over c-spine control as I continue the assessment.
PROCTOR: Noted.

Assess Circulation

Student: I am assessing the patient's circulation.
PROCTOR: Noted.

Assess for and Control Major Bleeding

Student: Do I find any major bleeding?
PROCTOR: No.

Assess the Pulse

Student: What are the rate and the quality of pulses?
PROCTOR: Rate: Tachycardic. Quality: Thready.

Assess the Skin

Student: I am assessing the skin. What are the color, temperature, and condition of the skin?
PROCTOR: Color: Pale. Temperature: Cool. Condition: Diaphoretic.

Identify Priority Patients/Make Transport Decision

Student: The patient is a high priority and is a load-and-go. I will rapidly extricate, begin packaging, and transport to a trauma center.
PROCTOR: Noted.

Critical Criteria:
- ❑ Did not provide high concentration of oxygen
- ❑ Did not find or manage problems associated with airway, breathing, hemorrhage or shock (hypoperfusion)
- ❑ Did not differentiate patient's need for transportation versus continued assessment at the scene
- ❑ Did other detailed examination before assessing the airway, breathing and circulation

Focused History and Physical Examination/Rapid Trauma Assessment

Select the Appropriate Assessment (Focused or Rapid)

Student: I am selecting the rapid physical exam to identify and treat life threats. I am checking for DCAP-BTLS. This acronym stands for deformities, contusions, abrasions, punctures, penetrations, and paradoxical motion in the chest, and burns, tenderness, lacerations, and swelling.
PROCTOR: Noted.

Head

Student: I am rapidly assessing the head.
PROCTOR: There are no obvious injuries.

Neck

Student: I am rapidly assessing the neck.
PROCTOR: There are no obvious injuries.

Student: I will apply a cervical collar.
PROCTOR: Noted.

▸ Chest

Student: I am rapidly assessing the chest. What are the lung sounds?
PROCTOR: There are no obvious injuries. Lung sounds are clear bilaterally.

▸ Abdomen/Pelvis

Student: I am rapidly assessing the abdomen.
PROCTOR: The liver is protruding out of the abdomen.
Student: I will recheck the dressing and assess for bleeding.
PROCTOR: The dressing is in place and there is no bleeding.
Student: I am rapidly assessing the pelvis.
PROCTOR: There are no obvious injuries.

▸ Extremities

Student: I am rapidly assessing the extremities.
PROCTOR: There are no obvious injuries.

▸ Assess Motor, Sensory, and Circulatory Function

Student: I am checking for DCAP-BTLS. I am also checking motor and sensory function, and pulses. Right leg?
PROCTOR: Negative DCAP-BTLS. Motor and sensory functions are present. Pulses are present.
Student: Left leg?
PROCTOR: Negative DCAP-BTLS. Motor and sensory functions are present. Pulses are present.
Student: Right arm?
PROCTOR: Negative DCAP-BTLS. Motor and sensory functions are present. Pulses are present.
Student: Left arm?
PROCTOR: Negative DCAP-BTLS. Motor and sensory functions are present. Pulses are present.

▸ Posterior

Student: I will rapidly assess the back. We will now log roll the patient as a unit to check the back. The person at the head will count to three and we will roll the patient.
PROCTOR: Noted.

▸ Assess the Thorax

Student: I am assessing the thorax. Do I find injuries?
PROCTOR: No.

▸ Assess the Lumbar Area

Student: I am assessing the flanks and lumbar area. Do I find injuries?
PROCTOR: No.

▸ Assess the Entire Backside

STUDENT: I am assessing the entire backside. Do I find injuries?
Proctor: No.

▸ Manage Secondary Injuries/Wounds

Student: We will apply a cervical collar and backboard with full immobilization per local protocol, if not yet done, at this time.
PROCTOR: Noted.
Student: Are there any changes in motor and sensory functions or pulses?
PROCTOR: No.
ALS Student: I will establish two large-bore IVs while en route to the hospital and maintain a systolic blood pressure of 90 mm Hg.
ALS Proctor: Noted.

▸ Reevaluate Transport Decision

Student: This patient is a load-and-go due to possible internal injuries.
PROCTOR: Noted.

▾ Baseline Vital Signs

Student: What are the patient's baseline vital signs, including blood pressure, pulse, respirations, pulse oximetry, and level of consciousness?
PROCTOR: Blood pressure, 154/90 mm Hg; pulse rate, 128 beats/min; respirations, 24 breaths/min; pulse oximetry reading, 97%; and the patient is alert.

▾ SAMPLE History

Student: At this time I will gather a SAMPLE history from the patient or family. What are the patient's signs and symptoms?
PROCTOR: Pain in the right side. Evisceration of the liver.
Student: Allergies?
PROCTOR: No allergies.
Student: Medications?
PROCTOR: Weight-loss pills.
Student: Pertinent past medical history?
PROCTOR: Obesity (the patient weighs 450 pounds).
Student: Last oral intake?
PROCTOR: 2 hours ago.
Student: Events leading up to the incident?
PROCTOR: The patient was not wearing a seat belt and her liver was eviscerated by the window crank during a motor vehicle collision.

Critical Criteria:
- ❑ Did not differentiate patient's need for transportation versus continued assessment at the scene
- ❑ Did not provide for spinal protection when indicated

Detailed Physical Examination

Student: I am conducting the detailed physical exam. I am looking for DCAP-BTLS.
PROCTOR: Noted. The detailed physical exam will be performed during transport.

▾ Assess the Head

Student: I am assessing the head. Do I find any DCAP-BTLS? Do I find any evidence of Battle's sign or raccoon eyes?
PROCTOR: No.

▸ Inspect and Palpate the Head and Ears

Student: I am assessing the head and ears.
PROCTOR: There are no obvious injuries.

▸ Assess the Eyes

Student: I am assessing the eyes. Are the pupils equal, round, and regular in size, and react properly to light (PEARRL)?
PROCTOR: They are PEARRL.

▸ Assess the Facial Area Including Oral and Nasal Areas

Student: I am assessing the face, nose, and mouth. Do I see any discharge or hear any obstructions?
PROCTOR: No.

▾ Assess the Neck

▸ Inspect and Palpate the Neck

Student: I am assessing the neck for DCAP-BTLS.
PROCTOR: There are no obvious injuries.

▸ Assess for Jugular Vein Distention

Student: Do I find any jugular vein distention (JVD)?
PROCTOR: No.

▸ Assess for Tracheal Deviation

Student: Do I see any tracheal deviation?
PROCTOR: No.

▾ Assess the Chest

Student: I am assessing the chest for DCAP-BTLS.
PROCTOR: Noted.

▸ Inspect

Student: What do I see when I look at the chest?
PROCTOR: There are no obvious injuries.
Student: Does the chest appear symmetric?
PROCTOR: Yes.

▸ Palpate

Student: When I touch the chest, do I feel crepitus or a flail segment?
PROCTOR: No.

▸ **Auscultate**

Student: Are lung sounds present in all fields?

PROCTOR: Yes.

Student: Do I hear any sucking sounds from the chest?

PROCTOR: No.

▼ Assess the Abdomen/Pelvis

▸ **Assess the Abdomen**

Student: I am assessing the abdomen for DCAP-BTLS. I am assessing all four quadrants. Do I find any problems?

PROCTOR: The liver is protruding out of the abdomen.

Student: I will recheck the dressing that was previously applied.

PROCTOR: Noted. Bleeding is controlled.

▸ **Assess the Pelvis**

Student: I am assessing the pelvis for DCAP-BTLS. Is the pelvis stable?

PROCTOR: Yes.

▸ **Assess the Genitalia/Perineum as Needed (Verbalize in Training)**

Student: I am assessing the genitalia/perineum for DCAP-BTLS.

PROCTOR: The area is unremarkable.

▼ Assess the Extremities

▸ **Inspect**

Student: I am assessing the lower and upper extremities for DCAP-BTLS. Do I find anything?

PROCTOR: No.

▸ **Palpate**

Student: Do I feel anything unusual?

PROCTOR: No.

▸ **Assess Motor, Sensory, and Circulatory Function**

Student: I am checking for DCAP-BTLS, motor and sensory function, and pulses. Right leg?

PROCTOR: Negative DCAP-BTLS. Motor and sensory functions are present. Pulses are present.

Student: Left leg?

PROCTOR: Negative DCAP-BTLS. Motor and sensory functions are present. Pulses are present.

Student: Right arm?

PROCTOR: Negative DCAP-BTLS. Motor and sensory functions are present. Pulses are present.

Student: Left arm?

PROCTOR: Negative DCAP-BTLS. Motor and sensory functions are present. Pulses are present.

▼ Assess the Posterior

Note: This portion of the detailed physical exam would not be done if the patient were previously backboarded per local protocol.

Student: We will not check the back since it was previously checked and the patient is backboarded.

PROCTOR: Noted.

▼ Manage Secondary Injuries/Wounds

Student: I would direct my partner to monitor the patient.

PROCTOR: Noted.

▼ Reassess Vital Signs

Student: I will reassess vital signs and mental status.

PROCTOR: Blood pressure, 150/90 mm Hg; pulse rate, 134 beats/min; respirations, 24 breaths/min; pulse oximetry reading, 98%; and the patient is alert.

Student: The vital signs have not changed significantly.

PROCTOR: Noted.

▼ Reassess Interventions

Student: I will reassess my interventions: oxygen, occlusive dressing, immobilization, straps, and treatment for shock.

PROCTOR: Noted.

ALS Student: I will reassess basic life support (BLS) interventions, plus the following: two large-bore IVs and cardiac monitor.

ALS Proctor: Noted. The cardiac monitor shows sinus tachycardia.

Critical Criteria:
❑ Did not find or manage problems associated with airway, breathing, hemorrhage or shock (hypoperfusion)

▼ Radio Report

(Provided by the student.)

PROCTOR: Noted.

▼ Ongoing Assessment

▼ Repeat Vital Signs

Student: I will reassess vital signs and mental status.

PROCTOR: Blood pressure, 144/88 mm Hg; pulse rate, 128 beats/min; respirations, 20 breaths/min; pulse oximetry reading, 98%; and the patient is alert.

Student: The vital signs have not changed significantly.

PROCTOR: Noted.

▼ Check Interventions

Student: I will check my interventions: oxygen, occlusive dressing, immobilization, straps, and treatment for shock.

PROCTOR: Noted.

ALS Student: I will check BLS interventions, plus the following: maintain two large-bore IVs and cardiac monitor.

ALS Proctor: Noted. The cardiac monitor shows sinus tachycardia.

Critical Criteria:
❑ Did not find or manage problems associated with airway, breathing, hemorrhage or shock (hypoperfusion)

▼ Handoff Report to Emergency Department Staff

Student: There was no change in the patient's condition during transport.

PROCTOR: Noted.

Critical Criteria:
❑ Did not transport patient within the (10) minute time limit

▼ Critical Criteria

(Inform the student of items missed, if any.)

❑ Pass ❑ Fail Date: ____________________

Proctor Comments: ____________________

Notes

Dispatch Information

PROCTOR: EMS 10, respond to a 59-year-old female who was struck in the head by the spring of a fold-down attic access ladder. She is conscious and breathing.

Pre-scene Action (BSI)

Student: I am wearing nonlatex gloves and safety glasses.
PROCTOR: Noted.

Critical Criteria:
- ❑ Did not take, or verbalize, body substance isolation (BSI) precautions when necessary

Scene Size-up

Scene Safety

Student: Is the scene safe?
PROCTOR: Yes.

Mechanism of Injury

Student: What was the mechanism of injury?
PROCTOR: Blunt head trauma. The patient was struck in the head by the spring of a fold-down attic ladder. She has arterial bleeding from the right temporal artery.

Number of Patients

Student: How many patients are there?
PROCTOR: One.

Additional Resources

Student: I would call for advanced life support (ALS) assistance.
PROCTOR: Noted.

C-Spine Stabilization

Student: On the basis of the mechanism of injury, I would stabilize the cervical spine (c-spine) in a neutral in-line position and immediately apply direct pressure.
PROCTOR: Noted.

Critical Criteria:
- ❑ Did not determine scene safety
- ❑ Did not assess for spinal protection
- ❑ Did not provide for spinal protection when indicated

Initial Assessment

Student: As I perform midline c-spine stabilization, I identify myself and ask the patient not to move.
PROCTOR: Noted.

General Impression

Student: My general impression is that the patient's condition is unstable.
PROCTOR: Noted.

Responsiveness/Level of Consciousness

Student: What is the patient's level of consciousness?
PROCTOR: Alert.

Chief Complaint/Apparent Life Threats

Student: What is the patient's chief complaint?
PROCTOR: The patient is complaining of pain in the side of the head and weakness.
Student: There are apparent life threats; the life threats are the mechanism of injury and arterial bleeding.
PROCTOR: Noted.

Assess the Airway and Breathing

Student: Is the airway open? Is the patient breathing?
PROCTOR: Yes, the airway is open and the patient is breathing.

Assessment

Student: What are the rate and the quality of breathing?
PROCTOR: Rate: Within normal limits. Quality: Normal.

Provide Oxygen

Student: I am applying oxygen at 15 L/min via nonrebreathing mask.
PROCTOR: Noted.

Ensure Adequate Ventilation

Student: The patient has adequate ventilations at this time.
PROCTOR: Noted.

Injury Management

Student: I will direct my partner to take over c-spine and control bleeding as I continue the assessment.
PROCTOR: Noted.

Assess Circulation

Student: I am assessing the patient's circulation.
PROCTOR: Noted.

Assess for and Control Major Bleeding

Student: Do I find any major bleeding?
PROCTOR: Yes, from the right side of the head.
Student: I would apply direct pressure and a dressing.
PROCTOR: Noted. The bleeding appears to be controlled.

Assess the Pulse

Student: What are the rate and the quality of pulses?
PROCTOR: Rate: Rapid. Quality: Strong.

Assess the Skin

Student: I am assessing the skin. What are the color, temperature, and condition of the skin?
PROCTOR: Color: Pale. Temperature: Cool. Condition: Moist.

Identify Priority Patients/Make Transport Decision

Student: The patient is a high priority and is a load-and-go. I will begin packaging and transport.
PROCTOR: Noted.

Critical Criteria:
- ❑ Did not provide high concentration of oxygen
- ❑ Did not find or manage problems associated with airway, breathing, hemorrhage or shock (hypoperfusion)
- ❑ Did not differentiate patient's need for transportation versus continued assessment at the scene
- ❑ Did other detailed examination before assessing the airway, breathing and circulation

Focused History and Physical Examination/Rapid Trauma Assessment

Select the Appropriate Assessment (Focused or Rapid)

Student: I am selecting the rapid physical exam to identify and treat life threats. I am checking for DCAP-BTLS. This acronym stands for deformities, contusions, abrasions, punctures, penetrations, and paradoxical motion in the chest, and burns, tenderness, lacerations, and swelling.
PROCTOR: Noted.

Head

Student: I am rapidly assessing the head.
PROCTOR: The patient's head has a large, gaping hole through which the skull is visible. The pressure dressing has successfully controlled the bleeding.

Neck

Student: I am rapidly assessing the neck.
PROCTOR: The patient complains of neck pain.
Student: I will apply a cervical collar.
PROCTOR: Noted.

▸ **Chest**

Student: I am rapidly assessing the chest. What are the lung sounds?

PROCTOR: There are no obvious injuries. Lung sounds are clear bilaterally.

▸ **Abdomen/Pelvis**

Student: I am rapidly assessing the abdomen.

PROCTOR: There are no obvious injuries.

Student: I am rapidly assessing the pelvis.

PROCTOR: There are no obvious injuries.

▸ **Extremities**

Student: I am rapidly assessing the extremities.

PROCTOR: The patient has a large laceration on the right arm.

Student: I will apply direct pressure and a dressing.

PROCTOR: Noted. Bleeding is controlled with the direct pressure and the dressing.

▸ **Assess Motor, Sensory, and Circulatory Function**

Student: I am checking for DCAP-BTLS. I am also checking motor and sensory function, and pulses. Right leg?

PROCTOR: Negative DCAP-BTLS. Motor and sensory functions are present. Pulses are present.

Student: Left leg?

PROCTOR: Negative DCAP-BTLS. Motor and sensory functions are present. Pulses are present.

Student: Right arm?

PROCTOR: Bleeding from a large laceration. Motor and sensory functions are present. Pulses are present.

Student: I will check the dressing.

PROCTOR: Noted. Bleeding is controlled.

Student: Left arm?

PROCTOR: Negative DCAP-BTLS. Motor and sensory functions are present. Pulses are present.

▸ **Posterior**

Student: I will rapidly assess the back. We will now log roll the patient as a unit to check the back. The person at the head will count to three and we will roll the patient.

PROCTOR: Noted.

▸ **Assess the Thorax**

Student: I am assessing the thorax. Do I find injuries?

PROCTOR: No.

▸ **Assess the Lumbar Area**

Student: I am assessing the flanks and lumbar area. Do I find injuries?

PROCTOR: No.

▸ **Assess the Entire Backside**

Student: I am assessing the entire backside. Do I find injuries?

PROCTOR: No.

▸ **Manage Secondary Injuries/Wounds**

Student: We will apply a cervical collar and backboard with full immobilization per local protocol, if not yet done, at this time.

PROCTOR: Noted.

Student: Are there any changes in motor and sensory functions or pulses?

PROCTOR: No.

ALS Student: I will establish two large-bore IVs en route to the hospital and administer a bolus of 20 mL/kg in order to maintain a systolic blood pressure of 90 mm Hg.

ALS Proctor: Noted.

▸ **Reevaluate Transport Decision**

Student: This patient is a load-and-go due to the mechanism of injury.

PROCTOR: Noted.

▾ Baseline Vital Signs

Student: What are the patient's baseline vital signs, including blood pressure, pulse, respirations, pulse oximetry, and level of consciousness?

PROCTOR: Blood pressure, 110/68 mm Hg; pulse rate, 136 beats/min; respirations, 20 breaths/min; pulse oximetry reading, 98%; and the patient is alert.

▾ SAMPLE History

Student: At this time I will gather a SAMPLE history from the patient or family. What are the patient's signs and symptoms?

PROCTOR: Pain in the head and feeling faint.

Student: Allergies?

PROCTOR: Penicillin (PCN).

Student: Medications?

PROCTOR: No medications.

Student: Pertinent past medical history?

PROCTOR: No pertinent medical history.

Student: Last oral intake?

PROCTOR: 2 hours ago.

Student: Events leading up to the incident?

PROCTOR: The patient was going to the attic to get Christmas decorations when the high-tension spring on the ladder broke free and struck her in the head and arm.

Student: Interventions?

PROCTOR: Her husband held a towel on her head to control the bleeding without applying much pressure.

Critical Criteria:

❑ Did not differentiate patient's need for transportation versus continued assessment at the scene

❑ Did not provide for spinal protection when indicated

▼ Detailed Physical Examination

Student: I am conducting the detailed physical exam. I am looking for DCAP-BTLS.

PROCTOR: Noted. The detailed physical exam will be performed during transport.

▾ Assess the Head

Student: I am assessing the head. Do I find any DCAP-BTLS? Do I find any evidence of Battle's sign or raccoon eyes?

PROCTOR: You find a large, gaping open wound to the head with arterial bleeding that is controlled with direct pressure.

Student: I will apply direct pressure and a dressing.

PROCTOR: Noted.

▸ **Inspect and Palpate the Head and Ears**

Student: I am assessing the head and ears.

PROCTOR: There is a large, gaping open wound to the head with arterial bleeding that is controlled with direct pressure.

▸ **Assess the Eyes**

Student: I am assessing the eyes. Are the pupils equal, round, and regular in size, and react properly to light (PEARRL)?

PROCTOR: They are PEARRL.

▸ **Assess the Facial Area Including Oral and Nasal Areas**

Student: I am assessing the face, nose, and mouth. Do I see any discharge or hear any obstructions?

PROCTOR: No.

▾ Assess the Neck

▸ **Inspect and Palpate the Neck**

Student: I am assessing the neck for DCAP-BTLS.

PROCTOR: There are no obvious injuries.

▸ **Assess for Jugular Vein Distention**

Student: Do I find any jugular vein distention (JVD)?

PROCTOR: No.

▸ **Assess for Tracheal Deviation**

Student: Do I see any tracheal deviation?

PROCTOR: No.

▾ Assess the Chest

Student: I am assessing the chest for DCAP-BTLS.

PROCTOR: Noted.

▸ Inspect

Student: What do I see when I look at the chest?

PROCTOR: There are no obvious injuries.

Student: Does the chest appear symmetric?

PROCTOR: Yes.

▸ Palpate

Student: When I touch the chest, do I feel crepitus or a flail segment?

PROCTOR: No.

▸ Auscultate

Student: Are lung sounds present in all fields?

PROCTOR: Yes.

Student: Do I hear any sucking sounds from the chest?

PROCTOR: No.

▼ Assess the Abdomen/Pelvis

▸ Assess the Abdomen

Student: I am assessing the abdomen for DCAP-BTLS. I am assessing all four quadrants. Do I find any problems?

PROCTOR: No.

▸ Assess the Pelvis

Student: I am assessing the pelvis for DCAP-BTLS. Is the pelvis stable?

PROCTOR: Yes.

▼ Assess the Genitalia/Perineum as Needed (Verbalize in Training)

Student: I am assessing the genitalia/perineum as necessary for DCAP-BTLS.

PROCTOR: The area is unremarkable.

▼ Assess the Extremities

▸ Inspect

Student: I am assessing the lower and upper extremities for DCAP-BTLS. Do I find anything?

PROCTOR: Yes.

▸ Palpate

Student: Do I feel anything unusual?

PROCTOR: No.

▸ Assess Motor, Sensory, and Circulatory Function

Student: I am checking for DCAP-BTLS, motor and sensory function, and pulses. Right leg?

PROCTOR: Negative DCAP-BTLS. Motor and sensory functions are present. Pulses are present.

Student: Left leg?

PROCTOR: Negative DCAP-BTLS. Motor and sensory functions are present. Pulses are present.

Student: Right arm?

PROCTOR: Bleeding from a large laceration. Motor and sensory functions are present. Pulses are present.

Student: I will apply direct pressure and a dressing.

PROCTOR: Noted. Bleeding is controlled with the direct pressure and the dressing.

Student: Left arm?

PROCTOR: Negative DCAP-BTLS. Motor and sensory functions are present. Pulses are present.

▼ Assess the Posterior

Note: This portion of the detailed physical exam would not be done if the patient were previously backboarded per local protocol.

Student: We will not check the back since it was previously checked and the patient is backboarded.

PROCTOR: Noted.

▼ Manage Secondary Injuries/Wounds

Student: I would direct my partner to maintain bleeding control.

PROCTOR: Noted.

▼ Reassess Vital Signs

Student: I will reassess vital signs and mental status.

PROCTOR: Blood pressure, 116/78 mm Hg; pulse rate, 130 beats/min; respirations, 20 breaths/min; pulse oximetry reading, 98%; and the patient is alert.

Student: The vital signs have not changed significantly.

PROCTOR: Noted.

▼ Reassess Interventions

Student: I will reassess my interventions: bleeding control, oxygen, immobilization, and straps.

PROCTOR: Noted.

ALS Student: I will reassess basic life support (BLS) interventions, plus the following: two large-bore IVs.

ALS Proctor: Noted.

Critical Criteria:

- ❑ Did not find or manage problems associated with airway, breathing, hemorrhage or shock (hypoperfusion)

▼ Radio Report

(Provided by the student.)

PROCTOR: Noted.

▼ Ongoing Assessment

▼ Repeat Vital Signs

Student: I will reassess vital signs and mental status.

PROCTOR: Blood pressure, 114/68 mm Hg; pulse rate, 126 beats/min; respirations, 20 breaths/min; pulse oximetry reading, 98%; and the patient is alert.

Student: The vital signs have not changed significantly.

PROCTOR: Noted.

▼ Check Interventions

Student: I will check my interventions: bleeding control, oxygen, immobilization, and straps.

PROCTOR: Noted.

ALS Student: I will check BLS interventions, plus the following: maintain two large-bore IVs.

ALS Proctor: Noted.

Critical Criteria:

- ❑ Did not find or manage problems associated with airway, breathing, hemorrhage or shock (hypoperfusion)

▼ Handoff Report to Emergency Department Staff

Student: There was no change in the patient's condition during transport.

PROCTOR: Noted.

Critical Criteria:

- ❑ Did not transport patient within the (10) minute time limit

▼ Critical Criteria

(Inform the student of items missed, if any.)

❑ Pass ❑ Fail Date: ______________________________

Proctor Comments: ______________________________

____

____

Notes

CASE 41

Dispatch Information

PROCTOR: EMS 10, respond to a motorcycle that has run into the rear of a car.

Pre-scene Action (BSI)

Student: I am wearing appropriate high-visibility personal protective equipment suitable for extrication, a helmet, extrication gloves, nonlatex gloves, safety glasses, and a mask.
PROCTOR: Noted.

Critical Criteria:
- ❑ Did not take, or verbalize, body substance isolation (BSI) precautions when necessary

Scene Size-up

Scene Safety

Student: Is the scene safe?
PROCTOR: Yes.

Mechanism of Injury

Student: What was the mechanism of injury?
PROCTOR: Motor vehicle collision. The 26-year-old patient was speeding on a motorcycle when the car in front of him stopped and he rear-ended the car. He flew through the rear window of the car. He was not wearing a helmet. He struck the back window with his shoulder and arm. He is lying on the trunk lid at this time.

Number of Patients

Student: How many patients are there?
PROCTOR: One.

Additional Resources

Student: I would call for advanced life support (ALS) assistance and additional resources: fire/rescue and police.
PROCTOR: Noted.

C-Spine Stabilization

Student: On the basis of the mechanism of injury, I would stabilize the cervical spine (c-spine) in a neutral in-line position.
PROCTOR: Noted.

Critical Criteria:
- ❑ Did not determine scene safety
- ❑ Did not assess for spinal protection
- ❑ Did not provide for spinal protection when indicated

Initial Assessment

Student: As I perform midline c-spine stabilization, I identify myself and ask the patient not to move.
PROCTOR: Noted.

General Impression

Student: My general impression is that the patient's condition is unstable.
PROCTOR: Noted.

Responsiveness/Level of Consciousness

Student: What is the patient's level of consciousness?
PROCTOR: Conscious and alert.

Chief Complaint/Apparent Life Threats

Student: What is the patient's chief complaint?
PROCTOR: The patient is complaining of right shoulder pain and difficulty breathing.
Student: There is an apparent life threat; the life threat is the mechanism of injury.
PROCTOR: Noted.

Assess the Airway and Breathing

Student: Is the airway open? Is the patient breathing?
PROCTOR: Yes, the airway is open and the patient is breathing.

Assessment

Student: What are the rate and the quality of breathing?
PROCTOR: Rate: Within normal limits. Quality: Guarded.

Provide Oxygen

Student: I am applying oxygen at 15 L/min via nonrebreathing mask.
PROCTOR: Noted.

Ensure Adequate Ventilation

Student: The patient has adequate ventilations at this time.
PROCTOR: Noted.

Injury Management

Student: I will direct my partner to take over c-spine control as I continue assessment.
PROCTOR: Noted.

Assess Circulation

Student: I am assessing the patient's circulation.
PROCTOR: Noted.

Assess for and Control Major Bleeding

Student: Do I find any major bleeding?
PROCTOR: No.

Assess the Pulse

Student: What are the rate and the quality of pulses?
PROCTOR: Rate: Tachycardic. Quality: Strong.

Assess the Skin

Student: I am assessing the skin. What are the color, temperature, and condition of the skin?
PROCTOR: Color: Flushed. Temperature: Warm. Condition: Moist.

Identify Priority Patients/Make Transport Decision

Student: The patient is a high priority and is a load-and-go. I will begin packaging and transport to a trauma center.
PROCTOR: Noted.

Critical Criteria:
- ❑ Did not provide high concentration of oxygen
- ❑ Did not find or manage problems associated with airway, breathing, hemorrhage or shock (hypoperfusion)
- ❑ Did not differentiate patient's need for transportation versus continued assessment at the scene
- ❑ Did other detailed examination before assessing the airway, breathing and circulation

Focused History and Physical Examination/Rapid Trauma Assessment

Select the Appropriate Assessment (Focused or Rapid)

Student: I am selecting the rapid physical exam to identify and treat life threats. I am checking for DCAP-BTLS. This acronym stands for deformities, contusions, abrasions, punctures, penetrations, and paradoxical motion in the chest, and burns, tenderness, lacerations, and swelling.
PROCTOR: Noted.

Head

Student: I am rapidly assessing the head.
PROCTOR: There is a contusion to the forehead.

Neck

Student: I am rapidly assessing the neck.
PROCTOR: There are no obvious injuries.
Student: I will apply a cervical collar.
PROCTOR: Noted.

▸ **Chest**

Student: I am rapidly assessing the chest.

PROCTOR: The right shoulder is dislocated, and the patient is complaining of pain to his right chest. There is a contusion on the right chest.

Student: Does the chest appear symmetric?

PROCTOR: Yes.

Student: When I touch the chest, do I feel crepitus or a flail segment?

PROCTOR: No crepitus, but the patient complains of pain and point tenderness around his rib on the right side. A contusion is present.

Student: I will treat the chest per local protocol.

PROCTOR: Noted.

Student: Are lung sounds present in all fields?

PROCTOR: Yes.

Student: Do I hear any sucking sounds from the chest?

PROCTOR: No.

▸ **Abdomen/Pelvis**

Student: I am rapidly assessing the abdomen.

PROCTOR: There are no obvious injuries.

Student: I am rapidly assessing the pelvis.

PROCTOR: There are no obvious injuries.

▸ **Extremities**

Student: I am rapidly assessing the extremities.

PROCTOR: The right arm is obviously deformed.

▸ **Assess Motor, Sensory, and Circulatory Function**

Student: I am checking for DCAP-BTLS. I am also checking motor and sensory function, and pulses. Right leg?

PROCTOR: Negative DCAP-BTLS. Motor and sensory functions are present. Pulses are present.

Student: Left leg?

PROCTOR: Negative DCAP-BTLS. Motor and sensory functions are present. Pulses are present.

Student: Right arm?

PROCTOR: There is a possible fracture to the right ulna/radius. Motor and sensory functions are present. Pulses are present.

Student: I will splint the arm per local protocol en route to the hospital.

PROCTOR: Noted.

Student: Left arm?

PROCTOR: Negative DCAP-BTLS. Motor and sensory functions are present. Pulses are present.

▸ **Posterior**

Student: I will rapidly assess the back. We will now log roll the patient as a unit to check the back. The person at the head will count to three and we will roll the patient.

PROCTOR: Noted.

▸ **Assess the Thorax**

Student: I am assessing the thorax. Do I find injuries?

PROCTOR: No.

▸ **Assess the Lumbar Area**

Student: I am assessing the flanks and lumbar area. Do I find injuries?

PROCTOR: No.

▸ **Assess the Entire Backside**

Student: I am assessing the entire backside. Do I find injuries?

PROCTOR: No.

▸ **Manage Secondary Injuries/Wounds**

Student: We will apply a cervical collar and backboard with full immobilization, if not yet done, at this time.

PROCTOR: Noted.

Student: Are there any changes in motor and sensory functions or pulses?

PROCTOR: No.

▸ **Reevaluate Transport Decision**

Student: This patient is a high priority and is a load-and-go due to the mechanism of injury.

PROCTOR: Noted.

▾ Baseline Vital Signs

Student: What are the patient's baseline vital signs, including blood pressure, pulse, respirations, pulse oximetry, and level of consciousness?

PROCTOR: Blood pressure, 136/88 mm Hg; pulse rate, 110 beats/min; respirations, 24 breaths/min; pulse oximetry reading, 99%; and the patient is alert.

▾ SAMPLE History

Student: At this time I will gather a SAMPLE history from the patient or family. What are the patient's signs and symptoms?

PROCTOR: He has pain in the right shoulder, arm, and chest.

Student: Allergies?

PROCTOR: No allergies.

Student: Medications?

PROCTOR: No medications.

Student: Pertinent past medical history?

PROCTOR: No pertinent medical history.

Student: Last oral intake?

PROCTOR: 3 hours ago.

Student: Events leading up to the incident?

PROCTOR: The patient was riding a motorcycle when the car in front of him stopped. He ran into the rear of the car and flew through its rear window.

Critical Criteria:
- ❑ Did not differentiate patient's need for transportation versus continued assessment at the scene
- ❑ Did not provide for spinal protection when indicated

Detailed Physical Examination

Student: I am conducting the detailed physical exam. I am looking for DCAP-BTLS.

PROCTOR: Noted. The detailed physical exam will be performed during transport.

▾ Assess the Head

Student: I am assessing the head. Do I find any DCAP-BTLS? Do I find any evidence of Battle's sign or raccoon eyes?

PROCTOR: There is a contusion to the forehead.

▸ **Inspect and Palpate the Head and Ears**

Student: I am assessing the head and ears.

PROCTOR: There is a bruise to the forehead.

▸ **Assess the Eyes**

Student: I am assessing the eyes. Are the pupils equal, round, and regular in size, and react properly to light (PEARRL)?

PROCTOR: They are PEARRL.

▸ **Assess the Facial Area Including Oral and Nasal Areas**

Student: I am assessing the face, nose, and mouth. Do I see any discharge or hear any obstructions?

PROCTOR: No.

▾ Assess the Neck

▸ **Inspect and Palpate the Neck**

Student: I am assessing the neck for DCAP-BTLS.

PROCTOR: There are no obvious injuries.

▸ **Assess for Jugular Vein Distention**

Student: Do I find any jugular vein distention (JVD)?

PROCTOR: No.

▸ **Assess for Tracheal Deviation**

Student: Do I see any tracheal deviation?

PROCTOR: No.

▾ Assess the Chest

Student: I am assessing the chest for DCAP-BTLS.

PROCTOR: Noted.

▸ **Inspect**

Student: What do I see when I look at the chest?

PROCTOR: A contusion is found on the right side.

Student: Does the chest appear symmetric?

PROCTOR: Yes.

▸ **Palpate**

Student: When I touch the chest, do I feel crepitus or a flail segment?

PROCTOR: No crepitus, but the patient complains of pain and point tenderness around his rib on the right side and a contusion is present.

Student: I will treat the chest per local protocol if not already done.

PROCTOR: Noted.

▸ **Auscultate**

Student: Are lung sounds present in all fields?

PROCTOR: Yes.

Student: Do I hear any sucking sounds from the chest?

PROCTOR: No.

▾ Assess the Abdomen/Pelvis

▸ **Assess the Abdomen**

Student: I am assessing the abdomen for DCAP-BTLS. I am assessing all four quadrants. Do I find any problems?

PROCTOR: No.

▸ **Assess the Pelvis**

Student: I am assessing the pelvis for DCAP-BTLS. Is the pelvis stable?

PROCTOR: Yes.

▾ Assess the Genitalia/Perineum as Needed (Verbalize in Training)

Student: I am assessing the genitalia/perineum as necessary for DCAP-BTLS.

PROCTOR: The area is unremarkable.

▾ Assess the Extremities

▸ **Inspect**

Student: I am assessing the lower and upper extremities for DCAP-BTLS. Do I find anything?

PROCTOR: Yes, the right arm is fractured.

▸ **Palpate**

Student: Do I feel anything unusual?

PROCTOR: The right shoulder is dislocated. There is a possible fracture to the right ulna/radius. Motor and sensory functions are present. Pulses are present.

Student: I will now splint the arm and sling and swathe the arm and shoulder.

PROCTOR: Noted.

▸ **Assess Motor, Sensory, and Circulatory Function**

Student: I am checking for DCAP-BTLS, motor and sensory function, and pulses. Right leg?

PROCTOR: Negative DCAP-BTLS. Motor and sensory functions are present. Pulses are present.

Student: Left leg?

PROCTOR: Negative DCAP-BTLS. Motor and sensory functions are present. Pulses are present.

Student: Right arm?

PROCTOR: The arm is splinted per local protocol. Motor and sensory functions are present. Pulses are present.

Student: Left arm?

PROCTOR: Negative DCAP-BTLS. Motor and sensory functions are present. Pulses are present.

▾ Assess the Posterior

Note: This portion of the detailed physical exam would not be done if the patient were previously backboarded per local protocol.

Student: We will not check the back because it was previously checked and the patient is backboarded.

PROCTOR: Noted.

▾ Manage Secondary Injuries/Wounds

Student: I would direct my partner to continuously monitor the patient.

PROCTOR: Noted.

▾ Reassess Vital Signs

Student: I will reassess vital signs and mental status.

PROCTOR: Blood pressure, 134/84 mm Hg; pulse rate, 108 beats/min; respirations, 20 breaths/min; pulse oximetry reading, 99%; and the patient is alert.

Student: The vital signs have not changed significantly.

PROCTOR: Noted.

▾ Reassess Interventions

Student: I will reassess my interventions: oxygen; assess the splint to the right arm and shoulder; immobilization and straps; and treatment for shock.

PROCTOR: Noted.

ALS Student: I will reassess basic life support (BLS) interventions, plus the following: two large-bore IVs and cardiac monitor.

ALS Proctor: Noted. The cardiac monitor shows sinus tachycardia.

Critical Criteria:

❑ Did not find or manage problems associated with airway, breathing, hemorrhage or shock (hypoperfusion)

▼ Radio Report

(Provided by the student.)

PROCTOR: Noted.

▼ Ongoing Assessment

▾ Repeat Vital Signs

Student: I will reassess vital signs and mental status.

PROCTOR: Blood pressure, 136/88 mm Hg; pulse rate, 110 beats/min; respirations, 24 breaths/min; pulse oximetry reading, 99%; and the patient is alert.

Student: The vital signs have not changed significantly.

PROCTOR: Noted.

▼ Check Interventions

Student: I will check my interventions: oxygen; splint to the right arm and shoulder; immobilization and straps; and treatment for shock.

PROCTOR: Noted.

ALS Student: I will check BLS interventions, plus the following: two large-bore IVs and cardiac monitor.

ALS Proctor: Noted. The cardiac monitor shows sinus tachycardia.

Critical Criteria:
❑ Did not find or manage problems associated with airway, breathing, hemorrhage or shock (hypoperfusion)

▼ Handoff Report to Emergency Department Staff

Student: There was no change in the patient's condition during transport.

PROCTOR: Noted.

Critical Criteria:
❑ Did not transport patient within the (10) minute time limit

▼ Critical Criteria

(Inform the student of items missed, if any.)

❑ Pass ❑ Fail Date: ______________________

Proctor Comments: ______________________

CASE 42

Dispatch Information

PROCTOR: EMS 10, respond to a 50-year-old male patient who was struck in the head with a thrown bat at a baseball game. He is not conscious and it is unknown if he is breathing.

Pre-scene Action (BSI)

Student: I am wearing nonlatex gloves and safety glasses.
PROCTOR: Noted.

Critical Criteria:
- ❑ Did not take, or verbalize, body substance isolation (BSI) precautions when necessary

Scene Size-up

Scene Safety

Student: Is the scene safe?
PROCTOR: Yes.

Mechanism of Injury

Student: What was the mechanism of injury?
PROCTOR: Direct blunt force trauma to the head. The patient was watching a baseball game. The patient was sitting in the stands behind the batter when the bat slipped from the batter's hands during his swing, striking the patient in the head.

Number of Patients

Student: How many patients are there?
PROCTOR: One.

Additional Resources

Student: I would call for advanced life support (ALS) assistance.
PROCTOR: Noted.

C-Spine Stabilization

Student: On the basis of the mechanism of injury, I would stabilize the cervical spine (c-spine) in a neutral in-line position.
PROCTOR: Noted.

Critical Criteria:
- ❑ Did not determine scene safety
- ❑ Did not assess for spinal protection
- ❑ Did not provide for spinal protection when indicated

Initial Assessment

Student: As I perform midline c-spine stabilization, I identify myself and ask the patient not to move.
PROCTOR: Noted.

General Impression

Student: My general impression is that the patient's condition is unstable.
PROCTOR: Noted.

Responsiveness/Level of Consciousness

Student: What is the patient's level of consciousness?
PROCTOR: Unresponsive.

Chief Complaint/Apparent Life Threats

Student: What is the patient's chief complaint?
PROCTOR: The patient is unresponsive, with an obvious depression on the right side of his head.
Student: There are apparent life threats; the life threats are the mechanism of injury and unresponsiveness with obvious head trauma.
PROCTOR: Noted.

Assess the Airway and Breathing

Student: I am opening the airway with the jaw-thrust maneuver. Is the patient breathing?
PROCTOR: Yes.

Assessment

Student: What are the rate and the quality of breathing?
PROCTOR: Rate: Slow. Quality: Deep.

Provide Oxygen

Student: I am assisting ventilations with a bag-valve device with 100% oxygen. I will insert an oral airway.
PROCTOR: Noted.

Ensure Adequate Ventilation

Student: I will assist ventilation with a bag-valve device.
PROCTOR: Noted.

Injury Management

Student: I will direct my partner to take over c-spine control and ventilation as I continue assessment.
PROCTOR: Noted.

Assess Circulation

Student: I am assessing the patient's circulation.
PROCTOR: Noted.

Assess for and Control Major Bleeding

Student: Do I find any major bleeding?
PROCTOR: No.

Assess the Pulse

Student: What are the rate and the quality of pulses?
PROCTOR: Rate: Within normal limits. Quality: Bounding.

Assess the Skin

Student: I am assessing the skin. What are the color, temperature, and condition of the skin?
PROCTOR: Color: Flushed. Temperature: Warm. Condition: Diaphoretic.

Identify Priority Patients/Make Transport Decision

Student: The patient is a high priority and is a load-and-go. I will begin packaging and transport.
PROCTOR: Noted.

Critical Criteria:
- ❑ Did not provide high concentration of oxygen
- ❑ Did not find or manage problems associated with airway, breathing, hemorrhage or shock (hypoperfusion)
- ❑ Did not differentiate patient's need for transportation versus continued assessment at the scene
- ❑ Did other detailed examination before assessing the airway, breathing and circulation

Focused History and Physical Examination/Rapid Trauma Assessment

Select the Appropriate Assessment (Focused or Rapid)

Student: I am selecting the rapid physical exam to identify and treat life threats. I am checking for DCAP-BTLS. This acronym stands for deformities, contusions, abrasions, punctures, penetrations, and paradoxical motion in the chest, and burns, tenderness, lacerations, and swelling.
PROCTOR: Noted.

Head

Student: I am rapidly assessing the head.
PROCTOR: There is a depressed area on the right side of the head that is consistent with the end of a baseball bat.
Student: I will have suction ready to protect the airway.
PROCTOR: Noted.

Neck

Student: I am rapidly assessing the neck.
PROCTOR: The neck is normal to palpation. The patient is unresponsive.
Student: I will apply a cervical collar.
PROCTOR: Noted.

▸ **Chest**

Student: I am rapidly assessing the chest. What are the lung sounds?
PROCTOR: There are no obvious injuries. Lung sounds are clear bilaterally.

▸ **Abdomen/Pelvis**

Student: I am rapidly assessing the abdomen.
PROCTOR: There are no obvious injuries.
Student: I am rapidly assessing the pelvis.
PROCTOR: There are no obvious injuries.

▸ **Extremities**

Student: I am rapidly assessing the extremities.
PROCTOR: There are no obvious injuries.

▸ **Assess Motor, Sensory, and Circulatory Function**

Student: I am checking for DCAP-BTLS. I am also checking motor and sensory function, and pulses. Right leg?
PROCTOR: Negative DCAP-BTLS. Motor and sensory functions are absent. Pulses are present.
Student: Left leg?
PROCTOR: Negative DCAP-BTLS. Motor and sensory functions are absent. Pulses are present.
Student: Right arm?
PROCTOR: Negative DCAP-BTLS. Motor and sensory functions are absent. Pulses are present.
Student: Left arm?
PROCTOR: Negative DCAP-BTLS. Motor and sensory functions are absent. Pulses are present.

▸ **Posterior**

Student: I will rapidly assess the back. We will now log roll the patient as a unit to check the back. The person at the head will count to three and we will roll the patient.
PROCTOR: Noted.

▸ **Assess the Thorax**

Student: I am assessing the thorax. Do I find injuries?
PROCTOR: No.

▸ **Assess the Lumbar Area**

Student: I am assessing the flanks and lumbar area. Do I find injuries?
PROCTOR: No.

▸ **Assess the Entire Backside**

Student: I am assessing the entire backside. Do I find injuries?
PROCTOR: No.

▸ **Manage Secondary Injuries/Wounds**

Student: We will apply a cervical collar and backboard with full immobilization per local protocol, if not yet done, at this time.
PROCTOR: Noted.
Student: Are there any changes in motor and sensory functions or pulses?
PROCTOR: No.
ALS Student: I will perform basic life support (BLS) interventions, plus the following: intubate the patient with spinal precautions and confirm lung sounds and end tidal CO_2.
ALS Proctor: Noted. End tidal CO_2 and lung sounds confirm endotracheal (ET) tube placement.

▸ **Reevaluate Transport Decision**

Student: This patient is a load-and-go due to the head injury and the mechanism of injury.
PROCTOR: Noted.

▾ Baseline Vital Signs

Student: What are the patient's baseline vital signs, including blood pressure, pulse, respirations, pulse oximetry, blood glucose level, and level of consciousness?
PROCTOR: Blood pressure, 190/100 mm Hg; pulse rate, 72 beats/min; respirations per bag-valve device; pulse oximetry reading, 97%; blood glucose level, 128 mg/dL; and the patient is unresponsive.

▾ SAMPLE History

Student: At this time I will gather a SAMPLE history from the patient or family. What are the patient's signs and symptoms?
PROCTOR: The patient is unresponsive, and you smell beer on his breath.
Student: Allergies?
PROCTOR: Unknown.
Student: Medications?
PROCTOR: Unknown.
Student: Pertinent past medical history?
PROCTOR: Unknown.
Student: Last oral intake?
PROCTOR: Unknown.
Student: Events leading up to the incident?
PROCTOR: The patient was sitting in the bleachers when he was struck in the head with an accidentally thrown bat.

Critical Criteria:
- ❑ Did not differentiate patient's need for transportation versus continued assessment at the scene
- ❑ Did not provide for spinal protection when indicated

Detailed Physical Examination

Student: I am conducting the detailed physical exam.
PROCTOR: Noted. The detailed physical exam will be performed during transport.

▾ Assess the Head

Student: I am assessing the head. Do I find any DCAP-BTLS? Do I find any evidence of Battle's sign or raccoon eyes?
PROCTOR: Yes, you see a depressed skull fracture on the right side. Battle's sign is noted.

▸ **Inspect and Palpate the Head and Ears**

Student: I am assessing the head and ears.
PROCTOR: There is blood and cerebrospinal fluid (CSF) in the right ear.

▸ **Assess the Eyes**

Student: I am assessing the eyes. Are the pupils equal, round, and regular in size, and react properly to light (PEARRL)?
PROCTOR: They are nonreactive and the right pupil is dilated.

▸ **Assess the Facial Area Including Oral and Nasal Areas**

Student: I am assessing the face, nose, and mouth. Do I see any discharge or hear any obstructions?
PROCTOR: Yes, you hear gurgling and occasionally there is projectile vomiting.
Student: I will suction the airway as needed.
PROCTOR: Noted.

▾ Assess the Neck

▸ **Inspect and Palpate the Neck**

Student: I am assessing the neck for DCAP-BTLS.
PROCTOR: There are no obvious injuries.

▸ **Assess for Jugular Vein Distention**

Student: Do I find any jugular vein distention (JVD)?
PROCTOR: No.

▸ **Assess for Tracheal Deviation**

Student: Do I see any tracheal deviation?
PROCTOR: No.

▾ Assess the Chest

Student: I am assessing the chest for DCAP-BTLS.
PROCTOR: Noted.

▸ **Inspect**

Student: What do I see when I look at the chest?
PROCTOR: There are no obvious injuries.
Student: Does the chest appear symmetric?
PROCTOR: Yes.

▸ Palpate

Student: When I touch the chest, do I feel crepitus or a flail segment?

PROCTOR: No.

▸ Auscultate

Student: Are lung sounds present in all fields?

PROCTOR: Yes.

Student: Do I hear any sucking sounds from the chest?

PROCTOR: No.

▼ Assess the Abdomen/Pelvis

▸ Assess the Abdomen

Student: I am assessing the abdomen for DCAP-BTLS. I am assessing all four quadrants. Do I find any problems?

PROCTOR: No.

▸ Assess the Pelvis

Student: I am assessing the pelvis for DCAP-BTLS. Is the pelvis stable?

PROCTOR: Yes.

▼ Assess the Genitalia/Perineum as Needed (Verbalize in Training)

Student: I am assessing the genitalia/perineum as necessary for DCAP-BTLS.

PROCTOR: The area is unremarkable.

▼ Assess the Extremities

▸ Inspect

Student: I am assessing the lower and upper extremities for DCAP-BTLS. Do I find anything?

PROCTOR: No.

▸ Palpate

Student: Do I feel anything unusual?

PROCTOR: No.

▸ Assess Motor, Sensory, and Circulatory Function

Student: I am checking for DCAP-BTLS, motor and sensory function, and pulses. Right leg?

PROCTOR: Negative DCAP-BTLS. Motor and sensory functions are absent. Pulses are present.

Student: Left leg?

PROCTOR: Negative DCAP-BTLS. Motor and sensory functions are absent. Pulses are present.

Student: Right arm?

PROCTOR: Negative DCAP-BTLS. Motor and sensory functions are absent. Pulses are present.

Student: Left arm?

PROCTOR: Negative DCAP-BTLS. Motor and sensory functions are absent. Pulses are present.

▼ Assess the Posterior

Note: This portion of the detailed physical exam would not be done if the patient were previously backboarded per local protocol.

Student: We will not check the back because it was previously checked and the patient is backboarded.

PROCTOR: Noted.

▼ Manage Secondary Injuries/Wounds

Student: I would direct my partner to maintain the airway.

PROCTOR: Noted.

▼ Reassess Vital Signs

Student: I will reassess vital signs and mental status.

PROCTOR: Blood pressure, 196/94 mm Hg; pulse rate, 68 beats/min; respirations per bag-valve device; pulse oximetry reading, 96%; and the patient is unresponsive.

Student: The vital signs are deteriorating.

PROCTOR: Noted.

▼ Reassess Interventions

Student: I will reassess my interventions: airway, breathing, bag-valve device and oxygen, oral airway (or advanced airway), suction, immobilization, and straps.

PROCTOR: Noted.

ALS Student: I will reassess BLS interventions, plus the following: maintain intubation, confirming lung sounds and end tidal CO_2, two large-bore IVs, and cardiac monitor.

ALS Proctor: Noted. End tidal CO_2 and lung sounds confirm placement of the ET tube. The cardiac monitor shows normal sinus rhythm.

Critical Criteria:

❑ Did not find or manage problems associated with airway, breathing, hemorrhage or shock (hypoperfusion)

Radio Report

(Provided by the student.)

PROCTOR: Noted.

Ongoing Assessment

▼ Repeat Vital Signs

Student: I will reassess vital signs and mental status.

PROCTOR: Blood pressure, 200/90 mm Hg; pulse rate, 66 beats/min; respirations per bag-valve device; pulse oximetry reading, 100%; and the patient is unresponsive.

Student: The vital signs have deteriorated.

PROCTOR: Noted.

▼ Check Interventions

Student: I will check my interventions: airway, breathing, bag-valve device and oxygen, oral airway (or advanced airway), suction, immobilization, and straps.

PROCTOR: Noted.

ALS Student: I will check BLS interventions, plus the following: maintain intubation, confirm end tidal CO_2 and lung sounds, two large-bore IVs, and cardiac monitor.

ALS Proctor: Noted. End tidal CO_2 and lung sounds confirm placement of the ET tube. The cardiac monitor shows normal sinus rhythm.

Critical Criteria:

❑ Did not find or manage problems associated with airway, breathing, hemorrhage or shock (hypoperfusion)

Handoff Report to Emergency Department Staff

Student: The patient's condition deteriorated during transport.

PROCTOR: Noted.

Critical Criteria:

❑ Did not transport patient within the (10) minute time limit

Critical Criteria

(Inform the student of items missed, if any.)

❑ Pass ❑ Fail Date: ____________________

Proctor Comments: ____________________

____

____

Notes

Dispatch Information

PROCTOR: EMS 10, respond to a motor vehicle collision. A tractor trailer has struck a passenger car. A 79-year-old male is pinned by his door in the car. He is conscious and breathing. Police are on scene.

Pre-scene Action (BSI)

Student: I am wearing the appropriate high visibility personal protective equipment with a helmet, extrication gloves, nonlatex gloves, and safety glasses.
PROCTOR: Noted.

Critical Criteria:
- ❑ Did not take, or verbalize, body substance isolation (BSI) precautions when necessary

Scene Size-up

Scene Safety

Student: Is the scene safe?
PROCTOR: Yes, the fire department has secured the vehicle and the police department has closed the roadway.

Mechanism of Injury

Student: What was the mechanism of injury?
PROCTOR: Motor vehicle collision. The patient was driving and ran a red light; his car was struck in the driver's-side door by a tractor trailer.
Student: I will allow fire/rescue to extricate the patient.
PROCTOR: Noted.

Number of Patients

Student: How many patients are there?
PROCTOR: One, and one who is refusing service. The refusal is being handled by another EMS crew.

Additional Resources

Student: I would call for advanced life support (ALS) assistance and additional resources: fire/rescue.
PROCTOR: Noted.

C-Spine Stabilization

Student: On the basis of the mechanism of injury, I would stabilize the cervical spine (c-spine) in a neutral in-line position.
PROCTOR: Noted.

Critical Criteria:
- ❑ Did not determine scene safety
- ❑ Did not assess for spinal protection
- ❑ Did not provide for spinal protection when indicated

Initial Assessment

Student: As I perform midline c-spine stabilization, I identify myself and ask the patient not to move.
PROCTOR: Noted.

General Impression

Student: My general impression is that the patient's condition is unstable.
PROCTOR: Noted.

Responsiveness/Level of Consciousness

Student: What is the patient's level of consciousness?
PROCTOR: Awake, but making inappropriate comments.

Chief Complaint/Apparent Life Threats

Student: What is the patient's chief compliant?
PROCTOR: The patient is complaining of hip and chest pain.
Student: There is an apparent life threat; the life threat is the mechanism of injury.
PROCTOR: Noted.

Assess the Airway and Breathing

Student: Is the airway open? Is the patient breathing?
PROCTOR: Yes, the airway is open and the patient is breathing.

Assessment

Student: What are the rate and the quality of breathing?
PROCTOR: Rate: Within normal limits. Quality: Shallow.

Provide Oxygen

Student: I am applying oxygen at 15 L/min via nonrebreathing mask.
PROCTOR: Noted.

Ensure Adequate Ventilation

Student: The patient has adequate ventilations at this time.
PROCTOR: Noted.

Injury Management

Student: I will direct my partner to take over c-spine control as I continue assessment.
PROCTOR: Noted.

Assess Circulation

Student: I am assessing the patient's circulation.
PROCTOR: Noted.

Assess for and Control Major Bleeding

Student: Do I find any major bleeding?
PROCTOR: No.

Assess the Pulse

Student: What are the rate and the quality of pulses?
PROCTOR: Rate: Within normal limits. Quality: Normal.

Assess the Skin

Student: I am assessing the skin. What are the color, temperature, and condition of the skin?
PROCTOR: Color: Pale. Temperature: Warm. Condition: Moist.

Identify Priority Patients/Make Transport Decision

Student: The patient is a high priority and is a load-and-go. I will begin packaging and transport.
PROCTOR: Noted.

Critical Criteria:
- ❑ Did not provide high concentration of oxygen
- ❑ Did not find or manage problems associated with airway, breathing, hemorrhage or shock (hypoperfusion)
- ❑ Did not differentiate patient's need for transportation versus continued assessment at the scene
- ❑ Did other detailed examination before assessing the airway, breathing and circulation

Focused History and Physical Examination/Rapid Trauma Assessment

Select the Appropriate Assessment (Focused or Rapid)

Student: I am selecting the rapid physical exam to identify and treat life threats. I am checking for DCAP-BTLS. This acronym stands for deformities, contusions, abrasions, punctures, penetrations, and paradoxical motion in the chest, and burns, tenderness, lacerations, and swelling.
PROCTOR: Noted.

Head

Student: I am rapidly assessing the head.
PROCTOR: There are no obvious injuries.

Neck

Student: I am rapidly assessing the neck.
PROCTOR: There are no obvious injuries.

Student: I will apply a cervical collar.
PROCTOR: Noted.

▸ **Chest**

Student: I am rapidly assessing the chest.
PROCTOR: The left chest has obvious significant bruising and deformity with paradoxical motion.
Student: I will stabilize the flail segment by taping a bulky pad or a pillow to the chest.
PROCTOR: Noted.
Student: What are his lung sounds?
PROCTOR: They are clear bilaterally.
Student: I will use a bag-valve device to ventilate the patient if necessary.
PROCTOR: Noted.
Student: I will assess the chest for tension pneumothorax by auscultation and assessment (for jugular vein distention [JVD], tracheal deviation, and decreased lung sounds).
PROCTOR: The lung sounds appear clear bilaterally, jugular vein distention is not present, and the trachea is midline.
ALS Student: I will assess the chest for hyperresonance to percussion.
ALS Proctor: Noted. There is no tension pneumothorax.
ALS Student: I will continuously reassess the chest.
ALS Proctor: Noted.
Student: I am anticipating other internal injuries.
PROCTOR: Noted.

▸ **Abdomen/Pelvis**

Student: I am rapidly assessing the abdomen.
PROCTOR: There are no obvious injuries.
Student: I am rapidly assessing the pelvis.
PROCTOR: The pelvis is unstable.
Student: I will stabilize it with a sheet tie or a commercial pelvic binder and the backboard.
PROCTOR: Noted.

▸ **Extremities**

Student: I am rapidly assessing the extremities.
PROCTOR: The left hip is deformed and the leg is shortened and externally rotated.
Student: I will treat this fracture with the long backboard and provide padding for comfort during transport.
PROCTOR: Noted.

▸ **Assess Motor, Sensory, and Circulatory Function**

Student: I am checking for DCAP-BTLS. I am also checking motor and sensory function, and pulses. Right leg?
PROCTOR: Negative DCAP-BTLS. Motor and sensory functions are present. Pulses are present.
Student: Left leg?
PROCTOR: Possible fracture to the hip. The left hip is deformed and the leg is shortened and externally rotated.
Student: I stabilized it with the backboard.
PROCTOR: Noted. Motor and sensory functions are present. Pulses are present.
Student: Right arm?
PROCTOR: Negative DCAP-BTLS. Motor and sensory functions are present. Pulses are present.
Student: Left arm?
PROCTOR: Negative DCAP-BTLS. Motor and sensory functions are present. Pulses are present.

▸ **Posterior**

Student: I will rapidly assess the back. We will now log roll the patient as a unit to check the back. The person at the head will count to three and we will roll the patient.
PROCTOR: Noted.

▸ **Assess the Thorax**

Student: I am assessing the thorax. Do I find injuries?
PROCTOR: No.

▸ **Assess the Lumbar Area**

Student: I am assessing the flanks and lumbar area. Do I find injuries?
PROCTOR: No.

▸ **Assess the Entire Backside**

Student: I am assessing the entire backside. Do I find injuries?
PROCTOR: No.

▸ **Manage Secondary Injuries/Wounds**

Student: We will apply a cervical collar and backboard with full immobilization with pelvic stabilization per local protocol, if not yet done, at this time.
PROCTOR: Noted.
ALS Student: I will apply basic life support (BLS) interventions, plus the following: establish two large-bore IVs in order to maintain a systolic blood pressure of 90 mm Hg en route to the hospital.
ALS Proctor: Noted.
Student: Are there any changes in motor and sensory functions or pulses?
PROCTOR: No.

▸ **Reevaluate Transport Decision**

Student: This patient is a load-and-go due to multiple trauma.
PROCTOR: Noted.

▾ Baseline Vital Signs

Student: What are the patient's baseline vital signs, including blood pressure, pulse, respirations, pulse oximetry, and level of consciousness?
PROCTOR: Blood pressure, 120/84 mm Hg; pulse rate, 70 beats/min; respirations, 20 breaths/min; pulse oximetry reading, 96%; and the patient is confused.

▾ SAMPLE History

Student: At this time I will gather a SAMPLE history from the patient or family. What are the patient's signs and symptoms?
PROCTOR: Pain in the left side of the chest.
Student: Allergies?
PROCTOR: Unknown.
Student: Medications?
PROCTOR: Beta blockers, insulin, dementia medications (per medic alert bracelet).
Student: I will check the patient's blood glucose level.
PROCTOR: Noted. It is 110 mg/dL.
Student: Pertinent past medical history?
PROCTOR: High blood pressure, diabetes, and dementia (per medic alert bracelet).
Student: Last oral intake?
PROCTOR: Unknown.
Student: Events leading up to the incident?
PROCTOR: The patient was driving and was confused. He ran a red light and his car was struck by a tractor-trailer.

Critical Criteria:
- ☐ Did not differentiate patient's need for transportation versus continued assessment at the scene
- ☐ Did not provide for spinal protection when indicated

▼ Detailed Physical Examination

Student: I am conducting the detailed physical exam.
PROCTOR: Noted. The detailed physical exam will be performed during transport.

▾ Assess the Head

Student: I am assessing the head. Do I find any DCAP-BTLS? Do I find any evidence of Battle's sign or raccoon eyes?
PROCTOR: No.

▸ **Inspect and Palpate the Head and Ears**

Student: I am assessing the head and ears.
PROCTOR: There are no obvious injuries.

▸ Assess the Eyes

Student: I am assessing the eyes. Are the pupils equal, round, and regular in size, and react properly to light (PEARRL)?

PROCTOR: They are PEARRL.

▸ Assess the Facial Area Including Oral and Nasal Areas

Student: I am assessing the face, nose, and mouth. Do I see any discharge or hear any obstructions?

PROCTOR: No.

▾ Assess the Neck

▸ Inspect and Palpate the Neck

Student: I am assessing the neck for DCAP-BTLS.

PROCTOR: There are no obvious injuries.

▸ Assess for Jugular Vein Distention

Student: Do I find any jugular vein distention (JVD)?

PROCTOR: No.

▸ Assess for Tracheal Deviation

Student: Do I see any tracheal deviation?

PROCTOR: No.

▾ Assess the Chest

Student: I am assessing the chest for DCAP-BTLS.

PROCTOR: Noted.

▸ Inspect

Student: What do I see when I look at the chest?

PROCTOR: The left chest has obvious severe trauma.

Student: Does the chest appear symmetric?

PROCTOR: No, but it was stabilized earlier.

▸ Palpate

Student: When I touch the chest, do I feel crepitus or a flail segment?

PROCTOR: The chest is stabilized. Crepitus palpated to the left side of the chest.

▸ Auscultate

Student: Are lung sounds present in all fields?

PROCTOR: Yes.

Student: Do I hear any sucking sounds from the chest?

PROCTOR: No.

ALS Student: I will assess the chest for hyperresonance to percussion.

ALS Proctor: Noted. There is no tension pneumothorax.

ALS Student: I will continuously reassess the chest.

ALS Proctor: Noted.

▾ Assess the Abdomen/Pelvis

▸ Assess the Abdomen

Student: I am assessing the abdomen for DCAP-BTLS. I am assessing all four quadrants. Do I find any problems?

PROCTOR: No.

▸ Assess the Pelvis

Student: I am assessing the pelvis for DCAP-BTLS. Is the pelvis stable?

PROCTOR: No, but it has been stablized.

▾ Assess the Genitalia/Perineum as Needed (Verbalize in Training)

Student: I am assessing the genitalia/perineum as necessary for DCAP-BTLS.

PROCTOR: The area is unremarkable.

▾ Assess the Extremities

▸ Inspect

Student: I am assessing the lower and upper extremities for DCAP-BTLS. Do I find anything?

PROCTOR: Yes, there is deformity and tenderness to the left hip area. The left hip is deformed and the leg is shortened and externally rotated.

▸ Palpate

Student: Do I feel anything unusual?

PROCTOR: Yes, deformity is noted to the left hip.

▸ Assess Motor, Sensory, and Circulatory Function

Student: I am checking for DCAP-BTLS, motor and sensory function, and pulses. Right leg?

PROCTOR: Negative DCAP-BTLS. Motor and sensory functions are present. Pulses are present.

Student: Left leg?

PROCTOR: Possible fracture to the hip.

Student: The hip has been previously stabilized.

PROCTOR: Noted. Motor and sensory functions are present. Pulses are present.

Student: Right arm?

PROCTOR: Negative DCAP-BTLS. Motor and sensory functions are present. Pulses are present.

Student: Left arm?

PROCTOR: Negative DCAP-BTLS. Motor and sensory functions are present. Pulses are present.

▾ Assess the Posterior

Note: This portion of the detailed physical exam would not be done if the patient were previously backboarded per local protocol.

Student: We will not check the back because it was previously checked and the patient is backboarded.

PROCTOR: Noted.

▾ Manage Secondary Injuries/Wounds

Student: I would direct my partner to continue providing oxygen, and maintain stabilization of the chest wall, pelvis, and left hip.

PROCTOR: Noted.

▾ Reassess Vital Signs

Student: I will reassess vital signs and mental status.

PROCTOR: Blood pressure, 118/82 mm Hg; pulse rate, 66 beats/min; respirations, 20 breaths/min; pulse oximetry reading, 97%; and the patient is confused.

Student: The vital signs have not changed significantly.

PROCTOR: Noted.

▾ Reassess Interventions

Student: I will reassess my interventions: oxygen and possible bag-valve ventilations if necessary; full immobilization; monitor the chest, pelvis, and hip en route to the hospital per local protocol; and treatment for shock.

PROCTOR: Noted.

ALS Student: I will reassess BLS interventions, plus the following: two large-bore IVs and cardiac monitor.

ALS Proctor: Noted. The cardiac monitor shows normal sinus rhythm.

Critical Criteria:

- ❑ Did not find or manage problems associated with airway, breathing, hemorrhage or shock (hypoperfusion)

▼ Radio Report

(Provided by the student.)

PROCTOR: Noted.

▼ Ongoing Assessment

▾ Repeat Vital Signs

Student: I will reassess vital signs and mental status.

PROCTOR: Blood pressure, 114/80 mm Hg; pulse rate, 68 beats/min; respirations, 20 breaths/min; pulse oximetry reading, 97%; and the patient is confused.

Student: The vital signs have not changed significantly.

PROCTOR: Noted.

▼Check Interventions

Student: I will check my interventions: oxygen and possible bag-valve ventilations if necessary; full immobilization; monitor the chest, pelvis, and hip en route to the hospital per local protocol; and treatment for shock.

PROCTOR: Noted.

ALS Student: I will check BLS interventions, plus the following: monitor the two large-bore IVs and cardiac monitor, and 12-lead ECG.

ALS Proctor: Noted. The cardiac monitor shows normal sinus rhythm.

Critical Criteria:
- ❑ Did not find or manage problems associated with airway, breathing, hemorrhage or shock (hypoperfusion)

▼ Handoff Report to Emergency Department Staff

Student: There was no change in the patient's condition during transport.

PROCTOR: Noted.

Critical Criteria:
- ❑ Did not transport patient within the (10) minute time limit

▼ Critical Criteria

(Inform the student of items missed, if any.)

❑ Pass ❑ Fail Date: ____________________

Proctor Comments: ____________________

____

____

CASE 44

Dispatch Information

PROCTOR: EMS 10, respond to a 4-year-old female who has been shot in the face. She is conscious and breathing. Police are en route.

Pre-scene Action (BSI)

Student: I am wearing nonlatex gloves, safety glasses, mask, and gown.
PROCTOR: Noted.

Critical Criteria:
- ❑ Did not take, or verbalize, body substance isolation (BSI) precautions when necessary

Scene Size-up

Scene Safety

Student: Is the scene safe?
PROCTOR: Yes, police are on scene and you are given clearance to enter.

Mechanism of Injury

Student: What was the mechanism of injury?
PROCTOR: Gunshot wound. The patient was playing in the front yard when she was shot. Her lower jaw is missing.

Number of Patients

Student: How many patients are there?
PROCTOR: One.

Additional Resources

Student: I would call for advanced life support (ALS) assistance.
PROCTOR: Noted.

C-Spine Stabilization

Student: On the basis of the mechanism of injury, I would stabilize the cervical spine (c-spine) in a neutral in-line position.
PROCTOR: Noted.

Critical Criteria:
- ❑ Did not determine scene safety
- ❑ Did not assess for spinal protection
- ❑ Did not provide for spinal protection when indicated

Initial Assessment

Student: As I perform midline c-spine stabilization, I identify myself and ask the patient not to move.
PROCTOR: Noted.

General Impression

Student: My general impression is that the patient's condition is unstable.
PROCTOR: Noted.

Responsiveness/Level of Consciousness

Student: What is the patient's level of consciousness?
PROCTOR: Alert.

Chief Complaint/Apparent Life Threats

Student: What is the patient's chief complaint?
PROCTOR: The jaw is obviously missing. She is visibly upset.
Student: There are apparent life threats; the life threats are related to airway involvement and blood loss.
PROCTOR: Noted.

Assess the Airway and Breathing

Student: I am opening the airway with a jaw-thrust maneuver. Is the patient breathing?
PROCTOR: Yes.
Student: I will suction the airway and apply direct pressure with dry, sterile dressings to the wound.
PROCTOR: Noted.
ALS Student: I will apply basic life support (BLS) interventions, plus the following: intubation per local protocol (rapid sequence intubation [RSI] if permitted) and confirm lung sounds and end tidal CO_2.
ALS Proctor: Noted. End tidal CO_2 and lung sounds confirm placement of the endotracheal (ET) tube.

Assessment

Student: What are the rate and the quality of breathing?
PROCTOR: Rate: Within normal limits. Quality: Normal.

Provide Oxygen

Student: I am applying oxygen at 15 L/min via nonrebreathing mask or blow-by method.
PROCTOR: Noted.
ALS Student: I will ventilate via the ET tube and control bleeding.
ALS Proctor: Noted.

Ensure Adequate Ventilation

Student: The patient has adequate ventilations at this time.
PROCTOR: Noted.

Injury Management

Student: I will direct my partner to take over c-spine control, ventilation or oxygenation, and bleeding control as I continue assessment.
PROCTOR: Noted.

Assess Circulation

Student: I am assessing the patient's circulation.
PROCTOR: Noted.

Assess for and Control Major Bleeding

Student: Do I find any major bleeding?
PROCTOR: Yes, some bleeding is noted through the dressings.
Student: I will have my partner control the bleeding with direct pressure and dressings.
PROCTOR: Noted.

Assess the Pulse

Student: What are the rate and the quality of pulses?
PROCTOR: Rate: Within normal limits. Quality: Bounding.

Assess the Skin

Student: I am assessing the skin. What are the color, temperature, and condition of the skin?
PROCTOR: Color: Flushed. Temperature: Normal. Condition: Moist.

Identify Priority Patients/Make Transport Decision

Student: The patient is a high priority and is a load-and-go. I will begin packaging and transport to a pediatric trauma center if available or to the nearest trauma center.
PROCTOR: Noted.

Critical Criteria:
- ❑ Did not provide high concentration of oxygen
- ❑ Did not find or manage problems associated with airway, breathing, hemorrhage or shock (hypoperfusion)
- ❑ Did not differentiate patient's need for transportation versus continued assessment at the scene
- ❑ Did other detailed examination before assessing the airway, breathing and circulation

Focused History and Physical Examination/Rapid Trauma Assessment

Select the Appropriate Assessment (Focused or Rapid)

Student: I am selecting the rapid physical exam to identify and treat life threats. I am checking for DCAP-BTLS. This acronym stands for deformities, contusions, abrasions, punctures, penetrations, and paradoxical motion in the chest, and burns, tenderness, lacerations, and swelling.
PROCTOR: Noted.

▸ Head

Student: I am rapidly assessing the head.
PROCTOR: The jaw is missing and there is bleeding noted in the area.
Student: I will continue to control the bleeding with direct pressure.
PROCTOR: Noted.

▸ Neck

Student: I am rapidly assessing the neck.
PROCTOR: There are no obvious injuries.
Student: I will apply a cervical collar.
PROCTOR: Noted.

▸ Chest

Student: I am rapidly assessing the chest. What are the lung sounds?
PROCTOR: There are no obvious injuries. Lung sounds are clear bilaterally.

▸ Abdomen/Pelvis

Student: I am rapidly assessing the abdomen.
PROCTOR: There are no obvious injuries.
Student: I am rapidly assessing the pelvis.
PROCTOR: There are no obvious injuries.

▸ Extremities

Student: I am rapidly assessing the extremities.
PROCTOR: There are no obvious injuries.
Student: Do I feel anything unusual?
PROCTOR: No.

▸ Assess Motor, Sensory, and Circulatory Function

Student: I am checking for DCAP-BTLS. I am also checking motor and sensory function, and pulses. Right leg?
PROCTOR: Negative DCAP-BTLS. Motor and sensory functions are present. Pulses are present.
Student: Left leg?
PROCTOR: Negative DCAP-BTLS. Motor and sensory functions are present. Pulses are present.
Student: Right arm?
PROCTOR: Negative DCAP-BTLS. Motor and sensory functions are present. Pulses are present.
Student: Left arm?
PROCTOR: Negative DCAP-BTLS. Motor and sensory functions are present. Pulses are present.

▸ Posterior

Student: I will rapidly assess the back. We will now log roll the patient as a unit to check the back. The person at the head will count to three and we will roll the patient.
PROCTOR: Noted.

▸ Assess the Thorax

Student: I am assessing the thorax. Do I find injuries?
PROCTOR: No.

▸ Assess the Lumbar Area

Student: I am assessing the flanks and lumbar area. Do I find injuries?
PROCTOR: No.

▸ Assess the Entire Backside

Student: I am assessing the entire backside. Do I find injuries?
PROCTOR: No.

▸ Manage Secondary Injuries/Wounds

Student: We will apply a cervical collar and backboard with full immobilization per local protocol, if not yet done, at this time.
PROCTOR: Noted.
Student: Are there any changes in motor and sensory functions or pulses?
PROCTOR: No.
ALS Student: I will establish two large-bore IVs en route to the hospital and administer a bolus of 20 mL/kg in order to maintain a systolic blood pressure of 90 mm Hg.
ALS Proctor: Noted.

▸ Reevaluate Transport Decision

Student: This patient is a high priority and is a load-and-go due to the mechanism of injury and airway involvement.
PROCTOR: Noted.

▼ Baseline Vital Signs

Student: What are the patient's baseline vital signs, including blood pressure, pulse, respirations, pulse oximetry, and level of consciousness?
PROCTOR: Blood pressure, 84/54 mm Hg; pulse rate, 110 beats/min; respirations, 24 breaths/min; pulse oximetry reading, 98%; and the patient is alert.

▼ SAMPLE History

Student: At this time I will gather a SAMPLE history from the patient or family. What are the patient's signs and symptoms?
PROCTOR: Pain and bleeding in the face.
Student: Allergies?
PROCTOR: No allergies.
Student: Medications?
PROCTOR: Seizure medications.
Student: Pertinent past medical history?
PROCTOR: Seizures.
Student: Last oral intake?
PROCTOR: 2 hours ago.
Student: Events leading up to the incident?
PROCTOR: The patient was playing in the yard when a car sped by and a man shot her.

Critical Criteria:
- ❑ Did not differentiate patient's need for transportation versus continued assessment at the scene
- ❑ Did not provide for spinal protection when indicated

▼ Detailed Physical Examination

Student: I am conducting the detailed physical exam.
PROCTOR: Noted. The detailed physical exam will be performed during transport.

▼ Assess the Head

Student: I am assessing the head. Do I find any DCAP-BTLS? Do I find any evidence of Battle's sign or raccoon eyes?
PROCTOR: No, you see only the jaw injury.

▸ Inspect and Palpate the Head and Ears

Student: I am assessing the head and ears.
PROCTOR: There are no obvious injuries to the rest of the head or ears, only the jaw injury.

▸ Assess the Eyes

Student: I am assessing the eyes. Are the pupils equal, round, and regular in size, and react properly to light (PEARRL)?
PROCTOR: They are PEARRL.

▸ Assess the Facial Area Including Oral and Nasal Areas

Student: I am assessing the face, nose, and mouth. Do I see any discharge or hear any obstructions?
PROCTOR: Yes, you hear occasional gurgling.
Student: I would suction as needed.
PROCTOR: Noted.

▼ Assess the Neck

▸ Inspect and Palpate the Neck

Student: I am assessing the neck for DCAP-BTLS.
PROCTOR: There are no obvious injuries.

▸ Assess for Jugular Vein Distention

Student: Do I find any jugular vein distention (JVD)?
PROCTOR: No.

Assess for Tracheal Deviation

Student: Do I see any tracheal deviation?

PROCTOR: No.

Assess the Chest

Student: I am assessing the chest for DCAP-BTLS.

PROCTOR: Noted.

Inspect

Student: What do I see when I look at the chest?

PROCTOR: There are no obvious injuries.

Student: Does the chest appear symmetric?

PROCTOR: Yes.

Palpate

Student: When I touch the chest, do I feel crepitus or a flail segment?

PROCTOR: No.

Auscultate

Student: Are lung sounds present in all fields?

PROCTOR: Yes.

Student: Do I hear any sucking sounds from the chest?

PROCTOR: No.

Assess the Abdomen/Pelvis

Assess the Abdomen

Student: I am assessing the abdomen for DCAP-BTLS. I am assessing all four quadrants. Do I find any problems?

PROCTOR: No.

Assess the Pelvis

Student: I am assessing the pelvis for DCAP-BTLS. Is the pelvis stable?

PROCTOR: Yes.

Assess the Genitalia/Perineum as Needed (Verbalize in Training)

Student: I am assessing the genitalia/perineum as necessary for DCAP-BTLS.

PROCTOR: The area is unremarkable.

Assess the Extremities

Inspect

Student: I am assessing the lower and upper extremities for DCAP-BTLS. Do I find anything?

PROCTOR: No.

Palpate

Student: Do I feel anything unusual?

PROCTOR: No.

Assess Motor, Sensory, and Circulatory Function

Student: I am checking for DCAP-BTLS, motor and sensory function, and pulses. Right leg?

PROCTOR: Negative DCAP-BTLS. Motor and sensory functions are present. Pulses are present.

Student: Left leg?

PROCTOR: Negative DCAP-BTLS. Motor and sensory functions are present. Pulses are present.

Student: Right arm?

PROCTOR: Negative DCAP-BTLS. Motor and sensory functions are present. Pulses are present.

Student: Left arm?

PROCTOR: Negative DCAP-BTLS. Motor and sensory functions are present. Pulses are present.

Assess the Posterior

Note: This portion of the detailed physical exam would not be done if the patient were previously backboarded per local protocol.

Student: We will not check the back because it was previously checked and the patient is backboarded.

PROCTOR: Noted.

Manage Secondary Injuries/Wounds

Student: I would direct my partner to reassess the dressings and maintain the airway.

PROCTOR: Noted.

Reassess Vital Signs

Student: I will reassess vital signs and mental status.

PROCTOR: Blood pressure, 82/52 mm Hg; pulse rate, 110 beats/min; respirations, 24 breaths/min; pulse oximetry reading, 98%; and the patient is alert.

Student: The vital signs have not changed significantly.

PROCTOR: Noted.

Reassess Interventions

Student: I will reassess my interventions: airway, suction, breathing, and oxygen; circulation and bleeding control; immobilization and straps; and treatment for shock.

PROCTOR: Noted.

ALS Student: I will reassess BLS interventions, plus the following: confirm ET tube placement with end tidal CO_2 and lung sounds if performed, two IVs, maintain blood pressure per local protocol, and cardiac monitor.

ALS Proctor: Noted. The lung sounds and end tidal CO_2 confirm ET tube placement. The cardiac monitor shows sinus tachycardia.

Critical Criteria:

- ❑ Did not find or manage problems associated with airway, breathing, hemorrhage or shock (hypoperfusion)

Radio Report

(Provided by the student.)

PROCTOR: Noted.

Ongoing Assessment

Repeat Vital Signs

Student: I will reassess vital signs and mental status.

PROCTOR: Blood pressure, 84/52 mm Hg; pulse rate, 108 beats/min; respirations, 22 breaths/min; pulse oximetry reading, 98%; and the patient is alert.

Student: The vital signs have not changed significantly.

PROCTOR: Noted.

Check Interventions

Student: I will check my interventions: airway, suction, breathing, and oxygen; circulation and bleeding control; immobilization and straps; and treatment for shock.

PROCTOR: Noted.

ALS Student: I will check BLS interventions, plus the following: maintain ET tube placement with end tidal CO_2 and lung sounds if performed, two IVs, maintain blood pressure per local protocol, and cardiac monitor.

ALS Proctor: Noted. The end tidal CO_2 confirms ET tube placement. The cardiac monitor shows sinus tachycardia.

Critical Criteria:
- ❑ Did not find or manage problems associated with airway, breathing, hemorrhage or shock (hypoperfusion)

Handoff Report to Emergency Department Staff

Student: There was no change in the patient's condition during transport.

PROCTOR: Noted.

Critical Criteria:
- ❑ Did not transport patient within the (10) minute time limit

Critical Criteria

(Inform the student of items missed, if any.)

❑ Pass ❑ Fail Date: ______________________

Proctor Comments: ______________________

____

____

CASE 45

Dispatch Information

PROCTOR: EMS 10, respond to a 27-year-old male who has been assaulted with a machete and a baseball bat. He is conscious and breathing. The police are en route.

Pre-scene Action (BSI)

Student: I am wearing nonlatex gloves, safety glasses, mask, and gown.
PROCTOR: Noted.

Critical Criteria:
- ❑ Did not take, or verbalize, body substance isolation (BSI) precautions when necessary

Scene Size-up

Scene Safety

Student: Is the scene safe?
PROCTOR: Yes, police are on scene and you are given clearance to enter.

Mechanism of Injury

Student: What was the mechanism of injury?
PROCTOR: Blunt and penetrating forces. The patient was beaten with a baseball bat and has lacerations from a machete. He is standing in the street calling out for help.

Number of Patients

Student: How many patients are there?
PROCTOR: One.

Additional Resources

Student: I would call for advanced life support (ALS) assistance.
PROCTOR: Noted.

C-Spine Stabilization

Student: On the basis of the mechanism of injury, I would stabilize the cervical spine (c-spine) in a neutral in-line position.
PROCTOR: Noted.

Critical Criteria:
- ❑ Did not determine scene safety
- ❑ Did not assess for spinal protection
- ❑ Did not provide for spinal protection when indicated

Initial Assessment

Student: As I perform midline c-spine stabilization, I identify myself and ask the patient not to move.
PROCTOR: Noted.

General Impression

Student: My general impression is that the patient's condition is unstable.
PROCTOR: Noted.

Responsiveness/Level of Consciousness

Student: What is the patient's level of consciousness?
PROCTOR: Alert.

Chief Complaint/Apparent Life Threats

Student: What is the patient's chief complaint?
PROCTOR: The patient is complaining of pain all over his body. His nose is hanging off, as are both of his thumbs. He has multiple injuries.
Student: There are apparent life threats; the life threats are potential airway obstruction from blood in the nose, blood loss, internal injuries, and shock.
PROCTOR: Noted.

Assess the Airway and Breathing

Student: Is the airway open? Is the patient breathing?
PROCTOR: Yes, the airway is open and the patient is breathing.

▸ Assessment

Student: What are the rate and the quality of breathing?
PROCTOR: Rate: Slightly fast. Quality: Guarded.

▸ Provide Oxygen

Student: I am applying oxygen at 15 L/min via nonrebreathing mask or the blow-by method. I will allow the patient to suction himself as necessary and apply manual pressure to the nose.
PROCTOR: Noted.

▸ Ensure Adequate Ventilation

Student: The patient has adequate ventilations at this time.
PROCTOR: Noted.

▸ Injury Management

Student: I will direct my partner to take over c-spine control as I continue assessment.
PROCTOR: Noted.

Assess Circulation

Student: I am assessing the patient's circulation.
PROCTOR: Noted.

▸ Assess for and Control Major Bleeding

Student: Do I find any major bleeding?
PROCTOR: Yes, the patient is bleeding from his nose, his thumbs, his chest, and his back.
Student: I would apply direct pressure and dressings to all wounds and continue to suction the airway as needed. I will use occlusive dressings on the chest and back.
PROCTOR: Noted.

▸ Assess the Pulse

Student: What are the rate and the quality of pulses?
PROCTOR: Rate: Tachycardic. Quality: Thready.

▸ Assess the Skin

Student: I am assessing the skin. What are the color, temperature, and condition of the skin?
PROCTOR: Color: Pale. Temperature: Cool. Condition: Diaphoretic.

Identify Priority Patients/Make Transport Decision

Student: The patient is a high priority and is a load-and-go. I will begin packaging and transport the patient to a trauma center.
PROCTOR: Noted.

Critical Criteria:
- ❑ Did not provide high concentration of oxygen
- ❑ Did not find or manage problems associated with airway, breathing, hemorrhage or shock (hypoperfusion)
- ❑ Did not differentiate patient's need for transportation versus continued assessment at the scene
- ❑ Did other detailed examination before assessing the airway, breathing and circulation

Focused History and Physical Examination/Rapid Trauma Assessment

Select the Appropriate Assessment (Focused or Rapid)

Student: I am selecting the rapid physical exam to identify and treat life threats. I am checking for DCAP-BTLS. This acronym stands for deformities, contusions, abrasions, punctures, penetrations, and paradoxical motion in the chest, and burns, tenderness, lacerations, and swelling.
PROCTOR: Noted.

▸ Head

Student: I am rapidly assessing the head.
PROCTOR: The patient's nose is barely hanging on. Bleeding is controlled.

Student: I would monitor the nose and have the patient suction the airway as needed.
PROCTOR: Noted.

- Neck

Student: I am rapidly assessing the neck.
PROCTOR: There are no obvious injuries.
Student: I will apply a cervical collar.
PROCTOR: Noted.

- Chest

Student: I am rapidly assessing the chest.
PROCTOR: The patient has a 7-inch-long gash to his chest and you can see his ribs.
Student: I will apply an occlusive dressing and tape it on three sides.
PROCTOR: Noted.
Student: I am listening to breath sounds.
PROCTOR: Noted. Breath sounds are present and equal on both sides.

- Abdomen/Pelvis

Student: I am rapidly assessing the abdomen.
PROCTOR: You see a bruise in the shape of a baseball bat across the belly. The abdomen is soft and tender at this time.

- Extremities

Student: I am rapidly assessing the extremities.
PROCTOR: Both of the thumbs have nearly been cut off.
Student: I will apply pressure dressings to both thumbs.
PROCTOR: Noted.

- Assess Motor, Sensory, and Circulatory Function

Student: I am checking for DCAP-BTLS. I am also checking motor and sensory function, and pulses. Right leg?
PROCTOR: Negative DCAP-BTLS. Motor and sensory functions are present. Pulses are weak.
Student: Left leg?
PROCTOR: Negative DCAP-BTLS. Motor and sensory functions are present. Pulses are weak.
Student: Right arm?
PROCTOR: A deglove injury to the right thumb. Motor and sensory functions are present. Pulses are weak.
Student: I will recheck the pressure dressing.
PROCTOR: Noted.
Student: Left arm?
PROCTOR: The bone of the left thumb has been sliced through and is just attached by skin. Motor and sensory functions are present. Pulses are weak.
Student: I will recheck the pressure dressing.
PROCTOR: Noted.

- Posterior

Student: I will rapidly assess the back. We will now log roll the patient as a unit to check the back. The person at the head will count to three and we will roll the patient.
PROCTOR: Noted.

  - Assess the Thorax

Student: I am assessing the thorax. Do I find injuries?
PROCTOR: You see an 11-inch laceration to the back.
Student: I will apply an occlusive dressing.
PROCTOR: Noted.

  - Assess the Lumbar Area

Student: I am assessing the flanks and lumbar area. Do I find injuries?
PROCTOR: No.

  - Assess the Entire Backside

Student: I am assessing the entire backside. Do I find injuries?
PROCTOR: No.

- Manage Secondary Injuries/Wounds

Student: We will apply a cervical collar and backboard with full immobilization per local protocol, if not yet done, at this time.
PROCTOR: Noted.
Student: Are there any changes in motor and sensory functions or pulses?
PROCTOR: No.
Student: I will rapidly control bleeding and begin transport to a trauma center.
PROCTOR: Noted.
ALS Student: I will apply basic life support (BLS) interventions, plus the following: establish two large-bore IVs and maintain the blood pressure.
ALS Proctor: Noted.

- Reevaluate Transport Decision

Student: This patient is a load-and-go due to multiple trauma.
PROCTOR: Noted.

Baseline Vital Signs

Student: What are the patient's baseline vital signs, including blood pressure, pulse, respirations, pulse oximetry, and level of consciousness?
PROCTOR: Blood pressure, 96/68 mm Hg; pulse, 134 beats/min; respirations, 18 breaths/min; pulse oximetry reading, 92%; and the patient is alert.

SAMPLE History

Student: At this time I will gather a SAMPLE history from the patient or family. What are the patient's signs and symptoms?
PROCTOR: Chest, back, nose, and thumb pain, and major bleeding.
Student: Allergies?
PROCTOR: No allergies.
Student: Medications?
PROCTOR: No medications.
Student: Pertinent past medical history?
PROCTOR: No pertinent medical history.
Student: Last oral intake?
PROCTOR: The patient has been drinking beer all night.
Student: Events leading up to the incident?
PROCTOR: The patient made a comment about someone else's wife, and then he was assaulted with a machete and a baseball bat.

Critical Criteria:
- ❑ Did not differentiate patient's need for transportation versus continued assessment at the scene
- ❑ Did not provide for spinal protection when indicated

Detailed Physical Examination

Student: I am conducting the detailed physical exam. I am looking for DCAP-BTLS.
PROCTOR: Noted. The detailed physical exam will be performed during transport.

Assess the Head

Student: I am assessing the head. Do I find any DCAP-BTLS? Do I find any evidence of Battle's sign or raccoon eyes?
PROCTOR: You see only the nose injury.

- Inspect and Palpate the Head and Ears

Student: I am assessing the head and ears.
PROCTOR: He has various bruises to his head.

- Assess the Eyes

Student: I am assessing the eyes. Are the pupils equal, round, and regular in size, and react properly to light (PEARRL)?
PROCTOR: They are sluggish.

▸ **Assess the Facial Area Including Oral and Nasal Areas**

Student: I am assessing the face, nose, and mouth. Do I see any discharge or hear any obstructions?
PROCTOR: No, bleeding is controlled.
Student: I will allow the patient to continue manual pressure to the nose and suction the airway as needed.
PROCTOR: Noted.

▾ Assess the Neck

▸ **Inspect and Palpate the Neck**

Student: I am assessing the neck for DCAP-BTLS.
PROCTOR: The patient has pain in the neck.

▸ **Assess for Jugular Vein Distention**

Student: Do I find any jugular vein distention (JVD)?
PROCTOR: No.

▸ **Assess for Tracheal Deviation**

Student: Do I see any tracheal deviation?
PROCTOR: No.

▾ Assess the Chest

Student: I am assessing the chest for DCAP-BTLS.
PROCTOR: Noted.

▸ **Inspect**

Student: What do I see when I look at the chest?
PROCTOR: A 7-inch laceration across the chest with the ribs exposed.
Student: I will recheck the occlusive dressing.
PROCTOR: Noted.
Student: Does the chest appear symmetric?
PROCTOR: Yes.

▸ **Palpate**

Student: When I touch the chest, do I feel crepitus or a flail segment?
PROCTOR: No.

▸ **Auscultate**

Student: Are lung sounds present in all fields?
PROCTOR: Yes.
Student: Do I hear any sucking sounds from the chest?
PROCTOR: No.

▾ Assess the Abdomen/Pelvis

▸ **Assess the Abdomen**

Student: I am assessing the abdomen for DCAP-BTLS. I am assessing all four quadrants. Do I find any problems?
PROCTOR: You see a bruise in the shape of a baseball bat to the belly. The abdomen is still soft and tender.

▸ **Assess the Pelvis**

Student: I am assessing the pelvis for DCAP-BTLS. Is the pelvis stable?
PROCTOR: Yes.

▸ **Assess the Genitalia/Perineum as Needed (Verbalize in Training)**

Student: I am assessing the genitalia as necessary for DCAP-BTLS.
PROCTOR: The area is unremarkable.

▾ Assess the Extremities

▸ **Inspect**

Student: I am assessing the lower and upper extremities for DCAP-BTLS. Do I find anything?
PROCTOR: Yes, the thumb injuries.
Student: I will treat the thumbs with pressure dressings.
PROCTOR: Noted.

▸ **Palpate**

Student: Do I feel anything unusual?
PROCTOR: No.

▸ **Assess Motor, Sensory, and Circulatory Function**

Student: I am checking for DCAP-BTLS, motor and sensory function, and pulses. Right leg?
PROCTOR: Negative DCAP-BTLS. Motor and sensory functions are present. Pulses are weak.
Student: Left leg?
PROCTOR: Negative DCAP-BTLS. Motor and sensory functions are present. Pulses are weak.
Student: Right arm?
PROCTOR: A deglove injury to the thumb. Motor and sensory functions are present. Pulses are weak.
Student: I will recheck the pressure dressing.
PROCTOR: Noted.
Student: Left arm?
PROCTOR: The bone has been sliced through on the thumb and the thumb is just attached by skin. Motor and sensory functions are present. Pulses are weak.
Student: I will recheck the pressure dressing.
PROCTOR: Noted.

▾ Assess the Posterior

Note: This portion of the detailed physical exam would not be done if the patient were previously backboarded per local protocol.
Student: We will not check the back because it was previously checked and the patient is backboarded.
PROCTOR: Noted.

▾ Manage Secondary Injuries/Wounds

Student: I would direct my partner to maintain the airway and check all bleeding areas.
PROCTOR: Noted.

▾ Reassess Vital Signs

Student: I will reassess vital signs and mental status.
PROCTOR: Blood pressure, 92/62 mm Hg; pulse, 144 beats/min; respirations, 24 breaths/min; pulse oximetry reading, 94%; and the patient is alert.
Student: The vital signs are deteriorating.
PROCTOR: Noted.

▾ Reassess Interventions

Student: I will reassess my interventions: airway, breathing, and oxygen; circulation and bleeding control; occlusive dressings; immobilization and straps; and treatment for shock.
PROCTOR: Noted.
ALS Student: I will reassess BLS interventions, plus the following: two large-bore IVs, cardiac monitor, and monitor the chest.
ALS Proctor: Noted. The cardiac monitor shows sinus tachycardia.

Critical Criteria:

- ❑ Did not find or manage problems associated with airway, breathing, hemorrhage or shock (hypoperfusion)

▾ Radio Report

(Provided by the student.)
PROCTOR: Noted.

▾ Ongoing Assessment

▾ Repeat Vital Signs

Student: I will reassess vital signs and mental status.
PROCTOR: Blood pressure, 88/56 mm Hg; pulse, 136 beats/min; respirations, 22 breaths/min; pulse oximetry reading, 93%; and the patient is alert.

Student: The vital signs have deteriorated.
PROCTOR: Noted.

Check Interventions

Student: I will check my interventions: airway, breathing, and oxygen; circulation and bleeding control; occlusive dressings; immobilization and straps; and treatment for shock.
PROCTOR: Noted.
ALS Student: I will check BLS interventions, plus the following: two large-bore IVs, cardiac monitor, and monitor the chest.
ALS Proctor: Noted. The cardiac monitor shows sinus tachycardia.

Critical Criteria:
- ❑ Did not find or manage problems associated with airway, breathing, hemorrhage or shock (hypoperfusion)

Handoff Report to Emergency Department Staff

Student: The patient's condition deteriorated during transport.
PROCTOR: Noted.

Critical Criteria:
- ❑ Did not transport patient within the (10) minute time limit

Critical Criteria

(Inform the student of items missed, if any.)

❑ Pass ❑ Fail Date: ______________________

Proctor Comments: ______________________

____

____

CASE 46

Dispatch Information

PROCTOR: EMS 10, respond to an 8-year-old female impaled through the chest with the handlebar from her bike. She is conscious and breathing.

Pre-scene Action (BSI)

Student: I am wearing appropriate high-visibility personal protective equipment, nonlatex gloves, and safety glasses.
PROCTOR: Noted.

Critical Criteria:
- ❑ Did not take, or verbalize, body substance isolation (BSI) precautions when necessary

Scene Size-up

Scene Safety

Student: Is the scene safe?
PROCTOR: Yes.

Mechanism of Injury

Student: What was the mechanism of injury?
PROCTOR: Penetrating force from a bike handlebar. The patient was riding her bike and struck a curb.

Number of Patients

Student: How many patients are there?
PROCTOR: One.

Additional Resources

Student: I would call for advanced life support (ALS) assistance and additional resources: fire/rescue.
PROCTOR: Noted.

C-Spine Stabilization

Student: On the basis of the mechanism of injury, I would stabilize the cervical spine (c-spine) in a neutral in-line position.
PROCTOR: Noted.

Critical Criteria:
- ❑ Did not determine scene safety
- ❑ Did not assess for spinal protection
- ❑ Did not provide for spinal protection when indicated

Initial Assessment

Student: As I perform midline c-spine stabilization, I identify myself and ask the patient not to move.
PROCTOR: Noted.

General Impression

Student: My general impression is that the patient's condition is unstable.
PROCTOR: Noted.

Responsiveness/Level of Consciousness

Student: What is the patient's level of consciousness?
PROCTOR: Alert.

Chief Complaint/Apparent Life Threats

Student: What is the patient's chief complaint?
PROCTOR: The patient is complaining of pain in the right chest. The handlebar does not have a grip and is impaled 3 or 4 inches into her chest.
Student: I will remove the handlebar from the bike, stabilize it to the patient's chest, apply an occlusive dressing, and consider air ambulance transport.
PROCTOR: Noted.

Assess the Airway and Breathing

Student: Is the airway open? Is the patient breathing?
PROCTOR: Yes, the airway is open and the patient is breathing.
Student: What are the lung sounds?
PROCTOR: Lung sounds are clear bilaterally.

Assessment

Student: What are the rate and the quality of breathing?
PROCTOR: Rate: Within normal limits. Quality: Guarded.

Provide Oxygen

Student: I am applying oxygen at 15 L/min via nonrebreathing mask.
PROCTOR: Noted.

Ensure Adequate Ventilation

Student: The patient has adequate ventilations at this time.
PROCTOR: Noted.

Injury Management

Student: I will direct my partner to take over c-spine control as I continue assessment.
PROCTOR: Noted.

Assess Circulation

Student: I am assessing the patient's circulation.
PROCTOR: Noted.

Assess for and Control Major Bleeding

Student: Do I find any major bleeding?
PROCTOR: No.

Assess the Pulse

Student: What are the rate and the quality of pulses?
PROCTOR: Rate: Tachycardic. Quality: Strong.

Assess the Skin

Student: I am assessing the skin. What are the color, temperature, and condition of the skin?
PROCTOR: Color: Flushed. Temperature: Warm. Condition: Moist.

Identify Priority Patients/Make Transport Decision

Student: The patient is a high priority and is a load-and-go. I will begin packaging and transport to a trauma center.
PROCTOR: Noted.

Critical Criteria:
- ❑ Did not provide high concentration of oxygen
- ❑ Did not find or manage problems associated with airway, breathing, hemorrhage or shock (hypoperfusion)
- ❑ Did not differentiate patient's need for transportation versus continued assessment at the scene
- ❑ Did other detailed examination before assessing the airway, breathing and circulation

Focused History and Physical Examination/Rapid Trauma Assessment

Select the Appropriate Assessment (Focused or Rapid)

Student: I am selecting the rapid physical exam to identify and treat life threats. I am checking for DCAP-BTLS. This acronym stands for deformities, contusions, abrasions, punctures, penetrations, and paradoxical motion in the chest, and burns, tenderness, lacerations, and swelling.
PROCTOR: Noted.

Head

Student: I am rapidly assessing the head.
PROCTOR: There are no obvious injuries.

Neck

Student: I am rapidly assessing the neck.
PROCTOR: There are no obvious injuries.
Student: I will apply a cervical collar.
PROCTOR: Noted.

Chest

Student: I am rapidly assessing the chest. What are the lung sounds?
PROCTOR: The handlebar is impaled through the chest wall between the ribs. It is stabilized. Lung sounds are clear bilaterally.

Student: I will assess the chest for tension pneumothorax by auscultation and assessment (for jugular vein distention [JVD], tracheal deviation, and decreased lung sounds).

PROCTOR: The lung sounds appear clear bilaterally, jugular vein distention is not present, and the trachea is midline.

ALS Student: I will assess the chest for hyperresonance to percussion.

ALS Proctor: Noted. There is no tension pneumothorax.

ALS Student: I will continuously reassess the chest.

ALS Proctor: Noted.

▸ **Abdomen/Pelvis**

Student: I am rapidly assessing the abdomen.

PROCTOR: There are no obvious injuries.

Student: I am rapidly assessing the pelvis.

PROCTOR: There are no obvious injuries.

▸ **Extremities**

Student: I am rapidly assessing the extremities.

PROCTOR: There are no obvious injuries.

▸ **Assess Motor, Sensory, and Circulatory Function**

Student: I am checking for DCAP-BTLS, motor and sensory function, and pulses. Right leg?

PROCTOR: Negative DCAP-BTLS. Motor and sensory functions are present. Pulses are present.

Student: Left leg?

PROCTOR: Negative DCAP-BTLS. Motor and sensory functions are present. Pulses are present.

Student: Right arm?

PROCTOR: Negative DCAP-BTLS. Motor and sensory functions are present. Pulses are present.

Student: Left arm?

PROCTOR: Negative DCAP-BTLS. Motor and sensory functions are present. Pulses are present.

▸ **Posterior**

Student: I will rapidly assess the back. We will now log roll the patient as a unit to check the back. The person at the head will count to three and we will roll the patient.

PROCTOR: Noted.

▸ **Assess the Thorax**

Student: I am assessing the thorax. Do I find injuries?

PROCTOR: No.

▸ **Assess the Lumbar Area**

Student: I am assessing the flanks and lumbar area. Do I find injuries?

PROCTOR: No.

▸ **Assess the Entire Backside**

Student: I am assessing the entire backside. Do I find injuries?

PROCTOR: No.

▸ **Manage Secondary Injuries/Wounds**

Student: We will apply a cervical collar and backboard with full immobilization per local protocol, if not yet done, at this time.

PROCTOR: Noted.

Student: Are there any changes in motor and sensory functions or pulses?

PROCTOR: No.

▸ **Reevaluate Transport Decision**

Student: This patient is a high priority and a load-and-go due to chest trauma.

PROCTOR: Noted.

▾ Baseline Vital Signs

Student: What are the patient's baseline vital signs, including blood pressure, pulse, respirations, pulse oximetry, and level of consciousness?

PROCTOR: Blood pressure, 110/72 mm Hg; pulse rate, 124 beats/min; respirations, 28 breaths/min; pulse oximetry reading, 98%; and the patient is alert.

▾ SAMPLE History

Student: At this time I will gather a SAMPLE history from the patient or family. What are the patient's signs and symptoms?

PROCTOR: Pain in the chest and mild difficulty breathing.

Student: Allergies?

PROCTOR: No allergies.

Student: Medications?

PROCTOR: No medications.

Student: Pertinent past medical history?

PROCTOR: No pertinent medical history.

Student: Last oral intake?

PROCTOR: 2 hours ago.

Student: Events leading up to the incident?

PROCTOR: The patient was riding her bike when she hit the curb and was impaled by the handlebar.

Critical Criteria:

- ❑ Did not differentiate patient's need for transportation versus continued assessment at the scene
- ❑ Did not provide for spinal protection when indicated

Detailed Physical Examination

Student: I am conducting the detailed physical exam. I am looking for DCAP-BTLS.

PROCTOR: Noted. The detailed physical exam will be performed during transport.

▾ Assess the Head

Student: I am assessing the head. Do I find any DCAP-BTLS? Do I find any evidence of Battle's sign or raccoon eyes?

PROCTOR: No.

▸ **Inspect and Palpate the Head and Ears**

Student: I am assessing the head and ears.

PROCTOR: There are no obvious injuries.

▸ **Assess the Eyes**

Student: I am assessing the eyes. Are the pupils equal, round, and regular in size, and react properly to light (PEARRL)?

PROCTOR: They are PEARRL.

▸ **Assess the Facial Area Including Oral and Nasal Areas**

Student: I am assessing the face, nose, and mouth. Do I see any discharge or hear any obstructions?

PROCTOR: No.

▾ Assess the Neck

▸ **Inspect and Palpate the Neck**

Student: I am assessing the neck for DCAP-BTLS.

PROCTOR: There are no obvious injuries.

▸ **Assess for Jugular Vein Distention**

Student: Do I find any jugular vein distention (JVD)?

PROCTOR: No.

▸ **Assess for Tracheal Deviation**

Student: Do I see any tracheal deviation?

PROCTOR: No.

▾ Assess the Chest

Student: I am assessing the chest for DCAP-BTLS.

PROCTOR: Noted.

▸ **Inspect**

Student: What do I see when I look at the chest?

PROCTOR: You see the handlebar impaled into the right chest between the ribs.

Student: Does the chest appear symmetric?

PROCTOR: Yes.

▸ **Palpate**

Student: When I touch the chest, do I feel crepitus or a flail segment?

PROCTOR: No.

▸ Auscultate

Student: Are lung sounds present in all fields?

PROCTOR: Yes.

Student: Do I hear any sucking sounds from the chest?

PROCTOR: No.

ALS Student: I will assess the chest for hyperresonance to percussion.

ALS Proctor: Noted. There is no tension pneumothorax.

ALS Student: I will continuously reassess the chest.

ALS Proctor: Noted.

▾ Assess the Abdomen/Pelvis

▸ Assess the Abdomen

Student: I am assessing the abdomen for DCAP-BTLS. I am assessing all four quadrants. Do I find any problems?

PROCTOR: No.

▸ Assess the Pelvis

Student: I am assessing the pelvis for DCAP-BTLS. Is the pelvis stable?

PROCTOR: Yes.

▾ Assess the Genitalia/Perineum as Needed (Verbalize in Training)

Student: I am assessing the genitalia/perineum as necessary for DCAP-BTLS.

PROCTOR: The area is unremarkable.

▾ Assess the Extremities

▸ Inspect

Student: I am assessing the lower and upper extremities for DCAP-BTLS. Do I find anything?

PROCTOR: No.

▸ Palpate

Student: Do I feel anything unusual?

PROCTOR: No.

▸ Assess Motor, Sensory, and Circulatory Function

Student: I am checking for DCAP-BTLS, motor and sensory function, and pulses. Right leg?

PROCTOR: Negative DCAP-BTLS. Motor and sensory functions are present. Pulses are present.

Student: Left leg?

PROCTOR: Negative DCAP-BTLS. Motor and sensory functions are present. Pulses are present.

Student: Right arm?

PROCTOR: Negative DCAP-BTLS. Motor and sensory functions are present. Pulses are present.

Student: Left arm?

PROCTOR: Negative DCAP-BTLS. Motor and sensory functions are present. Pulses are present.

▾ Assess the Posterior

Note: This portion of the detailed physical exam would not be done if the patient were previously backboarded per local protocol.

Student: We will not check the back because it was previously checked and the patient is backboarded.

PROCTOR: Noted.

▾ Manage Secondary Injuries/Wounds

Student: I would direct my partner to maintain control of the handlebar.

PROCTOR: Noted.

▾ Reassess Vital Signs

Student: I will reassess vital signs and mental status.

PROCTOR: Blood pressure, 112/70 mm Hg; pulse rate, 120 beats/min; respirations, 24 breaths/min; pulse oximetry reading, 99%; and the patient is alert.

Student: The vital signs have not changed significantly.

PROCTOR: Noted.

▾ Reassess Interventions

Student: I will reassess my interventions: airway, breathing, and oxygen; occlusive dressing and stabilization of the handlebar; immobilization and straps; and treatment for shock.

PROCTOR: Noted.

ALS Student: I will reassess basic life support (BLS) interventions, plus the following: two large-bore IVs and cardiac monitor.

ALS Proctor: Noted. The cardiac monitor shows sinus tachycardia.

> **Critical Criteria:**
> ❑ Did not find or manage problems associated with airway, breathing, hemorrhage or shock (hypoperfusion)

Radio Report

(Provided by the student.)

PROCTOR: Noted.

Ongoing Assessment

▾ Repeat Vital Signs

Student: I will reassess vital signs and mental status.

PROCTOR: Blood pressure, 108/72 mm Hg; pulse rate, 118 beats/min; respirations 24 breaths/min; pulse oximetry reading, 99%; and the patient is alert.

Student: The vital signs have not changed significantly.

PROCTOR: Noted.

▾ Check Interventions

Student: I will check my interventions: airway, breathing, and oxygen; occlusive dressing and stabilization of the handlebar; immobilization and straps; and treatment for shock.

PROCTOR: Noted.

ALS Student: I will check BLS interventions, plus the following: two large-bore IVs and cardiac monitor.

ALS Proctor: Noted. The cardiac monitor shows sinus tachycardia.

> **Critical Criteria:**
> ❑ Did not find or manage problems associated with airway, breathing, hemorrhage or shock (hypoperfusion)

Handoff Report to Emergency Department Staff

Student: There was no change in the patient's condition during transport.

PROCTOR: Noted.

> **Critical Criteria:**
> ❑ Did not transport patient within the (10) minute time limit

Critical Criteria

(Inform the student of items missed, if any.)

❑ Pass ❑ Fail Date: ______________________

Proctor Comments: ______________________

____

____

CASE 46

Notes

Dispatch Information

PROCTOR: EMS 10, respond to a 22-year-old male who has possibly been stabbed in the chest. He is conscious but is having difficulty breathing. Police officers are on scene.

Pre-scene Action (BSI)

Student: I am wearing nonlatex gloves, safety glasses, mask, and gown.
PROCTOR: Noted.

Critical Criteria:
- ❑ Did not take, or verbalize, body substance isolation (BSI) precautions when necessary

Scene Size-up

Scene Safety

Student: Is the scene safe?
PROCTOR: Yes, police are on scene and you are given clearance to enter.

Mechanism of Injury

Student: What was the mechanism of injury?
PROCTOR: Penetrating chest trauma. The patient was in a dark club and was dancing when he was stabbed twice in the chest and once in the back.

Number of Patients

Student: How many patients are there?
PROCTOR: One.

Additional Resources

Student: I would call for advanced life support (ALS) assistance.
PROCTOR: Noted.

C-Spine Stabilization

Student: On the basis of the mechanism of injury, I would stabilize the cervical spine (c-spine) in a neutral in-line position.
PROCTOR: Noted.

Critical Criteria:
- ❑ Did not determine scene safety
- ❑ Did not assess for spinal protection
- ❑ Did not provide for spinal protection when indicated

Initial Assessment

Student: As I perform midline c-spine stabilization, I identify myself and ask the patient not to move.
PROCTOR: Noted.

General Impression

Student: My general impression is that the patient's condition is unstable.
PROCTOR: Noted.

Responsiveness/Level of Consciousness

Student: What is the patient's level of consciousness?
PROCTOR: Conscious and alert.

Chief Complaint/Apparent Life Threats

Student: What is the patient's chief complaint?
PROCTOR: The patient is complaining of difficulty breathing.
Student: There are apparent life threats; the life threats are the chest wounds.
PROCTOR: Noted.

Assess the Airway and Breathing

Student: Is the airway open? Is the patient breathing?
PROCTOR: Yes, the airway is open and the patient is breathing.

▸ Assessment

Student: What are the rate and the quality of breathing?
PROCTOR: Rate: Tachypneic. Quality: Guarded.

▸ Provide Oxygen

Student: I am applying oxygen at 15 L/min via nonrebreathing mask.
PROCTOR: Noted.

▸ Ensure Adequate Ventilation

Student: The patient has adequate ventilations at this time.
PROCTOR: Noted.

Injury Management

Student: I will direct my partner to take over c-spine control as I continue assessment.
PROCTOR: Noted.

Assess Circulation

Student: I am assessing the patient's circulation.
PROCTOR: Noted.

▸ Assess for and Control Major Bleeding

Student: Do I find any major bleeding?
PROCTOR: No.

▸ Assess the Pulse

Student: What are the rate and the quality of pulses?
PROCTOR: Rate: Tachycardic. Quality: Bounding.

▸ Assess the Skin

Student: I am assessing the skin. What are the color, temperature, and condition of the skin?
PROCTOR: Color: Flushed. Temperature: Warm. Condition: Moist.

Identify Priority Patients/Make Transport Decision

Student: The patient is a high priority and is a load-and-go. I will begin packaging and transport to a trauma center.
PROCTOR: Noted.

Critical Criteria:
- ❑ Did not provide high concentration of oxygen
- ❑ Did not find or manage problems associated with airway, breathing, hemorrhage or shock (hypoperfusion)
- ❑ Did not differentiate patient's need for transportation versus continued assessment at the scene
- ❑ Did other detailed examination before assessing the airway, breathing and circulation

Focused History and Physical Examination/Rapid Trauma Assessment

Select the Appropriate Assessment (Focused or Rapid)

Student: I am selecting rapid physical exam to identify and treat life threats. I am checking for DCAP-BTLS. This acronym stands for deformities, contusions, abrasions, punctures, penetrations, and paradoxical motion in the chest, and burns, tenderness, lacerations, and swelling.
PROCTOR: Noted.

▸ Head

Student: I am rapidly assessing the head.
PROCTOR: There are no obvious injuries.

▸ Neck

Student: I am rapidly assessing the neck.
PROCTOR: There are no obvious injuries.
Student: I will apply a cervical collar.
PROCTOR: Noted.

▸ Chest

Student: I am rapidly assessing the chest.
PROCTOR: You see two small and narrow puncture wounds. There is one on each side of the chest.
Student: I would apply occlusive dressings to each wound.
PROCTOR: Noted.

Student: What are the lung sounds at this time?
PROCTOR: You hear some fluid on the left side, but sounds are equal.
Student: I will assess the chest for tension pneumothorax by auscultation and assessment (for jugular vein distention [JVD], tracheal deviation, and decreased lung sounds).
PROCTOR: The lung sounds appear equal but with some fluid heard on the left side, jugular vein distention is not present, and the trachea is midline.
ALS Student: I will assess the chest for hyperresonance to percussion.
ALS Proctor: Noted. There is no tension pneumothorax.
ALS Student: I will continuously reassess the chest.
ALS Proctor: Noted.

▸ **Abdomen/Pelvis**

Student: I am rapidly assessing the abdomen.
PROCTOR: There are no obvious injuries.
Student: I am rapidly assessing the pelvis.
PROCTOR: There are no obvious injuries.

▸ **Extremities**

Student: I am rapidly assessing the extremities.
PROCTOR: There are no obvious injuries.

▸ **Assess Motor, Sensory, and Circulatory Function**

Student: I am checking for DCAP-BTLS. I am also checking motor and sensory function, and pulses. Right leg?
PROCTOR: Negative DCAP-BTLS. Motor and sensory functions are present. Pulses are present.
Student: Left leg?
PROCTOR: Negative DCAP-BTLS. Motor and sensory functions are present. Pulses are present.
Student: Right arm?
PROCTOR: Negative DCAP-BTLS. Motor and sensory functions are present. Pulses are present.
Student: Left arm?
PROCTOR: Negative DCAP-BTLS. Motor and sensory functions are present. Pulses are present.

▸ **Posterior**

Student: I will rapidly assess the back. We will now log roll the patient as a unit to check the back. The person at the head will count to three and we will roll the patient.
PROCTOR: Noted.

▸ **Assess the Thorax**

Student: I am assessing the thorax. Do I find injuries?
PROCTOR: Yes, you see a puncture on the left side.
Student: I will apply an occlusive dressing.
PROCTOR: Noted.

▸ **Assess the Lumbar Area**

Student: I am assessing the flanks and lumbar area. Do I find injuries?
PROCTOR: No.

▸ **Assess the Entire Backside**

Student: I am assessing the entire backside. Do I find injuries?
PROCTOR: No.

▸ **Manage Secondary Injuries/Wounds**

Student: We will apply a cervical collar and backboard with full immobilization per local protocol, if not yet done, at this time.
PROCTOR: Noted.
Student: Are there any changes in motor and sensory functions or pulses?
PROCTOR: No.

ALS Student: I will apply basic life support (BLS) interventions, plus the following: establish two large-bore IVs and bolus of 20 mL/kg, maintain a systolic blood pressure of 90 mm Hg, a cardiac monitor, and treatment for pneumothorax if necessary.
ALS Proctor: Noted. The cardiac monitor shows normal sinus rhythm.

▸ **Reevaluate Transport Decision**

Student: This patient is a high priority and a load-and-go due to chest trauma.
PROCTOR: Noted.

▾ Baseline Vital Signs

Student: What are the patient's baseline vital signs, including blood pressure, pulse, respirations, pulse oximetry, and level of consciousness?
PROCTOR: Blood pressure, 128/80 mm Hg; pulse rate, 100 beats/min; respirations, 24 breaths/min; pulse oximetry reading, 97%; and the patient is alert.

▾ SAMPLE History

Student: At this time I will gather a SAMPLE history from the patient or family. What are the patient's signs and symptoms?
PROCTOR: He has pain in the chest and difficulty breathing.
Student: Allergies?
PROCTOR: No allergies.
Student: Medications?
PROCTOR: Insulin.
Student: Pertinent past medical history?
PROCTOR: Diabetes.
Student: Last oral intake?
PROCTOR: The patient has been drinking for 2 hours.
Student: Events leading up to the incident?
PROCTOR: He was dancing and another man tried to dance with his wife; the next thing he knew, he had been stabbed.

Critical Criteria:
- ❑ Did not differentiate patient's need for transportation versus continued assessment at the scene
- ❑ Did not provide for spinal protection when indicated

▼ Detailed Physical Examination

Student: I am conducting the detailed physical exam. I am looking for DCAP-BTLS.
PROCTOR: Noted. The detailed physical exam will be performed during transport.

▾ Assess the Head

Student: I am assessing the head. Do I find any DCAP-BTLS? Do I find any evidence of Battle's sign or raccoon eyes?
PROCTOR: No.

▸ **Inspect and Palpate the Head and Ears**

Student: I am assessing the head and ears.
PROCTOR: There are no obvious injuries.

▸ **Assess the Eyes**

Student: I am assessing the eyes. Are the pupils equal, round, and regular in size, and react properly to light (PEARRL)?
PROCTOR: They are PEARRL.

▸ **Assess the Facial Area Including Oral and Nasal Areas**

Student: I am assessing the face, nose, and mouth. Do I see any discharge or hear any obstructions?
PROCTOR: Yes, you see the patient spit up blood.
Student: I would suction as necessary.
PROCTOR: Noted.

Assess the Neck

Inspect and Palpate the Neck

Student: I am assessing the neck for DCAP-BTLS.
PROCTOR: There are no obvious injuries.

Assess for Jugular Vein Distention

Student: Do I find any jugular vein distention (JVD)?
PROCTOR: No.

Assess for Tracheal Deviation

Student: Do I see any tracheal deviation?
PROCTOR: No.

Assess the Chest

Student: I am assessing the chest for DCAP-BTLS.
PROCTOR: Noted.

Inspect

Student: What do I see when I look at the chest?
PROCTOR: You see a puncture wound on each side of the chest.
Student: Does the chest appear symmetric?
PROCTOR: Yes.

Palpate

Student: When I touch the chest, do I feel crepitus or a flail segment?
PROCTOR: No.

Auscultate

Student: Are lung sounds present in all fields?
PROCTOR: They are now diminished on the left side from what they were initially.
Student: Do I hear any sucking sounds from the chest?
PROCTOR: No.
ALS Student: I will assess the chest for hyperresonance to percussion.
ALS Proctor: Noted. There is a tension pneumothorax on the left side.
ALS Student: I will decompress the left chest.
ALS Proctor: Noted.

Assess the Abdomen/Pelvis

Assess the Abdomen

Student: I am assessing the abdomen for DCAP-BTLS. I am assessing all four quadrants. Do I find any problems?
PROCTOR: No.

Assess the Pelvis

Student: I am assessing the pelvis for DCAP-BTLS. Is the pelvis stable?
PROCTOR: Yes.

Assess the Genitalia/Perineum as Needed (Verbalize in Training)

Student: I am assessing the genitalia/perineum as necessary for DCAP-BTLS.
PROCTOR: The area is unremarkable.

Assess the Extremities

Inspect

Student: I am assessing the lower and upper extremities for DCAP-BTLS. Do I find anything?
PROCTOR: No.

Palpate

Student: Do I feel anything unusual?
PROCTOR: No.

Assess Motor, Sensory, and Circulatory Function

Student: I am checking for DCAP-BTLS, motor and sensory function, and pulses. Right leg?
PROCTOR: Negative DCAP-BTLS. Motor and sensory functions are present. Pulses are present.
Student: Left leg?
PROCTOR: Negative DCAP-BTLS. Motor and sensory functions are present. Pulses are present.
Student: Right arm?
PROCTOR: Negative DCAP-BTLS. Motor and sensory functions are present. Pulses are present.
Student: Left arm?
PROCTOR: Negative DCAP-BTLS. Motor and sensory functions are present. Pulses are present.

Assess the Posterior

Note: This portion of the detailed physical exam would not be done if the patient were previously backboarded per local protocol.
Student: We will not check the back because it was previously checked and the patient is backboarded.
PROCTOR: Noted.

Manage Secondary Injuries/Wounds

Student: I would direct my partner to monitor the airway, lung sounds, and pulse oximetry.
PROCTOR: Noted.

Reassess Vital Signs

Student: I will reassess vital signs and mental status.
PROCTOR: Blood pressure, 124/84 mm Hg; pulse rate, 104 beats/min; respirations, 24 breaths/min; pulse oximetry reading, 95%; and the patient is alert.
Student: The pulse oximetry reading has dropped. I will reassess the lungs.
PROCTOR: Noted.

Reassess Interventions

Student: I will reassess my interventions: airway, breathing, and oxygen; occlusive dressings; immobilization and straps; treatment for shock; and assess for tension pneumothorax.
PROCTOR: Noted.
ALS Student: I will reassess BLS interventions, plus the following: two large-bore IVs, a cardiac monitor, and treatment for pneumothorax if necessary.
ALS Proctor: Noted. The cardiac monitor shows sinus tachycardia.

Critical Criteria:
- ❑ Did not find or manage problems associated with airway, breathing, hemorrhage or shock (hypoperfusion)

Radio Report

(Provided by the student.)
PROCTOR: Noted.

Ongoing Assessment

Repeat Vital Signs

Student: I will reassess vital signs and mental status.
PROCTOR: Blood pressure, 120/76 mm Hg; pulse rate, 94 beats/min; respirations, 20 breaths/min; pulse oximetry reading, 96%; and the patient is alert.

Student: The vital signs have not changed significantly.
PROCTOR: Noted.

Check Interventions

Student: I will check my interventions: airway, breathing, and oxygen; occlusive dressings; immobilization and straps; treatment for shock; and assess for tension pneumothorax.
PROCTOR: Noted.
ALS Student: I will check BLS interventions, plus the following: two large-bore IVs, a cardiac monitor, and treatment for pneumothorax if necessary.
ALS Proctor: Noted. The cardiac monitor shows normal sinus rhythm.

Critical Criteria:
- ❑ Did not find or manage problems associated with airway, breathing, hemorrhage or shock (hypoperfusion)

Handoff Report to Emergency Department Staff

Student: There was no change during transport.
PROCTOR: Noted.

Critical Criteria:
- ❑ Did not transport patient within the (10) minute time limit

Critical Criteria

(Inform the student of items missed, if any.)

❑ Pass ❑ Fail Date: ____________________

Proctor Comments: ____________________

____

____

CASE 48

Dispatch Information

PROCTOR: EMS 10, respond to a 47-year-old male who has had his hands chopped off. He is conscious and breathing. Police have been notified and are en route.

Pre-scene Action (BSI)

Student: I am wearing nonlatex gloves, safety glasses, mask, and gown.
PROCTOR: Noted.

Critical Criteria:
- ❑ Did not take, or verbalize, body substance isolation (BSI) precautions when necessary

Scene Size-up

Scene Safety

Student: Is the scene safe?
PROCTOR: Yes, police are on scene and you are given clearance to enter. The patient is standing in his front yard.

Mechanism of Injury

Student: What was the mechanism of injury?
PROCTOR: Amputation from direct force. The patient was held down by gang members after not paying for his drugs. Both hands have been chopped off at the wrists.

Number of Patients

Student: How many patients are there?
PROCTOR: One.

Additional Resources

Student: I would call for advanced life support (ALS) assistance.
PROCTOR: Noted.

C-Spine Stabilization

Student: I would not stabilize the cervical spine (c-spine).
PROCTOR: Noted.

Critical Criteria:
- ❑ Did not determine scene safety
- ❑ Did not assess for spinal protection
- ❑ Did not provide for spinal protection when indicated

Initial Assessment

Student: As I approach the patient, I identify myself and ask the patient not to move.
PROCTOR: Noted.

General Impression

Student: My general impression is that the patient's condition is unstable.
PROCTOR: Noted.

Responsiveness/Level of Consciousness

Student: What is the patient's level of consciousness?
PROCTOR: Alert but anxious.

Chief Complaint/Apparent Life Threats

Student: What is the patient's chief complaint?
PROCTOR: The patient is complaining of his hands being cut off.
Student: The life threat is from possible blood loss.
PROCTOR: Noted.

Assess the Airway and Breathing

Student: Is the airway open? Is the patient breathing?
PROCTOR: Yes, the airway is open and the patient is breathing.

Assessment

Student: What are the rate and the quality of breathing?
PROCTOR: Rate: Rapid. Quality: Normal.

Provide Oxygen

Student: I am applying oxygen at 15 L/min via nonrebreathing mask.
PROCTOR: Noted.

Ensure Adequate Ventilation

Student: The patient has adequate ventilations at this time.
PROCTOR: Noted.

Injury Management

Student: I will direct my partner to quickly control bleeding as I continue assessment.
PROCTOR: Noted.

Assess Circulation

Student: I am assessing the patient's circulation.
PROCTOR: Noted.

Assess for and Control Major Bleeding

Student: Do I find any major bleeding?
PROCTOR: There is some bleeding noted from the stumps.
Student: I will control the bleeding with direct pressure and dressing. I will also splint the arms. I will wrap the hands in gauze and seal them in Ziplock bags keeping them cool without causing frost injuries.
PROCTOR: Noted.

Assess the Pulse

Student: What are the rate and the quality of pulses?
PROCTOR: Rate: Tachycardic. Quality: Strong.

Assess the Skin

Student: I am assessing the skin. What are the color, temperature, and condition of the skin?
PROCTOR: Color: Pale. Temperature: Warm. Condition: Moist.

Identify Priority Patients/Make Transport Decision

Student: The patient is a high priority and is a load-and-go. I will begin packaging and transport the patient and his hands to a trauma center.
PROCTOR: Noted.

Critical Criteria:
- ❑ Did not provide high concentration of oxygen
- ❑ Did not find or manage problems associated with airway, breathing, hemorrhage or shock (hypoperfusion)
- ❑ Did not differentiate patient's need for transportation versus continued assessment at the scene
- ❑ Did other detailed examination before assessing the airway, breathing and circulation

Focused History and Physical Examination/Rapid Trauma Assessment

Select the Appropriate Assessment (Focused or Rapid)

Student: I am selecting the rapid physical exam to identify and treat life threats. I am checking for DCAP-BTLS. This acronym stands for deformities, contusions, abrasions, punctures, penetrations, and paradoxical motion in the chest, and burns, tenderness, lacerations, and swelling.
PROCTOR: Noted.

Head

Student: I am rapidly assessing the head.
PROCTOR: There are no obvious injuries.

Neck

Student: I am rapidly assessing the neck.
PROCTOR: There are no obvious injuries.

Chest

Student: I am rapidly assessing the chest. What are the lung sounds?
PROCTOR: There are no obvious injuries. Lung sounds are clear bilaterally.

▸ **Abdomen/Pelvis**
Student: I am rapidly assessing the abdomen.
PROCTOR: There are no obvious injuries.
Student: I am rapidly assessing the pelvis.
PROCTOR: There are no obvious injuries.

▸ **Extremities**
Student: I am rapidly assessing the extremities.
PROCTOR: Both hands are chopped off but the bleeding is controlled.
Student: I will continuously reassess bleeding.
PROCTOR: Noted.

▸ **Posterior**
Student: I will rapidly assess the back.
PROCTOR: There are no obvious injuries.

▸ **Manage Secondary Injuries/Wounds**
ALS Student: I will establish two large-bore IVs en route to the hospital and administer a bolus of 20 mL/kg in order to maintain a systolic blood pressure of 90 mm Hg.
ALS Proctor: Noted.

▸ **Reevaluate Transport Decision**
Student: This patient is a load-and-go to a trauma center.
PROCTOR: Noted.

▾ Baseline Vital Signs
Student: What are the patient's baseline vital signs, including blood pressure, pulse, respirations, pulse oximetry, and level of consciousness?
PROCTOR: Blood pressure, 138/90 mm Hg, pulse rate, 124 beats/min; respirations, 28 breaths/min; pulse oximetry reading, 98%; and the patient is alert but starts to complain that he is light-headed.

▾ SAMPLE History
Student: At this time I will gather a SAMPLE history from the patient or family. What are the patient's signs and symptoms?
PROCTOR: He is experiencing pain in the stumps. His hands have been found.
Student: Allergies?
PROCTOR: Penicillin (PCN).
Student: Medications?
PROCTOR: Cocaine and other street drugs.
Student: Pertinent past medical history?
PROCTOR: None.
Student: Last oral intake?
PROCTOR: 2 hours ago.
Student: Events leading up to the incident?
PROCTOR: The patient was trying to take some drugs from a dealer, and gang members chopped off his hands with an axe.

Critical Criteria:
- ❑ Did not differentiate patient's need for transportation versus continued assessment at the scene
- ❑ Did not provide for spinal protection when indicated

▾ Detailed Physical Examination
Student: I am conducting the detailed physical exam. I am looking for DCAP-BTLS. This acronym stands for deformities, contusions, abrasions, punctures, penetrations, paradoxical motion in the chest, and burns, tenderness, lacerations, and swelling.
PROCTOR: Noted. The detailed physical exam will be performed during transport.

▾ Assess the Head
Student: I am assessing the head. Do I find any DCAP-BTLS? Do I find any evidence of Battle's sign or raccoon eyes?
PROCTOR: No.

▸ **Inspect and Palpate the Head and Ears**
Student: I am assessing the head and ears.
PROCTOR: There are no obvious injuries.

▸ **Assess the Eyes**
Student: I am assessing the eyes. Are the pupils equal, round, and regular in size, and react properly to light (PEARRL)?
PROCTOR: They are PEARRL.

▸ **Assess the Facial Area Including Oral and Nasal Areas**
Student: I am assessing the face, nose, and mouth. Do I see any discharge or hear any obstructions?
PROCTOR: No.

▾ Assess the Neck
▸ **Inspect and Palpate the Neck**
Student: I am assessing the neck for DCAP-BTLS.
PROCTOR: There are no obvious injuries.

▸ **Assess for Jugular Vein Distention**
Student: Do I find any jugular vein distention (JVD)?
PROCTOR: No.

▸ **Assess for Tracheal Deviation**
Student: Do I see any tracheal deviation?
PROCTOR: No.

▾ Assess the Chest
Student: I am assessing the chest for DCAP-BTLS.
PROCTOR: Noted.

▸ **Inspect**
Student: What do I see when I look at the chest?
PROCTOR: There are no obvious injuries.
Student: Does the chest appear symmetric?
PROCTOR: Yes.

▸ **Palpate**
Student: When I touch the chest, do I feel crepitus or a flail segment?
PROCTOR: No.

▸ **Auscultate**
Student: Are lung sounds present in all fields?
PROCTOR: Yes.
Student: Do I hear any sucking sounds from the chest?
PROCTOR: No.

▾ Assess the Abdomen/Pelvis
▸ **Assess the Abdomen**
Student: I am assessing the abdomen for DCAP-BTLS. I am assessing all four quadrants. Do I find any problems?
PROCTOR: No.

▸ **Assess the Pelvis**
Student: I am assessing the pelvis for DCAP-BTLS. Is the pelvis stable?
PROCTOR: Yes.

▾ Assess the Genitalia/Perineum as Needed (Verbalize in Training)
Student: I am assessing the genitalia/perineum as necessary for DCAP-BTLS.
PROCTOR: The area is unremarkable.

▾ Assess the Extremities
▸ **Inspect**
Student: I am assessing the lower and upper extremities for DCAP-BTLS. Do I find anything?
PROCTOR: Yes.

▸ **Palpate**
Student: Do I feel anything unusual?
PROCTOR: Both hands have been chopped off.

▸ **Assess Motor, Sensory, and Circulatory Function**
Student: I am checking for DCAP-BTLS, motor and sensory function, and pulses. Right leg?
PROCTOR: Negative DCAP-BTLS. Motor and sensory functions are present. Pulses are present.

Student: Left leg?
PROCTOR: Negative DCAP-BTLS. Motor and sensory functions are present. Pulses are present.
Student: Right arm?
PROCTOR: The stump is dressed and bleeding is controlled. Motor and sensory functions are absent. Radial pulses present.
Student: Left arm?
PROCTOR: The stump is dressed and bleeding is controlled. The hand appears to have been cleanly cut off. Motor and sensory functions are absent. Radial pulses present.
Student: I will reassess both stumps.
PROCTOR: Noted.

Assess the Posterior

Student: We will now check the back.
PROCTOR: Noted.

Assess the Thorax

Student: I am assessing the thorax. Do I find injuries?
PROCTOR: No.

Assess the Lumbar Area

Student: I am assessing the flanks and lumbar area. Do I find injuries?
PROCTOR: No.

Assess the Entire Backside

Student: I am assessing the entire backside. Do I find injuries?
PROCTOR: No.

Manage Secondary Injuries/Wounds

Student: I would direct my partner to maintain bleeding control.
PROCTOR: Noted.

Reassess Vital Signs

Student: I will reassess vital signs and mental status.
PROCTOR: Blood pressure, 124/84 mm Hg; pulse rate, 112 beats/min; respirations, 24 breaths/min; pulse oximetry reading, 99%; and the patient is alert and feeling less light-headed.
Student: The vital signs are improving.
PROCTOR: Noted.

Reassess Interventions

Student: I will reassess my interventions: airway, oxygen, circulation, and bleeding control, treating the hands per protocol, positioning for syncope, and treatment for shock. I also will protect the hands.
PROCTOR: Noted.
ALS Student: I will reassess basic life support (BLS) interventions, plus the following: establish two large-bore IVs and provide pain control per local protocol.
ALS Proctor: Noted.

Critical Criteria:
❑ Did not find or manage problems associated with airway, breathing, hemorrhage or shock (hypoperfusion)

Radio Report

(Provided by the student.)
PROCTOR: Noted.

Ongoing Assessment

Repeat Vital Signs

Student: I will reassess vital signs and mental status.
PROCTOR: Blood pressure, 128/82 mm Hg; pulse rate, 104 beats/min; respirations, 20 breaths/min; pulse oximetry reading, 99%; and the patient is alert.
Student: The vital signs have improved.
PROCTOR: Noted.

Check Interventions

Student: I will check my interventions: airway, oxygen, circulation, and bleeding control, treating the hands per protocol, positioning for syncope, and treatment for shock. I also will protect the hands.
PROCTOR: Noted.
ALS Student: I will check BLS interventions, plus the following: monitor IVs.
ALS Proctor: Noted.

Critical Criteria:
❑ Did not find or manage problems associated with airway, breathing, hemorrhage or shock (hypoperfusion)

Handoff Report to Emergency Department Staff

Student: The patient's condition improved during transport.
PROCTOR: Noted.

Critical Criteria:
❑ Did not transport patient within the (10) minute time limit

Critical Criteria

(Inform the student of items missed, if any.)

❑ Pass ❑ Fail Date: ____________________

Proctor Comments: ____________________

Notes

Dispatch Information

PROCTOR: EMS 10, respond to a motor vehicle head-on collision. There are two patients. I am sending EMS 12 as well.

Pre-scene Action (BSI)

Student: I am wearing appropriate high-visibility personal protective equipment suitable for extrication, a helmet, extrication gloves, nonlatex gloves, safety glasses, and a mask.
PROCTOR: Noted.

Critical Criteria:
- ❑ Did not take, or verbalize, body substance isolation (BSI) precautions when necessary

Scene Size-up

Scene Safety

Student: Is the scene safe?
PROCTOR: Yes.

Mechanism of Injury

Student: What was the mechanism of injury?
PROCTOR: Motor vehicle collision. The patient was driving and not wearing a seat belt. The car did not have an airbag and the steering wheel is displaced about 4 inches to the right. The windshield is intact. He is 19 years old and complaining of chest pain. EMS 12 is treating the other patient.

Number of Patients

Student: How many patients are there?
PROCTOR: One.

Additional Resources

Student: I would call for advanced life support (ALS) assistance and additional resources: fire/rescue and police.
PROCTOR: Noted.

C-Spine Stabilization

Student: On the basis of the mechanism of injury, I would stabilize the cervical spine (c-spine) in a neutral in-line position.
PROCTOR: Noted.

Critical Criteria:
- ❑ Did not determine scene safety
- ❑ Did not assess for spinal protection
- ❑ Did not provide for spinal protection when indicated

Initial Assessment

Student: As I perform midline c-spine stabilization, I identify myself and ask the patient not to move.
PROCTOR: Noted.

General Impression

Student: My general impression is that the patient's condition is unstable.
PROCTOR: Noted.

Responsiveness/Level of Consciousness

Student: What is the patient's level of consciousness?
PROCTOR: Alert.

Chief Complaint/Apparent Life Threats

Student: What is the patient's chief complaint?
PROCTOR: The patient is complaining of chest pain.
Student: There is an apparent life threat; the life threat is the mechanism of injury.
PROCTOR: Noted.

Assess the Airway and Breathing

Student: Is the airway open? Is the patient breathing?
PROCTOR: Yes, the airway is open and the patient is breathing.

Assessment

Student: What are the rate and the quality of breathing?
PROCTOR: Rate: Rapid. Quality: Shallow.

Provide Oxygen

Student: I am applying oxygen at 15 L/min via nonrebreathing mask.
PROCTOR: Noted.

Ensure Adequate Ventilation

Student: The patient has adequate ventilations at this time.
PROCTOR: Noted.

Injury Management

Student: I will direct my partner to take over c-spine control as I continue assessment.
PROCTOR: Noted.

Assess Circulation

Student: I am assessing the patient's circulation.
PROCTOR: Noted.

Assess for and Control Major Bleeding

Student: Do I find any major bleeding?
PROCTOR: No.

Assess the Pulse

Student: What are the rate and the quality of pulses?
PROCTOR: Rate: Tachycardic. Quality: Thready.

Assess the Skin

Student: I am assessing the skin. What are the color, temperature, and condition of the skin?
PROCTOR: Color: Pale. Temperature: Cool. Condition: Diaphoretic.

Identify Priority Patients/Make Transport Decision

Student: The patient is a high priority and is a load-and-go. I will begin packaging and transport.
PROCTOR: Noted.

Critical Criteria:
- ❑ Did not provide high concentration of oxygen
- ❑ Did not find or manage problems associated with airway, breathing, hemorrhage or shock (hypoperfusion)
- ❑ Did not differentiate patient's need for transportation versus continued assessment at the scene
- ❑ Did other detailed examination before assessing the airway, breathing and circulation

Focused History and Physical Examination/Rapid Trauma Assessment

Select the Appropriate Assessment (Focused or Rapid)

Student: I am selecting the rapid physical exam to identify and treat life threats. I am checking for DCAP-BTLS. This acronym stands for deformities, contusions, abrasions, punctures, penetrations, and paradoxical motion in the chest, and burns, tenderness, lacerations, and swelling.
PROCTOR: Noted.

Head

Student: I am rapidly assessing the head.
PROCTOR: There are no obvious injuries.

Neck

Student: I am rapidly assessing the neck.
PROCTOR: There are no obvious injuries.
Student: I will apply a cervical collar.
PROCTOR: Noted.

▸ **Chest**

Student: I am rapidly assessing the chest. What are the lung sounds?

PROCTOR: There is bruising across the chest. Lung sounds are clear bilaterally.

Student: I will assess the chest for tension pneumothorax by auscultation and assessment (for jugular vein distention [JVD], tracheal deviation, and decreased lung sounds).

PROCTOR: The lung sounds appear clear bilaterally, jugular vein distention is not present, and the trachea is midline.

ALS Student: I will assess the chest for hyperresonance to percussion.

ALS Proctor: Noted. There is no tension pneumothorax.

ALS Student: I will continuously reassess the chest.

ALS Proctor: Noted.

▸ **Abdomen/Pelvis**

Student: I am rapidly assessing the abdomen.

PROCTOR: There are no obvious injuries.

Student: I am rapidly assessing the pelvis.

PROCTOR: There are no obvious injuries.

▸ **Extremities**

Student: I am rapidly assessing the extremities.

PROCTOR: There are no obvious injuries.

▸ **Assess Motor, Sensory, and Circulatory Function**

Student: I am checking for DCAP-BTLS. I am also checking motor and sensory function, and pulses. Right leg?

PROCTOR: Negative DCAP-BTLS. Motor and sensory functions are present. Pulses are weak.

Student: Left leg?

PROCTOR: Negative DCAP-BTLS. Motor and sensory functions are present. Pulses are weak.

Student: Right arm?

PROCTOR: Negative DCAP-BTLS. Motor and sensory functions are present. Pulses are weak.

Student: Left arm?

PROCTOR: Negative DCAP-BTLS. Motor and sensory functions are present. Pulses are weak.

▸ **Posterior**

Student: I will rapidly assess the back. We will now log roll the patient as a unit to check the back. The person at the head will count to three and we will roll the patient.

PROCTOR: Noted.

▸ **Assess the Thorax**

Student: I am assessing the thorax. Do I find injuries?

PROCTOR: No.

▸ **Assess the Lumbar Area**

Student: I am assessing the flanks and lumbar area. Do I find injuries?

PROCTOR: No.

▸ **Assess the Entire Backside**

Student: I am assessing the entire backside. Do I find injuries?

PROCTOR: No.

▸ **Manage Secondary Injuries/Wounds**

Student: We will apply a cervical collar and backboard with full immobilization per local protocol, if not yet done, at this time.

PROCTOR: Noted.

Student: Are there any changes in motor and sensory functions or pulses?

PROCTOR: No.

ALS Student: I will apply basic life support (BLS) interventions, plus the following: establish two large-bore IVs while en route to the hospital, administer a bolus of 20 mL/kg, maintain a blood pressure of 90 mm Hg, and place him on a cardiac monitor.

ALS Proctor: Noted. The cardiac monitor shows sinus tachycardia.

▸ **Reevaluate Transport Decision**

Student: This patient is a load-and-go due to the chest trauma and the patient's condition.

PROCTOR: Noted.

▾ Baseline Vital Signs

Student: What are the patient's baseline vital signs, including blood pressure, pulse, respirations, pulse oximetry, and level of consciousness?

PROCTOR: Blood pressure, 90/66 mm Hg; pulse rate, 120 beats/min; respirations, 28 breaths/min; pulse oximetry reading, 97%; and the patient is anxious.

▾ SAMPLE History

Student: At this time I will gather a SAMPLE history from the patient or family. What are the patient's signs and symptoms?

PROCTOR: Pain in the chest.

Student: Allergies?

PROCTOR: No allergies.

Student: Medications?

PROCTOR: No medications.

Student: Pertinent past medical history?

PROCTOR: No pertinent medical history.

Student: Last oral intake?

PROCTOR: 5 hours ago.

Student: Events leading up to the incident?

PROCTOR: The patient was passing a car and hit an oncoming car head on.

Critical Criteria:

- ❑ Did not differentiate patient's need for transportation versus continued assessment at the scene
- ❑ Did not provide for spinal protection when indicated

▾ Detailed Physical Examination

Student: I am conducting the detailed physical exam. I am looking for DCAP-BTLS.

PROCTOR: Noted. The detailed physical exam will be performed during transport.

▾ Assess the Head

Student: I am assessing the head. Do I find any DCAP-BTLS? Do I find any evidence of Battle's sign or raccoon eyes?

PROCTOR: No.

▸ **Inspect and Palpate the Head and Ears**

Student: I am assessing the head and ears.

PROCTOR: There are no obvious injuries.

▸ **Assess the Eyes**

Student: I am assessing the eyes. Are the pupils equal, round, and regular in size, and react properly to light (PEARRL)?

PROCTOR: They are PEARRL.

▸ **Assess the Facial Area Including Oral and Nasal Areas**

Student: I am assessing the face, nose, and mouth. Do I see any discharge or hear any obstructions?

PROCTOR: No.

▾ Assess the Neck

▸ **Inspect and Palpate the Neck**

Student: I am assessing the neck for DCAP-BTLS.

PROCTOR: There are no obvious injuries.

▸ **Assess for Jugular Vein Distention**

Student: Do I find any jugular vein distention (JVD)?

PROCTOR: Yes.

▸ **Assess for Tracheal Deviation**

Student: Do I see any tracheal deviation?

PROCTOR: No.

▾ Assess the Chest

Student: I am assessing the chest for DCAP-BTLS.

PROCTOR: Noted.

▸ **Inspect**

Student: What do I see when I look at the chest?

PROCTOR: The contusion on the chest has expanded.

Student: Does the chest appear symmetric?
PROCTOR: Yes.

► Palpate

Student: When I touch the chest, do I feel crepitus or a flail segment?
PROCTOR: No.

► Auscultate

Student: Are lung sounds present in all fields?
PROCTOR: Yes.
Student: Do I hear any sucking sounds from the chest?
PROCTOR: No.
ALS Student: I will assess the chest for hyperresonance to percussion.
ALS Proctor: Noted. There is no tension pneumothorax.
ALS Student: I will continuously reassess the chest.
ALS Proctor: Noted.

▼ Assess the Abdomen/Pelvis

► Assess the Abdomen

Student: I am assessing the abdomen for DCAP-BTLS. I am assessing all four quadrants. Do I find any problems?
PROCTOR: No.

► Assess the Pelvis

Student: I am assessing the pelvis for DCAP-BTLS. Is the pelvis stable?
PROCTOR: Yes.

▼ Assess the Genitalia/Perineum as Needed (Verbalize in Training)

Student: I am assessing the genitalia/perineum as necessary for DCAP-BTLS.
PROCTOR: The area is unremarkable.

▼ Assess the Extremities

► Inspect

Student: I am assessing the lower and upper extremities for DCAP-BTLS. Do I find anything?
PROCTOR: No.

► Palpate

Student: Do I feel anything unusual?
PROCTOR: No.

► Assess Motor, Sensory, and Circulatory Function

Student: I am checking for DCAP-BTLS, motor and sensory function, and pulses. Right leg?
PROCTOR: Negative DCAP-BTLS. Motor and sensory functions are present. Pulses are weak.
Student: Left leg?
PROCTOR: Negative DCAP-BTLS. Motor and sensory functions are present. Pulses are weak.
Student: Right arm?
PROCTOR: Negative DCAP-BTLS. Motor and sensory functions are present. Pulses are weak.
Student: Left arm?
PROCTOR: Negative DCAP-BTLS. Motor and sensory functions are present. Pulses are weak.

▼ Assess the Posterior

Note: This portion of the detailed physical exam would not be done if the patient were previously backboarded per local protocol.
Student: We will not check the back because it was previously checked and the patient is backboarded.
PROCTOR: Noted.

▼ Manage Secondary Injuries/Wounds

Student: I would direct my partner to continue providing oxygen.
PROCTOR: Noted.

▼ Reassess Vital Signs

Student: I will reassess vital signs and mental status.
PROCTOR: Blood pressure, 86/66 mm Hg; pulse rate, 124 beats/min; respirations, 24 breaths/min; pulse oximetry reading, 96%; and the patient is anxious.
Student: The vital signs are deteriorating.
PROCTOR: Noted.

▼ Reassess Interventions

Student: I will reassess my interventions: oxygen, full immobilization, and treatment for shock.
PROCTOR: Noted.
ALS Student: I will reassess BLS interventions, plus the following: two large-bore IVs, a bolus of 20 mL/kg, maintain a systolic blood pressure of 90 mm Hg, and cardiac monitor.
ALS Proctor: Noted. The cardiac monitor shows sinus tachycardia.

Critical Criteria:
❑ Did not find or manage problems associated with airway, breathing, hemorrhage or shock (hypoperfusion)

▼ Radio Report

(Provided by the student.)
PROCTOR: Noted.

▼ Ongoing Assessment

▼ Repeat Vital Signs

Student: I will reassess vital signs and mental status.
PROCTOR: Blood pressure, 84/66 mm Hg; pulse rate, 128 beats/min; respirations, 28 breaths/min; pulse oximetry reading, 95%; and the patient is anxious.
Student: The vital signs have deteriorated.
PROCTOR: Noted.

▼ Check Interventions

Student: I will check my interventions: oxygen, full immobilization, and treatment for shock.
PROCTOR: Noted.
ALS Student: I will check BLS interventions, plus the following: two large-bore IVs, a bolus of 20 mL/kg, maintain a systolic blood pressure of 90 mm Hg, and cardiac monitor.
ALS Proctor: Noted. The cardiac monitor shows sinus tachycardia.

Critical Criteria:
❑ Did not find or manage problems associated with airway, breathing, hemorrhage or shock (hypoperfusion)

▼ Handoff Report to Emergency Department Staff

Student: The patient's condition deteriorated during transport.
PROCTOR: Noted.

Critical Criteria:
❑ Did not transport patient within the (10) minute time limit

▼ Critical Criteria

(Inform the student of items missed, if any.)

❑ Pass ❑ Fail Date: ____________________

Proctor Comments: ____________________

Notes

CASE 50

Dispatch Information

PROCTOR: EMS 10, respond to an 18-year-old male who has been shot. He is conscious and breathing and police are en route.

Pre-scene Action (BSI)

Student: I am wearing nonlatex gloves, safety glasses, mask, and gown.
PROCTOR: Noted.

Critical Criteria:
- ❑ Did not take, or verbalize, body substance isolation (BSI) precautions when necessary

Scene Size-up

Scene Safety

Student: Is the scene safe?
PROCTOR: Yes, police are on scene and you are given clearance to enter.

Mechanism of Injury

Student: What was the mechanism of injury?
PROCTOR: Gunshot wound. The patient was walking down the street when he heard shots and began running. He was shot twice.

Number of Patients

Student: How many patients are there?
PROCTOR: One.

Additional Resources

Student: I would call for advanced life support (ALS) assistance.
PROCTOR: Noted.

C-Spine Stabilization

Student: On the basis of the mechanism of injury, I would stabilize the cervical spine (c-spine) in a neutral in-line position.
PROCTOR: Noted.

Critical Criteria:
- ❑ Did not determine scene safety
- ❑ Did not assess for spinal protection
- ❑ Did not provide for spinal protection when indicated

Initial Assessment

Student: As I perform midline c-spine stabilization, I identify myself and ask the patient not to move.
PROCTOR: Noted.

General Impression

Student: My general impression is that the patient's condition is unstable.
PROCTOR: Noted.

Responsiveness/Level of Consciousness

Student: What is the patient's level of consciousness?
PROCTOR: Alert.

Chief Complaint/Apparent Life Threats

Student: What is the patient's chief complaint?
PROCTOR: The patient is complaining of being shot in the lower back and the thigh.
Student: There is an apparent life threat; the life threat is a gunshot wound in the lower back.
PROCTOR: Noted.

Assess the Airway and Breathing

Student: Is the airway open? Is the patient breathing?
PROCTOR: Yes, the airway is open and the patient is breathing.

Assessment

Student: What are the rate and the quality of breathing?
PROCTOR: Rate: Rapid. Quality: Shallow.

Provide Oxygen

Student: I am assisting ventilations with a bag-valve device with 100% oxygen.
PROCTOR: Noted.

Ensure Adequate Ventilation

Student: I will ensure adequate ventilation.
PROCTOR: Noted.

Injury Management

Student: I will direct my partner to take over c-spine control and bag-valve ventilations as I continue assessment.
PROCTOR: Noted.

Assess Circulation

Student: I am assessing the patient's circulation.
PROCTOR: Noted.

Assess for and Control Major Bleeding

Student: Do I find any major bleeding?
PROCTOR: Yes, from the right flank.
Student: I would apply direct pressure and an occlusive dressing per local protocol.
PROCTOR: Noted.

Assess the Pulse

Student: What are the rate and the quality of pulses?
PROCTOR: Rate: Tachycardic. Quality: Thready.

Assess the Skin

Student: I am assessing the skin. What are the color, temperature, and condition of the skin?
PROCTOR: Color: Pale. Temperature: Cold. Condition: Diaphoretic.

Identify Priority Patients/Make Transport Decision

Student: The patient is a high priority and is a load-and-go. I will begin packaging and transport.
PROCTOR: Noted.

Critical Criteria:
- ❑ Did not provide high concentration of oxygen
- ❑ Did not find or manage problems associated with airway, breathing, hemorrhage or shock (hypoperfusion)
- ❑ Did not differentiate patient's need for transportation versus continued assessment at the scene
- ❑ Did other detailed examination before assessing the airway, breathing and circulation

Focused History and Physical Examination/Rapid Trauma Assessment

Select the Appropriate Assessment (Focused or Rapid)

Student: I am selecting the rapid physical exam to identify and treat life threats. I am checking for DCAP-BTLS. This acronym stands for deformities, contusions, abrasions, punctures, penetrations, and paradoxical motion in the chest, and burns, tenderness, lacerations, and swelling.
PROCTOR: Noted.

Head

Student: I am rapidly assessing the head.
PROCTOR: There are no obvious injuries.

Neck

Student: I am rapidly assessing the neck.
PROCTOR: There are no obvious injuries.
Student: I will apply a cervical collar.
PROCTOR: Noted.

Chest

Student: I am rapidly assessing the chest. What are the lung sounds?
PROCTOR: There are no obvious injuries. Lung sounds are clear bilaterally.

Abdomen/Pelvis

Student: I am rapidly assessing the abdomen.
PROCTOR: The abdomen is board-like.

Student: I am rapidly assessing the pelvis.
PROCTOR: There are no obvious injuries.

▸ **Extremities**

Student: I am rapidly assessing the extremities.
PROCTOR: There is a puncture wound to the right posterior thigh.
Student: I would apply a pressure dressing.
PROCTOR: Noted. Exterior bleeding is now controlled.

▸ **Assess Motor, Sensory, and Circulatory Function**

Student: I am checking for DCAP-BTLS. I am also checking motor and sensory function, and pulses. Right leg?
PROCTOR: Bleeding from the posterior thigh, which was controlled with a pressure dressing. Motor and sensory functions are present. Pulses are weak.
Student: Left leg?
PROCTOR: Negative DCAP-BTLS. Motor and sensory functions are present. Pulses are weak.
Student: Right arm?
PROCTOR: Negative DCAP-BTLS. Motor and sensory functions are present. Pulses are weak.
Student: Left arm?
PROCTOR: Negative DCAP-BTLS. Motor and sensory functions are present. Pulses are weak.

▸ **Posterior**

Student: I will rapidly assess the back. We will now log roll the patient as a unit to check the back. The person at the head will count to three and we will roll the patient.
PROCTOR: Noted.

▸ **Assess the Thorax**

Student: I am assessing the thorax. Do I find injuries?
PROCTOR: No.

▸ **Assess the Lumbar Area**

Student: I am assessing the flanks and lumbar area. Do I find injuries?
PROCTOR: Yes, a puncture to the right flank. Exterior bleeding is controlled if treated with an occlusive dressing.
Student: I will check the occlusive pressure dressing.
PROCTOR: Noted.

▸ **Assess the Entire Backside**

Student: I am assessing the entire backside. Do I find injuries?
PROCTOR: Yes, to the right thigh.

▸ **Manage Secondary Injuries/Wounds**

Student: We will apply a cervical collar and backboard with full immobilization per local protocol, if not yet done, at this time.
PROCTOR: Noted.
Student: Are there any changes in motor and sensory functions or pulses?
PROCTOR: No.
ALS Student: I will apply basic life support (BLS) interventions, plus the following: establish two large-bore IVs while en route to the hospital, a bolus of 20 mL/kg, maintain a systolic blood pressure of 90 mm Hg, and a cardiac monitor.
ALS Proctor: Noted. The cardiac monitor shows sinus tachycardia.

▸ **Reevaluate Transport Decision**

Student: This patient is a high priority and is a load-and-go due to shock.
PROCTOR: Noted.

▾ Baseline Vital Signs

Student: What are the patient's baseline vital signs, including blood pressure, pulse, respirations, pulse oximetry, and level of consciousness?
PROCTOR: Blood pressure, 98/70 mm Hg; pulse rate, 140 beats/min; respirations per bag-valve device; pulse oximetry reading, 94%; and the patient responds to verbal instructions.

▾ SAMPLE History

Student: At this time I will gather a SAMPLE history from the patient or family. What are the patient's signs and symptoms?
PROCTOR: Pain in the back and leg.
Student: Allergies?
PROCTOR: No allergies.
Student: Medications?
PROCTOR: No medications.
Student: Pertinent past medical history?
PROCTOR: No pertinent medical history.
Student: Last oral intake?
PROCTOR: 4 hours ago.
Student: Events leading up to the incident?
PROCTOR: The patient was walking and heard shots. He began running when he was shot twice.

Critical Criteria:

- ❑ Did not differentiate patient's need for transportation versus continued assessment at the scene
- ❑ Did not provide for spinal protection when indicated

▼ Detailed Physical Examination

Student: I am conducting the detailed physical exam. I am looking for DCAP-BTLS.
PROCTOR: Noted. The detailed physical exam will be performed during transport.

▾ Assess the Head

Student: I am assessing the head. Do I find any DCAP-BTLS? Do I find any evidence of Battle's sign or raccoon eyes?
PROCTOR: No.

▸ **Inspect and Palpate the Head and Ears**

Student: I am assessing the head and ears.
PROCTOR: There are no obvious injuries.

▸ **Assess the Eyes**

Student: I am assessing the eyes. Are the pupils equal, round, and regular in size, and react properly to light (PEARRL)?
PROCTOR: They are PEARRL.

▸ **Assess the Facial Area Including Oral and Nasal Areas**

Student: I am assessing the face, nose, and mouth. Do I see any discharge or hear any obstructions?
PROCTOR: No.

▾ Assess the Neck

▸ **Inspect and Palpate the Neck**

Student: I am assessing the neck for DCAP-BTLS.
PROCTOR: There are no obvious injuries.

▸ **Assess for Jugular Vein Distention**

Student: Do I find any jugular vein distention (JVD)?
PROCTOR: No.

▸ **Assess for Tracheal Deviation**

Student: Do I see any tracheal deviation?
PROCTOR: No.

▾ Assess the Chest

Student: I am assessing the chest for DCAP-BTLS.
PROCTOR: Noted.

▸ **Inspect**

Student: What do I see when I look at the chest?
PROCTOR: There are no obvious injuries.
Student: Does the chest appear symmetric?
PROCTOR: Yes.

▸ **Palpate**

Student: When I touch the chest, do I feel crepitus or a flail segment?
PROCTOR: No.

▸ **Auscultate**

Student: Are lung sounds present in all fields?
PROCTOR: Yes.
Student: Do I hear any sucking sounds from the chest?
PROCTOR: No.

▼ **Assess the Abdomen/Pelvis**

▶ **Assess the Abdomen**

Student: I am assessing the abdomen for DCAP-BTLS. I am assessing all four quadrants. Do I find any problems?

PROCTOR: Yes, the abdomen is board-like.

▶ **Assess the Pelvis**

Student: I am assessing the pelvis for DCAP-BTLS. Is the pelvis stable?

PROCTOR: Yes.

▼ **Assess the Genitalia/Perineum as Needed (Verbalize in Training)**

Student: I am assessing the genitalia/perineum as necessary for DCAP-BTLS.

PROCTOR: The area is unremarkable.

▼ **Assess the Extremities**

▶ **Inspect**

Student: I am assessing the lower and upper extremities for DCAP-BTLS. Do I find anything?

PROCTOR: Yes, you see the entrance wound in the right thigh.

▶ **Palpate**

Student: Do I feel anything unusual?

PROCTOR: Yes, you feel the entrance wound in the right thigh.

▶ **Assess Motor, Sensory, and Circulatory Function**

Student: I am checking for DCAP-BTLS, motor and sensory function, and pulses. Right leg?

PROCTOR: Bleeding from the posterior thigh, which was controlled with a pressure dressing. Motor and sensory functions are present. Pulses are weak.

Student: Left leg?

PROCTOR: Negative DCAP-BTLS. Motor and sensory functions are present. Pulses are weak.

Student: Right arm?

PROCTOR: Negative DCAP-BTLS. Motor and sensory functions are present. Pulses are weak.

Student: Left arm?

PROCTOR: Negative DCAP-BTLS. Motor and sensory functions are present. Pulses are weak.

▼ **Assess the Posterior**

Note: This portion of the detailed physical exam would not be done if the patient were previously backboarded per local protocol.

Student: We will not check the back because it was previously checked and the patient is backboarded.

PROCTOR: Noted.

▼ **Manage Secondary Injuries/Wounds**

Student: I would direct my partner to check the dressings.

PROCTOR: Noted.

▼ **Reassess Vital Signs**

Student: I will reassess vital signs and mental status.

PROCTOR: Blood pressure, 94/66 mm Hg; pulse rate, 142 beats/min; respirations per bag-valve device; pulse oximetry reading, 90%; and the patient is responsive to painful stimuli.

Student: The vital signs are deteriorating.

PROCTOR: Noted.

▼ **Reassess Interventions**

Student: I will reassess my interventions: airway, breathing, and oxygen per bag-valve device; circulation and bleeding control; immobilization and straps; and treatment for shock per local protocol.

PROCTOR: Noted.

ALS Student: I will reassess BLS interventions, plus the following: I will intubate this patient and confirm placement with lung sounds and end tidal CO_2, two large-bore IVs, a bolus of 20 mL/kg, maintain a systolic blood pressure of 90 mm Hg, and cardiac monitor.

ALS Proctor: Noted. The lung sounds and end tidal CO_2 confirm ET tube placement. The cardiac monitor shows sinus tachycardia.

Critical Criteria:

❑ Did not find or manage problems associated with airway, breathing, hemorrhage or shock (hypoperfusion)

Radio Report

(Provided by the student.)

PROCTOR: Noted.

Ongoing Assessment

▼ **Repeat Vital Signs**

Student: I will reassess vital signs and mental status.

PROCTOR: Blood pressure, 88/60 mm Hg; pulse rate, 136 beats/min; respirations per bag-valve device; pulse oximetry reading, 89%; and the patient is unresponsive.

Student: The vital signs have deteriorated.

PROCTOR: Noted.

▼ **Check Interventions**

Student: I will check my interventions: airway, breathing, and oxygen per bag-valve device; circulation and bleeding control; immobilization and straps; and treatment for shock per local protocol.

PROCTOR: Noted.

ALS Student: I will check BLS interventions, plus the following: confirm ET tube placement, monitor the two large-bore IVs, a bolus of 20 mL/kg, maintain a systolic blood pressure of 90 mm Hg, and cardiac monitor.

ALS Proctor: Noted. The ET tube is still in place. The cardiac monitor shows sinus tachycardia.

Critical Criteria:

❑ Did not find or manage problems associated with airway, breathing, hemorrhage or shock (hypoperfusion)

Handoff Report to Emergency Department Staff

Student: The patient's condition deteriorated during transport.

PROCTOR: Noted.

Critical Criteria:

❑ Did not transport patient within the (10) minute time limit

Critical Criteria

(Inform the student of items missed, if any.)

❑ Pass ❑ Fail Date: ______________________

Proctor Comments: ______________________

____

____

CASE 50

Notes

Dispatch Information

PROCTOR: EMS 10, respond to a 21-year-old female who was thrown out of a van that was traveling at 65 miles per hour. She is conscious and breathing. Police are on the scene.

Pre-scene Action (BSI)

Student: I am wearing a high-visibility vest, nonlatex gloves, and safety glasses.
PROCTOR: Noted.

Critical Criteria:
- ❑ Did not take, or verbalize, body substance isolation (BSI) precautions when necessary

Scene Size-up

Scene Safety

Student: Is the scene safe?
PROCTOR: Yes, police are on scene and you are given clearance to enter.

Mechanism of Injury

Student: What was the mechanism of injury?
PROCTOR: Blunt trauma and gynecologic emergency. The patient was abducted and thrown out of a van after being raped.

Number of Patients

Student: How many patients are there?
PROCTOR: One.

Additional Resources

Student: I would call for advanced life support (ALS) assistance.
PROCTOR: Noted.

C-Spine Stabilization

Student: On the basis of the mechanism of injury, I would stabilize the cervical spine (c-spine) in a neutral in-line position.
PROCTOR: Noted.

Critical Criteria:
- ❑ Did not determine scene safety
- ❑ Did not assess for spinal protection
- ❑ Did not provide for spinal protection when indicated

Initial Assessment

Student: As I perform midline c-spine stabilization, I identify myself and ask the patient not to move.
PROCTOR: Noted.

General Impression

Student: My general impression is that the patient's condition is unstable.
PROCTOR: Noted.

Responsiveness/Level of Consciousness

Student: What is the patient's level of consciousness?
PROCTOR: Alert.

Chief Complaint/Apparent Life Threats

Student: What is the patient's chief complaint?
PROCTOR: The patient is complaining of broken ribs and legs.
Student: There are apparent life threats; the life threats are multiple trauma and possible shock.
PROCTOR: Noted.

Assess the Airway and Breathing

Student: Is the airway open? Is the patient breathing?
PROCTOR: Yes, the airway is open and the patient is breathing.

Assessment

Student: What are the rate and the quality of breathing?
PROCTOR: Rate: Within normal limits. Quality: Guarded.

Provide Oxygen

Student: I am applying oxygen at 15 L/min via nonrebreathing mask.
PROCTOR: Noted.

Ensure Adequate Ventilation

Student: The patient has adequate ventilations at this time.
PROCTOR: Noted.

Injury Management

Student: I will direct my partner to take over c-spine control as I continue assessment.
PROCTOR: Noted.

Assess Circulation

Student: I am assessing the patient's circulation.
PROCTOR: Noted.

Assess for and Control Major Bleeding

Student: Do I find any major bleeding?
PROCTOR: No.

Assess the Pulse

Student: What are the rate and the quality of pulses?
PROCTOR: Rate: Tachycardic. Quality: Thready.

Assess the Skin

Student: I am assessing the skin. What are the color, temperature, and condition of the skin?
PROCTOR: Color: Pale. Temperature: Cold. Condition: Moist.

Identify Priority Patients/Make Transport Decision

Student: The patient is a high priority and is a load-and-go. I will begin packaging and transport to a trauma center.
PROCTOR: Noted.

Critical Criteria:
- ❑ Did not provide high concentration of oxygen
- ❑ Did not find or manage problems associated with airway, breathing, hemorrhage or shock (hypoperfusion)
- ❑ Did not differentiate patient's need for transportation versus continued assessment at the scene
- ❑ Did other detailed examination before assessing the airway, breathing and circulation

Focused History and Physical Examination/Rapid Trauma Assessment

Select the Appropriate Assessment (Focused or Rapid)

Student: I am selecting the rapid physical exam to identify and treat life threats. I am checking for DCAP-BTLS. This acronym stands for deformities, contusions, abrasions, punctures, penetrations, paradoxical motion in the chest, and burns, tenderness, lacerations, and swelling.
PROCTOR: Noted.

Head

Student: I am rapidly assessing the head.
PROCTOR: You see abrasions with dried blood.

Neck

Student: I am rapidly assessing the neck.
PROCTOR: There are no obvious injuries.
Student: I will apply a cervical collar.
PROCTOR: Noted.

Chest

Student: I am rapidly assessing the chest. What are the lung sounds?
PROCTOR: The left chest has four ribs with paradoxical motion noted.
Student: I would immediately stabilize the chest with a bulky dressing, and assist ventilations with a bag-valve device if necessary.
PROCTOR: Noted.

Student: I will assess the chest for tension pneumothorax by auscultation and assessment (for jugular vein distention [JVD], tracheal deviation, and decreased lung sounds).

PROCTOR: The lung sounds appear clear bilaterally, jugular vein distention is not present, and the trachea is midline.

ALS Student: I will assess the chest for hyperresonance to percussion.

ALS Proctor: Noted. There is no tension pneumothorax.

ALS Student: I will continuously reassess the chest.

ALS Proctor: Noted.

▸ **Abdomen/Pelvis**

Student: I am rapidly assessing the abdomen.

PROCTOR: There are no obvious injuries.

Student: I am rapidly assessing the pelvis.

PROCTOR: There are no obvious injuries.

▸ **Extremities**

Student: I am rapidly assessing the extremities.

PROCTOR: There is obvious deformity to both femurs.

Student: I am rapidly assessing the lower and upper extremities for DCAP-BTLS. Do I find anything?

PROCTOR: Both femurs are fractured.

▸ **Assess Motor, Sensory, and Circulatory Function**

Student: I am checking for DCAP-BTLS, motor and sensory function, and pulses. Right leg?

PROCTOR: Obvious fracture to the femur. Motor and sensory functions are present. Pulses are weak.

Student: Left leg?

PROCTOR: Obvious fracture to the femur. Motor and sensory functions are present. Pulses are weak.

Student: Right arm?

PROCTOR: Minor cuts and abrasions. Motor and sensory functions are present. Pulses are weak.

Student: Left arm?

PROCTOR: Minor cuts and abrasions. Motor and sensory functions are present. Pulses are weak.

▸ **Posterior**

Student: I will rapidly assess the back. We will now log roll the patient as a unit to check the back. The person at the head will count to three and we will roll the patient.

PROCTOR: Noted.

▸ **Assess the Thorax**

Student: I am assessing the thorax. Do I find injuries?

PROCTOR: You find minor cuts and abrasions.

▸ **Assess the Lumbar Area**

Student: I am assessing the flanks and lumbar area. Do I find injuries?

PROCTOR: You find minor cuts and abrasions.

▸ **Assess the Entire Backside**

Student: I am assessing the entire backside. Do I find injuries?

PROCTOR: You find minor cuts and abrasions.

▸ **Manage Secondary Injuries/Wounds**

Student: We will apply a cervical collar and backboard with full immobilization per local protocol, if not yet done, at this time. We will treat the femurs using the backboard as a splint at this time. Traction splints would delay a load-and-go transport. Traction splints may be applied en route to the hospital on midshaft fractures per local protocol.

PROCTOR: Noted.

Student: Are there any changes in motor and sensory functions or pulses?

PROCTOR: No.

ALS Student: I will establish two large-bore IVs en route to the hospital and a bolus of 20 mL/kg, and maintain a systolic blood pressure of 90 mm Hg.

ALS Proctor: Noted.

▸ **Reevaluate Transport Decision**

Student: This patient is a load-and-go due to multiple trauma, the mechanism of injury, and shock.

PROCTOR: Noted.

▾ Baseline Vital Signs

Student: What are the patient's baseline vital signs, including blood pressure, pulse, respirations, pulse oximetry, and level of consciousness?

PROCTOR: Blood pressure, 90/68 mm Hg; pulse rate, 124 beats/min; respirations, 20 breaths/min; pulse oximetry reading, 96%; and the patient is alert.

▾ SAMPLE History

Student: At this time I will gather a SAMPLE history from the patient or family. What are the patient's signs and symptoms?

PROCTOR: Pain in the chest and legs.

Student: Allergies?

PROCTOR: No allergies.

Student: Medications?

PROCTOR: No medications.

Student: Pertinent past medical history?

PROCTOR: No pertinent medical history.

Student: Last oral intake?

PROCTOR: 10 hours ago.

Student: Events leading up to the incident?

PROCTOR: The patient was abducted from a club and raped repeatedly by four men. She was thrown out of a van that was traveling 65 miles per hour and fell to the bottom of a cliff. She has spent the last 6 hours climbing a hill (with her hands only); she was found by a passerby.

Critical Criteria:
- ☐ Did not differentiate patient's need for transportation versus continued assessment at the scene
- ☐ Did not provide for spinal protection when indicated

Detailed Physical Examination

Student: I am conducting the detailed physical exam. I am looking for DCAP-BTLS.

PROCTOR: Noted. The detailed physical exam will be performed during transport.

▾ Assess the Head

Student: I am assessing the head. Do I find any DCAP-BTLS? Do I find any evidence of Battle's sign or raccoon eyes?

PROCTOR: No.

▸ **Inspect and Palpate the Head and Ears**

Student: I am assessing the head and ears.

PROCTOR: You see dry abrasions.

▸ **Assess the Eyes**

Student: I am assessing the eyes. Are the pupils equal, round, and regular in size, and react properly to light (PEARRL)?

PROCTOR: They are PEARRL.

▸ **Assess the Facial Area Including Oral and Nasal Areas**

Student: I am assessing the face, nose, and mouth. Do I see any discharge or hear any obstructions?

PROCTOR: No.

▾ Assess the Neck

▸ **Inspect and Palpate the Neck**

Student: I am assessing the neck for DCAP-BTLS.

PROCTOR: There are no obvious injuries.

▸ **Assess for Jugular Vein Distention**

Student: Do I find any jugular vein distention (JVD)?

PROCTOR: No.

▸ Assess for Tracheal Deviation

Student: Do I see any tracheal deviation?
PROCTOR: No.

▾ Assess the Chest

Student: I am assessing the chest for DCAP-BTLS.
PROCTOR: Noted.

▸ Inspect

Student: What do I see when I look at the chest?
PROCTOR: You find four ribs with paradoxical motion on the left chest.
Student: I would check that my bulky dressing has stabilized the chest, and assist ventilations with a bag-valve device if necessary.
PROCTOR: Noted.
Student: Does the chest appear symmetric?
PROCTOR: No, there is paradoxical motion, which is stabilized at this time.

▸ Palpate

Student: When I touch the chest, do I feel crepitus or a flail segment?
PROCTOR: Yes, crepitus is palpated on the left side.

▸ Auscultate

Student: Are lung sounds present in all fields?
PROCTOR: Yes.
Student: Do I hear any sucking sounds from the chest?
PROCTOR: No.
ALS Student: I will assess the chest for hyperresonance to percussion.
ALS Proctor: Noted. There is no tension pneumothorax.
ALS Student: I will continuously reassess the chest.
ALS Proctor: Noted.

▾ Assess the Abdomen/Pelvis

▸ Assess the Abdomen

Student: I am assessing the abdomen for DCAP-BTLS. I am assessing all four quadrants. Do I find any problems?
PROCTOR: No.

▸ Assess the Pelvis

Student: I am assessing the pelvis for DCAP-BTLS. Is the pelvis stable?
PROCTOR: Yes.

▸ Assess the Genitalia/Perineum as Needed (Verbalize in Training)

Student: I am assessing the genitalia/perineum as necessary for DCAP-BTLS.
PROCTOR: The patient does not wish to be examined because she wishes to preserve evidence.

▾ Assess the Extremities

▸ Inspect

Student: I am assessing the lower and upper extremities for DCAP-BTLS. Do I find anything?
PROCTOR: Yes, both femurs are fractured (midshaft). They have been splinted by the backboard. They may be splinted using traction, per local protocol, at this time.

▸ Palpate

Student: Do I feel anything unusual?
PROCTOR: Yes, both femurs are fractured and have been splinted by the backboard.

▸ Assess Motor, Sensory, and Circulatory Function

Student: I am checking for DCAP-BTLS, motor and sensory function, and pulses. Right leg?
PROCTOR: Obvious fracture to the femur. Motor and sensory functions are present. Pulses are weak.
Student: Left leg?
PROCTOR: Obvious fracture to the femur. Motor and sensory functions are present. Pulses are weak.
Student: Right arm?
PROCTOR: Minor cuts and abrasions. Motor and sensory functions are present. Pulses are weak.
Student: Left arm?
PROCTOR: Minor cuts and abrasions. Motor and sensory functions are present. Pulses are weak.

▾ Assess the Posterior

Note: This portion of the detailed physical exam would not be done if the patient were previously backboarded per local protocol.
Student: We will not check the back because it was previously checked and the patient is backboarded.
PROCTOR: Noted.

▾ Manage Secondary Injuries/Wounds

Student: I would direct my partner to maintain the airway.
PROCTOR: Noted.

▾ Reassess Vital Signs

Student: I will reassess vital signs and mental status.
PROCTOR: Blood pressure, 90/70 mm Hg; pulse rate, 120 beats/min; respirations, 18 breaths/min; pulse oximetry reading, 97%; and the patient is alert.
Student: The vital signs have not changed significantly.
PROCTOR: Noted.

▾ Reassess Interventions

Student: I will reassess my interventions: airway, breathing, and oxygen (possible bag-valve ventilation); circulation; stabilization of the chest, bilateral Sager splints or local protocol, immobilization, and straps; warming efforts; and treatment for shock.
PROCTOR: Noted.
ALS Student: I will reassess basic life support (BLS) interventions, plus the following: maintain a systolic blood pressure of 90 mm Hg with two large-bore IVs and check the cardiac monitor.
ALS Proctor: Noted. The cardiac monitor shows sinus tachycardia.

Critical Criteria:
- ❑ Did not find or manage problems associated with airway, breathing, hemorrhage or shock (hypoperfusion)

Radio Report

(Provided by the student.)
PROCTOR: Noted.

Ongoing Assessment

▾ Repeat Vital Signs

Student: I will reassess vital signs and mental status.
PROCTOR: Blood pressure, 94/78 mm Hg; pulse rate, 118 beats/min; respirations, 16 breaths/min; pulse oximetry reading, 97%; and the patient is alert.
Student: The vital signs have not changed significantly.
PROCTOR: Noted.

▾ Check Interventions

Student: I will check my interventions: airway, breathing, and oxygen (possible bag-valve ventilation); circulation; stabilization of the chest, bilateral Sager splints or local protocol, immobilization, and straps; warming efforts; and treatment for shock.
PROCTOR: Noted.

ALS Student: I will check BLS interventions, plus the following: maintain a systolic blood pressure of 90 mm Hg with two large-bore IVs and check the cardiac monitor.

ALS Proctor: Noted. The cardiac monitor shows sinus tachycardia.

Critical Criteria:
- ❑ Did not find or manage problems associated with airway, breathing, hemorrhage or shock (hypoperfusion)

Handoff Report to Emergency Department Staff

Student: There was no change in the patient's condition during transport.

PROCTOR: Noted.

Critical Criteria:
- ❑ Did not transport patient within the (10) minute time limit

Critical Criteria

(Inform the student of items missed, if any.)

❑ Pass ❑ Fail Date: ____________________

Proctor Comments: ____________________

____

____

Dispatch Information

PROCTOR: EMS 10, respond to a 75-year-old male who has struck a power pole in his car. Wires are down across the car. He is calling from a cell phone.

Pre-scene Action (BSI)

Student: I am wearing extrication-level personal protective equipment and a helmet, nonlatex gloves, safety glasses, mask, and gown.
PROCTOR: Noted.

Critical Criteria:
- ❑ Did not take, or verbalize, body substance isolation (BSI) precautions when necessary

Scene Size-up

Scene Safety

Student: Is the scene safe?
PROCTOR: No, the power company has not arrived yet.

Mechanism of Injury

Student: What was the mechanism of injury?
PROCTOR: Motor vehicle collision. The patient was an unrestrained driver who struck a power pole. He is complaining of chest pain.

Number of Patients

Student: How many patients are there?
PROCTOR: One.

Additional Resources

Student: I would call for advanced life support (ALS) assistance and additional resources: fire/rescue, police, and the power company.
PROCTOR: Noted. The power company has a 45 minute ETA.
Student: I will wait for the power company to disconnect the power lines and make the area safe.
PROCTOR: Noted. The scene is now safe.

C-Spine Stabilization

Student: On the basis of the mechanism of injury, I would stabilize the cervical spine (c-spine) in a neutral in-line position.
PROCTOR: Noted.

Critical Criteria:
- ❑ Did not determine scene safety
- ❑ Did not assess for spinal protection
- ❑ Did not provide for spinal protection when indicated

Initial Assessment

Student: As I perform midline c-spine stabilization, I identify myself and ask the patient not to move.
PROCTOR: Noted.

General Impression

Student: My general impression is that the patient's condition is unstable.
PROCTOR: Noted.

Responsiveness/Level of Consciousness

Student: What is the patient's level of consciousness?
PROCTOR: Alert.

Chief Complaint/Apparent Life Threats

Student: What is the patient's chief complaint?
PROCTOR: The patient is complaining of chest pain. The steering wheel is deformed.
Student: There is an apparent life threat; the life threat is the mechanism of injury.
PROCTOR: Noted.

Assess the Airway and Breathing

Student: Is the airway open? Is the patient breathing?
PROCTOR: Yes, the airway is open and the patient is breathing.

Assessment

Student: What are the rate and the quality of breathing?
PROCTOR: Rate: Tachypneic. Quality: Shallow.

Provide Oxygen

Student: I am applying oxygen at 15 L/min via nonrebreathing mask.
PROCTOR: Noted.

Ensure Adequate Ventilation

Student: The patient has adequate ventilations at this time.
PROCTOR: Noted.

Injury Management

Student: I will direct my partner to take over c-spine control as I continue assessment.
PROCTOR: Noted.

Assess Circulation

Student: I am assessing the patient's circulation.
PROCTOR: Noted.

Assess for and Control Major Bleeding

Student: Do I find any major bleeding?
PROCTOR: No.

Assess the Pulse

Student: What are the rate and the quality of pulses?
PROCTOR: Rate: Tachycardic. Quality: Thready.

Assess the Skin

Student: I am assessing the skin. What are the color, temperature, and condition of the skin?
PROCTOR: Color: Pale. Temperature: Cool. Condition: Diaphoretic.

Identify Priority Patients/Make Transport Decision

Student: The patient is a high priority and is a load-and-go. I will begin packaging and transport.
PROCTOR: Noted.

Critical Criteria:
- ❑ Did not provide high concentration of oxygen
- ❑ Did not find or manage problems associated with airway, breathing, hemorrhage or shock (hypoperfusion)
- ❑ Did not differentiate patient's need for transportation versus continued assessment at the scene
- ❑ Did other detailed examination before assessing the airway, breathing and circulation

Focused History and Physical Examination/Rapid Trauma Assessment

Select the Appropriate Assessment (Focused or Rapid)

Student: I am selecting the rapid physical exam to identify and treat life threats. I am checking for DCAP-BTLS. This acronym stands for deformities, contusions, abrasions, punctures, penetrations, paradoxical motion in the chest, and burns, tenderness, lacerations, and swelling.
PROCTOR: Noted.

Head

Student: I am rapidly assessing the head.
PROCTOR: There are no obvious injuries.

Neck

Student: I am rapidly assessing the neck.
PROCTOR: There are no obvious injuries.
Student: I will apply a cervical collar.
PROCTOR: Noted.

Chest

Student: I am rapidly assessing the chest.
PROCTOR: The sternum appears to be a flail segment.

Student: I will stabilize the chest with a bulky dressing or a pillow. I will assist with ventilation if necessary.

PROCTOR: Noted.

Student: Are lung sounds present in all fields? Are they clear?

PROCTOR: Yes, lung sounds are present and clear.

Student: I will assess the chest for tension pneumothorax by auscultation and assessment (for jugular vein distention [JVD], tracheal deviation, and decreased lung sounds).

PROCTOR: The lung sounds appear clear bilaterally, jugular vein distention is not present, and the trachea is midline.

ALS Student: I will assess the chest for hyperresonance to percussion.

ALS Proctor: Noted. There is no tension pneumothorax.

ALS Student: I will continuously reassess the chest.

ALS Proctor: Noted.

▸ **Abdomen/Pelvis**

Student: I am rapidly assessing the abdomen.

PROCTOR: There are no obvious injuries.

Student: I am rapidly assessing the pelvis.

PROCTOR: There are no obvious injuries.

▸ **Extremities**

Student: I am rapidly assessing the extremities.

PROCTOR: There are no obvious injuries.

▸ **Assess Motor, Sensory, and Circulatory Function**

Student: I am checking for DCAP-BTLS, motor and sensory function, and pulses. Right leg?

PROCTOR: Negative DCAP-BTLS. Motor and sensory functions are present. Pulses are present.

Student: Left leg?

PROCTOR: Negative DCAP-BTLS. Motor and sensory functions are present. Pulses are present.

Student: Right arm?

PROCTOR: Negative DCAP-BTLS. Motor and sensory functions are present. Pulses are present.

Student: Left arm?

PROCTOR: Negative DCAP-BTLS. Motor and sensory functions are present. Pulses are present.

▸ **Posterior**

Student: I am assessing the backside prior to extricating the patient.

PROCTOR: Noted.

▸ **Assess the Thorax**

Student: I am assessing the thorax. Do I find injuries?

PROCTOR: No.

▸ **Assess the Lumbar Area**

Student: I am assessing the flanks and lumbar area. Do I find injuries?

PROCTOR: No.

▸ **Assess the Entire Backside**

Student: I am assessing the entire backside. Do I find injuries?

PROCTOR: No.

▸ **Manage Secondary Injuries/Wounds**

Student: I would direct my partner to maintain the flail sternum as we apply a cervical collar, perform a rapid extrication onto a long backboard, and fully immobilize the patient.

PROCTOR: Noted.

Student: Are there any changes in motor and sensory functions or pulses?

PROCTOR: No.

ALS Student: I will establish two large-bore IVs, cardiac monitor, and 12-lead ECG en route to the hospital.

ALS Proctor: Noted. The cardiac monitor shows sinus tachycardia.

▸ **Reevaluate Transport Decision**

Student: This patient is a high priority and a load-and-go due to the mechanism of injury and chest trauma.

PROCTOR: Noted.

▾ **Baseline Vital Signs**

Student: What are the patient's baseline vital signs, including blood pressure, pulse, respirations, pulse oximetry, and level of consciousness?

PROCTOR: Blood pressure, 142/82 mm Hg; pulse rate, 140 beats/min; respirations, 24 breaths/min; pulse oximetry reading, 95%; and the patient is anxious.

▾ **SAMPLE History**

Student: At this time I will gather a SAMPLE history from the patient or family. What are the patient's signs and symptoms?

PROCTOR: Pain in the chest.

Student: Allergies?

PROCTOR: No allergies.

Student: Medications?

PROCTOR: No medications.

Student: Pertinent past medical history?

PROCTOR: No pertinent medical history.

Student: Last oral intake?

PROCTOR: 3 hours ago.

Student: Events leading up to the incident?

PROCTOR: The patient was driving in the rain and struck a power pole. Extrication was delayed 45 minutes due to the response time of the power company.

Critical Criteria:
- ☐ Did not differentiate patient's need for transportation versus continued assessment at the scene
- ☐ Did not provide for spinal protection when indicated

Detailed Physical Examination

Student: I am conducting the detailed physical exam. I am looking for DCAP-BTLS.

PROCTOR: Noted. The detailed physical exam will be performed during transport.

▾ **Assess the Head**

Student: I am assessing the head. Do I find any DCAP-BTLS? Do I find any evidence of Battle's sign or raccoon eyes?

PROCTOR: No.

▸ **Inspect and Palpate the Head and Ears**

Student: I am assessing the head and ears.

PROCTOR: There are no obvious injuries.

▸ **Assess the Eyes**

Student: I am assessing the eyes. Are the pupils equal, round, and regular in size, and react properly to light (PEARRL)?

PROCTOR: They are PEARRL.

▸ **Assess the Facial Area Including Oral and Nasal Areas**

Student: I am assessing the face, nose, and mouth. Do I see any discharge or hear any obstructions?

PROCTOR: No.

▾ **Assess the Neck**

▸ **Inspect and Palpate the Neck**

Student: I am assessing the neck for DCAP-BTLS.

PROCTOR: There are no obvious injuries.

▸ **Assess for Jugular Vein Distention**

Student: Do I find any jugular vein distention (JVD)?

PROCTOR: No.

▸ Assess for Tracheal Deviation

Student: Do I see any tracheal deviation?

PROCTOR: No.

▾ Assess the Chest

Student: I am assessing the chest for DCAP-BTLS.

PROCTOR: Noted.

▸ Inspect

Student: What do I see when I look at the chest?

PROCTOR: There is a large bruise developing across the chest.

Student: Does the chest appear symmetric?

PROCTOR: No. There is paradoxical motion noted between the ribs and sternum. This area should have been stabilized previously.

Student: I will reassess the chest dressing.

PROCTOR: Noted. It is effective.

▸ Palpate

Student: When I touch the chest, do I feel crepitus or a flail segment?

PROCTOR: Yes.

▸ Auscultate

Student: Are lung sounds present in all fields?

PROCTOR: Yes.

Student: Do I hear any sucking sounds from the chest?

PROCTOR: No.

ALS Student: I will assess the chest for hyperresonance to percussion.

ALS Proctor: Noted. There is no tension pneumothorax.

ALS Student: I will continuously reassess the chest.

ALS Proctor: Noted.

▾ Assess the Abdomen/Pelvis

▸ Assess the Abdomen

Student: I am assessing the abdomen for DCAP-BTLS. I am assessing all four quadrants. Do I find any problems?

PROCTOR: No.

▸ Assess the Pelvis

Student: I am assessing the pelvis for DCAP-BTLS. Is the pelvis stable?

PROCTOR: Yes.

▾ Assess the Genitalia/Perineum as Needed (Verbalize in Training)

Student: I am assessing the genitalia/perineum as necessary for DCAP-BTLS.

PROCTOR: The area is unremarkable.

▾ Assess the Extremities

▸ Inspect

Student: I am assessing the lower and upper extremities for DCAP-BTLS. Do I find anything?

PROCTOR: No.

▸ Palpate

Student: Do I feel anything unusual?

PROCTOR: No.

▸ Assess Motor, Sensory, and Circulatory Function

Student: I am checking for DCAP-BTLS, motor and sensory function, and pulses. Right leg?

PROCTOR: Negative DCAP-BTLS. Motor and sensory functions are present. Pulses are present.

Student: Left leg?

PROCTOR: Negative DCAP-BTLS. Motor and sensory functions are present. Pulses are present.

Student: Right arm?

PROCTOR: Negative DCAP-BTLS. Motor and sensory functions are present. Pulses are present.

Student: Left arm?

PROCTOR: Negative DCAP-BTLS. Motor and sensory functions are present. Pulses are present.

▾ Assess the Posterior

Note: This portion of the detailed physical exam would not be done if the patient were previously backboarded per local protocol.

Student: We will not check the back because it was previously checked and the patient was extricated and backboarded.

PROCTOR: Noted.

▾ Manage Secondary Injuries/Wounds

Student: I would direct my partner to monitor the flail segment and the patient's respiratory status.

PROCTOR: Noted.

▾ Reassess Vital Signs

Student: I will reassess vital signs and mental status.

PROCTOR: Blood pressure, 134/80 mm Hg; pulse rate, 152 beats/min; respirations, 20 breaths/min; pulse oximetry reading, 97%; and the patient is anxious.

Student: The vital signs have not changed significantly.

PROCTOR: Noted.

▾ Reassess Interventions

Student: I will reassess my interventions: oxygen; stabilized the flail chest; immobilization and straps; and treatment for shock.

PROCTOR: Noted.

ALS Student: I will reassess basic life support (BLS) interventions, plus the following: two large-bore IVs, cardiac monitor, and 12-lead ECG.

ALS Proctor: Noted. The cardiac monitor shows sinus tachycardia.

Critical Criteria:

❑ Did not find or manage problems associated with airway, breathing, hemorrhage or shock (hypoperfusion)

Radio Report

(Provided by the student.)

PROCTOR: Noted.

Ongoing Assessment

▾ Repeat Vital Signs

Student: I will reassess vital signs and mental status.

PROCTOR: Blood pressure, 136/82 mm Hg; pulse rate, 146 beats/min; respirations, 20 breaths/min; pulse oximetry reading, 97%; and the patient is anxious.

Student: The vital signs have not changed significantly.

PROCTOR: Noted.

▾ Check Interventions

Student: I will check interventions: oxygen; assist with ventilation if necessary; stabilize the flail chest; immobilization and straps; and treatment for shock.

PROCTOR: Noted.

ALS Student: I will check BLS interventions, plus the following: two large-bore IVs, cardiac monitor, and 12-lead ECG.

ALS Proctor: Noted. The cardiac monitor shows sinus tachycardia.

Critical Criteria:
- ❑ Did not find or manage problems associated with airway, breathing, hemorrhage or shock (hypoperfusion)

Handoff Report to Emergency Department Staff

Student: There was no change in the patient's condition during transport.

PROCTOR: Noted.

Critical Criteria:
- ❑ Did not transport patient within the (10) minute time limit

Critical Criteria

(Inform the student of items missed, if any.)

❑ Pass ❑ Fail Date: ______________________________

Proctor Comments: ______________________________

____

____

Dispatch Information

PROCTOR: EMS 10, respond to a small aircraft crash involving a 55-year-old male pilot complaining of chest pain. He is conscious and breathing.

Pre-scene Action (BSI)

Student: I am wearing appropriate high-visibility personal protective equipment suitable for extrication, a helmet, extrication gloves, nonlatex gloves, safety glasses, and a mask.
PROCTOR: Noted.

Critical Criteria:
- ❑ Did not take, or verbalize, body substance isolation (BSI) precautions when necessary

Scene Size-up

Scene Safety

Student: Is the scene safe?
PROCTOR: Yes.

Mechanism of Injury

Student: What was the mechanism of injury?
PROCTOR: Blunt trauma. The patient was flying and ran out of fuel. He tried to land on a highway and crashed into a ditch.

Number of Patients

Student: How many patients are there?
PROCTOR: One.

Additional Resources

Student: I would call for advanced life support (ALS) assistance and additional resources: fire/rescue and police.
PROCTOR: Noted.

C-Spine Stabilization

Student: On the basis of the mechanism of injury I would stabilize the cervical spine (c-spine) in a neutral in-line position.
PROCTOR: Noted.

Critical Criteria:
- ❑ Did not determine scene safety
- ❑ Did not assess for spinal protection
- ❑ Did not provide for spinal protection when indicated

Initial Assessment

Student: As I perform midline c-spine stabilization, I identify myself and ask the patient not to move.
PROCTOR: Noted. The patient speaks a foreign language that is unknown to you.

General Impression

Student: My general impression is that the patient's condition is unstable.
PROCTOR: Noted.

Responsiveness/Level of Consciousness

Student: What is the patient's level of consciousness?
PROCTOR: Alert.

Chief Complaint/Apparent Life Threats

Student: What is the patient's chief complaint?
PROCTOR: The patient is pointing to his chest. You are able to see the bruised impression of the yoke (steering wheel) on his chest. The aircraft is an older model that is only equipped with a lap belt, which was being worn.
Student: There are apparent life threats; the life threats are the chest injury and the mechanism of injury.
PROCTOR: Noted.

Assess the Airway and Breathing

Student: Is the airway open? Is the patient breathing?
PROCTOR: Yes, the airway is open and the patient is breathing.

Assessment

Student: What are the rate and the quality of breathing?
PROCTOR: Rate: Rapid. Quality: Labored.

Provide Oxygen

Student: I am applying oxygen at 15 L/min via nonrebreathing mask.
PROCTOR: Noted.

Ensure Adequate Ventilation

Student: The patient has adequate ventilations at this time.
PROCTOR: Noted.

Injury Management

Student: I will direct my partner to take over c-spine control as I continue assessment.
PROCTOR: Noted.

Assess Circulation

Student: I am assessing the patient's circulation.
PROCTOR: Noted.

Assess for and Control Major Bleeding

Student: Do I find any major bleeding?
PROCTOR: No.

Assess the Pulse

Student: What are the rate and the quality of pulses?
PROCTOR: Rate: Fast. Quality: Bounding.

Assess the Skin

Student: I am assessing the skin. What are the color, temperature, and condition of the skin?
PROCTOR: Color: Flushed. Temperature: Warm. Condition: Moist.

Identify Priority Patients/Make Transport Decision

Student: The patient is a high priority and is a load-and-go. I will begin packaging and transport.
PROCTOR: Noted.

Critical Criteria:
- ❑ Did not provide high concentration of oxygen
- ❑ Did not find or manage problems associated with airway, breathing, hemorrhage or shock (hypoperfusion)
- ❑ Did not differentiate patient's need for transportation versus continued assessment at the scene
- ❑ Did other detailed examination before assessing the airway, breathing and circulation

Focused History and Physical Examination/Rapid Trauma Assessment

Select the Appropriate Assessment (Focused or Rapid)

Student: I am selecting the rapid physical exam to identify and treat life threats. I am checking for DCAP-BTLS. This acronym stands for deformities, contusions, abrasions, punctures, penetrations, paradoxical motion in the chest, and burns, tenderness, lacerations, and swelling.
PROCTOR: Noted.

Head

Student: I am rapidly assessing the head.
PROCTOR: There are no obvious injuries.

Neck

Student: I am rapidly assessing the neck.
PROCTOR: There are no obvious injuries.
Student: I will apply a cervical collar.
PROCTOR: Noted.

Chest

Student: I am rapidly assessing the chest.
PROCTOR: The yoke has left an imprint on the patient's chest.

Student: Does the chest appear symmetric?
PROCTOR: No, the ribs are depressed with paradoxical motion on the right side.
Student: I will stabilize the chest with a bulky dressing or a pillow.
PROCTOR: Noted.
Student: Are the lung sounds clear bilaterally?
PROCTOR: Yes.
Student: I will assist with ventilations if necessary.
PROCTOR: Noted.
Student: I will assess the chest for tension pneumothorax by auscultation and assessment (for jugular vein distention [JVD], tracheal deviation, and decreased lung sounds).
PROCTOR: The lung sounds appear clear bilaterally, jugular vein distention is not present, and the trachea is midline.
ALS Student: I will assess the chest for hyperresonance to percussion.
ALS Proctor: Noted. There is no tension pneumothorax.
ALS Student: I will continuously reassess the chest.
ALS Proctor: Noted.

▸ **Abdomen/Pelvis**

Student: I am rapidly assessing the abdomen.
PROCTOR: There are no obvious injuries.
Student: I am rapidly assessing the pelvis.
PROCTOR: There are no obvious injuries.

▸ **Extremities**

Student: I am rapidly assessing the extremities.
PROCTOR: There are no obvious injuries.

▸ **Assess Motor, Sensory, and Circulatory Function**

Student: I am checking for DCAP-BTLS, motor and sensory function, and pulses. Right leg?
PROCTOR: Negative DCAP-BTLS. Motor and sensory functions are present. Pulses are present.
Student: Left leg?
PROCTOR: Negative DCAP-BTLS. Motor and sensory functions are present. Pulses are present.
Student: Right arm?
PROCTOR: Negative DCAP-BTLS. Motor and sensory functions are present. Pulses are present.
Student: Left arm?
PROCTOR: Negative DCAP-BTLS. Motor and sensory functions are present. Pulses are present.

▸ **Posterior**

Student: I will rapidly assess the back. We will now log roll the patient as a unit to check the back. The person at the head will count to three and we will roll the patient.
PROCTOR: Noted.

▸ **Assess the Thorax**

Student: I am assessing the thorax. Do I find injuries?
PROCTOR: No.

▸ **Assess the Lumbar Area**

Student: I am assessing the flanks and lumbar area. Do I find injuries?
PROCTOR: No.

▸ **Assess the Entire Backside**

Student: I am assessing the entire backside. Do I find injuries?
PROCTOR: No.

▸ **Manage Secondary Injuries/Wounds**

Student: We will apply a cervical collar and backboard with full immobilization per local protocol, if not yet done, at this time.
PROCTOR: Noted.
Student: Are there any changes in motor and sensory functions or pulses?
PROCTOR: No.
ALS Student: I will establish two large-bore IVs en route to the hospital and administer a bolus of 20 mL/kg to maintain a systolic blood pressure of 90 mm Hg.
ALS Proctor: Noted.

▸ **Reevaluate Transport Decision**

Student: This patient is a load-and-go due to the mechanism of injury and chest trauma.
PROCTOR: Noted.

▾ Baseline Vital Signs

Student: What are the patient's baseline vital signs, including blood pressure, pulse, respirations, pulse oximetry, and level of consciousness?
PROCTOR: Blood pressure, 100/70 mm Hg; pulse rate, 110 beats/min; respirations, 24 breaths/min; pulse oximetry reading, 97%; and the patient is alert.

▾ SAMPLE History

Student: At this time I will gather a SAMPLE history from the patient or family. What are the patient's signs and symptoms?
PROCTOR: Pain in the chest made obvious by the patient.
Student: Allergies?
PROCTOR: Unknown.
Student: Medications?
PROCTOR: Unknown.
Student: Pertinent past medical history?
PROCTOR: Unknown.
Student: Last oral intake?
PROCTOR: Unknown.
Student: Events leading up to the incident?
PROCTOR: Unknown.

Critical Criteria:
- ☐ Did not differentiate patient's need for transportation versus continued assessment at the scene
- ☐ Did not provide for spinal protection when indicated

▼ Detailed Physical Examination

Student: I am conducting the detailed physical exam. I am looking for DCAP-BTLS.
PROCTOR: Noted. The detailed physical exam will be performed during transport.

▾ Assess the Head

Student: I am assessing the head. Do I find any DCAP-BTLS? Do I find any evidence of Battle's sign or raccoon eyes?
PROCTOR: No.

▸ **Inspect and Palpate the Head and Ears**

Student: I am assessing the head and ears.
PROCTOR: There are no obvious injuries.

▸ **Assess the Eyes**

Student: I am assessing the eyes. Are the pupils equal, round, and regular in size, and react properly to light (PEARRL)?
PROCTOR: They are PEARRL.

▸ **Assess the Facial Area Including Oral and Nasal Areas**

Student: I am assessing the face, nose, and mouth. Do I see any discharge or hear any obstructions?
PROCTOR: No.

▾ Assess the Neck

▸ **Inspect and Palpate the Neck**

Student: I am assessing the neck for DCAP-BTLS.
PROCTOR: There are no obvious injuries.

▸ **Assess for Jugular Vein Distention**

Student: Do I find any jugular vein distention (JVD)?

PROCTOR: No.

▸ **Assess for Tracheal Deviation**

Student: Do I see any tracheal deviation?

PROCTOR: No.

▼ Assess the Chest

Student: I am assessing the chest for DCAP-BTLS.

PROCTOR: Noted.

▸ **Inspect**

Student: What do I see when I look at the chest?

PROCTOR: The yoke print is visible on the chest.

Student: Does the chest appear symmetric?

PROCTOR: No, the ribs are depressed with paradoxical motion on the right side.

▸ **Palpate**

Student: When I touch the chest, do I feel crepitus or a flail segment?

PROCTOR: Yes.

Student: Was the previous treatment effective?

PROCTOR: Yes.

▸ **Auscultate**

Student: Are lung sounds present in all fields?

PROCTOR: Yes.

Student: Do I hear any sucking sounds from the chest?

PROCTOR: No.

ALS Student: I will assess the chest for hyperresonance to percussion.

ALS Proctor: Noted. There is no tension pneumothorax.

ALS Student: I will continuously reassess the chest.

ALS Proctor: Noted.

▼ Assess the Abdomen/Pelvis

▸ **Assess the Abdomen**

Student: I am assessing the abdomen for DCAP-BTLS. I am assessing all four quadrants. Do I find any problems?

PROCTOR: No.

▸ **Assess the Pelvis**

Student: I am assessing the pelvis for DCAP-BTLS. Is the pelvis stable?

PROCTOR: Yes.

▼ Assess the Genitalia/Perineum as Needed (Verbalize in Training)

Student: I am assessing the genitalia/perineum as necessary for DCAP-BTLS.

PROCTOR: The area is unremarkable.

▼ Assess the Extremities

▸ **Inspect**

Student: I am assessing the lower and upper extremities for DCAP-BTLS. Do I find anything?

PROCTOR: No.

▸ **Palpate**

Student: Do I feel anything unusual?

PROCTOR: No.

▸ **Assess Motor, Sensory, and Circulatory Function**

Student: I am checking for DCAP-BTLS, motor and sensory function, and pulses. Right leg?

PROCTOR: Negative DCAP-BTLS. Motor and sensory functions are present. Pulses are present.

Student: Left leg?

PROCTOR: Negative DCAP-BTLS. Motor and sensory functions are present. Pulses are present.

Student: Right arm?

PROCTOR: Negative DCAP-BTLS. Motor and sensory functions are present. Pulses are present.

Student: Left arm?

PROCTOR: Negative DCAP-BTLS. Motor and sensory functions are present. Pulses are present.

▼ Assess the Posterior

Note: This portion of the detailed physical exam would not be done if the patient were previously backboarded per local protocol.

Student: We will not check the back because it was previously checked and the patient is backboarded.

PROCTOR: Noted.

▼ Manage Secondary Injuries/Wounds

Student: I would direct my partner to monitor the airway.

PROCTOR: Noted.

▼ Reassess Vital Signs

Student: I will reassess vital signs and mental status.

PROCTOR: Blood pressure, 94/72 mm Hg; pulse rate, 112 beats/min; respirations, 24 breaths/min; pulse oximetry reading, 97%; and the patient is alert.

Student: The vital signs have deteriorated.

PROCTOR: Noted.

▼ Reassess Interventions

Student: I will reassess my interventions: oxygen, immobilization, straps, and treatment for shock.

PROCTOR: Noted.

ALS Student: I will reassess basic life support (BLS) interventions, plus the following: maintain two large-bore IVs and a systolic blood pressure of 90 mm Hg, and cardiac monitoring.

ALS Proctor: Noted. The cardiac monitor shows sinus tachycardia.

Critical Criteria:

❑ Did not find or manage problems associated with airway, breathing, hemorrhage or shock (hypoperfusion)

▼ Radio Report

(Provided by the student.)

PROCTOR: Noted.

▼ Ongoing Assessment

▼ Repeat Vital Signs

Student: I will reassess vital signs and mental status.

PROCTOR: Blood pressure, 88/74 mm Hg; pulse rate, 108 beats/min; respirations, 24 breaths/min; pulse oximetry reading, 96%; and the patient is alert.

Student: The vital signs have deteriorated.

PROCTOR: Noted.

▼ Check Interventions

Student: I will check my interventions: oxygen, immobilization, straps, and treatment for shock.

PROCTOR: Noted.

ALS Student: I will check BLS interventions, plus the following: maintain two large-bore IVs and a systolic blood pressure of 90 mm Hg, and cardiac monitoring.

ALS Proctor: Noted. The cardiac monitor shows sinus tachycardia.

Critical Criteria:

❑ Did not find or manage problems associated with airway, breathing, hemorrhage or shock (hypoperfusion)

Handoff Report to Emergency Department Staff

Student: The patient's condition deteriorated during transport.
PROCTOR: Noted.

Critical Criteria:
❑ Did not transport patient within the (10) minute time limit

Critical Criteria

(Inform the student of items missed, if any.)

❑ Pass ❑ Fail Date: ____________________

Proctor Comments: ____________________

____

____

CASE 54

Dispatch Information

PROCTOR: EMS 10, respond to a motor vehicle collision. The 18-year-old driver has been thrown through the windshield. Police officers are en route.

Pre-scene Action (BSI)

Student: I am wearing appropriate high-visibility personal protective equipment suitable for extrication, a helmet, extrication gloves, nonlatex gloves, safety glasses, and a mask.
PROCTOR: Noted.

Critical Criteria:
- ❑ Did not take, or verbalize, body substance isolation (BSI) precautions when necessary

Scene Size-up

Scene Safety

Student: Is the scene safe?
PROCTOR: Yes, police are on scene and you are given clearance to enter.

Mechanism of Injury

Student: What was the mechanism of injury?
PROCTOR: Motor vehicle collision. The patient was passing on the right and lost control of the vehicle, which struck a tree. He has been partially ejected through the windshield to his waist.

Number of Patients

Student: How many patients are there?
PROCTOR: One.

Additional Resources

Student: I would call for advanced life support (ALS) assistance and additional resources: fire/rescue.
PROCTOR: Noted.

C-Spine Stabilization

Student: On the basis of the mechanism of injury, I would stabilize the cervical spine (c-spine) in a neutral in-line position.
PROCTOR: Noted.

Critical Criteria:
- ❑ Did not determine scene safety
- ❑ Did not assess for spinal protection
- ❑ Did not provide for spinal protection when indicated

Initial Assessment

Student: As I perform midline c-spine stabilization, I identify myself and ask the patient not to move.
PROCTOR: Noted.

General Impression

Student: My general impression is that the patient's condition is unstable.
PROCTOR: Noted.

Responsiveness/Level of Consciousness

Student: What is the patient's level of consciousness?
PROCTOR: Alert.

Chief Complaint/Apparent Life Threats

Student: What is the patient's chief complaint?
PROCTOR: The patient is complaining of not being able to move.
Student: There is an apparent life threat; the life threat is the mechanism of injury.
PROCTOR: Noted.

Assess the Airway and Breathing

Student: Is the airway open? Is the patient breathing?
PROCTOR: Yes, the airway is open and the patient is breathing.

Assessment

Student: What are the rate and the quality of breathing?
PROCTOR: Rate: Within normal limits. Quality: Diaphragmatic.

Provide Oxygen

Student: We will rapidly extricate and begin assisting ventilations with a bag-valve device with 100% oxygen.
PROCTOR: Noted.

Ensure Adequate Ventilation

Student: As noted above, I am assisting ventilations with a bag-valve device.
PROCTOR: Noted.

Injury Management

Student: I will direct my partner to take over c-spine control and ventilations as I continue assessment.
PROCTOR: Noted.

Assess Circulation

Student: I am assessing the patient's circulation.
PROCTOR: Noted.

Assess for and Control Major Bleeding

Student: Do I find any major bleeding?
PROCTOR: Yes, the patient's clothing and large pieces of skin have been removed from the chest and abdomen by the glass.
Student: I would apply direct pressure and an occlusive dressing.
PROCTOR: Noted.

Assess the Pulse

Student: What are the rate and the quality of pulses?
PROCTOR: Rate: Within normal limits. Quality: Thready.

Assess the Skin

Student: I am assessing the skin. What are the color, temperature, and condition of the skin?
PROCTOR: Color: Pale. Temperature: Cool. Condition: Dry.

Identify Priority Patients/Make Transport Decision

Student: The patient is a high priority and is a load-and-go. I will begin packaging and transport.
PROCTOR: Noted.

Critical Criteria:
- ❑ Did not provide high concentration of oxygen
- ❑ Did not find or manage problems associated with airway, breathing, hemorrhage or shock (hypoperfusion)
- ❑ Did not differentiate patient's need for transportation versus continued assessment at the scene
- ❑ Did other detailed examination before assessing the airway, breathing and circulation

Focused History and Physical Examination/Rapid Trauma Assessment

Select the Appropriate Assessment (Focused or Rapid)

Student: I am selecting the rapid physical exam to identify and treat life threats. I am checking for DCAP-BTLS. This acronym stands for deformities, contusions, abrasions, punctures, penetrations, paradoxical motion in the chest, and burns, tenderness, lacerations, and swelling.
PROCTOR: Noted.

Head

Student: I am rapidly assessing the head.
PROCTOR: There is a large bruise across the forehead.

▸ Neck

Student: I am rapidly assessing the neck.
PROCTOR: It is painful.
Student: I will apply a cervical collar.
PROCTOR: Noted.

▸ Chest

Student: I am rapidly assessing the chest. What are the lung sounds?
PROCTOR: Skin is missing. The dressing was effective. Lung sounds are clear bilaterally.

▸ Abdomen/Pelvis

Student: I am rapidly assessing the abdomen.
PROCTOR: Skin is missing. The dressing was effective.
Student: I am rapidly assessing the pelvis.
PROCTOR: The pelvis is stable.

▸ Extremities

Student: I am rapidly assessing the extremities.
PROCTOR: Skin is missing from the arms.
Student: I will apply dressings to the areas where skin is missing.
PROCTOR: Noted.

▸ Assess Motor, Sensory, and Circulatory Function

Student: I am checking for DCAP-BTLS, motor and sensory function, and pulses. Right leg?
PROCTOR: Negative DCAP-BTLS. Motor and sensory functions are absent. Pulses are weak.
Student: Left leg?
PROCTOR: Negative DCAP-BTLS. Motor and sensory functions are absent. Pulses are weak.
Student: Right arm?
PROCTOR: Bleeding is controlled from the missing skin (dressings were applied earlier). Motor and sensory functions are absent. Pulses are weak.
Student: Left arm?
PROCTOR: Bleeding is controlled from the missing skin (dressings were applied earlier). Motor and sensory functions are absent. Pulses are weak.

▸ Posterior

Student: I will rapidly assess the back. We will now log roll the patient as a unit to check the back. The person at the head will count to three and we will roll the patient.
PROCTOR: Noted.

▸ Assess the Thorax

Student: I am assessing the thorax. Do I find injuries?
PROCTOR: No.

▸ Assess the Lumbar Area

Student: I am assessing the flanks and lumbar area. Do I find injuries?
PROCTOR: No.

▸ Assess the Entire Backside

Student: I am assessing the entire backside. Do I find injuries?
PROCTOR: No.

▸ Manage Secondary Injuries/Wounds

Student: We will apply a cervical collar and backboard with full immobilization per local protocol, if not yet done, at this time.
PROCTOR: Noted.
Student: Are there any changes in motor and sensory functions or pulses?
PROCTOR: No.

ALS Student: I will establish two large-bore IVs en route to the hospital and administer a bolus of 20 mL/kg to maintain a systolic blood pressure of 90 mm Hg.
ALS Proctor: Noted.

▸ Reevaluate Transport Decision

Student: This patient is a load-and-go due to the mechanism of injury and possible shock.
PROCTOR: Noted.

▾ Baseline Vital Signs

Student: What are the patient's baseline vital signs, including blood pressure, pulse, respirations, pulse oximetry, and level of consciousness?
PROCTOR: Blood pressure, 110/70 mm Hg; pulse rate, 88 beats/min; respirations per bag-valve device, 16 breaths/min; pulse oximetry reading, 95%; and the patient is alert.

▾ SAMPLE History

Student: At this time I will gather a SAMPLE history from the patient or family. What are the patient's signs and symptoms?
PROCTOR: Pain in the neck and not being able to move.
Student: Allergies?
PROCTOR: No allergies.
Student: Medications?
PROCTOR: No medications.
Student: Pertinent past medical history?
PROCTOR: No pertinent medical history.
Student: Last oral intake?
PROCTOR: 2 hours ago.
Student: Events leading up to the incident?
PROCTOR: He was passing on the right and lost control of the car, which struck a tree.

Critical Criteria:

- ❑ Did not differentiate patient's need for transportation versus continued assessment at the scene
- ❑ Did not provide for spinal protection when indicated

Detailed Physical Examination

Student: I am conducting the detailed physical exam. I am looking for DCAP-BTLS.
PROCTOR: Noted. The detailed physical exam will be performed during transport.

▾ Assess the Head

Student: I am assessing the head. Do I find any DCAP-BTLS? Do I find any evidence of Battle's sign or raccoon eyes?
PROCTOR: Yes, bruising is noted to the forehead.

▸ Inspect and Palpate the Head and Ears

Student: I am assessing the head and ears.
PROCTOR: You see only bruising to the forehead.

▸ Assess the Eyes

Student: I am assessing the eyes. Are the pupils equal, round, and regular in size, and react properly to light (PEARRL)?
PROCTOR: They are PEARRL.

▸ Assess the Facial Area Including Oral and Nasal Areas

Student: I am assessing the face, nose, and mouth. Do I see any discharge or hear any obstructions?
PROCTOR: No.

▼ Assess the Neck

▸ **Inspect and Palpate the Neck**

Student: I am assessing the neck for DCAP-BTLS.
PROCTOR: There are no obvious injuries.

▸ **Assess for Jugular Vein Distention**

Student: Do I find any jugular vein distention (JVD)?
PROCTOR: No.

▸ **Assess for Tracheal Deviation**

Student: Do I see any tracheal deviation?
PROCTOR: No.

▼ Assess the Chest

Student: I am assessing the chest for DCAP-BTLS.
PROCTOR: Noted.

▸ **Inspect**

Student: What do I see when I look at the chest?
PROCTOR: Skin is missing.
Student: Does the chest appear symmetric?
PROCTOR: Yes.
Student: Were the previous dressings effective?
PROCTOR: Yes.

▸ **Palpate**

Student: When I touch the chest, do I feel crepitus or a flail segment?
PROCTOR: No.

▸ **Auscultate**

Student: Are lung sounds present in all fields?
PROCTOR: Yes.
Student: Do I hear any sucking sounds from the chest?
PROCTOR: No.

▼ Assess the Abdomen/Pelvis

▸ **Assess the Abdomen**

Student: I am assessing the abdomen for DCAP-BTLS. I am assessing all four quadrants. Do I find any problems?
PROCTOR: Skin is missing.
Student: Were the previous dressings effective?
PROCTOR: Yes.

▸ **Assess the Pelvis**

Student: I am assessing the pelvis for DCAP-BTLS. Is the pelvis stable?
PROCTOR: Yes.

▼ Assess the Genitalia/Perineum as Needed (Verbalize in Training)

Student: I am assessing the genitalia/perineum as necessary for DCAP-BTLS.
PROCTOR: The area is unremarkable.

▼ Assess the Extremities

▸ **Inspect**

Student: I am assessing the lower and upper extremities for DCAP-BTLS. Do I find anything?
PROCTOR: No.

▸ **Palpate**

Student: Do I feel anything unusual?
PROCTOR: No.

▸ **Assess Motor, Sensory, and Circulatory Function**

Student: I am checking for DCAP-BTLS, motor and sensory function, and pulses. Right leg?
PROCTOR: Negative DCAP-BTLS. Motor and sensory functions are absent. Pulses are weak.
Student: Left leg?
PROCTOR: Negative DCAP-BTLS. Motor and sensory functions are absent. Pulses are weak.
Student: Right arm?
PROCTOR: Bleeding is controlled from the missing skin (dressings were applied earlier). Motor and sensory functions are absent. Pulses are weak.
Student: Left arm?
PROCTOR: Bleeding is controlled from the missing skin (dressings were applied earlier). Motor and sensory functions are absent. Pulses are weak.

▼ Assess the Posterior

Note: This portion of the detailed physical exam would not be done if the patient were previously backboarded per local protocol.
Student: We will not check the back because it was previously checked and the patient is backboarded.
PROCTOR: Noted.

▼ Manage Secondary Injuries/Wounds

Student: I would direct my partner to monitor the airway.
PROCTOR: Noted.

▼ Reassess Vital Signs

Student: I will reassess vital signs and mental status.
PROCTOR: Blood pressure, 100/68 mm Hg; pulse rate, 88 beats/min; respirations per bag-valve device; pulse oximetry reading, 93%; and the patient is alert.
Student: The vital signs are deteriorating.
PROCTOR: Noted.

▼ Reassess Interventions

Student: I will reassess my interventions: airway, bag-valve device, oxygen, bleeding control, full immobilization, and treatment for shock.
PROCTOR: Noted.
ALS Student: I will reassess basic life support (BLS) interventions, plus the following: maintain a systolic blood pressure of 90 mm Hg, and cardiac monitoring.
ALS Proctor: Noted. The cardiac monitor shows normal sinus rhythm.

Critical Criteria:
- ❑ Did not find or manage problems associated with airway, breathing, hemorrhage or shock (hypoperfusion)

▼ Radio Report

(Provided by the student.)
PROCTOR: Noted.

▼ Ongoing Assessment

▼ Repeat Vital Signs

Student: I will reassess vital signs and mental status.
PROCTOR: Blood pressure, 90/60 mm Hg; pulse rate, 84 beats/min; respirations per bag-valve device; pulse oximetry reading, 94%; and the patient is alert.
Student: The vital signs have deteriorated.
PROCTOR: Noted.

▼ Check Interventions

Student: I will check my interventions: airway, bag-valve device, oxygen, bleeding control, full immobilization, and treatment for shock.
PROCTOR: Noted.

ALS Student: I will check BLS interventions, plus the following: maintain a systolic blood pressure of 90 mm Hg, and cardiac monitoring.

ALS Proctor: Noted. The cardiac monitor shows normal sinus rhythm

Critical Criteria:
- ❑ Did not find or manage problems associated with airway, breathing, hemorrhage or shock (hypoperfusion)

Handoff Report to Emergency Department Staff

Student: The patient's condition deteriorated during transport.
PROCTOR: Noted.

Critical Criteria:
- ❑ Did not transport patient within the (10) minute time limit

Critical Criteria

(Inform the student of items missed, if any.)

❑ Pass ❑ Fail Date: ____________________

Proctor Comments: ____________________

____

____

CASE 55

Dispatch Information

PROCTOR: EMS 10, respond to a 40-year-old male who has been stabbed in the chest. He is conscious and breathing. Police are responding.

Pre-scene Action (BSI)

Student: I am wearing nonlatex gloves, safety glasses, mask, and gown.
PROCTOR: Noted.

Critical Criteria:
- ❑ Did not take, or verbalize, body substance isolation (BSI) precautions when necessary

Scene Size-up

Scene Safety

Student: Is the scene safe?
PROCTOR: Yes, police are on scene and you are given clearance to enter.

Mechanism of Injury

Student: What was the mechanism of injury?
PROCTOR: Penetrating trauma from a knife. The patient was stabbed by a family member at a family reunion.

Number of Patients

Student: How many patients are there?
PROCTOR: One.

Additional Resources

Student: I would call for advanced life support (ALS) assistance.
PROCTOR: Noted.

C-Spine Stabilization

Student: On the basis of the mechanism of injury, I would stabilize the cervical spine (c-spine) in a neutral in-line position.
PROCTOR: Noted.

Critical Criteria:
- ❑ Did not determine scene safety
- ❑ Did not assess for spinal protection
- ❑ Did not provide for spinal protection when indicated

Initial Assessment

Student: As I perform midline c-spine stabilization, I identify myself and ask the patient not to move.
PROCTOR: Noted.

General Impression

Student: My general impression is that the patient's condition is unstable.
PROCTOR: Noted.

Responsiveness/Level of Consciousness

Student: What is the patient's level of consciousness?
PROCTOR: Alert.

Chief Complaint/Apparent Life Threats

Student: What is the patient's chief complaint?
PROCTOR: The patient is complaining of extreme difficulty breathing.
Student: There are apparent life threats; the life threats are respiratory compromise and shock.
PROCTOR: Noted.

Assess the Airway and Breathing

Student: Is the airway open? Is the patient breathing?
PROCTOR: Yes, the airway is open and the patient is breathing.

▸ Assessment

Student: What are the rate and the quality of breathing?
PROCTOR: Rate: Tachypneic. Quality: Shallow and labored.

▸ Provide Oxygen

Student: I am assisting ventilations with a bag-valve device with 100% oxygen.
PROCTOR: Noted.

▸ Ensure Adequate Ventilation

Student: I am assisting ventilations with a bag-valve device.
PROCTOR: Noted.

Injury Management

Student: I will direct my partner to take over c-spine control and ventilations as I continue assessment.
PROCTOR: Noted.

Assess Circulation

Student: I am assessing the patient's circulation.
PROCTOR: Noted.

▸ Assess for and Control Major Bleeding

Student: Do I find any major bleeding?
PROCTOR: Yes, there is significant bleeding from a stab wound on his upper left chest.
Student: I will apply direct pressure and an occlusive dressing.
PROCTOR: Noted.

▸ Assess the Pulse

Student: What are the rate and the quality of pulses?
PROCTOR: Rate: Tachycardic. Quality: Bounding.

▸ Assess the Skin

Student: I am assessing the skin. What are the color, temperature, and condition of the skin?
PROCTOR: Color: Pale. Temperature: Cool. Condition: Diaphoretic.

Identify Priority Patients/Make Transport Decision

Student: The patient is a high priority and is a load-and-go. I will begin packaging and transport.
PROCTOR: Noted.

Critical Criteria:
- ❑ Did not provide high concentration of oxygen
- ❑ Did not find or manage problems associated with airway, breathing, hemorrhage or shock (hypoperfusion)
- ❑ Did not differentiate patient's need for transportation versus continued assessment at the scene
- ❑ Did other detailed examination before assessing the airway, breathing and circulation

Focused History and Physical Examination/Rapid Trauma Assessment

Select the Appropriate Assessment (Focused or Rapid)

Student: I am selecting the rapid physical exam to identify and treat life threats. I am checking for DCAP-BTLS. This acronym stands for deformities, contusions, abrasions, punctures, penetrations, paradoxical motion in the chest, and burns, tenderness, lacerations, and swelling.
PROCTOR: Noted.

▸ Head

Student: I am rapidly assessing the head.
PROCTOR: There are no obvious injuries.

▸ Neck

Student: I am rapidly assessing the neck.
PROCTOR: You see jugular vein distention (JVD) and tracheal deviation to the right.

Student: I would burp the occlusive dressing per protocol.
PROCTOR: Noted.
Student: I will apply a cervical collar.
PROCTOR: Noted.

▸ Chest

Student: I am rapidly assessing the chest.
PROCTOR: You see a puncture wound to the left upper chest that was treated with an occlusive dressing.
Student: Are the lung sounds clear bilaterally?
PROCTOR: No, they are diminished on the left.
Student: Did burping the occlusive dressing bring the trachea back to midline and relieve the tension?
PROCTOR: No.
Student: I will assess the chest for tension pneumothorax by auscultation and assessment of JVD, tracheal deviation, and decreased lung sounds.
PROCTOR: There are decreased lung sounds on the left side, JVD is present, and the trachea is deviated to the right.
ALS Student: I will assess the chest for hyperresonance to percussion.
ALS Proctor: Noted. There is a tension pneumothorax on the left side.
ALS Student: I will decompress the chest.
ALS Proctor: Noted. The decompression was effective.

▸ Abdomen/Pelvis

Student: I am rapidly assessing the abdomen.
PROCTOR: There are no obvious injuries.
Student: I am rapidly assessing the pelvis.
PROCTOR: There are no obvious injuries.

▸ Extremities

Student: I am rapidly assessing the extremities.
PROCTOR: There are no obvious injuries.

▸ Assess Motor, Sensory, and Circulatory Function

Student: I am checking for DCAP-BTLS, motor and sensory function, and pulses. Right leg?
PROCTOR: Negative DCAP-BTLS. Motor and sensory functions are present. Pulses are present.
Student: Left leg?
PROCTOR: Negative DCAP-BTLS. Motor and sensory functions are present. Pulses are present.
Student: Right arm?
PROCTOR: Negative DCAP-BTLS. Motor and sensory functions are present. Pulses are present.
Student: Left arm?
PROCTOR: Negative DCAP-BTLS. Motor and sensory functions are present. Pulses are present.

▸ Posterior

Student: I will rapidly assess the back. We will now log roll the patient as a unit to check the back. The person at the head will count to three and we will roll the patient.
PROCTOR: Noted.

▸ Assess the Thorax

Student: I am assessing the thorax. Do I find injuries?
PROCTOR: No.

▸ Assess the Lumbar Area

Student: I am assessing the flanks and lumbar area. Do I find injuries?
PROCTOR: No.

▸ Assess the Entire Backside

Student: I am assessing the entire backside. Do I find injuries?
PROCTOR: No.

▸ Manage Secondary Injuries/Wounds

Student: We will apply a cervical collar and backboard with full immobilization per local protocol, if not yet done, at this time.
PROCTOR: Noted.
Student: Are there any changes in motor and sensory functions or pulses?
PROCTOR: No.
ALS Student: I will establish two large-bore IVs and administer a bolus of 20 mL/kg in order to maintain a systolic blood pressure of 90 mm Hg, en route to the hospital.
ALS Proctor: Noted.

▸ Reevaluate Transport Decision

Student: This patient is a high priority and a load-and-go due to chest trauma, the mechanism of injury, and shock.
PROCTOR: Noted.

▼ Baseline Vital Signs

Student: What are the patient's baseline vital signs, including blood pressure, pulse, respirations, pulse oximetry, and level of consciousness?
PROCTOR: Blood pressure, 90/60 mm Hg; pulse rate, 130 beats/min; respirations per bag-valve device; pulse oximetry reading, 91%; and the patient is anxious.

▼ SAMPLE History

Student: At this time I will gather a SAMPLE history from the patient or family. What are the patient's signs and symptoms?
PROCTOR: Pain in the chest and difficulty breathing.
Student: Allergies?
PROCTOR: No allergies.
Student: Medications?
PROCTOR: Seizure medications.
Student: Pertinent past medical history?
PROCTOR: Seizures.
Student: Last oral intake?
PROCTOR: 1 hour ago.
Student: Events leading up to the incident?
PROCTOR: The patient was at a family reunion when a family member he had not seen in 10 years stabbed him in the chest.

Critical Criteria:
- ❑ Did not differentiate patient's need for transportation versus continued assessment at the scene
- ❑ Did not provide for spinal protection when indicated

▼ Detailed Physical Examination

Student: I am conducting the detailed physical exam. I am looking for DCAP-BTLS.
PROCTOR: Noted. The detailed physical exam will be performed during transport.

▼ Assess the Head

Student: I am assessing the head. Do I find any DCAP-BTLS? Do I find any evidence of Battle's sign or raccoon eyes?
PROCTOR: No.

▸ Inspect and Palpate the Head and Ears

Student: I am assessing the head and ears.
PROCTOR: There are no obvious injuries.

▸ Assess the Eyes

Student: I am assessing the eyes. Are the pupils equal, round, and regular in size, and react properly to light (PEARRL)?
PROCTOR: They are sluggish.

▸ **Assess the Facial Area Including Oral and Nasal Areas**

Student: I am assessing the face, nose, and mouth. Do I see any discharge or hear any obstructions?

PROCTOR: No.

Student: I will suction and maintain the airway if needed.

PROCTOR: Noted.

▾ Assess the Neck

▸ **Inspect and Palpate the Neck**

Student: I am assessing the neck for DCAP-BTLS.

PROCTOR: There are no obvious injuries.

▸ **Assess for Jugular Vein Distention**

Student: Do I find any jugular vein distention (JVD)?

PROCTOR: Yes. (No, if the chest was decompressed.)

▸ **Assess for Tracheal Deviation**

Student: Do I see any tracheal deviation?

PROCTOR: Yes. (No, if the chest was decompressed.)

▾ Assess the Chest

Student: I am assessing the chest for DCAP-BTLS.

PROCTOR: Noted.

▸ **Inspect**

Student: What do I see when I look at the chest?

PROCTOR: You see a puncture wound to the left chest.

Student: Does the chest appear symmetric?

PROCTOR: Yes.

▸ **Palpate**

Student: When I touch the chest, do I feel crepitus or a flail segment?

PROCTOR: No.

▸ **Auscultate**

Student: Are lung sounds present in all fields?

PROCTOR: Yes, but they are decreased on the left if the chest was not decompressed.

Student: Do I hear any sucking sounds from the chest?

PROCTOR: No. The wound has been treated with an occlusive dressing.

▾ Assess the Abdomen/Pelvis

▸ **Assess the Abdomen**

Student: I am assessing the abdomen for DCAP-BTLS. I am assessing all four quadrants. Do I find any problems?

PROCTOR: No.

▸ **Assess the Pelvis**

Student: I am assessing the pelvis for DCAP-BTLS. Is the pelvis stable?

PROCTOR: Yes.

▾ Assess the Genitalia/Perineum as Needed (Verbalize in Training)

Student: I am assessing the genitalia/perineum as necessary for DCAP-BTLS.

PROCTOR: The area is unremarkable.

▾ Assess the Extremities

▸ **Inspect**

Student: I am assessing the lower and upper extremities for DCAP-BTLS. Do I find anything?

PROCTOR: No.

▸ **Palpate**

Student: Do I feel anything unusual?

PROCTOR: No.

▸ **Assess Motor, Sensory, and Circulatory Function**

Student: I am checking for DCAP-BTLS, motor and sensory function, and pulses. Right leg?

PROCTOR: Negative DCAP-BTLS. Motor and sensory functions are present. Pulses are present.

Student: Left leg?

PROCTOR: Negative DCAP-BTLS. Motor and sensory functions are present. Pulses are present.

Student: Right arm?

PROCTOR: Negative DCAP-BTLS. Motor and sensory functions are present. Pulses are present.

Student: Left arm?

PROCTOR: Negative DCAP-BTLS. Motor and sensory functions are present. Pulses are present.

▾ Assess the Posterior

Note: This portion of the detailed physical exam would not be done if the patient were previously backboarded per local protocol.

Student: We will not check the back because it was previously checked and the patient is backboarded.

PROCTOR: Noted.

▾ Manage Secondary Injuries/Wounds

Student: I would direct my partner to monitor and maintain the airway and chest dressing.

PROCTOR: Noted.

▾ Reassess Vital Signs

Student: I will reassess vital signs and mental status.

PROCTOR: Blood pressure, 90 mm Hg by palpation; pulse rate, 132 beats/min; respirations per bag-valve device; pulse oximetry reading, 89%; and the patient is anxious.

Student: The vital signs are deteriorating.

PROCTOR: Noted.

▾ Reassess Interventions

Student: I will reassess my interventions: airway, breathing, bag-valve device, oxygen, and suctioning; maintain occlusive dressing; immobilization and straps; and treatment for shock.

PROCTOR: Noted.

ALS Student: I will reassess basic life support (BLS) interventions, plus the following: two large-bore IVs en route to the hospital, administer a bolus of 20 mL/kg to maintain a systolic blood pressure of 90 mm Hg, perform cardiac monitoring, monitor chest decompression (or rapid sequence intubation [RSI] depending on local protocol).

ALS Proctor: Noted. The cardiac monitor shows sinus tachycardia.

Critical Criteria:

- ❑ Did not find or manage problems associated with airway, breathing, hemorrhage or shock (hypoperfusion)

Radio Report

(Provided by the student.)

PROCTOR: Noted.

Ongoing Assessment

▾ Repeat Vital Signs

Student: I will reassess vital signs and mental status.

PROCTOR: Blood pressure, 100 mm Hg by palpation; pulse rate, 124 beats/min; respirations per bag-valve device; pulse oximetry reading, 88%; and the patient is anxious.

Student: The vital signs have deteriorated.

PROCTOR: Noted.

▾ Check Interventions

Student: I will check interventions: airway, breathing, bag-valve device, oxygen, and suctioning; maintain occlusive dressing; immobilization and straps; and treatment for shock.

PROCTOR: Noted.

ALS Student: I will check BLS interventions, plus the following: maintain a systolic blood pressure of 90 mm Hg, perform cardiac monitoring, monitor chest decompression, and consider RSI depending on local protocol.

ALS Proctor: Noted. The cardiac monitor shows sinus tachycardia.

Critical Criteria:
- ❑ Did not find or manage problems associated with airway, breathing, hemorrhage or shock (hypoperfusion)

Handoff Report to Emergency Department Staff

Student: The patient's condition deteriorated during transport.
PROCTOR: Noted.

Critical Criteria:
- ❑ Did not transport patient within the (10) minute time limit

Critical Criteria

(Inform the student of items missed, if any.)

❑ Pass ❑ Fail Date: ____________________

Proctor Comments: ____________________

____

____

CASE 56

Dispatch Information

PROCTOR: EMS 10, respond to a 60-year-old male who was cleaning his gun when it went off. He is conscious and breathing. Police are en route.

Pre-scene Action (BSI)

Student: I am wearing nonlatex gloves, safety glasses, mask, and gown.
PROCTOR: Noted.

Critical Criteria:
- ❑ Did not take, or verbalize, body substance isolation (BSI) precautions when necessary

Scene Size-up

Scene Safety

Student: Is the scene safe?
PROCTOR: Yes, police are on scene and you are given clearance to enter.

Mechanism of Injury

Student: What was the mechanism of injury?
PROCTOR: Gunshot wound. The patient was cleaning his gun when it went off.

Number of Patients

Student: How many patients are there?
PROCTOR: One.

Additional Resources

Student: I would call for advanced life support (ALS) assistance.
PROCTOR: Noted.

C-Spine Stabilization

Student: On the basis of the mechanism of injury, I would stabilize the cervical spine (c-spine) in a neutral in-line position.
PROCTOR: Noted.

Critical Criteria:
- ❑ Did not determine scene safety
- ❑ Did not assess for spinal protection
- ❑ Did not provide for spinal protection when indicated

Initial Assessment

Student: As I perform midline c-spine stabilization, I identify myself and ask the patient not to move.
PROCTOR: Noted.

General Impression

Student: My general impression is that the patient's condition is stable.
PROCTOR: Noted.

Responsiveness/Level of Consciousness

Student: What is the patient's level of consciousness?
PROCTOR: Alert.

Chief Complaint/Apparent Life Threats

Student: What is the patient's chief complaint?
PROCTOR: The patient is complaining of gunshot wounds and pain to his left hand, right leg, and right foot. He says he accidentally shot himself.
Student: There are no apparent life threats.
PROCTOR: Noted.

Assess the Airway and Breathing

Student: Is the airway open? Is the patient breathing?
PROCTOR: Yes, the airway is open and the patient is breathing.

▸ Assessment

Student: What are the rate and the quality of breathing?
PROCTOR: Rate: Within normal limits. Quality: Normal.

▸ Provide Oxygen

Student: I am applying oxygen at 15 L/min via nonrebreathing mask.
PROCTOR: Noted.

▸ Ensure Adequate Ventilation

Student: The patient has adequate ventilations at this time.
PROCTOR: Noted.

Injury Management

Student: I will direct my partner to take over c-spine control as I continue assessment.
PROCTOR: Noted.

Assess Circulation

Student: I am assessing the patient's circulation.
PROCTOR: Noted.

▸ Assess for and Control Major Bleeding

Student: Do I find any major bleeding?
PROCTOR: Yes, his left thumb is missing.
Student: I would apply direct pressure and a dressing.
PROCTOR: Noted.

▸ Assess the Pulse

Student: What are the rate and the quality of pulses?
PROCTOR: Rate: Within normal limits. Quality: Normal.

▸ Assess the Skin

Student: I am assessing the skin. What are the color, temperature, and condition of the skin?
PROCTOR: Color: Normal. Temperature: Normal. Condition: Normal.

Identify Priority Patients/Make Transport Decision

Student: The patient is a high priority due to hand involvement and should be transported immediately to the appropriate facility.
PROCTOR: Noted.

Critical Criteria:
- ❑ Did not provide high concentration of oxygen
- ❑ Did not find or manage problems associated with airway, breathing, hemorrhage or shock (hypoperfusion)
- ❑ Did not differentiate patient's need for transportation versus continued assessment at the scene
- ❑ Did other detailed examination before assessing the airway, breathing and circulation

Focused History and Physical Examination/Rapid Trauma Assessment

Select the Appropriate Assessment (Focused or Rapid)

Student: I am selecting the rapid physical exam to identify and treat life threats. I am checking for DCAP-BTLS. This acronym stands for deformities, contusions, abrasions, punctures, penetrations, paradoxical motion in the chest, and burns, tenderness, lacerations, and swelling.
PROCTOR: Noted.

▸ Head

Student: I am rapidly assessing the head.
PROCTOR: There are no obvious injuries.

▸ Neck

Student: I am rapidly assessing the neck.
PROCTOR: There are no obvious injuries.
Student: I will apply a cervical collar.
PROCTOR: Noted.

▸ Chest

Student: I am rapidly assessing the chest.
PROCTOR: There are no obvious injuries.

▸ Abdomen/Pelvis

Student: I am rapidly assessing the abdomen.
PROCTOR: There are no obvious injuries.

Student: I am rapidly assessing the pelvis.
PROCTOR: There are no obvious injuries.

▸ **Extremities**

Student: I am rapidly assessing the extremities.
PROCTOR: The left thumb is missing. There is a through-and-through injury to the right leg and an entrance in the top of the right foot.
Student: I will quickly attempt to recover the thumb and package it per local protocol.
PROCTOR: Noted.

▸ **Assess Motor, Sensory, and Circulatory Function**

Student: I am checking for DCAP-BTLS, motor and sensory function, and pulses. Right leg?
PROCTOR: Wounds to the medial flesh with an entrance and exit. Bleeding is minimal. There is an entrance wound to the top of the foot. Motor and sensory functions are present. Pulses are present.
Student: I will dress the injuries to the leg and foot with pressure dressings and splints.
PROCTOR: Noted.
Student: Left leg?
PROCTOR: Negative DCAP-BTLS. Motor and sensory functions are present. Pulses are present.
Student: Right arm?
PROCTOR: Negative DCAP-BTLS. Motor and sensory functions are present. Pulses are present.
Student: Left arm?
PROCTOR: The thumb is missing; the hand has been dressed. Motor and sensory functions are present. Pulses are present.

▸ **Posterior**

Student: I will rapidly assess the back. We will now log roll the patient as a unit to check the back. The person at the head will count to three and we will roll the patient.
PROCTOR: Noted.

▸ **Assess the Thorax**

Student: I am assessing the thorax. Do I find injuries?
PROCTOR: No.

▸ **Assess the Lumbar Area**

Student: I am assessing the flanks and lumbar area. Do I find injuries?
PROCTOR: No.

▸ **Assess the Entire Backside**

Student: I am assessing the entire backside. Do I find injuries?
PROCTOR: No.

▸ **Manage Secondary Injuries/Wounds**

Student: We will apply a cervical collar and backboard with full immobilization per local protocol, if not yet done, at this time.
PROCTOR: Noted.
Student: Are there any changes in motor and sensory functions or pulses?
PROCTOR: No.
ALS Student: I will establish two large-bore IVs en route to the hospital, cardiac monitoring, and pain management per local protocol.
ALS Proctor: Noted. The cardiac monitor shows normal sinus rhythm.

▸ **Reevaluate Transport Decision**

Student: The patient is a high priority due to hand involvement and should be transported immediately to the appropriate facility.
PROCTOR: Noted.

▾ Baseline Vital Signs

Student: What are the patient's baseline vital signs, including blood pressure, pulse, respirations, pulse oximetry, and level of consciousness?
PROCTOR: Blood pressure, 150/88 mm Hg; pulse rate, 98 beats/min; respirations, 16 breaths/min; pulse oximetry reading, 97%; and the patient is alert.

▾ SAMPLE History

Student: At this time I will gather a SAMPLE history from the patient or family. What are the patient's signs and symptoms?
PROCTOR: Pain in the thumb, leg, and foot.
Student: Allergies?
PROCTOR: Penicillin (PCN).
Student: Medications?
PROCTOR: Water pills.
Student: Pertinent past medical history?
PROCTOR: Heart problems.
Student: Last oral intake?
PROCTOR: 2 hours ago.
Student: Events leading up to the incident?
PROCTOR: The patient was cleaning a loaded gun when it fired. All wounds found are from the same bullet.
Student: Interventions?
PROCTOR: He wrapped the hand in an old T-shirt and has the thumb in a plastic bag.
Student: I would package and transport the thumb per local protocol.
PROCTOR: Noted.

Critical Criteria:

- ❑ Did not differentiate patient's need for transportation versus continued assessment at the scene
- ❑ Did not provide for spinal protection when indicated

▼ Detailed Physical Examination

Student: I am conducting the detailed physical exam. I am looking for DCAP-BTLS.
PROCTOR: Noted. The detailed physical exam will be performed during transport.

▾ Assess the Head

Student: I am assessing the head. Do I find any DCAP-BTLS? Do I find any evidence of Battle's sign or raccoon eyes?
PROCTOR: No.

▸ **Inspect and Palpate the Head and Ears**

Student: I am assessing the head and ears.
PROCTOR: There are no obvious injuries.

▸ **Assess the Eyes**

Student: I am assessing the eyes. Are the pupils equal, round, and regular in size, and react properly to light (PEARRL)?
PROCTOR: They are PEARRL.

▸ **Assess the Facial Area Including Oral and Nasal Areas**

Student: I am assessing the face, nose, and mouth. Do I see any discharge or hear any obstructions?
PROCTOR: No.

▾ Assess the Neck

▸ **Inspect and Palpate the Neck**

Student: I am assessing the neck for DCAP-BTLS.
PROCTOR: There are no obvious injuries.

▸ **Assess for Jugular Vein Distention**

Student: Do I find any jugular vein distention (JVD)?
PROCTOR: No.

▸ **Assess for Tracheal Deviation**

Student: Do I see any tracheal deviation?
PROCTOR: No.

▾ Assess the Chest

Student: I am assessing the chest for DCAP-BTLS.
PROCTOR: Noted.

▸ **Inspect**

Student: What do I see when I look at the chest?
PROCTOR: There are no obvious injuries.
Student: Does the chest appear symmetric?
PROCTOR: Yes.

▸ Palpate

Student: When I touch the chest, do I feel crepitus or a flail segment?

PROCTOR: No.

▸ Auscultate

Student: Are lung sounds present in all fields?

PROCTOR: Yes.

Student: Do I hear any sucking sounds from the chest?

PROCTOR: No.

▾ **Assess the Abdomen/Pelvis**

▸ Assess the Abdomen

Student: I am assessing the abdomen for DCAP-BTLS. I am assessing all four quadrants. Do I find any problems?

PROCTOR: No.

▸ Assess the Pelvis

Student: I am assessing the pelvis for DCAP-BTLS. Is the pelvis stable?

PROCTOR: Yes.

▾ **Assess the Genitalia/Perineum as Needed (Verbalize in Training)**

Student: I am assessing the genitalia/perineum as necessary for DCAP-BTLS.

PROCTOR: The area is unremarkable.

▾ **Assess the Extremities**

▸ Inspect

Student: I am assessing the lower and upper extremities for DCAP-BTLS. Do I find anything?

PROCTOR: Yes. The left thumb is missing. There is a through-and-through injury to the right leg and an entrance in the top of the right foot, which have all been effectively treated.

▸ Palpate

Student: Do I feel anything unusual?

PROCTOR: No.

▸ Assess Motor, Sensory, and Circulatory Function

Student: I am checking for DCAP-BTLS, motor and sensory function, and pulses. Right leg?

PROCTOR: Wounds to the medial flesh with an entrance and exit. Bleeding is minimal. There is an entrance wound to the top of the foot. Motor and sensory functions are present. Pulses are present. These were treated with dressings and splints.

Student: Left leg?

PROCTOR: Negative DCAP-BTLS. Motor and sensory functions are present. Pulses are present.

Student: Right arm?

PROCTOR: Negative DCAP-BTLS. Motor and sensory functions are present. Pulses are present.

Student: Left arm?

PROCTOR: The thumb is missing. Motor and sensory functions are present. Pulses are present.

▾ **Assess the Posterior**

Note: This portion of the detailed physical exam would not be done if the patient were previously backboarded per local protocol.

Student: We will not check the back because it was previously checked and the patient is backboarded.

PROCTOR: Noted.

▾ **Manage Secondary Injuries/Wounds**

Student: We will monitor blood loss and treat for shock.

PROCTOR: Noted.

▾ **Reassess Vital Signs**

Student: I will reassess vital signs and mental status.

PROCTOR: Blood pressure, 140/78 mm Hg; pulse rate, 88 beats/min; respirations, 16 breaths/min; pulse oximetry reading, 98%; and the patient is alert.

Student: The vital signs are improving.

PROCTOR: Noted.

▾ **Reassess Interventions**

Student: I will reassess my interventions: airway, breathing, and oxygen; circulation and bleeding control; splints, immobilization, and straps; and treatment for shock.

PROCTOR: Noted.

ALS Student: I will reassess basic life support (BLS) interventions, plus the following: two large-bore IVs, cardiac monitoring, and pain management per local protocol.

ALS Proctor: Noted. The cardiac monitor shows normal sinus rhythm.

Critical Criteria:

❑ Did not find or manage problems associated with airway, breathing, hemorrhage or shock (hypoperfusion)

Radio Report

(Provided by the student.)

PROCTOR: Noted.

Ongoing Assessment

▾ **Repeat Vital Signs**

Student: I will reassess vital signs and mental status.

PROCTOR: Blood pressure, 136/76 mm Hg; pulse rate, 84 beats/min; respirations, 16 breaths/min; pulse oximetry reading, 98%; and the patient is alert.

Student: The vital signs have improved.

PROCTOR: Noted.

▾ **Check Interventions**

Student: I will check my interventions: airway, breathing, and oxygen; circulation and bleeding control; splints, immobilization, and straps; and treatment for shock.

PROCTOR: Noted.

ALS Student: I will check BLS interventions, plus the following: two large-bore IVs, cardiac monitor, and pain management per local protocol.

ALS Proctor: Noted. The cardiac monitor shows normal sinus rhythm.

Critical Criteria:

❑ Did not find or manage problems associated with airway, breathing, hemorrhage or shock (hypoperfusion)

Handoff Report to Emergency Department Staff

Student: The patient's condition improved during transport.

PROCTOR: Noted.

Critical Criteria:

❑ Did not transport patient within the (10) minute time limit

Critical Criteria

(Inform the student of items missed, if any.)

❑ Pass ❑ Fail Date: ____________________

Proctor Comments: ____________________

____

____

CASE 56

Notes

CASE 57

Dispatch Information

PROCTOR: EMS 10, respond to an 81-year-old male who has fallen down the basement stairs. He is conscious and breathing.

Pre-scene Action (BSI)

Student: I am wearing nonlatex gloves and safety glasses.
PROCTOR: Noted.

Critical Criteria:
- ❑ Did not take, or verbalize, body substance isolation (BSI) precautions when necessary

Scene Size-up

Scene Safety

Student: Is the scene safe?
PROCTOR: Yes.

Mechanism of Injury

Student: What was the mechanism of injury?
PROCTOR: Fall. The patient tripped and fell down the basement stairs. He has a head injury.

Number of Patients

Student: How many patients are there?
PROCTOR: One.

Additional Resources

Student: I would call for advanced life support (ALS) assistance and additional resources: fire/rescue.
PROCTOR: Noted.

C-Spine Stabilization

Student: On the basis of the mechanism of injury, I would stabilize the cervical spine (c-spine) in a neutral in-line position.
PROCTOR: Noted.

Critical Criteria:
- ❑ Did not determine scene safety
- ❑ Did not assess for spinal protection
- ❑ Did not provide for spinal protection when indicated

Initial Assessment

Student: As I perform midline c-spine stabilization, I identify myself and ask the patient not to move.
PROCTOR: Noted.

General Impression

Student: My general impression is that the patient's condition is unstable.
PROCTOR: Noted.

Responsiveness/Level of Consciousness

Student: What is the patient's level of consciousness?
PROCTOR: Unresponsive. He was conscious per dispatch but is now unresponsive.

Chief Complaint/Apparent Life Threats

Student: What is the patient's chief complaint?
PROCTOR: The patient is unresponsive.
Student: There are apparent life threats; the life threats are the head injury and the mechanism of injury.
PROCTOR: Noted.

Assess the Airway and Breathing

Student: I am opening the airway using the jaw-thrust maneuver. Is the patient breathing?
PROCTOR: Yes.

Assessment

Student: What are the rate and the quality of breathing?
PROCTOR: Rate: Occasional. Quality: Shallow.

Provide Oxygen

Student: I am assisting ventilations with a bag-valve device with 100% oxygen and inserting an oral airway or an advanced airway.
PROCTOR: Noted.

Ensure Adequate Ventilation

Student: I am assisting ventilation with the bag-valve device.
PROCTOR: Noted.

Injury Management

Student: I will direct my partner to take over c-spine control and hyperventilate the patient per local head injury protocol as I continue assessment.
PROCTOR: Noted.

Assess Circulation

Student: I am assessing the patient's circulation.
PROCTOR: Noted.

Assess for and Control Major Bleeding

Student: Do I find any major bleeding?
PROCTOR: No.

Assess the Pulse

Student: What are the rate and the quality of pulses?
PROCTOR: Rate: Within normal limits. Quality: Bounding.

Assess the Skin

Student: I am assessing the skin. What are the color, temperature, and condition of the skin?
PROCTOR: Color: Flushed. Temperature: Warm. Condition: Dry.

Identify Priority Patients/Make Transport Decision

Student: The patient is a high priority and is a load-and-go. I will begin packaging and transport.
PROCTOR: Noted.

Critical Criteria:
- ❑ Did not provide high concentration of oxygen
- ❑ Did not find or manage problems associated with airway, breathing, hemorrhage or shock (hypoperfusion)
- ❑ Did not differentiate patient's need for transportation versus continued assessment at the scene
- ❑ Did other detailed examination before assessing the airway, breathing and circulation

Focused History and Physical Examination/Rapid Trauma Assessment

Select the Appropriate Assessment (Focused or Rapid)

Student: I am selecting the rapid physical exam to identify and treat life threats. I am checking for DCAP-BTLS. This acronym stands for deformities, contusions, abrasions, punctures, penetrations, paradoxical motion in the chest, and burns, tenderness, lacerations, and swelling.
PROCTOR: Noted.

Head

Student: I am rapidly assessing the head.
PROCTOR: There is bruising to the forehead.
Student: I am assessing the eyes. Are the pupils equal, round, and regular in size, and react properly to light (PEARRL)?
PROCTOR: They are equal and nonreactive.

Neck

Student: I am rapidly assessing the neck.
PROCTOR: There are no obvious injuries.
Student: I will apply a cervical collar.
PROCTOR: Noted.

Chest

Student: I am rapidly assessing the chest.
PROCTOR: There are no obvious injuries.
Student: Are lung sounds present in all fields?
PROCTOR: Yes, they are clear bilaterally.

▸ **Abdomen/Pelvis**

Student: I am rapidly assessing the abdomen.
PROCTOR: There are no obvious injuries.
Student: I am rapidly assessing the pelvis.
PROCTOR: There are no obvious injuries.

▸ **Extremities**

Student: I am rapidly assessing the extremities.
PROCTOR: There are skin tears and bruises.

▸ **Assess Motor, Sensory, and Circulatory Function**

Student: I am checking for DCAP-BTLS, motor and sensory function, and pulses. Right leg?
PROCTOR: Negative DCAP-BTLS. Motor and sensory functions are absent. Pulses are present.
Student: Left leg?
PROCTOR: Negative DCAP-BTLS. Motor and sensory functions are absent. Pulses are present.
Student: Right arm?
PROCTOR: Open skin tears (minor). Motor and sensory functions are absent. Pulses are present.
Student: Left arm?
PROCTOR: Open skin tears (minor). Motor and sensory functions are absent. Pulses are present.

▸ **Posterior**

Student: I will rapidly assess the back. We will now log roll the patient as a unit to check the back. The person at the head will count to three and we will roll the patient.
PROCTOR: Noted.

▸ **Assess the Thorax**

Student: I am assessing the thorax. Do I find injuries?
PROCTOR: No.

▸ **Assess the Lumbar Area**

Student: I am assessing the flanks and lumbar area. Do I find injuries?
PROCTOR: No.

▸ **Assess the Entire Backside**

Student: I am assessing the entire backside. Do I find injuries?
PROCTOR: No.

▸ **Manage Secondary Injuries/Wounds**

Student: We will apply a cervical collar and backboard with full immobilization per local protocol, if not yet done, at this time. We will also manage the airway.
PROCTOR: Noted.
Student: Are there any changes in motor and sensory functions or pulses?
PROCTOR: No.
ALS Student: I will intubate and confirm end tidal CO_2 and lung sounds.
ALS Proctor: Noted. End tidal CO_2 and lung sounds confirm placement of the endotrachael (ET) tube.

▸ **Reevaluate Transport Decision**

Student: This patient is a load-and-go due to head trauma.
PROCTOR: Noted.

▾ Baseline Vital Signs

Student: What are the patient's baseline vital signs, including blood pressure, pulse, respirations, pulse oximetry, blood glucose level, and level of consciousness?
PROCTOR: Blood pressure, 170/80 mm Hg; pulse rate, 60 beats/min; respirations, per bag-valve device; pulse oximetry reading, 96%; blood glucose level, 112 mg/dL; and the patient is unresponsive.

▾ SAMPLE History

Student: At this time I will gather a SAMPLE history from the patient or family. What are the patient's signs and symptoms?
PROCTOR: The patient is unresponsive.
Student: Allergies?
PROCTOR: Bee stings.
Student: Medications?
PROCTOR: EpiPen.
Student: Pertinent past medical history?
PROCTOR: Arthritis.
Student: Last oral intake?
PROCTOR: 2 hours ago.
Student: Events leading up to the incident?
PROCTOR: The patient tripped and fell down the stairs, landing on his head.

Critical Criteria:
- ❑ Did not differentiate patient's need for transportation versus continued assessment at the scene
- ❑ Did not provide for spinal protection when indicated

Detailed Physical Examination

Student: I am conducting the detailed physical exam. I am looking for DCAP-BTLS.
PROCTOR: Noted. The detailed physical exam will be performed during transport.

▾ Assess the Head

Student: I am assessing the head. Do I find any DCAP-BTLS? Do I find any evidence of Battle's sign or raccoon eyes?
PROCTOR: Yes, Battle's sign is present.

▸ **Inspect and Palpate the Head and Ears**

Student: I am assessing the head and ears.
PROCTOR: There are no obvious injuries.

▸ **Assess the Eyes**

Student: I am assessing the eyes. Are the eyes PEARRL?
PROCTOR: They are equal and nonreactive.

▸ **Assess the Facial Area Including Oral and Nasal Areas**

Student: I am assessing the face, nose, and mouth. Do I see any discharge or hear any obstructions?
PROCTOR: Yes, the patient begins to projectile vomit.
Student: I will suction the airway. If the patient is intubated, I will suction the mouth.
PROCTOR: Noted.

▾ Assess the Neck

▸ **Inspect and Palpate the Neck**

Student: I am assessing the neck for DCAP-BTLS.
PROCTOR: There are no obvious injuries.

▸ **Assess for Jugular Vein Distention**

Student: Do I find any jugular vein distention (JVD)?
PROCTOR: Yes.

▸ **Assess for Tracheal Deviation**

Student: Do I see any tracheal deviation?
PROCTOR: No.

▾ Assess the Chest

Student: I am assessing the chest for DCAP-BTLS.
PROCTOR: Noted.

▸ **Inspect**

Student: What do I see when I look at the chest?
PROCTOR: There are no obvious injuries.
Student: Does the chest appear symmetric?
PROCTOR: Yes.

▸ **Palpate**

Student: When I touch the chest, do I feel crepitus or a flail segment?
PROCTOR: No.

▸ **Auscultate**

Student: Are lung sounds present in all fields?
PROCTOR: Yes.
Student: Do I hear any sucking sounds from the chest?
PROCTOR: No.

▼ **Assess the Abdomen/Pelvis**

▸ **Assess the Abdomen**

Student: I am assessing the abdomen for DCAP-BTLS. I am assessing all four quadrants. Do I find any problems?

PROCTOR: No.

▸ **Assess the Pelvis**

Student: I am assessing the pelvis for DCAP-BTLS. Is the pelvis stable?

PROCTOR: Yes.

▸ **Assess the Genitalia/Perineum as Needed (Verbalize in Training)**

Student: I am assessing the genitalia/perineum as necessary for DCAP-BTLS.

PROCTOR: The area is unremarkable.

▼ **Assess the Extremities**

▸ **Inspect**

Student: I am assessing the lower and upper extremities for DCAP-BTLS. Do I find anything?

PROCTOR: Yes, there are minor skin tears to both arms.

▸ **Palpate**

Student: Do I feel anything unusual?

PROCTOR: No.

▸ **Assess Motor, Sensory, and Circulatory Function**

Student: I am checking for DCAP-BTLS, motor and sensory function, and pulses. Right leg?

PROCTOR: Negative DCAP-BTLS. Motor and sensory functions are absent. Pulses are present.

Student: Left leg?

PROCTOR: Negative DCAP-BTLS. Motor and sensory functions are absent. Pulses are present.

Student: Right arm?

PROCTOR: Open skin tears (minor). Motor and sensory functions are absent. Pulses are present.

Student: Left arm?

PROCTOR: Open skin tears (minor). Motor and sensory functions are absent. Pulses are present.

▼ **Assess the Posterior**

Note: This portion of the detailed physical exam would not be done if the patient were previously backboarded per local protocol.

Student: We will not check the back because it was previously checked and the patient is backboarded.

PROCTOR: Noted.

▼ **Manage Secondary Injuries/Wounds**

Student: I would direct my partner to maintain the airway.

PROCTOR: Noted.

▼ **Reassess Vital Signs**

Student: I will reassess vital signs and mental status.

PROCTOR: Blood pressure, 166/84 mm Hg; pulse rate, 58 beats/min; respirations, per bag-valve device; pulse oximetry reading, 98%; and the patient is unresponsive.

Student: The vital signs have not changed significantly.

PROCTOR: Noted.

▼ **Reassess Interventions**

Student: I will reassess my interventions: maintain the airway, suction as necessary, bag-valve device, and oxygen; oral airway/advanced airway; bleeding control; blood glucose level monitoring; head injury treatment per local protocol; and full immobilization.

PROCTOR: Noted. The blood glucose level is 112 mg/dL.

ALS Student: I will reassess basic life support (BLS) interventions, plus the following: intubation, confirm end tidal CO_2 and lung sounds, IVs, cardiac monitoring, and local protocol.

ALS Proctor: Noted. The cardiac monitor shows sinus bradycardia. End tidal CO_2 and lung sounds confirm ET tube placement.

Critical Criteria:

❑ Did not find or manage problems associated with airway, breathing, hemorrhage or shock (hypoperfusion)

Radio Report

(Provided by the student.)

PROCTOR: Noted.

Ongoing Assessment

▼ **Repeat Vital Signs**

Student: I will reassess vital signs and mental status.

PROCTOR: Blood pressure, 170/80 mm Hg; pulse, 56 beats/min; respirations, per bag-valve device; pulse oximetry reading, N/A; and the patient is unresponsive.

Student: The vital signs have not changed significantly.

PROCTOR: Noted.

▼ **Check Interventions**

Student: I will check my interventions: maintain the airway, suction as necessary, bag-valve device, and oxygen; oral airway/advanced airway; bleeding control; blood glucose level monitoring; head injury treatment per local protocol; and full immobilization.

PROCTOR: Noted. The blood glucose level is 112 mg/dL.

ALS Student: I will check BLS interventions, plus the following: intubation, confirm end tidal CO_2 and lung sounds, IVs, cardiac monitoring, and local protocol.

ALS Proctor: Noted. The cardiac monitor shows sinus bradycardia. End tidal CO_2 and lung sounds confirm ET tube placement.

Critical Criteria:

❑ Did not find or manage problems associated with airway, breathing, hemorrhage or shock (hypoperfusion)

Handoff Report to Emergency Department Staff

Student: There was no change in the patient's condition during transport.

PROCTOR: Noted.

Critical Criteria:

❑ Did not transport patient within the (10) minute time limit

Critical Criteria

(Inform the student of items missed, if any.)

❑ Pass ❑ Fail Date: ______________________

Proctor Comments: ______________________

____

____

Notes

Dispatch Information

PROCTOR: EMS 10, respond to a one-vehicle rollover on the interstate. The 19-year-old male driver has been ejected. It is not known if he is conscious or breathing.

Pre-scene Action (BSI)

Student: I am wearing appropriate high-visibility personal protective equipment suitable for extrication, a helmet, extrication gloves, nonlatex gloves, safety glasses, and a mask.

PROCTOR: Noted.

Critical Criteria:

- ❑ Did not take, or verbalize, body substance isolation (BSI) precautions when necessary

Scene Size-up

Scene Safety

Student: Is the scene safe?

PROCTOR: Yes.

Mechanism of Injury

Student: What was the mechanism of injury?

PROCTOR: Motor vehicle collision. The patient was street racing a small pickup truck when he lost control and rolled the truck. He was unrestrained in the cab and was ejected onto the street.

Number of Patients

Student: How many patients are there?

PROCTOR: One.

Additional Resources

Student: I would call for advanced life support (ALS) assistance and additional resources: fire/rescue.

PROCTOR: Noted.

C-Spine Stabilization

Student: On the basis of the mechanism of injury, I would stabilize the cervical spine (c-spine) in a neutral in-line position.

PROCTOR: Noted.

Critical Criteria:

- ❑ Did not determine scene safety
- ❑ Did not assess for spinal protection
- ❑ Did not provide for spinal protection when indicated

Initial Assessment

Student: As I perform midline c-spine stabilization, I identify myself and ask the patient not to move.

PROCTOR: Noted.

General Impression

Student: My general impression is that the patient's condition is unstable.

PROCTOR: Noted.

Responsiveness/Level of Consciousness

Student: What is the patient's level of consciousness?

PROCTOR: Conscious and alert.

Chief Complaint/Apparent Life Threats

Student: What is the patient's chief complaint?

PROCTOR: The patient is complaining of difficulty breathing and is in obvious distress.

Student: There are apparent life threats; the life threats are the mechanism of injury and the respiratory compromise.

PROCTOR: Noted.

Assess the Airway and Breathing

Student: Is the airway open? Is the patient breathing?

PROCTOR: Yes, the airway is open and the patient is breathing.

Assessment

Student: What are the rate and the quality of breathing?

PROCTOR: Rate: Bradypneic. Quality: Shallow.

Provide Oxygen

Student: I am assisting ventilations with a bag-valve device with 100% oxygen.

PROCTOR: Noted.

Ensure Adequate Ventilation

Student: As noted, I am assisting ventilation with a bag-valve device.

PROCTOR: Noted.

Injury Management

Student: I will direct my partner to take over c-spine control and ventilations as I continue assessment.

PROCTOR: Noted.

Assess Circulation

Student: I am assessing the patient's circulation.

PROCTOR: Noted.

Assess for and Control Major Bleeding

Student: Do I find any major bleeding?

PROCTOR: No.

Assess the Pulse

Student: What are the rate and the quality of pulses?

PROCTOR: Rate: Tachycardic. Quality: Thready.

Assess the Skin

Student: I am assessing the skin. What are the color, temperature, and condition of the skin?

PROCTOR: Color: Cyanotic. Temperature: Cool. Condition: Diaphoretic.

Identify Priority Patients/Make Transport Decision

Student: The patient is a high priority and a load-and-go. I will begin packaging and transport to a trauma center.

PROCTOR: Noted.

Critical Criteria:

- ❑ Did not provide high concentration of oxygen
- ❑ Did not find or manage problems associated with airway, breathing, hemorrhage or shock (hypoperfusion)
- ❑ Did not differentiate patient's need for transportation versus continued assessment at the scene
- ❑ Did other detailed examination before assessing the airway, breathing and circulation

Focused History and Physical Examination/Rapid Trauma Assessment

Select the Appropriate Assessment (Focused or Rapid)

Student: I am selecting the rapid physical exam to identify and treat life threats. I am checking for DCAP-BTLS. This acronym stands for deformities, contusions, abrasions, punctures, penetrations, paradoxical motion in the chest, and burns, tenderness, lacerations, and swelling.

PROCTOR: Noted.

Head

Student: I am rapidly assessing the head.

PROCTOR: The patient has small pieces of tempered glass in his face.

Neck

Student: I am rapidly assessing the neck.

PROCTOR: There are no obvious injuries.

Student: I will apply a cervical collar.

PROCTOR: Noted.

▸ Chest

Student: I am rapidly assessing the chest.
PROCTOR: There is significant bruising to the chest.
Student: I will assess the chest for tension pneumothorax by auscultation and assessment of jugular vein distention (JVD), tracheal deviation, and decreased lung sounds.
PROCTOR: There are decreased lung sounds on the left side, JVD is present, and the trachea is deviated to the right.
ALS Student: I will assess the chest for hyperresonance to percussion.
ALS Proctor: Noted. There is a tension pneumothorax on the left side.
ALS Student: I will decompress the chest.
ALS Proctor: Noted. The decompression was effective.

▸ Abdomen/Pelvis

Student: I am rapidly assessing the abdomen.
PROCTOR: There are no obvious injuries.
Student: I am rapidly assessing the pelvis.
PROCTOR: There are no obvious injuries.

▸ Extremities

Student: I am rapidly assessing the extremities.
PROCTOR: There are multiple fractures to both arms and legs.

▸ Assess Motor, Sensory, and Circulatory Function

Student: I am checking for DCAP-BTLS, motor and sensory function, and pulses. Right leg?
PROCTOR: Deformity and crepitation are found to the tibia/fibula. Motor and sensory functions are present. Pulses are weak.
Student: Left leg?
PROCTOR: Deformity and crepitation are found to the femur. Motor and sensory functions are present. Pulses are weak.
Student: Right arm?
PROCTOR: Deformity and crepitation are found to the humerus. Motor and sensory functions are present. Pulses are weak.
Student: Left arm?
PROCTOR: Deformity and crepitation are found to the wrist. Motor and sensory functions are present. Pulses are weak.

▸ Posterior

Student: I will rapidly assess the back. We will now log roll the patient as a unit to check the back. The person at the head will count to three and we will roll the patient.
PROCTOR: Noted.

▸ Assess the Thorax

Student: I am assessing the thorax. Do I find injuries?
PROCTOR: No.

▸ Assess the Lumbar Area

Student: I am assessing the flanks and lumbar area. Do I find injuries?
PROCTOR: No.

▸ Assess the Entire Backside

Student: I am assessing the entire backside. Do I find injuries?
PROCTOR: No.

▸ Manage Secondary Injuries/Wounds

Student: We will apply a cervical collar and backboard with full immobilization per local protocol, if not yet done, at this time. I will use the backboard to splint the right tibia/fibula and the left femur. Other splints will be administered during transport.
PROCTOR: Noted.
Student: Are there any changes in motor and sensory functions or pulses?
PROCTOR: No.

ALS Student: I will establish two large-bore IVs en route to the hospital and administer a bolus of 20 mL/kg in order to maintain a systolic blood pressure of 90 mm Hg.
ALS Proctor: Noted.

▸ Reevaluate Transport Decision

Student: This patient is a high priority due to multiple trauma.
PROCTOR: Noted.

▾ Baseline Vital Signs

Student: What are the patient's baseline vital signs, including blood pressure, pulse, respirations, pulse oximetry, and level of consciousness?
PROCTOR: Blood pressure, 110/72 mm Hg; pulse rate, 134 beats/min; respirations per bag-valve device; pulse oximetry reading, 93%; and the patient is anxious.

▾ SAMPLE History

Student: At this time I will gather a SAMPLE history from the patient or family. What are the patient's signs and symptoms?
PROCTOR: Pain in the left chest, and to the right lower leg, the left leg, the right arm, and the left wrist.
Student: Allergies?
PROCTOR: No allergies.
Student: Medications?
PROCTOR: No medications.
Student: Pertinent past medical history?
PROCTOR: No pertinent medical history.
Student: Last oral intake?
PROCTOR: 3 hours ago.
Student: Events leading up to the incident?
PROCTOR: The patient was street racing, rolled his pickup truck, and was ejected to the street.

Critical Criteria:
- ❑ Did not differentiate patient's need for transportation versus continued assessment at the scene
- ❑ Did not provide for spinal protection when indicated

▾ Detailed Physical Examination

Student: I am conducting the detailed physical exam. I am looking for DCAP-BTLS.
PROCTOR: Noted. The detailed physical exam will be performed during transport.

▾ Assess the Head

Student: I am assessing the head. Do I find any DCAP-BTLS? Do I find any evidence of Battle's sign or raccoon eyes?
PROCTOR: You see bruising to his forehead.

▸ Inspect and Palpate the Head and Ears

Student: I am assessing the head and ears.
PROCTOR: You see bruising to his forehead.

▸ Assess the Eyes

Student: I am assessing the eyes. Are the pupils equal, round, and regular in size, and react properly to light (PEARRL)?
PROCTOR: They are PEARRL.

▸ Assess the Facial Area Including Oral and Nasal Areas

Student: I am assessing the face, nose, and mouth. Do I see any discharge or hear any obstructions?
PROCTOR: No.

▼ Assess the Neck

▸ **Inspect and Palpate the Neck**

Student: I am assessing the neck for DCAP-BTLS.
PROCTOR: There are no obvious injuries.

▸ **Assess for Jugular Vein Distention**

Student: Do I find any jugular vein distention (JVD)?
PROCTOR: Not if the chest was decompressed by ALS.

▸ **Assess for Tracheal Deviation**

Student: Do I see any tracheal deviation?
PROCTOR: Not if the chest was decompressed by ALS.

▼ Assess the Chest

Student: I am assessing the chest for DCAP-BTLS.
PROCTOR: Noted.

▸ **Inspect**

Student: What do I see when I look at the chest?
PROCTOR: There is significant bruising to the chest.
Student: Does the chest appear symmetric?
PROCTOR: Yes.

▸ **Palpate**

Student: When I touch the chest, do I feel crepitus or a flail segment?
PROCTOR: No.

▸ **Auscultate**

Student: Are lung sounds present in all fields?
PROCTOR: Yes, if decompressed by ALS.
Student: Do I hear any sucking sounds from the chest?
PROCTOR: No.
Student: I will reassess the chest for tension pneumothorax by auscultation and assessment of JVD, tracheal deviation, and decreased lung sounds.
PROCTOR: The lung sounds are present bilaterally, JVD is not present, and the trachea is midline.
ALS Student: I will assess the chest for hyperresonance to percussion.
ALS Proctor: Noted. There is no tension pneumothorax noted. The decompression was effective.

▼ Assess the Abdomen/Pelvis

▸ **Assess the Abdomen**

Student: I am assessing the abdomen for DCAP-BTLS. I am assessing all four quadrants. Do I find any problems?
PROCTOR: No.

▸ **Assess the Pelvis**

Student: I am assessing the pelvis for DCAP-BTLS. Is the pelvis stable?
PROCTOR: Yes.

▼ Assess the Genitalia/Perineum as Needed (Verbalize in Training)

Student: I am assessing the genitalia/perineum as necessary for DCAP-BTLS.
PROCTOR: The area is unremarkable.

▼ Assess the Extremities

▸ **Inspect**

Student: I am assessing the lower and upper extremities for DCAP-BTLS. Do I find anything?
PROCTOR: Yes. There are multiple fractures to both arms and legs.

▸ **Palpate**

Student: Do I feel anything unusual?
PROCTOR: Yes.

▸ **Assess Motor, Sensory, and Circulatory Function**

Student: I am checking for DCAP-BTLS, motor and sensory function, and pulses. Right leg?
PROCTOR: Deformity and crepitation are found to the tibia/fibula. Motor and sensory functions are present. Pulses are weak.
Student: Left leg?
PROCTOR: Deformity and crepitation are found to the femur. Motor and sensory functions are present. Pulses are weak.
Student: Right arm?
PROCTOR: Deformity and crepitation are found to the humerus. Motor and sensory functions are present. Pulses are weak.
Student: Left arm?
PROCTOR: Deformity and crepitation are found to the wrist. Motor and sensory functions are present. Pulses are weak.

▼ Assess the Posterior

Note: This portion of the detailed physical exam would not be done if the patient were previously backboarded per local protocol.
Student: We will not check the back because it was previously checked and the patient is backboarded.
PROCTOR: Noted.

▼ Manage Secondary Injuries/Wounds

Student: I would direct my partner to maintain the airway. I will splint the arm and wrist fractures.
PROCTOR: Noted.

▼ Reassess Vital Signs

Student: I will reassess vital signs and mental status.
PROCTOR: Blood pressure, 108/70 mm Hg; pulse rate, 130 beats/min; respirations per bag-valve device; pulse oximetry reading, 94%; and the patient is anxious.
Student: The vital signs have not changed significantly.
PROCTOR: Noted.

▼ Reassess Interventions

Student: I will reassess my interventions: airway, bag-valve device ventilations, and oxygen; bleeding control; immobilization, straps, and splints to all extremities; and treatment for shock.
PROCTOR: Noted.
ALS Student: I will reassess basic life support (BLS) interventions, plus the following: monitor the left chest, maintain a systolic blood pressure of 90 mm Hg, and cardiac monitoring.
ALS Proctor: Noted. The cardiac monitor shows sinus tachycardia.

Critical Criteria:
- ❑ Did not find or manage problems associated with airway, breathing, hemorrhage or shock (hypoperfusion)

▼ Radio Report

(Provided by the student.)
PROCTOR: Noted.

Ongoing Assessment

Repeat Vital Signs

Student: I will reassess vital signs and mental status.

PROCTOR: Blood pressure, 104/68 mm Hg; pulse rate, 134 beats/min; respirations per bag-valve device; pulse oximetry reading, 94%; and the patient is anxious.

Student: The vital signs have not changed significantly.

PROCTOR: Noted.

Check Interventions

Student: I will check my interventions: airway, bag-valve device ventilations, and oxygen; bleeding control; immobilization, straps, and splints to all extremities; and treatment for shock.

PROCTOR: Noted.

ALS Student: I will check BLS interventions, plus the following: monitor the left chest, maintain a systolic blood pressure of 90 mm Hg, and cardiac monitoring.

ALS Proctor: Noted. The cardiac monitor shows sinus tachycardia.

Critical Criteria:
- ❑ Did not find or manage problems associated with airway, breathing, hemorrhage or shock (hypoperfusion)

Handoff Report to Emergency Department Staff

Student: There was no change in the patient's condition during transport.

PROCTOR: Noted.

Critical Criteria:
- ❑ Did not transport patient within the (10) minute time limit

Critical Criteria

(Inform the student of items missed, if any.)

❑ Pass ❑ Fail Date: ______________________

Proctor Comments: ______________________

____

____

CASE 59

Dispatch Information

PROCTOR: EMS 10, respond to a hunting injury. A 17-year-old male was shot in the left shoulder with bird shot. He is conscious and breathing but is dizzy.

Pre-scene Action (BSI)

Student: I am wearing nonlatex gloves, safety glasses, mask, and gown.
PROCTOR: Noted.

Critical Criteria:
- ☐ Did not take, or verbalize, body substance isolation (BSI) precautions when necessary

Scene Size-up

Scene Safety

Student: Is the scene safe?
PROCTOR: Yes.

Mechanism of Injury

Student: What was the mechanism of injury?
PROCTOR: Gunshot wound. The patient was hunting and was accidentally shot by his uncle.

Number of Patients

Student: How many patients are there?
PROCTOR: One.

Additional Resources

Student: I would call for advanced life support (ALS) assistance.
PROCTOR: Noted.

C-Spine Stabilization

Student: On the basis of the mechanism of injury, I would stabilize the cervical spine (c-spine) in a neutral in-line position.
PROCTOR: Noted.

Critical Criteria:
- ☐ Did not determine scene safety
- ☐ Did not assess for spinal protection
- ☐ Did not provide for spinal protection when indicated

Initial Assessment

Student: As I perform midline c-spine stabilization, I identify myself and ask the patient not to move.
PROCTOR: Noted.

General Impression

Student: My general impression is that the patient's condition is unstable.
PROCTOR: Noted.

Responsiveness/Level of Consciousness

Student: What is the patient's level of consciousness?
PROCTOR: Alert.

Chief Complaint/Apparent Life Threats

Student: What is the patient's chief complaint?
PROCTOR: The patient is complaining of pain in the shoulder and dizziness.
Student: There is an apparent life threat; the life threat is the mechanism of injury.
PROCTOR: Noted.

Assess the Airway and Breathing

Student: Is the airway open? Is the patient breathing?
PROCTOR: Yes, the airway is open and the patient is breathing.

Assessment

Student: What are the rate and the quality of breathing?
PROCTOR: Rate: A little fast. Quality: Normal.

Provide Oxygen

Student: I am applying oxygen at 15 L/min via nonrebreathing mask.
PROCTOR: Noted.

Ensure Adequate Ventilation

Student: The patient has adequate ventilations at this time.
PROCTOR: Noted.

Injury Management

Student: I will direct my partner to take over c-spine control as I continue assessment.
PROCTOR: Noted.

Assess Circulation

Student: I am assessing the patient's circulation.
PROCTOR: Noted.

Assess for and Control Major Bleeding

Student: Do I find any major bleeding?
PROCTOR: Nothing major, but there is some minor bleeding noted in the area of the left shoulder.
Student: I would apply dry, sterile dressings to the area.
PROCTOR: Noted.

Assess the Pulse

Student: What are the rate and the quality of pulses?
PROCTOR: Rate: Tachycardic. Quality: Bounding.

Assess the Skin

Student: I am assessing the skin. What are the color, temperature, and condition of the skin?
PROCTOR: Color: Pale. Temperature: Normal. Condition: Moist.

Identify Priority Patients/Make Transport Decision

Student: The patient is a high priority and is a load-and-go due to the mechanism of injury. I will begin packaging and transport.
PROCTOR: Noted.

Critical Criteria:
- ☐ Did not provide high concentration of oxygen
- ☐ Did not find or manage problems associated with airway, breathing, hemorrhage or shock (hypoperfusion)
- ☐ Did not differentiate patient's need for transportation versus continued assessment at the scene
- ☐ Did other detailed examination before assessing the airway, breathing and circulation

Focused History and Physical Examination/Rapid Trauma Assessment

Select the Appropriate Assessment (Focused or Rapid)

Student: I am selecting the rapid physical exam to identify and treat life threats. I am checking for DCAP-BTLS. This acronym stands for deformities, contusions, abrasions, punctures, penetrations, paradoxical motion in the chest, and burns, tenderness, lacerations, and swelling.
PROCTOR: Noted.

Head

Student: I am rapidly assessing the head.
PROCTOR: There are no obvious injuries.

Neck

Student: I am rapidly assessing the neck.
PROCTOR: There are no obvious injuries.
Student: I will apply a cervical collar.
PROCTOR: Noted.

Chest

Student: I am rapidly assessing the chest.
PROCTOR: You see multiple small BB holes to the left shoulder area. Bleeding has been controlled.

Abdomen/Pelvis

Student: I am rapidly assessing the abdomen.
PROCTOR: There are no obvious injuries.

Student: I am rapidly assessing the pelvis.
PROCTOR: There are no obvious injuries.

▸ **Extremities**

Student: I am rapidly assessing the extremities.
PROCTOR: You see multiple small BB holes to the left shoulder. Bleeding has been controlled.

▸ **Assess Motor, Sensory, and Circulatory Function**

Student: I am checking for DCAP-BTLS, motor and sensory function, and pulses. Right leg?
PROCTOR: Negative DCAP-BTLS. Motor and sensory functions are present. Pulses are present.
Student: Left leg?
PROCTOR: Negative DCAP-BTLS. Motor and sensory functions are present. Pulses are present.
Student: Right arm?
PROCTOR: Negative DCAP-BTLS. Motor and sensory functions are present. Pulses are present.
Student: Left arm?
PROCTOR: Small BB holes are seen at the shoulder. Motor and sensory functions are present. Pulses are present.

▸ **Posterior**

Student: I will rapidly assess the back. We will now log roll the patient as a unit to check the back. The person at the head will count to three and we will roll the patient.
PROCTOR: Noted.

▸ **Assess the Thorax**

Student: I am assessing the thorax. Do I find injuries?
PROCTOR: No.

▸ **Assess the Lumbar Area**

Student: I am assessing the flanks and lumbar area. Do I find injuries?
PROCTOR: No.

▸ **Assess the Entire Backside**

Student: I am assessing the entire backside. Do I find injuries?
PROCTOR: No.

▸ **Manage Secondary Injuries/Wounds**

Student: We will apply a cervical collar and backboard with full immobilization per local protocol, if not yet done, at this time.
PROCTOR: Noted.
Student: Are there any changes in motor and sensory functions or pulses?
PROCTOR: No.
ALS Student: I will establish two large-bore IVs en route to the hospital and cardiac monitoring.
ALS Proctor: Noted. The cardiac monitor shows normal sinus rhythm.

▸ **Reevaluate Transport Decision**

Student: This patient is a high priority due to the mechanism of injury.
PROCTOR: Noted.

▾ Baseline Vital Signs

Student: What are the patient's baseline vital signs, including blood pressure, pulse, respirations, pulse oximetry, blood glucose level, and level of consciousness?
PROCTOR: Blood pressure, 130/88 mm Hg; pulse rate, 120 beats/min; respirations, 22 breaths/min; pulse oximetry reading, 98%; blood glucose level, 116 mg/dL; and the patient is alert.

▾ SAMPLE History

Student: At this time I will gather a SAMPLE history from the patient or family. What are the patient's signs and symptoms?
PROCTOR: Pain in the left shoulder.
Student: Allergies?
PROCTOR: No allergies.
Student: Medications?
PROCTOR: Insulin.
Student: Pertinent past medical history?
PROCTOR: Diabetes.
Student: Last oral intake?
PROCTOR: 3 hours ago.
Student: Events leading up to the incident?
PROCTOR: The patient was hunting when he was accidentally shot by his uncle.

Critical Criteria:
- ❑ Did not differentiate patient's need for transportation versus continued assessment at the scene
- ❑ Did not provide for spinal protection when indicated

▼ Detailed Physical Examination

Student: I am conducting the detailed physical exam. I am looking for DCAP-BTLS.
PROCTOR: Noted. The detailed physical exam will be performed during transport.

▾ Assess the Head

Student: I am assessing the head. Do I find any DCAP-BTLS? Do I find any evidence of Battle's sign or raccoon eyes?
PROCTOR: No.

▸ **Inspect and Palpate the Head and Ears**

Student: I am assessing the head and ears.
PROCTOR: There are no obvious injuries.

▸ **Assess the Eyes**

Student: I am assessing the eyes. Are the pupils equal, round, and regular in size, and react properly to light (PEARRL)?
PROCTOR: They are PEARRL.

▸ **Assess the Facial Area Including Oral and Nasal Areas**

Student: I am assessing the face, nose, and mouth. Do I see any discharge or hear any obstructions?
PROCTOR: No.

▾ Assess the Neck

▸ **Inspect and Palpate the Neck**

Student: I am assessing the neck for DCAP-BTLS.
PROCTOR: There are no obvious injuries.

▸ **Assess for Jugular Vein Distention**

Student: Do I find any jugular vein distention (JVD)?
PROCTOR: No.

▸ **Assess for Tracheal Deviation**

Student: Do I see any tracheal deviation?
PROCTOR: No.

▾ Assess the Chest

Student: I am assessing the chest for DCAP-BTLS.
PROCTOR: Noted.

▸ **Inspect**

Student: What do I see when I look at the chest?
PROCTOR: You see small BB holes to the upper left shoulder area.
Student: Does the chest appear symmetric?
PROCTOR: Yes.

▸ **Palpate**

Student: When I touch the chest, do I feel crepitus or a flail segment?
PROCTOR: No.

▸ **Auscultate**

Student: Are lung sounds present in all fields?
PROCTOR: Yes.
Student: Do I hear any sucking sounds from the chest?
PROCTOR: No.

▾ Assess the Abdomen/Pelvis

▸ **Assess the Abdomen**

Student: I am assessing the abdomen for DCAP-BTLS. I am assessing all four quadrants. Do I find any problems?
PROCTOR: No.

▸ **Assess the Pelvis**

Student: I am assessing the pelvis for DCAP-BTLS. Is the pelvis stable?

PROCTOR: Yes.

▾ Assess the Genitalia/Perineum as Needed (Verbalize in Training)

Student: I am assessing the genitalia/perineum as necessary for DCAP-BTLS.

PROCTOR: The area is unremarkable.

▾ Assess the Extremities

▸ **Inspect**

Student: I am assessing the lower and upper extremities for DCAP-BTLS. Do I find anything?

PROCTOR: Yes.

▸ **Palpate**

Student: Do I feel anything unusual?

PROCTOR: No.

▸ **Assess Motor, Sensory, and Circulatory Function**

Student: I am checking for DCAP-BTLS, motor and sensory function, and pulses. Right leg?

PROCTOR: Negative DCAP-BTLS. Motor and sensory functions are present. Pulses are present.

Student: Left leg?

PROCTOR: Negative DCAP-BTLS. Motor and sensory functions are present. Pulses are present.

Student: Right arm?

PROCTOR: Negative DCAP-BTLS. Motor and sensory functions are present. Pulses are present.

Student: Left arm?

PROCTOR: Small BB holes are seen at the shoulder. Motor and sensory functions are present. Pulses are present.

▾ Assess the Posterior

Note: This portion of the detailed physical exam would not be done if the patient were previously backboarded per local protocol.

Student: We will not check the back because it was previously checked and the patient is backboarded.

PROCTOR: Noted.

▾ Manage Secondary Injuries/Wounds

Student: I would direct my partner to reassess the dressing and splint the arm with a sling and swathe.

PROCTOR: Noted.

▾ Reassess Vital Signs

Student: I will reassess vital signs and mental status.

PROCTOR: Blood pressure, 124/86 mm Hg; pulse rate, 110 beats/min; respirations, 18 breaths/min; pulse oximetry reading, 99%; and the patient is alert.

Student: The vital signs are improving.

PROCTOR: Noted.

▾ Reassess Interventions

Student: I will reassess my interventions: airway, breathing, and oxygen; circulation and bleeding control; immobilization and straps; sling and swathe; and treatment for shock.

PROCTOR: Noted.

ALS Student: I will reassess basic life support (BLS) interventions, plus the following: two large-bore IVs and cardiac monitor.

ALS Proctor: Noted. The cardiac monitor shows normal sinus rhythm.

Critical Criteria:
- ❑ Did not find or manage problems associated with airway, breathing, hemorrhage or shock (hypoperfusion)

▼ Radio Report

(Provided by the student.)

PROCTOR: Noted.

▼ Ongoing Assessment

▾ Repeat Vital Signs

Student: I will reassess vital signs and mental status.

PROCTOR: Blood pressure, 124/80 mm Hg; pulse rate, 104 beats/min; respirations, 16 breaths/min; pulse oximetry reading, 99%; and the patient is alert.

Student: The vital signs have improved.

PROCTOR: Noted.

▾ Check Interventions

Student: I will check my interventions: airway, breathing, and oxygen; circulation and bleeding control; immobilization and straps; sling and swathe; and treatment for shock.

PROCTOR: Noted.

ALS Student: I will check BLS interventions, plus the following: two large-bore IVs and cardiac monitor.

ALS Proctor: Noted. The cardiac monitor shows normal sinus rhythm.

Critical Criteria:
- ❑ Did not find or manage problems associated with airway, breathing, hemorrhage or shock (hypoperfusion)

▼ Handoff Report to Emergency Department Staff

Student: The patient's condition improved during transport. He began to relax.

PROCTOR: Noted.

Critical Criteria:
- ❑ Did not transport patient within the (10) minute time limit

▼ Critical Criteria

(Inform the student of items missed, if any.)

❑ Pass ❑ Fail Date: ______________________________

Proctor Comments: ______________________________

____

____

CASE 59

Notes

CASE 60

Dispatch Information

PROCTOR: EMS 10, respond to a 40-year-old iron worker who was working with a tape measure that came in contact with a high-voltage wire. He is conscious and breathing.

Pre-scene Action (BSI)

Student: I am wearing appropriate high-visibility personal protective equipment suitable for extrication, a helmet, extrication gloves, nonlatex gloves, safety glasses, and a mask.
PROCTOR: Noted.

Critical Criteria:
- ❑ Did not take, or verbalize, body substance isolation (BSI) precautions when necessary

Scene Size-up

Scene Safety

Student: Is the scene safe?
PROCTOR: Yes.

Mechanism of Injury

Student: What was the mechanism of injury?
PROCTOR: Electric shock. The patient was measuring a beam when the wind blew his tape measure into a power line.

Number of Patients

Student: How many patients are there?
PROCTOR: One.

Additional Resources

Student: I would call for advanced life support (ALS) assistance and additional resources: fire/rescue and the power company. I would request a medical helicopter if one is available.
PROCTOR: Noted.

C-Spine Stabilization

Student: On the basis of the mechanism of injury, I would stabilize the cervical spine (c-spine) in a neutral in-line position.
PROCTOR: Noted.

Critical Criteria:
- ❑ Did not determine scene safety
- ❑ Did not assess for spinal protection
- ❑ Did not provide for spinal protection when indicated

Initial Assessment

Student: As I perform midline c-spine stabilization, I identify myself and ask the patient not to move.
PROCTOR: Noted.

General Impression

Student: My general impression is that the patient's condition is unstable.
PROCTOR: Noted.

Responsiveness/Level of Consciousness

Student: What is the patient's level of consciousness?
PROCTOR: Alert and anxious.

Chief Complaint/Apparent Life Threats

Student: What is the patient's chief complaint?
PROCTOR: The patient is complaining of feeling burned and a pins-and-needles sensation all over his body.
Student: There are apparent life threats; the life threats are the mechanism of injury and internal burns.
PROCTOR: Noted.

Assess the Airway and Breathing

Student: Is the airway open? Is the patient breathing?
PROCTOR: Yes, the airway is open and the patient is breathing.

▸ Assessment

Student: What are the rate and the quality of breathing?
PROCTOR: Rate: Tachypneic. Quality: Deep.

▸ Provide Oxygen

Student: I am applying oxygen at 15 L/min via nonrebreathing mask.
PROCTOR: Noted.

▸ Ensure Adequate Ventilation

Student: The patient has adequate ventilations at this time.
PROCTOR: Noted.

Injury Management

Student: I will direct my partner to maintain c-spine control as I continue assessment.
PROCTOR: Noted.

Assess Circulation

Student: I am assessing the patient's circulation.
PROCTOR: Noted.

▸ Assess for and Control Major Bleeding

Student: Do I find any major bleeding?
PROCTOR: No.

▸ Assess the Pulse

Student: What are the rate and the quality of pulses?
PROCTOR: Rate: Tachycardic. Quality: Bounding.

▸ Assess the Skin

Student: I am assessing the skin. What are the color, temperature, and condition of the skin?
PROCTOR: Color: Pale. Temperature: Warm. Condition: Diaphoretic.

Identify Priority Patients/Make Transport Decision

Student: The patient is a high priority and is a load-and-go. I will begin packaging and transport.
PROCTOR: Noted.

Critical Criteria:
- ❑ Did not provide high concentration of oxygen
- ❑ Did not find or manage problems associated with airway, breathing, hemorrhage or shock (hypoperfusion)
- ❑ Did not differentiate patient's need for transportation versus continued assessment at the scene
- ❑ Did other detailed examination before assessing the airway, breathing and circulation

Focused History and Physical Examination/Rapid Trauma Assessment

Select the Appropriate Assessment (Focused or Rapid)

Student: I am selecting the rapid physical exam to identify and treat life threats. I am checking for DCAP-BTLS. This acronym stands for deformities, contusions, abrasions, punctures, penetrations, paradoxical motion in the chest, and burns, tenderness, lacerations, and swelling.
PROCTOR: Noted.

▸ Head

Student: I am rapidly assessing the head.
PROCTOR: There are no obvious injuries.

▸ Neck

Student: I am rapidly assessing the neck.
PROCTOR: There are no obvious injuries.
Student: I will apply a cervical collar.
PROCTOR: Noted.

▸ Chest

Student: I am rapidly assessing the chest.
PROCTOR: There are no obvious injuries.
Student: What are the lung sounds?
PROCTOR: They are clear bilaterally.

▸ Abdomen/Pelvis

Student: I am rapidly assessing the abdomen.

PROCTOR: There are no obvious injuries.

Student: I am rapidly assessing the pelvis.

PROCTOR: There are no obvious injuries.

▸ Extremities

Student: I am rapidly assessing the extremities.

PROCTOR: The patient has an entrance wound to the right hand and exit wounds to both feet.

▸ Assess Motor, Sensory, and Circulatory Function

Student: I am checking for DCAP-BTLS, motor and sensory function, and pulses. Right leg?

PROCTOR: An explosive electrical burn injury is found to the toes. Motor and sensory functions are present. Pulses are present.

Student: Left leg?

PROCTOR: An explosive electrical burn injury is found to the heel of the foot. Pulses are present.

Student: Right arm?

PROCTOR: An explosive electrical burn injury is found to the palm and fingers of the hand. Motor and sensory functions are present. Pulses are present.

Student: Left arm?

PROCTOR: Negative DCAP-BTLS. Motor and sensory functions are present. Pulses are present.

▸ Posterior

Student: I will rapidly assess the back. We will now log roll the patient as a unit to check the back. The person at the head will count to three and we will roll the patient.

PROCTOR: Noted.

▸ Assess the Thorax

Student: I am assessing the thorax. Do I find injuries?

PROCTOR: No.

▸ Assess the Lumbar Area

Student: I am assessing the flanks and lumbar area. Do I find injuries?

PROCTOR: No.

▸ Assess the Entire Backside

Student: I am assessing the entire backside. Do I find injuries?

PROCTOR: No.

▸ Manage Secondary Injuries/Wounds

Student: We will apply a cervical collar and backboard with full immobilization per local protocol, if not yet done, at this time. I will treat the wounds with dry dressings en route to the hospital.

PROCTOR: Noted.

Student: Are there any changes in motor and sensory functions or pulses?

PROCTOR: No.

ALS Student: I will establish two large-bore IVs en route to the hospital and administer a bolus of 20 mL/kg in order to maintain a systolic blood pressure of 90 mm Hg. I also will monitor the heart and perform a 12-lead ECG en route.

ALS Proctor: Noted.

▸ Reevaluate Transport Decision

Student: This patient is a load-and-go due to the mechanism of injury.

PROCTOR: Noted.

▾ Baseline Vital Signs

Student: What are the patient's baseline vital signs, including blood pressure, pulse, respirations, pulse oximetry, and level of consciousness?

PROCTOR: Blood pressure, 150/90 mm Hg; pulse rate, 150 beats/min; respirations, 24 breaths/min; pulse oximetry reading, 98%; and the patient is alert.

▾ SAMPLE History

Student: At this time I will gather a SAMPLE history from the patient or family. What are the patient's signs and symptoms?

PROCTOR: Pain and a feeling of being burned all over the body.

Student: Allergies?

PROCTOR: No allergies.

Student: Medications?

PROCTOR: No medications.

Student: Pertinent past medical history?

PROCTOR: No pertinent medical history.

Student: Last oral intake?

PROCTOR: 3 hours ago.

Student: Events leading up to the incident?

PROCTOR: The patient was measuring an I-beam when the wind caught his tape measure and blew it into a power line.

Critical Criteria:
- ❑ Did not differentiate patient's need for transportation versus continued assessment at the scene
- ❑ Did not provide for spinal protection when indicated

Detailed Physical Examination

Student: I am conducting the detailed physical exam. I am looking for DCAP-BTLS.

PROCTOR: Noted. The detailed physical exam will be performed during transport.

▾ Assess the Head

Student: I am assessing the head. Do I find any DCAP-BTLS? Do I find any evidence of Battle's sign or raccoon eyes?

PROCTOR: No.

▸ Inspect and Palpate the Head and Ears

Student: I am assessing the head and ears.

PROCTOR: There are no obvious injuries.

▸ Assess the Eyes

Student: I am assessing the eyes. Are the pupils equal, round, and regular in size, and react properly to light (PEARRL)?

PROCTOR: They are PEARRL.

▸ Assess the Facial Area Including Oral and Nasal Areas

Student: I am assessing the face, nose, and mouth. Do I see any discharge or hear any obstructions?

PROCTOR: No.

▾ Assess the Neck

▸ Inspect and Palpate the Neck

Student: I am assessing the neck for DCAP-BTLS.

PROCTOR: There are no obvious injuries.

▸ Assess for Jugular Vein Distention

Student: Do I find any jugular vein distention (JVD)?

PROCTOR: No.

▸ **Assess for Tracheal Deviation**
Student: Do I see any tracheal deviation?
PROCTOR: No.

▾ Assess the Chest
Student: I am assessing the chest for DCAP-BTLS.
PROCTOR: Noted.

▸ **Inspect**
Student: What do I see when I look at the chest?
PROCTOR: There are no obvious injuries.
Student: Does the chest appear symmetric?
PROCTOR: Yes.

▸ **Palpate**
Student: When I touch the chest, do I feel crepitus or a flail segment?
PROCTOR: No.

▸ **Auscultate**
Student: Are lung sounds present in all fields?
PROCTOR: Yes.
Student: Do I hear any sucking sounds from the chest?
PROCTOR: No.

▾ Assess the Abdomen/Pelvis
▸ **Assess the Abdomen**
Student: I am assessing the abdomen for DCAP-BTLS. I am assessing all four quadrants. Do I find any problems?
PROCTOR: No.

▸ **Assess the Pelvis**
Student: I am assessing the pelvis for DCAP-BTLS. Is the pelvis stable?
PROCTOR: Yes.

▾ Assess the Genitalia/Perineum as Needed (Verbalize in Training)
Student: I am assessing the genitalia/perineum as necessary for DCAP-BTLS.
PROCTOR: The area is unremarkable.

▾ Assess the Extremities
▸ **Inspect**
Student: I am assessing the lower and upper extremities for DCAP-BTLS. Do I find anything?
PROCTOR: Yes.

▸ **Palpate**
Student: Do I feel anything unusual?
PROCTOR: No.

▸ **Assess Motor, Sensory, and Circulatory Function**
Student: I am checking for DCAP-BTLS, motor and sensory function, and pulses. Right leg?
PROCTOR: There is an explosive exit wound to the toes. Motor and sensory functions are absent. Pulses are present. Bleeding is minimal.
Student: I will dress the injury with a dry sterile dressing.
PROCTOR: Noted.
Student: Left leg?
PROCTOR: There is an explosive exit wound to the heel of the foot. Motor and sensory functions are absent. Pulses are present. Bleeding is minimal.
Student: I will dress the injury with a dry sterile dressing.
PROCTOR: Noted.
Student: Right arm?
PROCTOR: There is an entrance wound to the hand. It is smoking and the bone appears cooked. Motor and sensory functions are absent. Pulses are present. Bleeding is minimal.
Student: I will dress the injury with a dry sterile dressing.
PROCTOR: Noted.
Student: Left arm?
PROCTOR: Negative DCAP-BTLS. Motor and sensory functions are absent. Pulses are present.

▾ Assess the Posterior
Note: This portion of the detailed physical exam would not be done if the patient were previously backboarded per local protocol.
Student: We will not check the back because it was previously checked and the patient is backboarded.
PROCTOR: Noted.

▾ Manage Secondary Injuries/Wounds
Student: I would direct my partner to monitor the patient.
PROCTOR: Noted.

▾ Reassess Vital Signs
Student: I will reassess vital signs and mental status.
PROCTOR: Blood pressure, 146/90 mm Hg; pulse rate, 144 beats/min; respirations, 20 breaths/min; pulse oximetry reading, 98%; and the patient is alert.
Student: The vital signs have not changed significantly.
PROCTOR: Noted.

▾ Reassess Interventions
Student: I will reassess my interventions: oxygen, wound dressings, assessment, and reassurance. I will confirm Medivac transport.
PROCTOR: Noted.
ALS Student: I will reassess basic life support (BLS) interventions, plus the following: two large-bore IVs, cardiac monitor, 12-lead ECG, advanced cardiac life support (ACLS), and regional protocol for possible pain management.
ALS Proctor: Noted. The cardiac monitor shows sinus tachycardia.

Critical Criteria:
❑ Did not find or manage problems associated with airway, breathing, hemorrhage or shock (hypoperfusion)

▾ Radio Report
(Provided by the student.)
PROCTOR: Noted.

▾ Ongoing Assessment
▾ Repeat Vital Signs
Student: I will reassess vital signs and mental status.
PROCTOR: Blood pressure, 140/82 mm Hg; pulse rate, 138 beats/min; respirations, 20 breaths/min; pulse oximetry reading, 98%; and the patient is alert.
Student: The vital signs have not changed significantly.
PROCTOR: Noted.

Check Interventions

Student: I will check my interventions: oxygen, wound dressings, assessment, and reassurance. I will hand the patient over to Medivac as soon as possible.

PROCTOR: Noted.

ALS Student: I will check BLS interventions, plus the following: IVs, cardiac monitor, 12-lead ECG, ACLS, and regional protocol.

ALS Proctor: Noted. The cardiac monitor shows sinus tachycardia.

Critical Criteria:

- ❑ Did not find or manage problems associated with airway, breathing, hemorrhage or shock (hypoperfusion)

Handoff Report to Emergency Department Staff

Student: There was no change in the patient's condition during transport.

PROCTOR: Noted.

Critical Criteria:

- ❑ Did not transport patient within the (10) minute time limit

Critical Criteria

(Inform the student of items missed, if any.)

❑ Pass ❑ Fail Date: ______________________________

Proctor Comments: ______________________________

____

____

CASE 61

Dispatch Information

PROCTOR: EMS 10, respond to a motor vehicle collision. A small car has driven under the trailer of a semi-truck. Police on the scene are requesting that you expedite your arrival. The patient is critical.

Pre-scene Action (BSI)

Student: I am wearing appropriate high-visibility personal protective equipment suitable for extrication, a helmet, extrication gloves, nonlatex gloves, safety glasses, and a mask.
PROCTOR: Noted.

Critical Criteria:
- ❑ Did not take, or verbalize, body substance isolation (BSI) precautions when necessary

Scene Size-up

Scene Safety

Student: Is the scene safe?
PROCTOR: Yes, police are on scene and you are given clearance to enter.

Mechanism of Injury

Student: What was the mechanism of injury?
PROCTOR: Penetrating head trauma. The patient drove his small car under the trailer of a semi-truck. He is impaled through the head by a solid steel bar that was hanging down from the trailer.

Number of Patients

Student: How many patients are there?
PROCTOR: One.

Additional Resources

Student: I would call for advanced life support (ALS) assistance and additional resources: fire/rescue.
PROCTOR: Noted.

C-Spine Stabilization

Student: On the basis of the mechanism of injury, I would stabilize the cervical spine (c-spine) in a neutral in-line position.
PROCTOR: Noted.

Critical Criteria:
- ❑ Did not determine scene safety
- ❑ Did not assess for spinal protection
- ❑ Did not provide for spinal protection when indicated

Initial Assessment

Student: As I perform midline c-spine stabilization, I identify myself and ask the patient not to move.
PROCTOR: Noted.

General Impression

Student: My general impression is that the patient's condition is unstable.
PROCTOR: Noted.

Responsiveness/Level of Consciousness

Student: What is the patient's level of consciousness?
PROCTOR: The patient is unresponsive.

Chief Complaint/Apparent Life Threats

Student: What is the patient's chief complaint?
PROCTOR: The patient is unresponsive.
Student: There are apparent life threats; the life threats are the impaled object and the mechanism of injury.
PROCTOR: Noted.

Assess the Airway and Breathing

Student: I am opening the airway using the jaw-thrust maneuver. Is the patient breathing?
PROCTOR: Yes.

Assessment

Student: What are the rate and the quality of breathing?
PROCTOR: Rate: 6 breaths/min. Quality: See-saw.

Provide Oxygen

Student: I am assisting ventilations with a bag-valve device with 100% oxygen.
PROCTOR: Noted. You are unable to get a seal because the bar entered the left side of the patient's head and came out his mouth.
Student: I will attempt to seal the wound and continue to ventilate while using an oral/advanced airway.
PROCTOR: Noted. You are unable to get a seal on a bag-valve due to the steel bar exiting through the mouth. A Combitube® or a King LT® airway will allow ventilation.
ALS Student: I will apply basic life support (BLS) interventions, plus the following: intubate and confirm endotracheal (ET) tube placement.
ALS Proctor: Noted. ET tube placement is confirmed by end tidal CO_2 and lung sounds.

Ensure Adequate Ventilation

Student: I will suction and supply oxygen as best I can by nonrebreathing mask or blow-by method, if an advanced airway is not available.
PROCTOR: Noted.

Injury Management

Student: I will direct my partner to take over c-spine control and ventilation as I continue assessment.
PROCTOR: Noted.

Assess Circulation

Student: I am assessing the patient's circulation.
PROCTOR: Noted.

Assess for and Control Major Bleeding

Student: Do I find any major bleeding?
PROCTOR: Yes, in the mouth.
Student: I will suction and apply direct pressure and a dressing.
PROCTOR: Noted.

Assess the Pulse

Student: What are the rate and the quality of pulses?
PROCTOR: Rate: Within normal limits. Quality: Bounding.

Assess the Skin

Student: I am assessing the skin. What are the color, temperature, and condition of the skin?
PROCTOR: Color: Flushed. Temperature: Warm. Condition: Moist.

Identify Priority Patients/Make Transport Decision

Student: The patient is a high priority and is a load-and-go. I will begin packaging and transport.
PROCTOR: Noted.

Critical Criteria:
- ❑ Did not provide high concentration of oxygen
- ❑ Did not find or manage problems associated with airway, breathing, hemorrhage or shock (hypoperfusion)
- ❑ Did not differentiate patient's need for transportation versus continued assessment at the scene
- ❑ Did other detailed examination before assessing the airway, breathing and circulation

Focused History and Physical Examination/Rapid Trauma Assessment

Select the Appropriate Assessment (Focused or Rapid)

Student: I am selecting the rapid physical exam to identify and treat life threats. I am checking for DCAP-BTLS. This acronym stands for deformities, contusions, abrasions, punctures, penetrations, paradoxical motion in the chest, and burns, tenderness, lacerations, and swelling.

PROCTOR: Noted.

Head

Student: I am rapidly assessing the head.

PROCTOR: There is a ½-inch, solid steel bar impaling the patient through the left side of the head and exiting the mouth.

Student: I will allow the fire/rescue department to cut the bar from the truck and extricate the patient from the car. I will stabilize the bar to the patient's head, control bleeding into the mouth, and maintain the airway.

PROCTOR: Noted.

Neck

Student: I am rapidly assessing the neck.

PROCTOR: There are no obvious injuries.

Student: I will apply a cervical collar.

PROCTOR: Noted.

Chest

Student: I am rapidly assessing the chest. What are the lung sounds?

PROCTOR: There are no obvious injuries. Lung sounds are clear bilaterally.

Abdomen/Pelvis

Student: I am rapidly assessing the abdomen.

PROCTOR: There are no obvious injuries.

Student: I am rapidly assessing the pelvis.

PROCTOR: There are no obvious injuries.

Extremities

Student: I am rapidly assessing the extremities.

PROCTOR: There are no obvious injuries.

Assess Motor, Sensory, and Circulatory Function

Student: I am checking for DCAP-BTLS, motor and sensory function, and pulses. Right leg?

PROCTOR: Negative DCAP-BTLS. Motor and sensory functions are absent. Pulses are present.

Student: Left leg?

PROCTOR: Negative DCAP-BTLS. Motor and sensory functions are absent. Pulses are present.

Student: Right arm?

PROCTOR: Negative DCAP-BTLS. Motor and sensory functions are absent. Pulses are present.

Student: Left arm?

PROCTOR: Negative DCAP-BTLS. Motor and sensory functions are absent. Pulses are present.

Posterior

Student: I will rapidly assess the back. We will now log roll the patient as a unit to check the back. The person at the head will count to three and we will roll the patient.

PROCTOR: Noted.

Assess the Thorax

Student: I am assessing the thorax. Do I find injuries?

PROCTOR: No.

Assess the Lumbar Area

Student: I am assessing the flanks and lumbar area. Do I find injuries?

PROCTOR: No. The fire/rescue department has now cut the bar from the underside of the trailer and freed the driver.

Assess the Entire Backside

Student: I am assessing the entire backside. Do I find injuries?

PROCTOR: No.

Manage Secondary Injuries/Wounds

Student: We will apply a cervical collar and backboard with full immobilization per local protocol, and rapidly extricate the patient. We will continue airway management.

PROCTOR: Noted. The patient was able to lie flat on the backboard despite the bar.

ALS Student: I will establish two large-bore IVs en route to the hospital and maintain a systolic blood pressure of 90 mm Hg.

ALS Proctor: Noted.

Student: Are there any changes in motor and sensory functions or pulses?

PROCTOR: No.

Reevaluate Transport Decision

Student: This patient is a load-and-go due to head trauma.

PROCTOR: Noted.

Baseline Vital Signs

Student: What are the patient's baseline vital signs, including blood pressure, pulse, respirations, pulse oximetry, blood glucose level, and level of consciousness?

PROCTOR: Blood pressure, 172/90 mm Hg; pulse, 88 beats/min; respirations, 6 breaths/min or per bag-valve device; pulse oximetry reading, 95%; blood glucose level, 156 mg/dL; and the patient is unresponsive.

SAMPLE History

Student: At this time I will gather a SAMPLE history from the patient or family. What are the patient's signs and symptoms?

PROCTOR: The patient is unresponsive.

Student: Allergies?

PROCTOR: Unknown.

Student: Medications?

PROCTOR: Unknown.

Student: Pertinent past medical history?

PROCTOR: Unknown.

Student: Last oral intake?

PROCTOR: Unknown.

Student: Events leading up to the incident?

PROCTOR: Unknown.

Critical Criteria:

- ❑ Did not differentiate patient's need for transportation versus continued assessment at the scene
- ❑ Did not provide for spinal protection when indicated

Detailed Physical Examination

Student: I am conducting the detailed physical exam. I am looking for DCAP-BTLS.

PROCTOR: Noted. The detailed physical exam will be performed during transport.

Assess the Head

Student: I am assessing the head. Do I find any DCAP-BTLS? Do I find any evidence of Battle's sign or raccoon eyes?

PROCTOR: There is a ½-inch thick, solid steel bar impaling the patient through the left side of the head and exiting the mouth. The bar was cut from the trailer after being stabilized to the patient's head.

Student: I will control bleeding into the mouth, maintain the airway, and suction as necessary.

PROCTOR: Noted.

▸ **Inspect and Palpate the Head and Ears**

Student: I am assessing the head and ears.

PROCTOR: Some bleeding and cerebrospinal fluid (CSF) are noted to the left side of the head, just below the ear, where the bar entered. The bar extends about two inches out of the head to the left-rear side of the head, just below the occiput. The bar is protruding out of the mouth about seven inches.

Student: I will control bleeding, suction as necessary, provide oxygen (ventilate with an advanced airway), and maintain stabilization of the bar.

PROCTOR: Noted.

▸ **Assess the Eyes**

Student: I am assessing the eyes. Are the pupils equal, round, and regular in size, and react properly to light (PEARRL)?

PROCTOR: They are nonreactive.

▸ **Assess the Facial Area Including Oral and Nasal Areas**

Student: I am assessing the face, nose, and mouth. Do I see any discharge or hear any obstructions?

PROCTOR: Yes, you hear occasional gurgling. The bar extends out of the mouth about seven inches. It has been stabilized.

Student: I will suction the airway as needed.

PROCTOR: Noted.

▼ Assess the Neck

▸ **Inspect and Palpate the Neck**

Student: I am assessing the neck for DCAP-BTLS.

PROCTOR: The bar is extended out two inches from the left side of the head at the top of the neck and just below the occipital region. The bar is stabilized.

▸ **Assess for Jugular Vein Distention**

Student: Do I find any jugular vein distention (JVD)?

PROCTOR: No.

▸ **Assess for Tracheal Deviation**

Student: Do I see any tracheal deviation?

PROCTOR: No.

▼ Assess the Chest

Student: I am assessing the chest for DCAP-BTLS.

PROCTOR: Noted.

▸ **Inspect**

Student: What do I see when I look at the chest?

PROCTOR: There are no obvious injuries.

Student: Does the chest appear symmetric?

PROCTOR: Yes.

▸ **Palpate**

Student: When I touch the chest, do I feel crepitus or a flail segment?

PROCTOR: No.

▸ **Auscultate**

Student: Are lung sounds present in all fields?

PROCTOR: Yes.

Student: Do I hear any sucking sounds from the chest?

PROCTOR: No.

▼ Assess the Abdomen/Pelvis

▸ **Assess the Abdomen**

Student: I am assessing the abdomen for DCAP-BTLS. I am assessing all four quadrants. Do I find any problems?

PROCTOR: No.

▸ **Assess the Pelvis**

Student: I am assessing the pelvis for DCAP-BTLS. Is the pelvis stable?

PROCTOR: Yes.

▼ Assess the Genitalia/Perineum as Needed (Verbalize in Training)

Student: I am assessing the genitalia/perineum as necessary for DCAP-BTLS.

PROCTOR: The area is unremarkable.

▼ Assess the Extremities

▸ **Inspect**

Student: I am assessing the lower and upper extremities for DCAP-BTLS. Do I find anything?

PROCTOR: No.

▸ **Palpate**

Student: Do I feel anything unusual?

PROCTOR: No.

▸ **Assess Motor, Sensory, and Circulatory Function**

Student: I am checking for DCAP-BTLS, motor and sensory function, and pulses. Right leg?

PROCTOR: Negative DCAP-BTLS. Motor and sensory functions are absent. Pulses are present.

Student: Left leg?

PROCTOR: Negative DCAP-BTLS. Motor and sensory functions are absent. Pulses are present.

Student: Right arm?

PROCTOR: Negative DCAP-BTLS. Motor and sensory functions are absent. Pulses are present.

Student: Left arm?

PROCTOR: Negative DCAP-BTLS. Motor and sensory functions are absent. Pulses are present.

▼ Assess the Posterior

Note: This portion of the detailed physical exam would not be done if the patient were previously backboarded per local protocol.

Student: We will not check the back because it was previously checked and the patient is backboarded.

PROCTOR: Noted.

▼ Manage Secondary Injuries/Wounds

Student: I would direct my partner to maintain the airway and ventilation if an advanced airway is in place.

PROCTOR: Noted.

▼ Reassess Vital Signs

Student: I will reassess vital signs and mental status.

PROCTOR: Blood pressure, 178/94 mm Hg; pulse, 88 beats/min; respirations, 6 breaths/min if not intubated or advanced airway in place, and per bag-valve device if advanced airway is in place; pulse oximetry reading, 96%; and the patient is unresponsive.

Student: The vital signs have not changed significantly.

PROCTOR: Noted.

▼ Reassess Interventions

Student: I will reassess my interventions: airway, oxygen, suction, ventilation if possible, bleeding control, full immobilization, and immobilization of the impaled object.

PROCTOR: Noted.

ALS Student: I will reassess BLS interventions, plus the following: intubation, confirm end tidal CO_2, check lung sounds, two large-bore IVs, and cardiac monitor.

ALS Proctor: Noted. The cardiac monitor shows normal sinus rhythm. End tidal CO_2 and lung sounds confirm ET tube placement.

Critical Criteria:

❑ Did not find or manage problems associated with airway, breathing, hemorrhage or shock (hypoperfusion)

Radio Report

(Provided by the student.)

PROCTOR: Noted.

Ongoing Assessment

Repeat Vital Signs

Student: I will reassess vital signs and mental status.

PROCTOR: Blood pressure, 172/90 mm Hg; pulse, 92 beats/min; respirations, 6 breaths/min if not intubated or advanced airway in place, and per bag-valve device if advanced airway is not in place; pulse oximetry reading, 96%; and the patient is unresponsive.

Student: The vital signs have not changed significantly.

PROCTOR: Noted.

Check Interventions

Student: I will check my interventions: airway, oxygen, suction, ventilation if possible, bleeding control, full immobilization, and immobilization of the impaled object.

PROCTOR: Noted.

ALS Student: I will check BLS interventions, plus the following: intubation, confirm end tidal CO_2, check lung sounds, two large-bore IVs, and cardiac monitor.

ALS Proctor: Noted. The cardiac monitor shows normal sinus rhythm. End tidal CO_2 and lung sounds confirm ET tube placement.

Critical Criteria:

❑ Did not find or manage problems associated with airway, breathing, hemorrhage or shock (hypoperfusion)

Handoff Report to Emergency Department Staff

Student: There was no change in the patient's condition during transport.

PROCTOR: Noted.

Critical Criteria:

❑ Did not transport patient within the (10) minute time limit

Critical Criteria

(Inform the student of items missed, if any.)

❑ Pass ❑ Fail Date: ____________________

Proctor Comments: ____________________

Dispatch Information

PROCTOR: EMS 10, respond to a 75-year-old male who has been stabbed through the hand and the knife is stuck in a table. He is conscious and breathing. Police officers are en route.

Pre-scene Action (BSI)

Student: I am wearing nonlatex gloves, safety glasses, mask, and gown.
PROCTOR: Noted.

Critical Criteria:
- ❑ Did not take, or verbalize, body substance isolation (BSI) precautions when necessary

Scene Size-up

Scene Safety

Student: Is the scene safe?
PROCTOR: Yes, police are on scene and you are given clearance to enter.

Mechanism of Injury

Student: What was the mechanism of injury?
PROCTOR: Penetrating trauma. The patient was robbed at his meat market and stabbed in the hand. The knife is through his hand and is stuck in the table.

Number of Patients

Student: How many patients are there?
PROCTOR: One.

Additional Resources

Student: I would not call for additional assistance.
PROCTOR: Noted.

C-Spine Stabilization

Student: I would not stabilize the cervical spine (c-spine).
PROCTOR: Noted.

Critical Criteria:
- ❑ Did not determine scene safety
- ❑ Did not assess for spinal protection
- ❑ Did not provide for spinal protection when indicated

Initial Assessment

General Impression

Student: My general impression is that the patient's condition is stable.
PROCTOR: Noted.

Responsiveness/Level of Consciousness

Student: What is the patient's level of consciousness?
PROCTOR: Alert.

Chief Complaint/Apparent Life Threats

Student: What is the patient's chief complaint?
PROCTOR: The patient is complaining of pain in the hand.
Student: There are no apparent life threats.
PROCTOR: Noted.

Assess the Airway and Breathing

Student: Is the airway open? Is the patient breathing?
PROCTOR: Yes, the airway is open and the patient is breathing.

Assessment

Student: What are the rate and the quality of breathing?
PROCTOR: Rate: Within normal limits. Quality: Normal.

Provide Oxygen

Student: I am applying oxygen at 15 L/min via nonrebreathing mask.
PROCTOR: Noted.

Ensure Adequate Ventilation

Student: The patient has adequate ventilations at this time.
PROCTOR: Noted.

Injury Management

Student: There is no airway or c-spine injury management necessary so I will continue assessment.
PROCTOR: Noted.

Assess Circulation

Student: I am assessing the patient's circulation.
PROCTOR: Noted.

Assess for and Control Major Bleeding

Student: Do I find any major bleeding?
PROCTOR: Yes, from the hand. There is a sharp kitchen knife all the way through the left hand and it is stuck in the table below.
Student: I would apply direct pressure and a dressing to control bleeding.
PROCTOR: Noted.

Assess the Pulse

Student: What are the rate and the quality of pulses?
PROCTOR: Rate: Within normal limits. Quality: Normal.

Assess the Skin

Student: I am assessing the skin. What are the color, temperature, and condition of the skin?
PROCTOR: Color: Flushed. Temperature: Warm. Condition: Normal.

Identify Priority Patients/Make Transport Decision

Student: The patient is a low priority and does not need immediate transport.
PROCTOR: Noted.

Critical Criteria:
- ❑ Did not provide high concentration of oxygen
- ❑ Did not find or manage problems associated with airway, breathing, hemorrhage or shock (hypoperfusion)
- ❑ Did not differentiate patient's need for transportation versus continued assessment at the scene
- ❑ Did other detailed examination before assessing the airway, breathing and circulation

Focused History and Physical Examination/Rapid Trauma Assessment

Select the Appropriate Assessment (Focused or Rapid)

Student: I am selecting the focused physical exam to identify and treat life threats.
PROCTOR: Noted.
Student: I am assessing the left hand for DCAP-BTLS. This acronym stands for deformities, contusions, abrasions, punctures, penetrations, paradoxical motion in the chest, and burns, tenderness, lacerations, and swelling. Do I find anything?
PROCTOR: Yes, there is a knife all the way through the patient's left hand and it is stuck in the tabletop.
Student: I will check for motor and sensory functions and pulses.
PROCTOR: Motor and sensory functions are present. Pulses are present.
Student: I will stabilize the knife to the hand with a cut-to-fit Sam® splint over a dressing. I will then gently remove the knife from the table without removing it from the hand.
PROCTOR: Noted. The knife is now removed from the table but is still through the hand.

Student: I will now splint the bottom of the hand using the rest of the Sam® splint to protect the sharp end of the knife over a bulky dressing.
PROCTOR: Noted.

Reevaluate Transport Decision

Student: The patient is a low priority and does not require immediate transport.
PROCTOR: Noted.

Baseline Vital Signs

Student: What are the patient's baseline vital signs, including blood pressure, pulse, respirations, pulse oximetry, and level of consciousness?
PROCTOR: Blood pressure, 150/100 mm Hg; pulse rate, 96 beats/min; respirations, 18 breaths/min; pulse oximetry reading, 97%; and the patient is alert.

SAMPLE History

Student: At this time I will gather a SAMPLE history from the patient or family. What are the patient's signs and symptoms?
PROCTOR: Pain in the hand.
Student: Allergies?
PROCTOR: Penicillin (PCN).
Student: Medications?
PROCTOR: Water pills and nitroglycerin; others are unknown.
Student: Pertinent past medical history?
PROCTOR: Heart problems and high blood pressure.
Student: Last oral intake?
PROCTOR: 2 hours ago.
Student: Events leading up to the incident?
PROCTOR: The patient was stabbed through the hand during a robbery.

Critical Criteria:
- ❑ Did not differentiate patient's need for transportation versus continued assessment at the scene
- ❑ Did not provide for spinal protection when indicated

Detailed Physical Examination

Student: I am conducting the detailed physical exam. I am looking for DCAP-BTLS.
PROCTOR: Noted. The detailed physical exam will be performed during transport.

Assess the Head

Student: I am assessing the head. Do I find any DCAP-BTLS? Do I find any evidence of Battle's sign or raccoon eyes?
PROCTOR: No.

Inspect and Palpate the Head and Ears

Student: I am assessing the head and ears.
PROCTOR: There are no obvious injuries.

Assess the Eyes

Student: I am assessing the eyes. Are the pupils equal, round, and regular in size, and react properly to light (PEARRL)?
PROCTOR: They are PEARRL.

Assess the Facial Area Including Oral and Nasal Areas

Student: I am assessing the face, nose, and mouth. Do I see any discharge or hear any obstructions?
PROCTOR: No.

Assess the Neck

Inspect and Palpate the Neck

Student: I am assessing the neck for DCAP-BTLS.
PROCTOR: There are no obvious injuries.

Assess for Jugular Vein Distention

Student: Do I find any jugular vein distention (JVD)?
PROCTOR: No.

Assess for Tracheal Deviation

Student: Do I see any tracheal deviation?
PROCTOR: No.

Assess the Chest

Student: I am assessing the chest for DCAP-BTLS.
PROCTOR: Noted.

Inspect

Student: What do I see when I look at the chest?
PROCTOR: There are no obvious injuries.
Student: Does the chest appear symmetric?
PROCTOR: Yes.

Palpate

Student: When I touch the chest, do I feel crepitus or a flail segment?
PROCTOR: No.

Auscultate

Student: Are lung sounds present in all fields?
PROCTOR: Yes.
Student: Do I hear any sucking sounds from the chest?
PROCTOR: No.

Assess the Abdomen/Pelvis

Assess the Abdomen

Student: I am assessing the abdomen for DCAP-BTLS. I am assessing all four quadrants. Do I find any problems?
PROCTOR: No.

Assess the Pelvis

Student: I am assessing the pelvis for DCAP-BTLS. Is the pelvis stable?
PROCTOR: Yes.

Assess the Genitalia/Perineum as Needed (Verbalize in Training)

Student: I am assessing the genitalia/perineum as necessary for DCAP-BTLS.
PROCTOR: The area is unremarkable.

Assess the Extremities

Inspect

Student: I am assessing the lower and upper extremities for DCAP-BTLS. Do I find anything?
PROCTOR: Yes, there is a knife in the patient's left hand. Bleeding is controlled and the knife is stabilized in position.

Palpate

Student: Do I feel anything unusual?
PROCTOR: Yes, the knife in the left hand.

Assess Motor, Sensory, and Circulatory Function

Student: I am checking for DCAP-BTLS, motor and sensory function, and pulses. Right leg?
PROCTOR: Negative DCAP-BTLS. Motor and sensory functions are present. Pulses are present.
Student: Left leg?
PROCTOR: Negative DCAP-BTLS. Motor and sensory functions are present. Pulses are present.
Student: Right arm?
PROCTOR: Negative DCAP-BTLS. Motor and sensory functions are present. Pulses are present.
Student: Left arm?
PROCTOR: Bleeding from the stabbing injury to the hand is controlled and the knife has been stabilized. Motor and sensory functions are present. Pulses are present.

Assess the Posterior

Student: We will check the back.
PROCTOR: Noted.

Assess the Thorax

Student: I am assessing the thorax. Do I find injuries?
PROCTOR: No.

▸ Assess the Lumbar Area

Student: I am assessing the flanks and lumbar area. Do I find injuries?

PROCTOR: No.

▸ Assess the Entire Backside

Student: I am assessing the entire backside. Do I find injuries?

PROCTOR: No.

▼ Manage Secondary Injuries/Wounds

Student: I would direct my partner to sling and swathe the left arm.

PROCTOR: Noted.

▼ Reassess Vital Signs

Student: I will reassess vital signs and mental status.

PROCTOR: Blood pressure, 144/96 mm Hg; pulse rate, 94 beats/min; respirations, 18 breaths/min; pulse oximetry reading, 97%; and the patient is alert.

Student: The vital signs have not changed significantly.

PROCTOR: Noted.

▼ Reassess Interventions

Student: I will reassess my interventions: oxygen, circulation, and bleeding control, stabilization of the impaled knife, and a sling and swathe.

PROCTOR: Noted.

ALS Student: I will reassess basic life support (BLS) interventions, plus the following: administer IV and pain management per local protocol if needed.

ALS Proctor: Noted.

Critical Criteria:
- ❑ Did not find or manage problems associated with airway, breathing, hemorrhage or shock (hypoperfusion)

▼ Radio Report

(Provided by the student.)

PROCTOR: Noted.

▼ Ongoing Assessment

▼ Repeat Vital Signs

Student: I will reassess vital signs and mental status.

PROCTOR: Blood pressure, 140/90 mm Hg; pulse rate, 92 beats/min; respirations, 18 breaths/min; pulse oximetry reading, 97%; and the patient is alert.

Student: The vital signs have not changed significantly.

PROCTOR: Noted.

▼ Check Interventions

Student: I will check my interventions: oxygen, circulation, and bleeding control, stabilization of the impaled knife, and a sling and swathe.

PROCTOR: Noted.

ALS Student: I will check BLS interventions, plus the following: administer IV and pain management per local protocol if needed.

ALS Proctor: Noted.

Critical Criteria:
- ❑ Did not find or manage problems associated with airway, breathing, hemorrhage or shock (hypoperfusion)

▼ Handoff Report to Emergency Department Staff

Student: There was no change in the patient's condition during transport.

PROCTOR: Noted.

Critical Criteria:
- ❑ Did not transport patient within the (10) minute time limit

▼ Critical Criteria

(Inform the student of items missed, if any.)

❑ Pass ❑ Fail Date: ______________________

Proctor Comments: ______________________

____

____

Notes

CASE 63

Dispatch Information

PROCTOR: EMS 10, respond to a head-on collision involving four patients. All patients are trapped. Police and fire/rescue are responding.

Pre-scene Action (BSI)

Student: I am wearing appropriate high-visibility personal protective equipment suitable for extrication, a helmet, extrication gloves, nonlatex gloves, safety glasses, and a mask.
PROCTOR: Noted.

Critical Criteria:
- ❑ Did not take, or verbalize, body substance isolation (BSI) precautions when necessary

Scene Size-up

Scene Safety

Student: Is the scene safe?
PROCTOR: Yes, police are on scene and have blocked traffic. Fire/rescue has stabilized the vehicle and is now completing extrication.

Mechanism of Injury

Student: What was the mechanism of injury?
PROCTOR: Motor vehicle collision. Your patient is a 32-year-old female who was a front-seat passenger. An unrestrained, obese rear-seat passenger flew forward and crushed her.

Number of Patients

Student: How many patients are there?
PROCTOR: There are four patients, but you have only this one. She has been removed from the vehicle by fire/rescue first responders and is secured to a backboard with four straps, cervical collar, and a Headbed®. First responders have given a quick handoff report that her most significant injury is the head trauma. They have stated that her backside was clear of obvious injury when she was placed on the board.

Additional Resources

Student: I would call for advanced life support (ALS) assistance.
PROCTOR: Noted.

C-Spine Stabilization

Student: The patient has already been immobilized by first responders.
PROCTOR: Noted.

Critical Criteria:
- ❑ Did not determine scene safety
- ❑ Did not assess for spinal protection
- ❑ Did not provide for spinal protection when indicated

Initial Assessment

Student: I identify myself and ask the patient not to move.
PROCTOR: Noted.

General Impression

Student: My general impression is that the patient's condition is unstable.
PROCTOR: Noted.

Responsiveness/Level of Consciousness

Student: What is the patient's level of consciousness?
PROCTOR: The patient responds to painful stimuli.

Chief Complaint/Apparent Life Threats

Student: What is the patient's chief complaint?
PROCTOR: The patient has an altered level of consciousness. She has obvious facial trauma with many teeth missing, and the face is crushed. You do see blood in the nose and mouth.
Student: There are apparent life threats; the life threats are the mechanism of injury, the altered level of consciousness, and the head trauma. I will immediately suction the mouth and remove any teeth in the airway.
PROCTOR: Noted.

Assess the Airway and Breathing

Student: I am opening the airway using the jaw-thrust maneuver. Is the patient breathing?
PROCTOR: Yes.

Assessment

Student: What are the rate and the quality of breathing?
PROCTOR: Rate: 4 breaths/min. Quality: Deep.

Provide Oxygen

Student: I am assisting ventilations with a bag-valve device with 100% oxygen and an oral/advanced airway if there is no gag reflex.
PROCTOR: Noted.
ALS Student: I will perform rapid intubation and confirm tube placement with lung sounds and end tidal CO_2.
ALS Proctor: Noted. Lung sounds and end tidal CO_2 confirm endotracheal (ET) tube placement.

Ensure Adequate Ventilation

Student: As noted earlier, I am assisting ventilation with a bag-valve device.
PROCTOR: Noted.

Injury Management

Student: I will direct my partner to take over ventilation as I continue assessment.
PROCTOR: Noted.

Assess Circulation

Student: I am assessing the patient's circulation.
PROCTOR: Noted.

Assess for and Control Major Bleeding

Student: Do I find any major bleeding?
PROCTOR: Yes, she is bleeding from her face. She has an open laceration across her forehead that is just above her eyes and is about four inches long. The skull and a skull fracture are visible.
Student: I will apply a dressing.
PROCTOR: Noted.

Assess the Pulse

Student: What are the rate and the quality of pulses?
PROCTOR: Rate: Within normal limits. Quality: Bounding.

Assess the Skin

Student: I am assessing the skin. What are the color, temperature, and condition of the skin?
PROCTOR: Color: Cyanotic. Temperature: Cool. Condition: Diaphoretic.

Identify Priority Patients/Make Transport Decision

Student: The patient is a high priority and is a load-and-go. I will complete the rapid trauma assessment and transport.
PROCTOR: Noted.

Critical Criteria:
- ❑ Did not provide high concentration of oxygen
- ❑ Did not find or manage problems associated with airway, breathing, hemorrhage or shock (hypoperfusion)
- ❑ Did not differentiate patient's need for transportation versus continued assessment at the scene
- ❑ Did other detailed examination before assessing the airway, breathing and circulation

Focused History and Physical Examination/Rapid Trauma Assessment

Select the Appropriate Assessment (Focused or Rapid)

Student: I am selecting the rapid physical exam to identify and treat life threats. I will be looking at the patient's face for a reaction to painful stimuli. I am checking for DCAP-BTLS. This acronym stands for deformities, contusions, abrasions, punctures, penetrations, paradoxical motion in the chest, and burns, tenderness, lacerations, and swelling.

PROCTOR: Noted.

Head

Student: I am rapidly assessing the head.

PROCTOR: The patient's face is crushed and many teeth are missing.

Student: I will suction the airway and insert an oral/advanced airway per local protocol.

PROCTOR: Noted.

ALS Student: I will apply basic life support (BLS) interventions, plus the following: intubation, confirm end tidal CO_2, and check lung sounds per local protocol if not already completed.

ALS Proctor: Noted. End tidal CO_2 and lung sounds confirm placement of the ET tube.

Neck

Student: I am rapidly assessing the neck.

PROCTOR: There are no obvious injuries.

Chest

Student: I am rapidly assessing the chest. What are the lung sounds?

PROCTOR: There are no obvious injuries. Lung sounds are clear bilaterally.

Abdomen/Pelvis

Student: I am rapidly assessing the abdomen.

PROCTOR: There are no obvious injuries.

Student: I am rapidly assessing the pelvis.

PROCTOR: There are no obvious injuries.

Extremities

Student: I am rapidly assessing the extremities.

PROCTOR: There are no obvious injuries.

Assess Motor, Sensory, and Circulatory Function

Student: I am checking for DCAP-BTLS, motor and sensory function, and pulses. Right leg?

PROCTOR: Negative DCAP-BTLS. Motor and sensory functions are absent. Pulses are present.

Student: Left leg?

PROCTOR: Negative DCAP-BTLS. Motor and sensory functions are absent. Pulses are present.

Student: Right arm?

PROCTOR: Negative DCAP-BTLS. Motor and sensory functions are absent. Pulses are present.

Student: Left arm?

PROCTOR: Negative DCAP-BTLS. Motor and sensory functions are absent. Pulses are present.

Posterior

Student: We will not check the back since it was previously checked and the patient is backboarded.

PROCTOR: Noted.

Manage Secondary Injuries/Wounds

Student: We will maintain the airway, ventilate, suction as needed, control bleeding, and treat for shock.

PROCTOR: Noted.

Student: Are there any changes in motor and sensory functions or pulses?

PROCTOR: No.

ALS Student: I will establish two large-bore IVs en route to the hospital and maintain a systolic blood pressure of 90 mm Hg.

ALS Proctor: Noted.

Reevaluate Transport Decision

Student: This patient is a high priority and a load-and-go due to head trauma. I will transport to a trauma center and call for a medivac per local protocol.

PROCTOR: Noted.

Baseline Vital Signs

Student: What are the patient's baseline vital signs, including blood pressure, pulse, respirations, pulse oximetry, blood glucose level, and level of consciousness?

PROCTOR: Blood pressure, 188/92 mm Hg; pulse rate, 62 beats/min; respirations per bag-valve device; pulse oximetry reading, 94%; blood glucose level, 112 mg/dL; and the patient is unresponsive.

SAMPLE History

Student: At this time I will gather a SAMPLE history from the patient or family. What are the patient's signs and symptoms?

PROCTOR: The patient is unresponsive.

Student: Allergies?

PROCTOR: Unknown.

Student: Medications?

PROCTOR: Unknown.

Student: Pertinent past medical history?

PROCTOR: Unknown.

Student: Last oral intake?

PROCTOR: Unknown.

Student: Events leading up to the incident?

PROCTOR: The patient was an unrestrained front-seat passenger. An unrestrained, obese rear-seat passenger flew forward and crushed/pinned her to the dashboard during a collision.

Critical Criteria:
- ❑ Did not differentiate patient's need for transportation versus continued assessment at the scene
- ❑ Did not provide for spinal protection when indicated

Detailed Physical Examination

Student: I am conducting the detailed physical exam. I am looking for DCAP-BTLS. I will look at the patient's face for a reaction to painful stimuli.

PROCTOR: Noted. The detailed physical exam will be performed during transport.

Assess the Head

Student: I am assessing the head. Do I find any DCAP-BTLS? Do I find any evidence of Battle's sign or raccoon eyes?

PROCTOR: You see Battle's sign.

Inspect and Palpate the Head and Ears

Student: I am assessing the head and ears.

PROCTOR: The face is deformed and depressed. Facial injuries have been addressed.

Assess the Eyes

Student: I am assessing the eyes. Are the pupils equal, round, and regular in size, and react properly to light (PEARRL)?

PROCTOR: They are nonreactive.

Assess the Facial Area Including Oral and Nasal Areas

Student: I am assessing the face, nose, and mouth. Do I see any discharge or hear any obstructions?

PROCTOR: Yes, you hear occasional gurgling.

Student: I will continue to suction the airway as needed.

PROCTOR: Noted.

ALS Student: I will reconfirm ET tube placement per end tidal CO_2, and check lung sounds.

ALS Proctor: Noted. End tidal CO_2 and lung sounds confirm placement of the ET tube.

Assess the Neck

Inspect and Palpate the Neck

Student: I am assessing the neck for DCAP-BTLS.

PROCTOR: There are no obvious injuries.

Assess for Jugular Vein Distention

Student: Do I find any jugular vein distention (JVD)?

PROCTOR: Yes.

Assess for Tracheal Deviation

Student: Do I see any tracheal deviation?

PROCTOR: No.

Assess the Chest

Student: I am assessing the chest for DCAP-BTLS.

PROCTOR: Noted.

Inspect

Student: What do I see when I look at the chest?

PROCTOR: There are no obvious injuries.

Student: Does the chest appear symmetric?

PROCTOR: Yes.

Palpate

Student: When I touch the chest, do I feel crepitus or a flail segment?

PROCTOR: No.

Auscultate

Student: Are lung sounds present in all fields?

PROCTOR: Yes.

Student: Do I hear any sucking sounds from the chest?

PROCTOR: No.

Assess the Abdomen/Pelvis

Assess the Abdomen

Student: I am assessing the abdomen for DCAP-BTLS. I am assessing all four quadrants. Do I find any problems?

PROCTOR: No.

Assess the Pelvis

Student: I am assessing the pelvis for DCAP-BTLS. Is the pelvis stable?

PROCTOR: Yes.

Assess the Genitalia/Perineum as Needed (Verbalize in Training)

Student: I am assessing the genitalia/perineum as necessary for DCAP-BTLS.

PROCTOR: The area is unremarkable.

Assess the Extremities

Inspect

Student: I am assessing the lower and upper extremities for DCAP-BTLS. Do I find anything?

PROCTOR: No.

Palpate

Student: Do I feel anything unusual?

PROCTOR: No.

Assess Motor, Sensory, and Circulatory Function

Student: I am checking for DCAP-BTLS, motor and sensory function, and pulses. Right leg?

PROCTOR: Negative DCAP-BTLS. Motor and sensory functions are absent. Pulses are present.

Student: Left leg?

PROCTOR: Negative DCAP-BTLS. Motor and sensory functions are absent. Pulses are present.

Student: Right arm?

PROCTOR: Negative DCAP-BTLS. Motor and sensory functions are absent. Pulses are present.

Student: Left arm?

PROCTOR: Negative DCAP-BTLS. Motor and sensory functions are absent. Pulses are present.

Assess the Posterior

Note: This portion of the detailed physical exam would not be done if the patient was previously backboarded per local protocol.

Student: We will not check the back because it was previously checked and the patient is backboarded.

PROCTOR: Noted.

Manage Secondary Injuries/Wounds

Student: I would direct my partner to maintain the airway, ventilate, suction as needed, and control facial bleeding.

PROCTOR: Noted.

Reassess Vital Signs

Student: I will reassess vital signs and mental status.

PROCTOR: Blood pressure, 190/94 mm Hg; pulse rate, 56 beats/min; respirations per bag-valve device; pulse oximetry reading, 96%; and the patient is unresponsive.

Student: The vital signs have not changed significantly.

PROCTOR: Noted.

Reassess Interventions

Student: I will reassess my interventions: airway, oxygen, suction, bag-valve device, oral airway/advanced airway, and immobilization and straps.

PROCTOR: Noted.

ALS Student: I will reassess BLS interventions, plus the following: ET tube placement, confirm end tidal CO_2, and lung sounds, monitor two large-bore IVs, and cardiac monitor.

ALS Proctor: Noted. The cardiac monitor shows normal sinus rhythm and end tidal CO_2 and lung sounds confirm placement of the ET tube.

Critical Criteria:

- ❑ Did not find or manage problems associated with airway, breathing, hemorrhage or shock (hypoperfusion)

Radio Report

(Provided by the student.)

PROCTOR: Noted.

Ongoing Assessment

Repeat Vital Signs

Student: I will reassess vital signs and mental status.

PROCTOR: Blood pressure, 182/86 mm Hg; pulse rate, 52 beats/min; respirations per bag-valve device; pulse oximetry reading, 97%; and the patient is unresponsive.

Student: The vital signs have not changed significantly.

PROCTOR: Noted.

Check Interventions

Student: I will check interventions: airway, oxygen, suction, bag-valve device, oral airway/advanced airway, and immobilization and straps.

PROCTOR: Noted.

ALS Student: I will check BLS interventions, plus the following: ET tube placement, confirm end tidal CO_2 and lung sounds, monitor IVs, and cardiac monitor.

ALS Proctor: Noted. The cardiac monitor shows normal sinus rhythm and end tidal CO_2 and lung sounds confirm placement of the ET tube.

Critical Criteria:

❑ Did not find or manage problems associated with airway, breathing, hemorrhage or shock (hypoperfusion)

Handoff Report to Emergency Department Staff

Student: There was no change in the patient's condition during transport.

PROCTOR: Noted.

Critical Criteria:

❑ Did not transport patient within the (10) minute time limit

Critical Criteria

(Inform the student of items missed, if any.)

❑ Pass ❑ Fail Date: ______________________

Proctor Comments: ______________________

____

____

CASE 64

Dispatch Information

PROCTOR: EMS 10, respond to 36-year-old female who has fallen from a second-story window. She is conscious and breathing.

Pre-scene Action (BSI)

Student: I am wearing nonlatex gloves and safety glasses.
PROCTOR: Noted.

Critical Criteria:
- ❑ Did not take, or verbalize, body substance isolation (BSI) precautions when necessary

Scene Size-up

Scene Safety

Student: Is the scene safe?
PROCTOR: Yes.

Mechanism of Injury

Student: What was the mechanism of injury?
PROCTOR: Fall. The patient was standing on a window air conditioner when it fell out of the window. She fell to the sidewalk, landing on her face.

Number of Patients

Student: How many patients are there?
PROCTOR: One.

Additional Resources

Student: I would call for advanced life support (ALS) assistance.
PROCTOR: Noted.

C-Spine Stabilization

Student: On the basis of the mechanism of injury, I would stabilize the cervical spine (c-spine) in a neutral in-line position.
PROCTOR: Noted.

Critical Criteria:
- ❑ Did not determine scene safety
- ❑ Did not assess for spinal protection
- ❑ Did not provide for spinal protection when indicated

Initial Assessment

Student: As I perform midline c-spine stabilization, I identify myself and ask the patient not to move.
PROCTOR: Noted.

General Impression

Student: My general impression is that the patient's condition is unstable.
PROCTOR: Noted.

Responsiveness/Level of Consciousness

Student: What is the patient's level of consciousness?
PROCTOR: Alert but combative.

Chief Complaint/Apparent Life Threats

Student: What is the patient's chief complaint?
PROCTOR: The patient is very combative and her jaw is obviously dislocated.
Student: I would call for police assistance.
PROCTOR: Noted. The police are on the scene and it is safe at this time.
Student: There are apparent life threats; the life threats are altered mental status and possible head injury.
PROCTOR: Noted.

Assess the Airway and Breathing

Student: Is the airway open? Is the patient breathing?
PROCTOR: Yes, the mouth is open and the jaw is displaced to the right side. The patient is breathing.

Assessment

Student: What are the rate and the quality of breathing?
PROCTOR: Rate: Difficult to assess due to crying. Quality: Labored with obvious drooling.
Student: I will suction as necessary.
PROCTOR: Noted.

Provide Oxygen

Student: I am applying oxygen at 15 L/min via nonrebreathing mask or by blow-by method.
PROCTOR: Noted.

Ensure Adequate Ventilation

Student: The patient has adequate ventilations at this time.
PROCTOR: Noted.

Injury Management

Student: I will direct my partner to take over c-spine control as I continue assessment.
PROCTOR: Noted.

Assess Circulation

Student: I am assessing the patient's circulation.
PROCTOR: Noted.

Assess for and Control Major Bleeding

Student: Do I find any major bleeding?
PROCTOR: No.

Assess the Pulse

Student: What are the rate and the quality of pulses?
PROCTOR: Rate: Tachycardic. Quality: Bounding.

Assess the Skin

Student: I am assessing the skin. What are the color, temperature, and condition of the skin?
PROCTOR: Color: Jaundice. Temperature: Cool. Condition: Diaphoretic.

Identify Priority Patients/Make Transport Decision

Student: The patient is a high priority and is a load-and-go. I will begin packaging and transport.
PROCTOR: Noted.

Critical Criteria:
- ❑ Did not provide high concentration of oxygen
- ❑ Did not find or manage problems associated with airway, breathing, hemorrhage or shock (hypoperfusion)
- ❑ Did not differentiate patient's need for transportation versus continued assessment at the scene
- ❑ Did other detailed examination before assessing the airway, breathing and circulation

Focused History and Physical Examination/Rapid Trauma Assessment

Select the Appropriate Assessment (Focused or Rapid)

Student: I am selecting the rapid physical exam to identify and treat life threats. I am checking for DCAP-BTLS. This acronym stands for deformities, contusions, abrasions, punctures, penetrations, paradoxical motion in the chest, and burns, tenderness, lacerations, and swelling.
PROCTOR: Noted.

Head

Student: I am rapidly assessing the head.
PROCTOR: The patient's jaw is dislocated to the right. She is breathing, crying, and drooling.

Student: I will suction as needed.
PROCTOR: Noted.

▸ **Neck**

Student: I am rapidly assessing the neck.
PROCTOR: The patient has pain in her neck.
Student: I will apply a cervical collar.
PROCTOR: Noted.

▸ **Chest**

Student: I am rapidly assessing the chest.
PROCTOR: There are no obvious injuries.

▸ **Abdomen/Pelvis**

Student: I am rapidly assessing the abdomen.
PROCTOR: There are no obvious injuries.
Student: I am rapidly assessing the pelvis.
PROCTOR: There are no obvious injuries.

▸ **Extremities**

Student: I am rapidly assessing the extremities.
PROCTOR: Minor injuries are noted.

▸ **Assess Motor, Sensory, and Circulatory Function**

Student: I am checking for DCAP-BTLS, motor and sensory function, and pulses. Right leg?
PROCTOR: The patient has bruises in various stages of healing. Motor and sensory functions are present. Pulses are present.
Student: Left leg?
PROCTOR: She has bruises in various stages of healing. Motor and sensory functions are present. Pulses are present.
Student: Right arm?
PROCTOR: She has bruises in various stages of healing. Motor and sensory functions are present. Pulses are present.
Student: Left arm?
PROCTOR: She has bruises in various stages of healing. Motor and sensory functions are present. Pulses are present.

▸ **Posterior**

Student: I will rapidly assess the back. We will now log roll the patient as a unit to check the back. The person at the head will count to three and we will roll the patient.
PROCTOR: She has bruises in various stages of healing.

▸ **Assess the Thorax**

Student: I am assessing the thorax. Do I find injuries?
PROCTOR: She has pain in her back. She has bruises in various stages of healing.

▸ **Assess the Lumbar Area**

Student: I am assessing the flanks and lumbar area. Do I find injuries?
PROCTOR: She has bruises in various stages of healing.

▸ **Assess the Entire Backside**

Student: I am assessing the entire backside. Do I find injuries?
PROCTOR: She has bruises in various stages of healing.

▸ **Manage Secondary Injuries/Wounds**

Student: We will apply a cervical collar and backboard with full immobilization per local protocol, if not yet done, at this time.
PROCTOR: Noted.
Student: Are there any changes in motor and sensory functions or pulses?
PROCTOR: No.

▸ **Reevaluate Transport Decision**

Student: This patient is a high priority and a load-and-go due to airway compromise and altered level of consciousness.
PROCTOR: Noted.

▾ Baseline Vital Signs

Student: What are the patient's baseline vital signs, including blood pressure, pulse, respirations, pulse oximetry, blood glucose level, and level of consciousness?
PROCTOR: Blood pressure, 134/82 mm Hg; pulse rate, 124 beats/min; respirations, 24 breaths/min; pulse oximetry reading, 96%; blood glucose level, 102 mg/dL; and the patient is combative.

▾ SAMPLE History

Student: At this time I will gather a SAMPLE history from the patient or family. What are the patient's signs and symptoms?
PROCTOR: She has a dislocated jaw and is complaining of neck and back pain.
Student: Allergies?
PROCTOR: No allergies.
Student: Medications?
PROCTOR: Liver pills.
Student: Pertinent past medical history?
PROCTOR: Liver disease and alcoholism.
Student: Last oral intake?
PROCTOR: 15 minutes ago.
Student: Events leading up to the incident?
PROCTOR: The patient has been drinking beer for two days. Her boyfriend was preventing her from leaving for more beer when she went out the window of the house and stood on the air conditioner. She fell to the sidewalk (about 12 feet).

Critical Criteria:
- ❑ Did not differentiate patient's need for transportation versus continued assessment at the scene
- ❑ Did not provide for spinal protection when indicated

Detailed Physical Examination

Student: I am conducting the detailed physical exam. I am looking for DCAP-BTLS.
PROCTOR: Noted. The detailed physical exam will be performed during transport.

▾ Assess the Head

Student: I am assessing the head. Do I find any DCAP-BTLS? Do I find any evidence of Battle's sign or raccoon eyes?
PROCTOR: The patient's jaw is dislocated and she is drooling heavily.
Student: I will continue to suction as needed.
PROCTOR: Noted.

▸ **Inspect and Palpate the Head and Ears**

Student: I am assessing the head and ears.
PROCTOR: She has bruises.

▸ **Assess the Eyes**

Student: I am assessing the eyes. Are the pupils equal, round, and regular in size, and react properly to light (PEARRL)?
PROCTOR: They are sluggish.

▸ **Assess the Facial Area Including Oral and Nasal Areas**

Student: I am assessing the face, nose, and mouth. Do I see any discharge or hear any obstructions?
PROCTOR: Yes, you hear occasional gurgling.
Student: I will suction as necessary.
PROCTOR: Noted.

▾ Assess the Neck

▸ **Inspect and Palpate the Neck**

Student: I am assessing the neck for DCAP-BTLS.
PROCTOR: There are no obvious injuries.

▸ **Assess for Jugular Vein Distention**

Student: Do I find any jugular vein distention (JVD)?
PROCTOR: Yes.

▸ **Assess for Tracheal Deviation**

Student: Do I see any tracheal deviation?
PROCTOR: No.

▾ Assess the Chest

Student: I am assessing the chest for DCAP-BTLS.
PROCTOR: Noted.

▸ **Inspect**

Student: What do I see when I look at the chest?
PROCTOR: She has bruises in various stages of healing.

Student: Does the chest appear symmetric?
PROCTOR: Yes.

▸ Palpate

Student: When I touch the chest, do I feel crepitus or a flail segment?
PROCTOR: No.

▸ Auscultate

Student: Are lung sounds present in all fields?
PROCTOR: Yes.
Student: Do I hear any sucking sounds from the chest?
PROCTOR: No.

▼ Assess the Abdomen/Pelvis

▸ Assess the Abdomen

Student: I am assessing the abdomen for DCAP-BTLS. I am assessing all four quadrants. Do I find any problems?
PROCTOR: No.

▸ Assess the Pelvis

Student: I am assessing the pelvis for DCAP-BTLS. Is the pelvis stable?
PROCTOR: Yes.

▼ Assess the Genitalia/Perineum as Needed (Verbalize in Training)

Student: I am assessing the genitalia/perineum as necessary for DCAP-BTLS.
PROCTOR: The area is unremarkable.

▼ Assess the Extremities

▸ Inspect

Student: I am assessing the lower and upper extremities for DCAP-BTLS. Do I find anything?
PROCTOR: The patient has bruises in various stages of healing.

▸ Palpate

Student: Do I feel anything unusual?
PROCTOR: No.

▸ Assess Motor, Sensory, and Circulatory Function

Student: I am checking for DCAP-BTLS, motor and sensory function, and pulses. Right leg?
PROCTOR: The patient has bruises in various stages of healing. Motor and sensory functions are present. Pulses are present.
Student: Left leg?
PROCTOR: She has bruises in various stages of healing. Motor and sensory functions are present. Pulses are present.
Student: Right arm?
PROCTOR: She has bruises in various stages of healing. Motor and sensory functions are present. Pulses are present.
Student: Left arm?
PROCTOR: She has bruises in various stages of healing. Motor and sensory functions are present. Pulses are present.

▼ Assess the Posterior

Note: This portion of the detailed physical exam would not be done if the patient were previously backboarded per local protocol.
Student: We will not check the back because it was previously checked and the patient is backboarded.
PROCTOR: Noted.

▼ Manage Secondary Injuries/Wounds

Student: I would direct my partner to maintain the airway, provide oxygen, and suction as necessary.
PROCTOR: Noted.

▼ Reassess Vital Signs

Student: I will reassess vital signs and mental status.
PROCTOR: Blood pressure, 130/84 mm Hg; pulse rate, 120 beats/min; respirations, 20 breaths/min; pulse oximetry reading, 97%; blood glucose level, 102 mg/dL; and the patient is combative.
Student: The vital signs have not changed significantly.
PROCTOR: Noted.

▼ Reassess Interventions

Student: I will reassess my interventions: suction, airway, breathing, and oxygen; circulation; immobilization and straps; and treat the jaw per medical control/protocol.
PROCTOR: Noted.
ALS Student: I will reassess basic life support (BLS) interventions, plus the following: establish two large-bore IVs.
ALS Proctor: Noted.

Critical Criteria:
❑ Did not find or manage problems associated with airway, breathing, hemorrhage or shock (hypoperfusion)

Radio Report

(Provided by the student.)
PROCTOR: Noted.

Ongoing Assessment

▼ Repeat Vital Signs

Student: I will reassess vital signs and mental status.
PROCTOR: Blood pressure, 132/84 mm Hg; pulse rate, 116 beats/min; respirations, 20 breaths/min; pulse oximetry reading, 97%; blood glucose level, 102 mg/dL; and the patient is combative.
Student: The vital signs have not changed significantly.
PROCTOR: Noted.

▼ Check Interventions

Student: I will check my interventions: suction, airway, breathing, and oxygen; immobilization, and straps; and treat the jaw per medical control/protocol.
PROCTOR: Noted.
ALS Student: I will check BLS interventions, plus the following: two large-bore IVs.
ALS Proctor: Noted.

Critical Criteria:
❑ Did not find or manage problems associated with airway, breathing, hemorrhage or shock (hypoperfusion)

Handoff Report to Emergency Department Staff

Student: There was no change in the patient's condition during transport.
PROCTOR: Noted.

Critical Criteria:
❑ Did not transport patient within the (10) minute time limit

Critical Criteria

(Inform the student of items missed, if any.)

❑ Pass ❑ Fail Date: ____________________

Proctor Comments: ____________________

CASE 64

Notes

CASE 65

Dispatch Information

PROCTOR: EMS 10, respond to a drive-by shooting. The patient is a 24-year-old male. He is conscious and breathing. Police are on the scene.

Pre-scene Action (BSI)

Student: I am wearing nonlatex gloves, safety glasses, mask, and gown.
PROCTOR: Noted.

Critical Criteria:
- ❑ Did not take, or verbalize, body substance isolation (BSI) precautions when necessary

Scene Size-up

Scene Safety

Student: Is the scene safe?
PROCTOR: Yes, police are on scene and you are given clearance to enter.

Mechanism of Injury

Student: What was the mechanism of injury?
PROCTOR: Gunshot wound. The patient was waiting on tables when a drive-by shooting occurred.

Number of Patients

Student: How many patients are there?
PROCTOR: One.

Additional Resources

Student: I would call for advanced life support (ALS) assistance.
PROCTOR: Noted.

C-Spine Stabilization

Student: On the basis of the mechanism of injury, I would stabilize the cervical spine (c-spine) in a neutral in-line position.
PROCTOR: Noted.

Critical Criteria:
- ❑ Did not determine scene safety
- ❑ Did not assess for spinal protection
- ❑ Did not provide for spinal protection when indicated

Initial Assessment

Student: As I perform midline c-spine stabilization, I identify myself and ask the patient not to move.
PROCTOR: Noted.

General Impression

Student: My general impression is that the patient's condition is unstable.
PROCTOR: Noted.

Responsiveness/Level of Consciousness

Student: What is the patient's level of consciousness?
PROCTOR: Alert.

Chief Complaint/Apparent Life Threats

Student: What is the patient's chief complaint?
PROCTOR: The patient is complaining of a gunshot wound to his shoulder.
Student: There is an apparent life threat; the life threat is the mechanism of injury.
PROCTOR: Noted.

Assess the Airway and Breathing

Student: Is the airway open? Is the patient breathing?
PROCTOR: Yes, the airway is open and the patient is breathing.

▸ Assessment

Student: What are the rate and the quality of breathing?
PROCTOR: Rate: Within normal limits. Quality: Normal.

▸ Provide Oxygen

Student: I am applying oxygen at 15 L/min via nonrebreathing mask.
PROCTOR: Noted.

▸ Ensure Adequate Ventilation

Student: The patient has adequate ventilations at this time.
PROCTOR: Noted.

Injury Management

Student: I will direct my partner to take over c-spine control as I continue assessment.
PROCTOR: Noted.

Assess Circulation

Student: I am assessing the patient's circulation.
PROCTOR: Noted.

▸ Assess for and Control Major Bleeding

Student: Do I find any major bleeding?
PROCTOR: No.

▸ Assess the Pulse

Student: What are the rate and the quality of pulses?
PROCTOR: Rate: Tachycardic. Quality: Normal.

▸ Assess the Skin

Student: I am assessing the skin. What are the color, temperature, and condition of the skin?
PROCTOR: Color: Normal. Temperature: Cool. Condition: Moist.

Identify Priority Patients/Make Transport Decision

Student: The patient is a high priority and is a load-and-go. I will begin packaging and transport.
PROCTOR: Noted.

Critical Criteria:
- ❑ Did not provide high concentration of oxygen
- ❑ Did not find or manage problems associated with airway, breathing, hemorrhage or shock (hypoperfusion)
- ❑ Did not differentiate patient's need for transportation versus continued assessment at the scene
- ❑ Did other detailed examination before assessing the airway, breathing and circulation

Focused History and Physical Examination/Rapid Trauma Assessment

Select the Appropriate Assessment (Focused or Rapid)

Student: I am selecting the rapid physical exam to identify and treat life threats. I am checking for DCAP-BTLS. This acronym stands for deformities, contusions, abrasions, punctures, penetrations, paradoxical motion in the chest, and burns, tenderness, lacerations, and swelling.
PROCTOR: Noted.

▸ Head

Student: I am rapidly assessing the head.
PROCTOR: He has small pieces of glass in his face from a window that was shot out.

▸ Neck

Student: I am rapidly assessing the neck.
PROCTOR: There are no obvious injuries.
Student: I will apply a cervical collar.
PROCTOR: Noted.

▸ Chest

Student: I am rapidly assessing the chest.
PROCTOR: There are no obvious injuries.

▸ Abdomen/Pelvis

Student: I am rapidly assessing the abdomen.
PROCTOR: There are no obvious injuries.
Student: I am rapidly assessing the pelvis.
PROCTOR: There are no obvious injuries.

▸ Extremities

Student: I am rapidly assessing the extremities.
PROCTOR: He has an entrance wound to the anterior right shoulder and an exit would to the posterior shoulder.

▸ Assess Motor, Sensory, and Circulatory Function

Student: I am checking for DCAP-BTLS, motor and sensory function, and pulses. Right leg?
PROCTOR: Negative DCAP-BTLS. Motor and sensory functions are present. Pulses are present.
Student: Left leg?
PROCTOR: Negative DCAP-BTLS. Motor and sensory functions are present. Pulses are present.
Student: Right arm?
PROCTOR: He has a through-and-through puncture wound to the right shoulder. The entrance is about ½ inch in diameter and the exit is about an inch in diameter. Bleeding is minimal. Motor and sensory functions are present. Pulses are present.
Student: I will apply a dressing to both the entrance and the exit wounds and sling and swathe the arm.
PROCTOR: Noted. Bleeding is controlled.
Student: Left arm?
PROCTOR: Negative DCAP-BTLS. Motor and sensory functions are present. Pulses are present.

▸ Posterior

Student: I will rapidly assess the back. We will now log roll the patient as a unit to check the back. The person at the head will count to three and we will roll the patient.
PROCTOR: Noted.

▸ Assess the Thorax

Student: I am assessing the thorax. Do I find injuries?
PROCTOR: No.

▸ Assess the Lumbar Area

Student: I am assessing the flanks and lumbar area. Do I find injuries?
PROCTOR: No.

▸ Assess the Entire Backside

Student: I am assessing the entire backside. Do I find injuries?
PROCTOR: No.

▸ Manage Secondary Injuries/Wounds

Student: We will apply a cervical collar and backboard with full immobilization per local protocol, if not yet done, at this time.
PROCTOR: Noted.
Student: Are there any changes in motor and sensory functions or pulses?
PROCTOR: No.
Student: My interventions include: oxygen; bleeding control; and immobilization and straps.
PROCTOR: Noted.
ALS Student: I will establish two large-bore IVs en route to the hospital, maintain a systolic blood pressure of 90 mm Hg, and check the cardiac monitor.
ALS Proctor: Noted. The cardiac monitor shows normal sinus rhythm.

▸ Reevaluate Transport Decision

Student: This patient is a load-and-go due to the mechanism of injury.
PROCTOR: Noted.

▾ Baseline Vital Signs

Student: What are the patient's baseline vital signs, including blood pressure, pulse, respirations, pulse oximetry, and level of consciousness?
PROCTOR: Blood pressure, 124/84 mm Hg; pulse, 100 beats/min; respirations, 18 breaths/min; pulse oximetry reading, 98%; and the patient is alert.

▾ SAMPLE History

Student: At this time I will gather a SAMPLE history from the patient or family. What are the patient's signs and symptoms?
PROCTOR: A gunshot wound to the right shoulder.
Student: Allergies?
PROCTOR: Penicillin (PCN).
Student: Medications?
PROCTOR: Asthma medications.
Student: Pertinent past medical history?
PROCTOR: Asthma.
Student: Last oral intake?
PROCTOR: 1 hour ago.
Student: Events leading up to the incident?
PROCTOR: The patient was leaning over to serve a customer when someone drove by and shot him.

Critical Criteria:
- ❑ Did not differentiate patient's need for transportation versus continued assessment at the scene
- ❑ Did not provide for spinal protection when indicated

Detailed Physical Examination

Student: I am conducting the detailed physical exam. I am looking for DCAP-BTLS.
PROCTOR: Noted. The detailed physical exam will be performed during transport.

▾ Assess the Head

Student: I am assessing the head. Do I find any DCAP-BTLS? Do I find any evidence of Battle's sign or raccoon eyes?
PROCTOR: No.

▸ Inspect and Palpate the Head and Ears

Student: I am assessing the head and ears.
PROCTOR: There are no obvious injuries.

▸ Assess the Eyes

Student: I am assessing the eyes. Are the pupils equal, round, and regular in size, and react properly to light (PEARRL)?
PROCTOR: They are PEARRL.

▸ Assess the Facial Area Including Oral and Nasal Areas

Student: I am assessing the face, nose, and mouth. Do I see any discharge or hear any obstructions?
PROCTOR: He has some minor glass fragments on his face from the window.

▾ Assess the Neck

▸ Inspect and Palpate the Neck

Student: I am assessing the neck for DCAP-BTLS.
PROCTOR: There are no obvious injuries.

▸ Assess for Jugular Vein Distention

Student: Do I find any jugular vein distention (JVD)?
PROCTOR: No.

▸ Assess for Tracheal Deviation

Student: Do I see any tracheal deviation?
PROCTOR: No.

▾ Assess the Chest

Student: I am assessing the chest for DCAP-BTLS.
PROCTOR: Noted.

▸ Inspect

Student: What do I see when I look at the chest?
PROCTOR: There are no obvious injuries.
Student: Does the chest appear symmetric?
PROCTOR: Yes.

▸ Palpate

Student: When I touch the chest, do I feel crepitus or a flail segment?
PROCTOR: No.

▸ Auscultate

Student: Are lung sounds present in all fields?
PROCTOR: Yes.
Student: Do I hear any sucking sounds from the chest?
PROCTOR: No.

▼ Assess the Abdomen/Pelvis

▸ Assess the Abdomen

Student: I am assessing the abdomen for DCAP-BTLS. I am assessing all four quadrants. Do I find any problems?
PROCTOR: No.

▸ Assess the Pelvis

Student: I am assessing the pelvis for DCAP-BTLS. Is the pelvis stable?
PROCTOR: Yes.

▼ Assess the Genitalia/Perineum as Needed (Verbalize in Training)

Student: I am assessing the genitalia/perineum as necessary for DCAP-BTLS.
PROCTOR: The area is unremarkable.

▼ Assess the Extremities

▸ Inspect

Student: I am assessing the lower and upper extremities for DCAP-BTLS. Do I find anything?
PROCTOR: No.

▸ Palpate

Student: Do I feel anything unusual?
PROCTOR: No.

▸ Assess Motor, Sensory, and Circulatory Function

Student: I am checking for DCAP-BTLS, motor and sensory function, and pulses. Right leg?
PROCTOR: Negative DCAP-BTLS. Motor and sensory functions are present. Pulses are present.
Student: Left leg?
PROCTOR: Negative DCAP-BTLS. Motor and sensory functions are present. Pulses are present.
Student: Right arm?
PROCTOR: He has a through-and-through puncture wound to the right shoulder. The entrance is about ½ inch in diameter and the exit is about an inch in diameter. Bleeding is controlled. Motor and sensory functions are present. Pulses are present.
Student: Left arm?
PROCTOR: Negative DCAP-BTLS. Motor and sensory functions are present. Pulses are present.

▼ Assess the Posterior

Note: This portion of the detailed physical exam would not be done if the patient were previously backboarded per local protocol.
Student: We will not check the back because it was previously checked and the patient is backboarded.
PROCTOR: Noted.

▼ Manage Secondary Injuries/Wounds

Student: I would direct my partner to reassess the patient's dressings.
PROCTOR: Noted.

▼ Reassess Vital Signs

Student: I will reassess vital signs and mental status.
PROCTOR: Blood pressure, 120/82 mm Hg; pulse, 96 beats/min; respirations, 18 breaths/min; pulse oximetry reading, 97%; and the patient is anxious.
Student: The vital signs have not changed significantly.
PROCTOR: Noted.

▼ Reassess Interventions

Student: I will reassess my interventions: oxygen; circulation; bleeding control; and immobilization and straps.
PROCTOR: Noted.
ALS Student: I will reassess basic life support (BLS) interventions, plus the following: monitor the two large-bore IVs and cardiac monitor.
ALS Proctor: Noted. The cardiac monitor shows normal sinus rhythm.

Critical Criteria:
❑ Did not find or manage problems associated with airway, breathing, hemorrhage or shock (hypoperfusion)

▼ Radio Report

(Provided by the student.)
PROCTOR: Noted.

▼ Ongoing Assessment

▼ Repeat Vital Signs

Student: I will reassess vital signs and mental status.
PROCTOR: Blood pressure, 122/84 mm Hg; pulse, 94 beats/min; respirations, 18 breaths/min; pulse oximetry reading, 98%; and the patient is anxious.
Student: The vital signs have not changed significantly.
PROCTOR: Noted.

▼ Check Interventions

Student: I will check my interventions: oxygen; bleeding control; and immobilization and straps.
PROCTOR: Noted.
ALS Student: I will check BLS interventions, plus the following: monitor the two large-bore IVs and cardiac monitor.
ALS Proctor: Noted. The cardiac monitor shows normal sinus rhythm.

Critical Criteria:
❑ Did not find or manage problems associated with airway, breathing, hemorrhage or shock (hypoperfusion)

▼ Handoff Report to Emergency Department Staff

Student: There was no change in the patient's condition during transport.
PROCTOR: Noted.

Critical Criteria:
❑ Did not transport patient within the (10) minute time limit

▼ Critical Criteria

(Inform the student of items missed, if any.)

❑ Pass ❑ Fail Date: ____________________

Proctor Comments: ____________________

____

____

Notes

Dispatch Information

PROCTOR: EMS 10, respond to a man shot at the mall. He has possibly been shot numerous times. It is unknown if the patient is conscious or breathing. Police have captured the suspect.

Pre-scene Action (BSI)

Student: I am wearing nonlatex gloves, safety glasses, mask, and gown.
PROCTOR: Noted.

Critical Criteria:
- ❑ Did not take, or verbalize, body substance isolation (BSI) precautions when necessary

Scene Size-up

Scene Safety

STUDENT: Is the scene safe?
PROCTOR: Yes, police are on scene and you are given clearance to enter.

Mechanism of Injury

Student: What was the mechanism of injury?
PROCTOR: Gunshot wound. The patient is a store manager who had an argument with a customer who came back with a gun.

Number of Patients

Student: How many patients are there?
PROCTOR: One.

Additional Resources

Student: I would call for advanced life support (ALS) assistance.
PROCTOR: Noted.

C-Spine Stabilization

Student: On the basis of the mechanism of injury, I would stabilize the cervical spine (c-spine) in a neutral in-line position.
PROCTOR: Noted.

Critical Criteria:
- ❑ Did not determine scene safety
- ❑ Did not assess for spinal protection
- ❑ Did not provide for spinal protection when indicated

Initial Assessment

Student: As I perform midline c-spine stabilization, I identify myself and ask the patient not to move.
PROCTOR: Noted.

General Impression

Student: My general impression is that the patient's condition is unstable.
PROCTOR: Noted.

Responsiveness/Level of Consciousness

Student: What is the patient's level of consciousness?
PROCTOR: Alert.

Chief Complaint/Apparent Life Threats

Student: What is the patient's chief complaint?
PROCTOR: The patient is complaining of blood in the mouth and difficulty breathing.
Student: I would suction the mouth and manage the airway.
PROCTOR: Noted.
Student: There are apparent life threats; the life threats are multiple gunshot wounds and airway involvement.
PROCTOR: Noted.

Assess the Airway and Breathing

Student: Is the airway open? Is the patient breathing?
PROCTOR: Yes, the airway is open and the patient is breathing.

Assessment

Student: What are the rate and the quality of breathing?
PROCTOR: Rate: He is upset and the respirations are hard to count. Quality: Shallow.

Provide Oxygen

Student: I am applying oxygen at 15 L/min via nonrebreathing mask.
PROCTOR: Noted.

Ensure Adequate Ventilation

Student: The patient has adequate ventilations at this time.
PROCTOR: Noted.

Injury Management

Student: I will direct my partner to take over c-spine control as I continue assessment.
PROCTOR: Noted.

Assess Circulation

Student: I am assessing the patient's circulation.
PROCTOR: Noted.

Assess for and Control Major Bleeding

Student: Do I find any major bleeding?
PROCTOR: Yes, the entrance wound is just above the mouth.
Student: I will apply direct pressure and a dressing to the wound.
PROCTOR: Noted.
Student: I will suction as necessary.
PROCTOR: Noted.

Assess the Pulse

Student: What are the rate and the quality of pulses?
PROCTOR: Rate: Tachycardic. Quality: Thready.

Assess the Skin

Student: I am assessing the skin. What are the color, temperature, and condition of the skin?
PROCTOR: Color: Ashen. Temperature: Cool. Condition: Diaphoretic.

Identify Priority Patients/Make Transport Decision

Student: The patient is a high priority and is a load-and-go. I will begin packaging and transport.
PROCTOR: Noted.

Critical Criteria:
- ❑ Did not provide high concentration of oxygen
- ❑ Did not find or manage problems associated with airway, breathing, hemorrhage or shock (hypoperfusion)
- ❑ Did not differentiate patient's need for transportation versus continued assessment at the scene
- ❑ Did other detailed examination before assessing the airway, breathing and circulation

Focused History and Physical Examination/Rapid Trauma Assessment

Select the Appropriate Assessment (Focused or Rapid)

Student: I am selecting the rapid physical exam to identify and treat life threats. I am checking for DCAP-BTLS. This acronym stands for deformities, contusions, abrasions, punctures, penetrations, paradoxical motion in the chest, and burns, tenderness, lacerations, and swelling.
PROCTOR: Noted.

Head

Student: I am rapidly assessing the head.
PROCTOR: You see a small puncture wound just below the nose with bleeding in the mouth.

Student: I would dress the wound, apply direct pressure, and suction the mouth as needed.
PROCTOR: Noted.

▸ Neck

Student: I am rapidly assessing the neck.
PROCTOR: There are no obvious injuries.
Student: I will apply a cervical collar.
PROCTOR: Noted.

▸ Chest

Student: I am rapidly assessing the chest.
PROCTOR: There is a small puncture wound to the right chest.
Student: I will apply an occlusive dressing to the chest.
PROCTOR: Noted.
Student: I will reassess the chest for tension pneumothorax by auscultation, and assessment (jugular vein distention [JVD], tracheal deviation, and decreased lung sounds).
PROCTOR: The lung sounds are present bilaterally, jugular vein distension is not present, and the trachea is midline.
ALS Student: I will assess the chest for hyperresonance to percussion.
ALS Proctor: Noted. There is no tension pneumothorax noted.

▸ Abdomen/Pelvis

Student: I am rapidly assessing the abdomen.
PROCTOR: There are two small puncture wounds noted.
Student: I will apply occlusive dressings.
PROCTOR: Noted.
Student: I am rapidly assessing the pelvis.
PROCTOR: There are no obvious injuries.

▸ Extremities

Student: I am rapidly assessing the extremities.
PROCTOR: There are no obvious injuries.

▸ Assess Motor, Sensory, and Circulatory Function

Student: I am checking for DCAP-BTLS. I am also checking for motor and sensory function and pulses. Right leg?
PROCTOR: Negative DCAP-BTLS. Motor and sensory functions are present. Pulses are present.
Student: Left leg?
PROCTOR: Negative DCAP-BTLS. Motor and sensory functions are present. Pulses are present.
Student: Right arm?
PROCTOR: Negative DCAP-BTLS. Motor and sensory functions are present. Pulses are present.
Student: Left arm?
PROCTOR: Negative DCAP-BTLS. Motor and sensory functions are present. Pulses are present.

▸ Posterior

Student: I will rapidly assess the back. We will now log roll the patient as a unit to check the back. The person at the head will count to three and we will roll the patient.
PROCTOR: Noted.

▸ Assess the Thorax

Student: I am assessing the thorax. Do I find injuries?
PROCTOR: No.

▸ Assess the Lumbar Area

Student: I am assessing the flanks and lumbar area. Do I find injuries?
PROCTOR: No.

▸ Assess the Entire Backside

Student: I am assessing the entire backside. Do I find injuries?
PROCTOR: No.

▸ Manage Secondary Injuries/Wounds

Student: We will apply a cervical collar and backboard with full immobilization per local protocol, if not yet done, at this time.
PROCTOR: Noted.
Student: Are there any changes in motor and sensory functions or pulses?
PROCTOR: No.
ALS Student: I will intubate and confirm tube placement with lung sounds and end tidal CO_2. I will establish two large-bore IVs en route to the hospital and maintain a systolic blood pressure of 90 mm Hg.
ALS Proctor: Noted. Lung sounds and end tidal CO_2 confirm endotracheal (ET) tube placement.

▸ Reevaluate Transport Decision

Student: This patient is a load-and-go due to airway trauma and the mechanism of injury.
PROCTOR: Noted.

▾ Baseline Vital Signs

Student: What are the patient's baseline vital signs, including blood pressure, pulse, respirations, pulse oximetry, and level of consciousness?
PROCTOR: Blood pressure, 160/100 mm Hg; pulse, 100 beats/min; respirations, 24 breaths/min; pulse oximetry reading, 98%; and the patient is alert.

▾ SAMPLE History

Student: At this time I will gather a SAMPLE history from the patient or family. What are the patient's signs and symptoms?
PROCTOR: The blood is making him sick.
Student: Allergies?
PROCTOR: Sulfa medications.
Student: Medications?
PROCTOR: Blood pressure medications that he has not been taking.
Student: Pertinent past medical history?
PROCTOR: High blood pressure.
Student: Last oral intake?
PROCTOR: 2 hours ago.
Student: Events leading up to the incident?
PROCTOR: The patient had an argument with a customer, and the customer came back to the store with a gun.

Critical Criteria:
- ❑ Did not differentiate patient's need for transportation versus continued assessment at the scene
- ❑ Did not provide for spinal protection when indicated

▾ Detailed Physical Examination

Student: I am conducting the detailed physical exam. I am looking for DCAP-BTLS.
PROCTOR: Noted. The detailed physical exam will be performed during transport.

▾ Assess the Head

Student: I am assessing the head. Do I find any DCAP-BTLS? Do I find any evidence of Battle's sign or raccoon eyes?
PROCTOR: No.

▸ Inspect and Palpate the Head and Ears

Student: I am assessing the head and ears.
PROCTOR: You see the small entrance wound just above the mouth.

▸ Assess the Eyes

Student: I am assessing the eyes. Are the pupils equal, round, and regular in size, and react properly to light (PEARRL)?
PROCTOR: They are PEARRL.

▸ Assess the Facial Area Including Oral and Nasal Areas

Student: I am assessing the face, nose, and mouth. Do I see any discharge or hear any obstructions?
PROCTOR: Bleeding is now minimal.
Student: I will suction as necessary.
PROCTOR: Noted.

▼ Assess the Neck

▸ **Inspect and Palpate the Neck**

Student: I am assessing the neck for DCAP-BTLS.

PROCTOR: There are no obvious injuries.

▸ **Assess for Jugular Vein Distention**

Student: Do I find any jugular vein distention (JVD)?

PROCTOR: No.

▸ **Assess for Tracheal Deviation**

Student: Do I see any tracheal deviation?

PROCTOR: No.

▼ Assess the Chest

Student: I am assessing the chest for DCAP-BTLS.

PROCTOR: Noted.

▸ **Inspect**

Student: What do I see when I look at the chest?

PROCTOR: You see the small puncture wound on the right chest. It has been treated with an occlusive dressing.

Student: Does the chest appear symmetric?

PROCTOR: Yes.

▸ **Palpate**

Student: When I touch the chest, do I feel crepitus or a flail segment?

PROCTOR: No.

▸ **Auscultate**

Student: Are lung sounds present in all fields?

PROCTOR: Yes.

Student: Do I hear any sucking sounds from the chest?

PROCTOR: No.

Student: I will reassess the chest for tension pneumothorax by auscultation, and assessment (jugular vein distention [JVD], tracheal deviation, and decreased lung sounds).

PROCTOR: The lung sounds are present bilaterally, jugular vein distension is not present, and the trachea is midline.

ALS Student: I will assess the chest for hyperresonance to percussion.

ALS Proctor: Noted. There is no tension pneumothorax noted.

▼ Assess the Abdomen/Pelvis

▸ **Assess the Abdomen**

Student: I am assessing the abdomen for DCAP-BTLS. I am assessing all four quadrants. Do I find any problems?

PROCTOR: You see the two small puncture wounds with minimal bleeding, but the abdomen is tender upon palpation. The patient is nauseated.

▸ **Assess the Pelvis**

Student: I am assessing the pelvis for DCAP-BTLS. Is the pelvis stable?

PROCTOR: Yes.

▼ Assess the Genitalia/Perineum as Needed (Verbalize in Training)

Student: I am assessing the genitalia/perineum as necessary for DCAP-BTLS.

PROCTOR: The area is unremarkable.

▼ Assess the Extremities

▸ **Inspect**

Student: I am assessing the lower and upper extremities for DCAP-BTLS. Do I find anything?

PROCTOR: No.

▸ **Palpate**

Student: Do I feel anything unusual?

PROCTOR: No.

▸ **Assess Motor, Sensory, and Circulatory Function**

Student: I am checking for DCAP-BTLS, motor and sensory function, and pulses. Right leg?

PROCTOR: Negative DCAP-BTLS. Motor and sensory functions are present. Pulses are present.

Student: Left leg?

PROCTOR: Negative DCAP-BTLS. Motor and sensory functions are present. Pulses are present.

Student: Right arm?

PROCTOR: Negative DCAP-BTLS. Motor and sensory functions are present. Pulses are present.

Student: Left arm?

PROCTOR: Negative DCAP-BTLS. Motor and sensory functions are present. Pulses are present.

▼ Assess the Posterior

Note: This portion of the detailed physical exam would not be done if the patient were previously backboarded per local protocol.

Student: We will not check the back because it was previously checked and the patient is backboarded.

PROCTOR: Noted.

▼ Manage Secondary Injuries/Wounds

Student: I would direct my partner to reassess the dressings and continue managing the airway.

PROCTOR: Noted.

▼ Reassess Vital Signs

Student: I will reassess vital signs and mental status.

PROCTOR: Blood pressure, 152/92 mm Hg; pulse, 110 beats/min; respirations, 24 breaths/min; pulse oximetry reading, 97%; and the patient is alert.

Student: The vital signs have not changed significantly.

PROCTOR: Noted.

▼ Reassess Interventions

Student: I will reassess my interventions: airway, breathing, and oxygen; occlusive dressings; circulation and bleeding control; and immobilization and straps.

PROCTOR: Noted.

ALS Student: I will reassess basic life support (BLS) interventions, plus the following: two large-bore IVs, cardiac monitor, and intubate and confirm end tidal CO_2 and lung sounds if necessary.

ALS Proctor: Noted. The cardiac monitor shows sinus tachycardia and end tidal CO_2 and lung sounds confirm placement of the endotracheal (ET) tube.

Critical Criteria:

❑ Did not find or manage problems associated with airway, breathing, hemorrhage or shock (hypoperfusion)

▼ Radio Report

(Provided by the student.)

PROCTOR: Noted.

Ongoing Assessment

Repeat Vital Signs

Student: I will reassess vital signs and mental status.

PROCTOR: Blood pressure, 144/80 mm Hg; pulse, 120 beats/min; respirations, 20 breaths/min; pulse oximetry reading, 94%; and the patient is alert.

Student: The vital signs have deteriorated.

PROCTOR: Noted.

Check Interventions

Student: I will check my interventions: airway, breathing, and oxygen; occlusive dressings; circulation and bleeding control; and immobilization and straps.

PROCTOR: Noted.

ALS Student: I will check BLS interventions, plus the following: two large-bore IVs, cardiac monitor, and intubate and confirm end tidal CO_2 and lung sounds if necessary.

ALS Proctor: Noted. The cardiac monitor shows sinus tachycardia and end tidal CO_2 and lung sounds confirm placement of the ET tube.

Critical Criteria:
- ❑ Did not find or manage problems associated with airway, breathing, hemorrhage or shock (hypoperfusion)

Handoff Report to Emergency Department Staff

Student: The patient's condition deteriorated during transport.

PROCTOR: Noted.

Critical Criteria:
- ❑ Did not transport patient within the (10) minute time limit

Critical Criteria

(Inform the student of items missed, if any.)

❑ Pass ❑ Fail Date: ____________________

Proctor Comments: ____________________

Dispatch Information

PROCTOR: EMS 10, respond to a tractor that has rolled over on a farm. The 50-year-old farmer appears to be under the tractor. The status of his breathing and consciousness is unknown.

Pre-scene Action (BSI)

Student: I am wearing appropriate high-visibility personal protective equipment suitable for extrication, a helmet, extrication gloves, nonlatex gloves, safety glasses, and a mask.
PROCTOR: Noted.

Critical Criteria:
- ❑ Did not take, or verbalize, body substance isolation (BSI) precautions when necessary

Scene Size-up

▼ Scene Safety

Student: Is the scene safe?
PROCTOR: Yes.

▼ Mechanism of Injury

Student: What was the mechanism of injury?
PROCTOR: Blunt and penetrating trauma. The patient was cutting grass on a hill when the tractor rolled over. The yoke of the tractor has impaled the farmer through the head.

▼ Number of Patients

Student: How many patients are there?
PROCTOR: One.

▼ Additional Resources

Student: I would call for advanced life support (ALS) assistance and additional resources: fire/rescue (heavy rescue).
PROCTOR: Noted.

▼ C-Spine Stabilization

Student: On the basis of the mechanism of injury, I would stabilize the cervical spine (c-spine) in a neutral in-line position.
PROCTOR: Noted.

Critical Criteria:
- ❑ Did not determine scene safety
- ❑ Did not assess for spinal protection
- ❑ Did not provide for spinal protection when indicated

Initial Assessment

Student: As I perform midline c-spine stabilization, I identify myself and ask the patient not to move.
PROCTOR: Noted.

▼ General Impression

Student: My general impression is that the patient's condition is unstable.
PROCTOR: Noted.

▼ Responsiveness/Level of Consciousness

Student: What is the patient's level of consciousness?
PROCTOR: Unresponsive.

▼ Chief Complaint/Apparent Life Threats

Student: What is the patient's chief complaint?
PROCTOR: The patient is unresponsive.
Student: There are apparent life threats; the life threats are head and spinal injuries and the mechanism of injury.
PROCTOR: Noted.

▼ Assess the Airway and Breathing

Student: Is the airway open? Is the patient breathing?
PROCTOR: Yes, the airway is open and the patient is breathing. You hear some gurgling.
Student: I will suction as necessary.
PROCTOR: Noted.

▸ Assessment

Student: What are the rate and the quality of breathing?
PROCTOR: Rate: Bradypneic. Quality: Diaphragmatic.

▸ Provide Oxygen

Student: I am inserting an oral/advanced airway and assisting ventilations with a bag-valve device with 100% oxygen.
PROCTOR: Noted.
ALS Student: I will intubate and confirm tube placement with lung sounds and end tidal CO_2.
ALS Proctor: Noted. Lung sounds and end tidal CO_2 confirm endotracheal (ET) tube placement.

▸ Ensure Adequate Ventilation

Student: As noted earlier, I am assisting ventilation with a bag-valve device.
PROCTOR: Noted.

▼ Injury Management

Student: I will direct my partner to take over ventilation, suction, and c-spine control as I continue assessment.
PROCTOR: Noted.

▼ Assess Circulation

Student: I am assessing the patient's circulation.
PROCTOR: Noted.

▸ Assess for and Control Major Bleeding

Student: Do I find any major bleeding?
PROCTOR: No.

▸ Assess the Pulse

Student: What are the rate and the quality of pulses?
PROCTOR: Rate: Within normal limits. Quality: Bounding.

▸ Assess the Skin

Student: I am assessing the skin. What are the color, temperature, and condition of the skin?
PROCTOR: Color: Cyanotic. Temperature: Cool. Condition: Diaphoretic.

▼ Identify Priority Patients/Make Transport Decision

Student: The patient is a high priority and is a load-and-go. I will begin packaging and transport to a trauma center.
PROCTOR: Noted.

Critical Criteria:
- ❑ Did not provide high concentration of oxygen
- ❑ Did not find or manage problems associated with airway, breathing, hemorrhage or shock (hypoperfusion)
- ❑ Did not differentiate patient's need for transportation versus continued assessment at the scene
- ❑ Did other detailed examination before assessing the airway, breathing and circulation

Focused History and Physical Examination/Rapid Trauma Assessment

▼ Select the Appropriate Assessment (Focused or Rapid)

Student: I am selecting the rapid physical exam to identify and treat life threats. I am checking for DCAP-BTLS. This acronym stands for deformities, contusions, abrasions, punctures, penetrations, paradoxical motion in the chest, and burns, tenderness, lacerations, and swelling.
PROCTOR: Noted.

▸ **Head**

Student: I am rapidly assessing the head.

PROCTOR: The yoke entered the right side of the head in the temporal region.

Student: I will stabilize the yoke to the head while protecting the c-spine. I will have the fire/rescue team remove the yoke from the tractor.

PROCTOR: Noted.

▸ **Neck**

Student: I am rapidly assessing the neck.

PROCTOR: There is deformity to the base of the neck.

Student: I will apply a cervical collar.

PROCTOR: Noted.

▸ **Chest**

Student: I am rapidly assessing the chest.

PROCTOR: The breathing is diaphragmatic, but clear.

Student: My partner is ventilating with a bag-valve device.

PROCTOR: Noted.

▸ **Abdomen/Pelvis**

Student: I am rapidly assessing the abdomen.

PROCTOR: There are no obvious injuries.

Student: I am rapidly assessing the pelvis.

PROCTOR: There are no obvious injuries.

▸ **Extremities**

Student: I am rapidly assessing the extremities.

PROCTOR: There are no obvious injuries.

▸ **Assess Motor, Sensory, and Circulatory Function**

Student: I am checking for DCAP-BTLS, motor and sensory function, and pulses. Right leg?

PROCTOR: Negative DCAP-BTLS. Motor and sensory functions are absent. Pulses are present.

Student: Left leg?

PROCTOR: Negative DCAP-BTLS. Motor and sensory functions are absent. Pulses are present.

Student: Right arm?

PROCTOR: Negative DCAP-BTLS. Motor and sensory functions are absent. Pulses are present.

Student: Left arm?

PROCTOR: Negative DCAP-BTLS. Motor and sensory functions are absent. Pulses are present.

▸ **Posterior**

Student: I will rapidly assess the back. We will now log roll the patient as a unit to check the back. The person at the head will count to three and we will roll the patient.

PROCTOR: Noted.

▸ **Assess the Thorax**

Student: I am assessing the thorax. Do I find injuries?

PROCTOR: Yes, there is a deformity to the base of the neck/top of the rib cage.

▸ **Assess the Lumbar Area**

Student: I am assessing the flanks and lumbar area. Do I find injuries?

PROCTOR: Yes, there appears to be a deformity to the spine of the lumbar region.

▸ **Assess the Entire Backside**

Student: I am assessing the entire backside. Do I find injuries?

PROCTOR: You see the deformity to the base of the neck and the lumbar region.

▸ **Manage Secondary Injuries/Wounds**

Student: We have inserted an oral/advanced airway and are providing ventilation with a bag-valve device. We will suction as necessary. We have stabilized the yoke to the head and removed the yoke from the tractor. We will apply a cervical collar and backboard with full immobilization per local protocol, if not yet done, at this time.

PROCTOR: Noted.

ALS Student: I will reassess the placement of the ET tube through lung sounds and end tidal CO_2. I will establish two large-bore IVs en route to the hospital to maintain a systolic blood pressure of 90 mm Hg.

ALS Proctor: Noted. The lung sounds and end tidal CO_2 confirm tube placement.

Student: Are there any changes in motor and sensory functions or pulses?

PROCTOR: No.

▸ **Reevaluate Transport Decision**

Student: This patient is a load-and-go due to head trauma. I will transport to a trauma center if available and/or via medical helicopter.

PROCTOR: Noted.

▾ Baseline Vital Signs

Student: What are the patient's baseline vital signs, including blood pressure, pulse, respirations, pulse oximetry, blood glucose level, and level of consciousness?

PROCTOR: Blood pressure, 180/98 mm Hg; pulse rate, 78 beats/min; respirations per bag-valve device; pulse oximetry reading, 92%; blood glucose level, 122 mg/dL; and the patient is unresponsive.

▾ SAMPLE History

Student: At this time I will gather a SAMPLE history from the patient or family. What are the patient's signs and symptoms?

PROCTOR: The patient is unresponsive.

Student: Allergies?

PROCTOR: Unknown.

Student: Medications?

PROCTOR: Unknown.

Student: Pertinent past medical history?

PROCTOR: Unknown.

Student: Last oral intake?

PROCTOR: Unknown.

Student: Events leading up to the incident?

PROCTOR: Unknown.

Critical Criteria:

- ❑ Did not differentiate patient's need for transportation versus continued assessment at the scene
- ❑ Did not provide for spinal protection when indicated

▼ Detailed Physical Examination

Student: I am conducting the detailed physical exam. I am looking for DCAP-BTLS.

PROCTOR: Noted. The detailed physical exam will be performed during transport.

▾ Assess the Head

Student: I am assessing the head. Do I find any DCAP-BTLS? Do I find any evidence of Battle's sign or raccoon eyes?

PROCTOR: You see the yoke entering the right temple area and impaled to a depth of about 4 inches. It has been stabilized to the head and bleeding is controlled.

▸ **Inspect and Palpate the Head and Ears**

Student: I am assessing the head and ears.

PROCTOR: The skull is depressed. It has been adequately treated.

▸ **Assess the Eyes**

Student: I am assessing the eyes. Are the pupils equal, round, and regular in size, and react properly to light (PEARRL)?

PROCTOR: They are nonreactive.

▸ **Assess the Facial Area Including Oral and Nasal Areas**

Student: I am assessing the face, nose, and mouth. Do I see any discharge or hear any obstructions?

PROCTOR: Yes, you hear gurgling.

Student: I will suction the airway as needed and reassess the oral airway or advanced airway.

PROCTOR: Noted.

ALS Student: I will apply basic life support (BLS) interventions, plus the following: confirm end tidal CO_2, and check lung sounds.

ALS Proctor: Noted. End tidal CO_2 and lung sounds confirm placement of the ET tube.

▾ Assess the Neck

▸ **Inspect and Palpate the Neck**

Student: I am assessing the neck for DCAP-BTLS.

PROCTOR: There was a deformity to the base of the neck. A cervical collar is in place.

▸ **Assess for Jugular Vein Distention**

Student: Do I find any jugular vein distention (JVD)?

PROCTOR: Yes.

▸ **Assess for Tracheal Deviation**

Student: Do I see any tracheal deviation?

PROCTOR: No.

▾ Assess the Chest

Student: I am assessing the chest for DCAP-BTLS.

PROCTOR: Noted.

▸ **Inspect**

Student: What do I see when I look at the chest?

PROCTOR: You see diaphragmatic breathing.

Student: Does the chest appear symmetric?

PROCTOR: Yes.

▸ **Palpate**

Student: When I touch the chest, do I feel crepitus or a flail segment?

PROCTOR: No.

▸ **Auscultate**

Student: Are lung sounds present in all fields?

PROCTOR: Yes.

Student: Do I hear any sucking sounds from the chest?

PROCTOR: No.

▾ Assess the Abdomen/Pelvis

▸ **Assess the Abdomen**

Student: I am assessing the abdomen for DCAP-BTLS. I am assessing all four quadrants. Do I find any problems?

PROCTOR: No.

▸ **Assess the Pelvis**

Student: I am assessing the pelvis for DCAP-BTLS. Is the pelvis stable?

PROCTOR: Yes.

▾ Assess the Genitalia/Perineum as Needed (Verbalize in Training)

Student: I am assessing the genitalia/perineum as necessary for DCAP-BTLS.

PROCTOR: The area is unremarkable.

▾ Assess the Extremities

▸ **Inspect**

Student: I am assessing the lower and upper extremities for DCAP-BTLS. Do I find anything?

PROCTOR: No.

▸ **Palpate**

Student: Do I feel anything unusual?

PROCTOR: No.

▸ **Assess Motor, Sensory, and Circulatory Function**

Student: I am checking for DCAP-BTLS, motor and sensory function, and pulses. Right leg?

PROCTOR: Negative DCAP-BTLS. Motor and sensory functions are absent. Pulses are present.

Student: Left leg?

PROCTOR: Negative DCAP-BTLS. Motor and sensory functions are absent. Pulses are present.

Student: Right arm?

PROCTOR: Negative DCAP-BTLS. Motor and sensory functions are absent. Pulses are present.

Student: Left arm?

PROCTOR: Negative DCAP-BTLS. Motor and sensory functions are absent. Pulses are present.

▾ Assess the Posterior

Note: This portion of the detailed physical exam would not be done if the patient were previously backboarded per local protocol.

Student: We will not check the back because it was previously checked and the patient is backboarded.

PROCTOR: Noted.

▾ Manage Secondary Injuries/Wounds

Student: I would direct my partner to monitor the airway and provide ventilation.

PROCTOR: Noted.

▾ Reassess Vital Signs

Student: I will reassess vital signs and mental status.

PROCTOR: Blood pressure, 176/92 mm Hg; pulse rate, 70 beats/min; respirations per bag-valve device; pulse oximetry reading, 94%; and the patient is unresponsive.

Student: The vital signs have not changed significantly.

PROCTOR: Noted.

▾ Reassess Interventions

Student: I will reassess my interventions: airway, oral airway/advanced airway, bag-valve device ventilations, and oxygen; suction and bleeding control; stabilization of the impaled object; and immobilization and straps.

PROCTOR: Noted.

ALS Student: I will reassess BLS interventions, plus the following: confirm ET tube placement with end tidal CO_2, check lung sounds, monitor the two large-bore IVs, and cardiac monitor.

ALS Proctor: Noted. The cardiac monitor shows normal sinus rhythm and end tidal CO_2 and lung sounds confirm placement of the ET tube.

Critical Criteria:

❑ Did not find or manage problems associated with airway, breathing, hemorrhage or shock (hypoperfusion)

▾ Radio Report

(Provided by the student.)

PROCTOR: Noted.

Ongoing Assessment

Repeat Vital Signs

Student: I will reassess vital signs and mental status.

PROCTOR: Blood pressure, 182/94 mm Hg; pulse rate, 74 beats/min; respirations per bag-valve device; pulse oximetry reading, 95%; and the patient is unresponsive.

Student: The vital signs have not changed significantly.

PROCTOR: Noted.

Check Interventions

Student: I will check my interventions: airway, oral airway/advanced airway, bag-valve device ventilations, and oxygen; suction and bleeding control; stabilization of the impaled object; and immobilization and straps.

PROCTOR: Noted.

ALS Student: I will check BLS interventions, plus the following: intubate, confirm ET tube placement with end tidal CO_2, check lung sounds, monitor the two large-bore IVs, and cardiac monitor.

ALS Proctor: Noted. The cardiac monitor shows normal sinus rhythm and end tidal CO_2 and lung sounds confirm placement of the ET tube.

Critical Criteria:

❑ Did not find or manage problems associated with airway, breathing, hemorrhage or shock (hypoperfusion)

Handoff Report to Emergency Department Staff

Student: There was no change in the patient's condition during transport.

PROCTOR: Noted.

Critical Criteria:

❑ Did not transport patient within the (10) minute time limit

Critical Criteria

(Inform the student of items missed, if any.)

❑ Pass ❑ Fail Date: ____________________

Proctor Comments: ____________________

____

____

Dispatch Information

PROCTOR: EMS 10, respond to a 24-year-old factory worker who has been shocked by high voltage. He is conscious and breathing.

Pre-scene Action (BSI)

Student: I am wearing nonlatex gloves and safety glasses.
PROCTOR: Noted.

Critical Criteria:
- ❑ Did not take, or verbalize, body substance isolation (BSI) precautions when necessary

Scene Size-up

Scene Safety

Student: Is the scene safe?
PROCTOR: Yes.

Mechanism of Injury

Student: What was the mechanism of injury?
PROCTOR: Electric shock. The patient was activating a high-voltage knife throw switch without the required gloves or safety pole when it arced and shocked him.

Number of Patients

Student: How many patients are there?
PROCTOR: One.

Additional Resources

Student: I would call for advanced life support (ALS) assistance.
PROCTOR: Noted.

C-Spine Stabilization

Student: On the basis of the mechanism of injury, I would stabilize the cervical spine (c-spine) in a neutral in-line position.
PROCTOR: Noted.

Critical Criteria:
- ❑ Did not determine scene safety
- ❑ Did not assess for spinal protection
- ❑ Did not provide for spinal protection when indicated

Initial Assessment

Student: As I perform midline c-spine stabilization, I identify myself and ask the patient not to move.
PROCTOR: Noted.

General Impression

Student: My general impression is that the patient's condition is unstable.
PROCTOR: Noted.

Responsiveness/Level of Consciousness

Student: What is the patient's level of consciousness?
PROCTOR: Alert and anxious.

Chief Complaint/Apparent Life Threats

Student: What is the patient's chief complaint?
PROCTOR: The patient is complaining of extreme pain in the hand, uncontrolled shaking, chest pain, and a feeling of impending doom.
Student: There is an apparent life threat; the life threat is electrocution.
PROCTOR: Noted.

Assess the Airway and Breathing

Student: Is the airway open? Is the patient breathing?
PROCTOR: Yes, the airway is open and the patient is breathing.

Assessment

Student: What are the rate and the quality of breathing?
PROCTOR: Rate: Tachypneic. Quality: Deep.

Provide Oxygen

Student: I am applying oxygen at 15 L/min via nonrebreathing mask.
PROCTOR: Noted.

Ensure Adequate Ventilation

Student: The patient has adequate ventilations at this time.
PROCTOR: Noted.

Injury Management

Student: I will direct my partner to maintain c-spine control as I continue assessment.
PROCTOR: Noted.

Assess Circulation

Student: I am assessing the patient's circulation.
PROCTOR: Noted.

Assess for and Control Major Bleeding

Student: Do I find any major bleeding?
PROCTOR: No.

Assess the Pulse

Student: What are the rate and the quality of pulses?
PROCTOR: Rate: Tachycardic. Quality: Bounding and irregular.

Assess the Skin

Student: I am assessing the skin. What are the color, temperature, and condition of the skin?
PROCTOR: Color: Pasty white. Temperature: Cool. Condition: Diaphoretic.

Identify Priority Patients/Make Transport Decision

Student: The patient is a high priority and is a load-and-go. I will begin packaging and transport.
PROCTOR: Noted.

Critical Criteria:
- ❑ Did not provide high concentration of oxygen
- ❑ Did not find or manage problems associated with airway, breathing, hemorrhage or shock (hypoperfusion)
- ❑ Did not differentiate patient's need for transportation versus continued assessment at the scene
- ❑ Did other detailed examination before assessing the airway, breathing and circulation

Focused History and Physical Examination/Rapid Trauma Assessment

Select the Appropriate Assessment (Focused or Rapid)

Student: I am selecting the rapid physical exam to identify and treat life threats. I will remove all of the patient's clothing to find exit wounds. I am checking for DCAP-BTLS. This acronym stands for deformities, contusions, abrasions, punctures, penetrations, paradoxical motion in the chest, and burns, tenderness, lacerations, and swelling.
PROCTOR: Noted.

Head

Student: I am rapidly assessing the head.
PROCTOR: There are no obvious injuries.

Neck

Student: I am rapidly assessing the neck.
PROCTOR: There are no obvious injuries.
Student: I will apply a cervical collar.
PROCTOR: Noted.

Chest

Student: I am rapidly assessing the chest. What are the lung sounds?
PROCTOR: There are no obvious injuries. Lung sounds are clear bilaterally.

▸ Abdomen/Pelvis

Student: I am rapidly assessing the abdomen.
PROCTOR: There are no obvious injuries.
Student: I am rapidly assessing the pelvis.
PROCTOR: There are no obvious injuries.

▸ Extremities

Student: I am rapidly assessing the extremities.
PROCTOR: There is an entrance wound on the palm of the right hand and an explosive exit on the back of the right hand. There is no bleeding noted. The hand looks cooked.
Student: I will treat this injury while en route to the hospital.
PROCTOR: Noted.

▸ Assess Motor, Sensory, and Circulatory Function

Student: I am checking for DCAP-BTLS, motor and sensory function, and pulses. Right leg?
PROCTOR: Negative DCAP-BTLS. Motor and sensory functions are present. Pulses are present.
Student: Left leg?
PROCTOR: Negative DCAP-BTLS. Motor and sensory functions are present. Pulses are present.
Student: Right arm?
PROCTOR: The entrance wound is on the palm and the explosive exit wound is on the back of the hand. The bones of the hand are visible and appear "cooked." Motor and sensory functions are present. Pulses are present.
Student: I would dress the injuries with dry dressings per local protocol.
PROCTOR: Noted.
Student: Left arm?
PROCTOR: Negative DCAP-BTLS. Motor and sensory functions are present. Pulses are present.

▸ Posterior

Student: I will rapidly assess the back. We will now log roll the patient as a unit to check the back. The person at the head will count to three and we will roll the patient.
PROCTOR: Noted.

▸ Assess the Thorax

Student: I am assessing the thorax. Do I find injuries?
PROCTOR: No.

▸ Assess the Lumbar Area

Student: I am assessing the flanks and lumbar area. Do I find injuries?
PROCTOR: No.

▸ Assess the Entire Backside

Student: I am assessing the entire backside. Do I find injuries?
PROCTOR: No.

▸ Manage Secondary Injuries/Wounds

Student: We will apply a cervical collar and backboard with full immobilization per local protocol, if not yet done, at this time.
PROCTOR: Noted.
Student: Are there any changes in motor and sensory functions or pulses?
PROCTOR: No.
ALS Student: I will establish two large-bore IVs en route to the hospital and maintain a systolic blood pressure of 90 mm Hg. I will also establish cardiac monitoring and a 12-lead ECG.
ALS Proctor: Noted. The cardiac monitor shows sinus tachycardia.

▸ Reevaluate Transport Decision

Student: This patient is a high priority and a load-and-go due to the mechanism of injury.
PROCTOR: Noted.

▾ Baseline Vital Signs

Student: What are the patient's baseline vital signs, including blood pressure, pulse, respirations, pulse oximetry, blood glucose level, and level of consciousness?
PROCTOR: Blood pressure, 200/90 mm Hg; pulse rate, 136 beats/min; respirations, 24 breaths/min; pulse oximetry reading, 97%; blood glucose level, 114 mg/dL; and the patient is anxious.

▾ SAMPLE History

Student: At this time I will gather a SAMPLE history from the patient or family. What are the patient's signs and symptoms?
PROCTOR: Chest pain, pins and needles sensation all over, muscle tremors, and burns to the right hand.
Student: Allergies?
PROCTOR: No allergies.
Student: Medications?
PROCTOR: No medications.
Student: Pertinent past medical history?
PROCTOR: No pertinent medical history.
Student: Last oral intake?
PROCTOR: 5 hours ago.
Student: Events leading up to the incident?
PROCTOR: The patient was turning on a 700-volt knife-type switch when it flashed and shocked him.

Critical Criteria:
- ❑ Did not differentiate patient's need for transportation versus continued assessment at the scene
- ❑ Did not provide for spinal protection when indicated

Detailed Physical Examination

Student: I am conducting the detailed physical exam. I am looking for DCAP-BTLS.
PROCTOR: Noted. The detailed physical exam will be performed during transport.

▾ Assess the Head

Student: I am assessing the head. Do I find any DCAP-BTLS? Do I find any evidence of Battle's sign or raccoon eyes?
PROCTOR: No.

▸ Inspect and Palpate the Head and Ears

Student: I am assessing the head and ears.
PROCTOR: There are no obvious injuries.

▸ Assess the Eyes

Student: I am assessing the eyes. Are the pupils equal, round, and regular in size, and react properly to light (PEARRL)?
PROCTOR: They are PEARRL.

▸ Assess the Facial Area Including Oral and Nasal Areas

Student: I am assessing the face, nose, and mouth. Do I see any discharge or hear any obstructions?
PROCTOR: No.

▾ Assess the Neck

▸ Inspect and Palpate the Neck

Student: I am assessing the neck for DCAP-BTLS.
PROCTOR: There are no obvious injuries.

▸ Assess for Jugular Vein Distention

Student: Do I find any jugular vein distention (JVD)?
PROCTOR: Yes.

▸ Assess for Tracheal Deviation

Student: Do I see any tracheal deviation?
PROCTOR: No.

▼ Assess the Chest

Student: I am assessing the chest for DCAP-BTLS.

PROCTOR: Noted.

▸ **Inspect**

Student: What do I see when I look at the chest?

PROCTOR: There are no obvious injuries.

Student: Does the chest appear symmetric?

PROCTOR: Yes.

▸ **Palpate**

Student: When I touch the chest, do I feel crepitus or a flail segment?

PROCTOR: No.

▸ **Auscultate**

Student: Are lung sounds present in all fields?

PROCTOR: Yes.

Student: Do I hear any sucking sounds from the chest?

PROCTOR: No.

▼ Assess the Abdomen/Pelvis

▸ **Assess the Abdomen**

Student: I am assessing the abdomen for DCAP-BTLS. I am assessing all four quadrants. Do I find any problems?

PROCTOR: No.

▸ **Assess the Pelvis**

Student: I am assessing the pelvis for DCAP-BTLS. Is the pelvis stable?

PROCTOR: Yes.

▼ Assess the Genitalia/Perineum as Needed (Verbalize in Training)

Student: I am assessing the genitalia/perineum as necessary for DCAP-BTLS.

PROCTOR: The area is unremarkable.

▼ Assess the Extremities

▸ **Inspect**

Student: I am assessing the lower and upper extremities for DCAP-BTLS. Do I find anything?

PROCTOR: The right hand has an entrance wound on the palm and an explosive exit wound on the back of the hand. The bones of the hand are visible and appear "cooked."

▸ **Palpate**

Student: Do I feel anything unusual?

PROCTOR: No.

▸ **Assess Motor, Sensory, and Circulatory Function**

Student: I am checking for DCAP-BTLS, motor and sensory function, and pulses. Right leg?

PROCTOR: Negative DCAP-BTLS. Motor and sensory functions are present. Pulses are present.

Student: Left leg?

PROCTOR: Negative DCAP-BTLS. Motor and sensory functions are present. Pulses are present.

Student: Right arm?

PROCTOR: The entrance wound on the palm and the explosive exit wound on the back of the hand. Motor and sensory functions are present. Pulses are present.

Student: I will dress the hand with a dry sterile dressing and apply a splint, sling, and swathe.

PROCTOR: Noted.

Student: Left arm?

PROCTOR: Negative DCAP-BTLS. Motor and sensory functions are present. Pulses are present.

▼ Assess the Posterior

Note: This portion of the detailed physical exam would not be done if the patient were previously backboarded per local protocol.

Student: We will not check the back because it was previously checked and the patient is backboarded.

PROCTOR: Noted.

▼ Manage Secondary Injuries/Wounds

Student: I would direct my partner to monitor the patient.

PROCTOR: Noted.

▼ Reassess Vital Signs

Student: I will reassess vital signs and mental status.

PROCTOR: Blood pressure, 190/82 mm Hg; pulse rate, 124 beats/min; respirations, 24 breaths/min; pulse oximetry reading, 98%; and the patient is alert.

Student: The vital signs have not changed significantly.

PROCTOR: Noted.

▼ Reassess Interventions

Student: I will reassess my interventions: oxygen, burn dressing per protocol, and reassurance.

PROCTOR: Noted.

ALS Student: I will reassess basic life support (BLS) interventions, plus the following: two large-bore IVs, cardiac monitor, and 12-lead ECG, and pain management per local protocol.

ALS Proctor: Noted. The cardiac monitor shows sinus tachycardia with occasional premature ventricular complexes.

Critical Criteria:
- ❑ Did not find or manage problems associated with airway, breathing, hemorrhage or shock (hypoperfusion)

▼ Radio Report

(Provided by the student.)

PROCTOR: Noted.

▼ Ongoing Assessment

▼ Repeat Vital Signs

Student: I will reassess vital signs and mental status.

PROCTOR: Blood pressure, 178/78 mm Hg; pulse rate, 118 beats/min; respirations, 24 breaths/min; pulse oximetry reading, 98%; and the patient is alert.

Student: The vital signs have improved.

PROCTOR: Noted.

▼ Check Interventions

Student: I will check interventions: oxygen, burn dressing per protocol, and reassurance.

PROCTOR: Noted.

ALS Student: I will check BLS interventions, plus the following: two large-bore IVs, cardiac monitor, 12-lead ECG, and pain management per local protocol.

ALS Proctor: Noted. The cardiac monitor shows sinus tachycardia with occasional premature ventricular complexes.

Critical Criteria:
- ❑ Did not find or manage problems associated with airway, breathing, hemorrhage or shock (hypoperfusion)

Handoff Report to Emergency Department Staff

Student: The patient's condition improved during transport.
PROCTOR: Noted.

Critical Criteria:
❑ Did not transport patient within the (10) minute time limit

Critical Criteria

(Inform the student of items missed, if any.)

❑ Pass ❑ Fail Date: ____________________

Proctor Comments: ____________________

____

____

Dispatch Information

PROCTOR: EMS 10, respond to a 17-year-old male who was struck in the head with a baseball bat. He is unconscious. It is unknown if he is breathing. Police officers are en route.

Pre-scene Action (BSI)

Student: I am wearing nonlatex gloves, safety glasses, mask, and gown.
PROCTOR: Noted.

Critical Criteria:
- ❑ Did not take, or verbalize, body substance isolation (BSI) precautions when necessary

Scene Size-up

Scene Safety

Student: Is the scene safe?
PROCTOR: Yes, police are on scene and you are given clearance to enter.

Mechanism of Injury

Student: What was the mechanism of injury?
PROCTOR: Blunt head trauma. The patient was breaking into a home. He had broken a window and was climbing in when the elderly homeowner struck him with a baseball bat and knocked the patient into the yard.

Number of Patients

Student: How many patients are there?
PROCTOR: One.

Additional Resources

Student: I would call for advanced life support (ALS) assistance.
PROCTOR: Noted.

C-Spine Stabilization

Student: On the basis of the mechanism of injury, I would stabilize the cervical spine (c-spine) in a neutral in-line position.
PROCTOR: Noted.

Critical Criteria:
- ❑ Did not determine scene safety
- ❑ Did not assess for spinal protection
- ❑ Did not provide for spinal protection when indicated

Initial Assessment

Student: As I perform midline c-spine stabilization, I identify myself and ask the patient not to move.
PROCTOR: Noted.

General Impression

Student: My general impression is that the patient's condition is unstable.
PROCTOR: Noted.

Responsiveness/Level of Consciousness

Student: What is the patient's level of consciousness?
PROCTOR: Unresponsive.

Chief Complaint/Apparent Life Threats

Student: What is the patient's chief complaint?
PROCTOR: The patient is unresponsive.
Student: There are apparent life threats; the life threats are the mechanism of injury and the head trauma.
PROCTOR: Noted.

Assess the Airway and Breathing

Student: Is the airway open? Is the patient breathing?
PROCTOR: Yes, the airway is open and the patient is breathing.

Assessment

Student: What are the rate and the quality of breathing?
PROCTOR: Rate: Slow. Quality: Labored.

Provide Oxygen

Student: I am assisting ventilations with a bag-valve device with 100% oxygen and an oral airway if the patient does not have a gag reflex.
PROCTOR: The patient accepts the oral airway.
ALS Student: I will intubate (midline with trauma precaution) and confirm tube placement with lung sounds and end tidal CO_2.
ALS Proctor: Noted. Lung sounds and end tidal CO_2 confirm endotracheal (ET) tube placement.

Ensure Adequate Ventilation

Student: As noted earlier, I am assisting ventilations with a bag-valve device.
PROCTOR: Noted.

Injury Management

Student: I will direct my partner to take over c-spine control and ventilation as I continue assessment.
PROCTOR: Noted.

Assess Circulation

Student: I am assessing the patient's circulation.
PROCTOR: Noted.

Assess for and Control Major Bleeding

Student: Do I find any major bleeding?
PROCTOR: No.

Assess the Pulse

Student: What are the rate and the quality of pulses?
PROCTOR: Rate: Within normal limits. Quality: Bounding.

Assess the Skin

Student: I am assessing the skin. What are the color, temperature, and condition of the skin?
PROCTOR: Color: Pale. Temperature: Warm. Condition: Moist.

Identify Priority Patients/Make Transport Decision

Student: The patient is a high priority and is a load-and-go. I will begin packaging and transport to a trauma center.
PROCTOR: Noted.

Critical Criteria:
- ❑ Did not provide high concentration of oxygen
- ❑ Did not find or manage problems associated with airway, breathing, hemorrhage or shock (hypoperfusion)
- ❑ Did not differentiate patient's need for transportation versus continued assessment at the scene
- ❑ Did other detailed examination before assessing the airway, breathing and circulation

Focused History and Physical Examination/Rapid Trauma Assessment

Select the Appropriate Assessment (Focused or Rapid)

Student: I am selecting the rapid physical exam to identify and treat life threats. I am checking for DCAP-BTLS. This acronym stands for deformities, contusions, abrasions, punctures, penetrations, paradoxical motion in the chest, and burns, tenderness, lacerations, and swelling.
PROCTOR: Noted.

Head

Student: I am rapidly assessing the head.
PROCTOR: You feel a large deformity to the top of the head, consistent with a depressed skull fracture. Minor bleeding is noted from the ears.
Student: I would apply a dressing to any open wounds.
PROCTOR: Noted.

▸ **Neck**

Student: I am rapidly assessing the neck.
PROCTOR: There are no obvious injuries.
Student: I will apply a cervical collar.
PROCTOR: Noted.

▸ **Chest**

Student: I am rapidly assessing the chest. What are the lung sounds?
PROCTOR: There are no obvious injuries. Lung sounds are clear bilaterally.

▸ **Abdomen/Pelvis**

Student: I am rapidly assessing the abdomen.
PROCTOR: There are no obvious injuries.
Student: I am rapidly assessing the pelvis.
PROCTOR: There are no obvious injuries.

▸ **Extremities**

Student: I am rapidly assessing the extremities.
PROCTOR: There are no obvious injuries.

▸ **Assess Motor, Sensory, and Circulatory Function**

Student: I am checking for DCAP-BTLS, motor and sensory function, and pulses. Right leg?
PROCTOR: Negative DCAP-BTLS. Motor and sensory functions are absent. Pulses are present.
Student: Left leg?
PROCTOR: Negative DCAP-BTLS. Motor and sensory functions are absent. Pulses are present.
Student: Right arm?
PROCTOR: Negative DCAP-BTLS. Motor and sensory functions are absent. Pulses are present.
Student: Left arm?
PROCTOR: Negative DCAP-BTLS. Motor and sensory functions are absent. Pulses are present.

▸ **Posterior**

Student: I will rapidly assess the back. We will now log roll the patient as a unit to check the back. The person at the head will count to three and we will roll the patient.
PROCTOR: Noted.

▸ **Assess the Thorax**

Student: I am assessing the thorax. Do I find injuries?
PROCTOR: No.

▸ **Assess the Lumbar Area**

Student: I am assessing the flanks and lumbar area. Do I find injuries?
PROCTOR: No.

▸ **Assess the Entire Backside**

Student: I am assessing the entire backside. Do I find injuries?
PROCTOR: No.

▸ **Manage Secondary Injuries/Wounds**

Student: We will apply a cervical collar and backboard with full immobilization per local protocol, if not yet done, at this time.
PROCTOR: Noted.
Student: Are there any changes in motor and sensory functions or pulses?
PROCTOR: No.

▸ **Reevaluate Transport Decision**

Student: This patient is a high priority and is a load-and-go due to head trauma.
PROCTOR: Noted.

▾ Baseline Vital Signs

Student: What are the patient's baseline vital signs, including blood pressure, pulse, respirations, pulse oximetry, blood glucose level, and level of consciousness?
PROCTOR: Blood pressure, 160/90 mm Hg; pulse rate, 84 beats/min; respirations, per bag-valve device; pulse oximetry reading, 94%; blood glucose level, 120 mg/dL, and the patient is unresponsive.

▾ SAMPLE History

Student: At this time I will gather a SAMPLE history from the patient or family. What are the patient's signs and symptoms?
PROCTOR: He is unresponsive.
Student: Allergies?
PROCTOR: Unknown.
Student: Medications?
PROCTOR: Unknown.
Student: Pertinent past medical history?
PROCTOR: Unknown.
Student: Last oral intake?
PROCTOR: Unknown.
Student: Events leading up to the incident?
PROCTOR: The patient was breaking into a home and was entering through a first-floor window when the homeowner struck him in the head with a baseball bat. The patient was knocked into the yard.

Critical Criteria:

- ❑ Did not differentiate patient's need for transportation versus continued assessment at the scene
- ❑ Did not provide for spinal protection when indicated

Detailed Physical Examination

Student: I am conducting the detailed physical exam. I am looking for DCAP-BTLS.
PROCTOR: Noted. The detailed physical exam will be performed during transport.

▾ Assess the Head

Student: I am assessing the head. Do I find any DCAP-BTLS? Do I find any evidence of Battle's sign or raccoon eyes?
PROCTOR: Yes, you see Battle's signs to both sides of the head.

▸ **Inspect and Palpate the Head and Ears**

Student: I am assessing the head and ears.
PROCTOR: Minor bleeding is noted from the ears.

▸ **Assess the Eyes**

Student: I am assessing the eyes. Are the pupils equal, round, and regular in size, and react properly to light (PEARRL)?
PROCTOR: The left pupil is dilated.

▸ **Assess the Facial Area Including Oral and Nasal Areas**

Student: I am assessing the face, nose, and mouth. Do I see any discharge or hear any obstructions?
PROCTOR: No.

▾ Assess the Neck

▸ **Inspect and Palpate the Neck**

Student: I am assessing the neck for DCAP-BTLS.
PROCTOR: There are no obvious injuries.

▸ **Assess for Jugular Vein Distention**

Student: Do I find any jugular vein distention (JVD)?
PROCTOR: No.

▸ **Assess for Tracheal Deviation**

Student: Do I see any tracheal deviation?
PROCTOR: No.

▾ Assess the Chest

Student: I am assessing the chest for DCAP-BTLS.
PROCTOR: Noted.

▸ **Inspect**

Student: What do I see when I look at the chest?
PROCTOR: There are no obvious injuries.
Student: Does the chest appear symmetric?
PROCTOR: Yes.

▸ **Palpate**

Student: When I touch the chest, do I feel crepitus or a flail segment?

PROCTOR: No.

▸ **Auscultate**

Student: Are lung sounds present in all fields?

PROCTOR: Yes.

Student: Do I hear any sucking sounds from the chest?

PROCTOR: No.

▾ Assess the Abdomen/Pelvis

▸ **Assess the Abdomen**

Student: I am assessing the abdomen for DCAP-BTLS. I am assessing all four quadrants. Do I find any problems?

PROCTOR: No.

▸ **Assess the Pelvis**

Student: I am assessing the pelvis for DCAP-BTLS. Is the pelvis stable?

PROCTOR: Yes.

▾ Assess the Genitalia/Perineum as Needed (Verbalize in Training)

Student: I am assessing the genitalia/perineum as necessary for DCAP-BTLS.

PROCTOR: The area is unremarkable.

▾ Assess the Extremities

▸ **Inspect**

Student: I am assessing the lower and upper extremities for DCAP-BTLS. Do I find anything?

PROCTOR: No.

▸ **Palpate**

Student: Do I feel anything unusual?

PROCTOR: No.

▸ **Assess Motor, Sensory, and Circulatory Function**

Student: I am checking for DCAP-BTLS, motor and sensory function, and pulses. Right leg?

PROCTOR: Negative DCAP-BTLS. Motor and sensory functions are absent. Pulses are present.

Student: Left leg?

PROCTOR: Negative DCAP-BTLS. Motor and sensory functions are absent. Pulses are present.

Student: Right arm?

PROCTOR: Negative DCAP-BTLS. Motor and sensory functions are absent. Pulses are present.

Student: Left arm?

PROCTOR: Negative DCAP-BTLS. Motor and sensory functions are absent. Pulses are present.

▾ Assess the Posterior

Note: This portion of the detailed physical exam would not be done if the patient were previously backboarded per local protocol.

Student: We will not check the back because it was previously checked and the patient is backboarded.

PROCTOR: Noted.

▾ Manage Secondary Injuries/Wounds

Student: I would direct my partner to maintain the airway.

PROCTOR: Noted.

▾ Reassess Vital Signs

Student: I will reassess vital signs and mental status.

PROCTOR: Blood pressure, 162/84 mm Hg; pulse rate, 78 beats/min; respirations per bag-valve device; pulse oximetry reading, 97%; blood glucose level, 120 mg/dL; and the patient is unresponsive.

Student: The vital signs have not changed significantly.

PROCTOR: Noted.

▾ Reassess Interventions

Student: I will reassess my interventions: airway, breathing, oral airway, bag-valve ventilation for the head injury, and oxygen; circulation and bleeding control; and immobilization and straps.

PROCTOR: Noted.

ALS Student: I will reassess basic life support (BLS) interventions, plus the following: confirm ET tube placement with end tidal CO_2, check lung sounds, monitor two large-bore IVs, and cardiac monitor.

ALS Proctor: Noted. The cardiac monitor shows normal sinus rhythm and end tidal CO_2 and lung sounds confirm placement of the ET tube.

Critical Criteria:
- ❑ Did not find or manage problems associated with airway, breathing, hemorrhage or shock (hypoperfusion)

Radio Report

(Provided by the student.)

PROCTOR: Noted.

Ongoing Assessment

▾ Repeat Vital Signs

Student: I will reassess vital signs and mental status.

PROCTOR: Blood pressure, 170/82 mm Hg; pulse rate, 74 beats/min; respirations per bag-valve device; pulse oximetry reading, 96%; and the patient is unresponsive.

Student: The vital signs have deteriorated.

PROCTOR: Noted.

▾ Check Interventions

Student: I will check my interventions: airway, breathing, oral airway, bag-valve ventilation for the head injury, and oxygen; circulation and bleeding control; and immobilization and straps.

PROCTOR: Noted.

ALS Student: I will check BLS interventions, plus the following: confirm ET tube placement with end tidal CO_2, check lung sounds, two large-bore IVs, and cardiac monitor.

ALS Proctor: Noted. The cardiac monitor shows normal sinus rhythm and end tidal CO_2 and lung sounds confirm placement of the ET tube.

Critical Criteria:
- ❑ Did not find or manage problems associated with airway, breathing, hemorrhage or shock (hypoperfusion)

Handoff Report to Emergency Department Staff

Student: The patient's condition deteriorated during transport.

PROCTOR: Noted.

Critical Criteria:
- ❑ Did not transport patient within the (10) minute time limit

Critical Criteria

(Inform the student of items missed, if any.)

❑ Pass ❑ Fail Date: ____________________

Proctor Comments: ____________________

Notes

Dispatch Information

PROCTOR: EMS 10, respond to a 24-year-old female who was shot in the neck and the chest. She is conscious but barely breathing. Police are en route.

Pre-scene Action (BSI)

Student: I am wearing nonlatex gloves, safety glasses, mask, and gown.
PROCTOR: Noted.

> **Critical Criteria:**
> - ❑ Did not take, or verbalize, body substance isolation (BSI) precautions when necessary

Scene Size-up

Scene Safety

Student: Is the scene safe?
PROCTOR: Yes, police are on scene and you are given clearance to enter.

Mechanism of Injury

Student: What was the mechanism of injury?
PROCTOR: Gunshot wound. The patient was shot by her ex-boyfriend.

Number of Patients

Student: How many patients are there?
PROCTOR: One.

Additional Resources

Student: I would call for advanced life support (ALS) assistance.
PROCTOR: Noted.

C-Spine Stabilization

Student: On the basis of the mechanism of injury, I would stabilize the cervical spine (c-spine) in a neutral in-line position.
PROCTOR: Noted.

> **Critical Criteria:**
> - ❑ Did not determine scene safety
> - ❑ Did not assess for spinal protection
> - ❑ Did not provide for spinal protection when indicated

Initial Assessment

Student: As I perform midline c-spine stabilization, I identify myself and ask the patient not to move.
PROCTOR: Noted.

General Impression

Student: My general impression is that the patient's condition is unstable.
PROCTOR: Noted.

Responsiveness/Level of Consciousness

Student: What is the patient's level of consciousness?
PROCTOR: Alert.

Chief Complaint/Apparent Life Threats

Student: What is the patient's chief complaint?
PROCTOR: The patient is complaining of difficulty breathing.
Student: There is an apparent life threat; the life threat is the mechanism of injury.
PROCTOR: Noted.

Assess the Airway and Breathing

Student: Is the airway open? Is the patient breathing?
PROCTOR: Yes, the airway is open and the patient is breathing.

Assessment

Student: What are the rate and the quality of breathing?
PROCTOR: Rate: Tachypneic. Quality: Labored.

Provide Oxygen

Student: I am assisting ventilations with a bag-valve device with 100% oxygen.
PROCTOR: Noted.

Ensure Adequate Ventilation

Student: I will ensure adequate ventilation. I will suction the airway as needed.
PROCTOR: Noted.
ALS Student: I will consider rapid sequence intubation (RSI) per local protocol to intubate the patient, confirm end tidal CO_2, and check lung sounds.
ALS Proctor: Noted. End tidal CO_2 and lung sounds confirm endotracheal (ET) tube placement.

Injury Management

Student: I will direct my partner to take over c-spine control and ventilation as I continue assessment.
PROCTOR: Noted.

Assess Circulation

Student: I am assessing the patient's circulation.
PROCTOR: Noted.

Assess for and Control Major Bleeding

Student: Do I find any major bleeding?
PROCTOR: Yes, from the neck and chest.
Student: I would apply direct pressure and an occlusive dressing.
PROCTOR: Noted.

Assess the Pulse

Student: What are the rate and the quality of pulses?
PROCTOR: Rate: Tachycardic. Quality: Thready.

Assess the Skin

Student: I am assessing the skin. What are the color, temperature, and condition of the skin?
PROCTOR: Color: Pasty white. Temperature: Cold. Condition: Diaphoretic.

Identify Priority Patients/Make Transport Decision

Student: The patient is a high priority and is a load-and-go. I will begin packaging and transport.
PROCTOR: Noted.

> **Critical Criteria:**
> - ❑ Did not provide high concentration of oxygen
> - ❑ Did not find or manage problems associated with airway, breathing, hemorrhage or shock (hypoperfusion)
> - ❑ Did not differentiate patient's need for transportation versus continued assessment at the scene
> - ❑ Did other detailed examination before assessing the airway, breathing and circulation

Focused History and Physical Examination/Rapid Trauma Assessment

Select the Appropriate Assessment (Focused or Rapid)

Student: I am selecting the rapid physical exam to identify and treat life threats. I am checking for DCAP-BTLS. This acronym stands for deformities, contusions, abrasions, punctures, penetrations, paradoxical motion in the chest, and burns, tenderness, lacerations, and swelling.
PROCTOR: Noted.

Head

Student: I am rapidly assessing the head.
PROCTOR: There are no obvious injuries.

▸ **Neck**

Student: I am rapidly assessing the neck.
PROCTOR: There are multiple small punctures to the neck.
Student: I would use direct pressure to control the bleeding and apply occlusive dressings.
PROCTOR: Noted.
Student: I will apply a cervical collar.
PROCTOR: Noted.

▸ **Chest**

Student: I am rapidly assessing the chest.
PROCTOR: There are multiple small puncture wounds to the upper chest.
Student: I would apply occlusive dressings if not already done.
PROCTOR: Noted.
Student: I will assess the chest for tension pneumothorax by auscultation, and assessment (jugular vein distention [JVD], tracheal deviation, and decreased lung sounds).
PROCTOR: Lung sounds are present, jugular vein distension is not present, and the trachea is midline.
Student: Do I hear any sucking sounds from the chest?
PROCTOR: No (if an occlusive dressing was used).
ALS Student: I will assess the chest for hyperresonance to percussion.
ALS Proctor: Noted. There is no tension noted.
ALS Student: I will monitor the chest.
ALS Proctor: Noted.

▸ **Abdomen/Pelvis**

Student: I am rapidly assessing the abdomen.
PROCTOR: There are no obvious injuries.
Student: I am rapidly assessing the pelvis.
PROCTOR: There are no obvious injuries.

▸ **Extremities**

Student: I am rapidly assessing the extremities.
PROCTOR: There are no obvious injuries.

▸ **Assess Motor, Sensory, and Circulatory Function**

Student: I am checking for DCAP-BTLS, motor and sensory function, and pulses. Right leg?
PROCTOR: Negative DCAP-BTLS. Motor and sensory functions are present. Pulses are weak.
Student: Left leg?
PROCTOR: Negative DCAP-BTLS. Motor and sensory functions are present. Pulses are weak.
Student: Right arm?
PROCTOR: Negative DCAP-BTLS. Motor and sensory functions are present. Pulses are weak.
Student: Left arm?
PROCTOR: Negative DCAP-BTLS. Motor and sensory functions are present. Pulses are weak.

▸ **Posterior**

Student: I will rapidly assess the back. We will now log roll the patient as a unit to check the back. The person at the head will count to three and we will roll the patient.
PROCTOR: Noted.

▸ **Assess the Thorax**

Student: I am assessing the thorax. Do I find injuries?
PROCTOR: No.

▸ **Assess the Lumbar Area**

Student: I am assessing the flanks and lumbar area. Do I find injuries?
PROCTOR: No.

▸ **Assess the Entire Backside**

Student: I am assessing the entire backside. Do I find injuries?
PROCTOR: No.

▸ **Manage Secondary Injuries/Wounds**

Student: We will apply a cervical collar and backboard with full immobilization per local protocol, if not yet done, at this time.
PROCTOR: Noted.
Student: Are there any changes in motor and sensory functions or pulses?
PROCTOR: No.
ALS Student: I will maintain the ET tube. I will establish two large-bore IVs en route to the hospital and administer a bolus of 20 mL/kg to maintain a systolic blood pressure of 90 mm Hg.
ALS Proctor: Noted.

▸ **Reevaluate Transport Decision**

Student: This patient is a load-and-go due to neck and chest gunshot wounds.
PROCTOR: Noted.

▾ **Baseline Vital Signs**

Student: What are the patient's baseline vital signs, including blood pressure, pulse, respirations, pulse oximetry, blood glucose level, and level of consciousness?
PROCTOR: Blood pressure, 100/70 mm Hg; pulse, 120 beats/min; respirations, per bag-valve device; pulse oximetry reading, 95%; blood glucose level, 99 mg/dL; and the patient is tired.
ALS Proctor: If RSI was used, the patient's level of consciousness is unresponsive.

▾ **SAMPLE History**

Student: At this time I will gather a SAMPLE history from the patient or family. What are the patient's signs and symptoms?
PROCTOR: Gunshot wound to the neck and chest.
Student: Allergies?
PROCTOR: No allergies.
Student: Medications?
PROCTOR: No medications.
Student: Pertinent past medical history?
PROCTOR: No pertinent past medical history.
Student: Last oral intake?
PROCTOR: 2 hours ago.
Student: Events leading up to the incident?
PROCTOR: The patient opened her front door and was shot by her ex-boyfriend.

Critical Criteria:
- ☐ Did not differentiate patient's need for transportation versus continued assessment at the scene
- ☐ Did not provide for spinal protection when indicated

Detailed Physical Examination

Student: I am conducting the detailed physical exam. I am looking for DCAP-BTLS.
PROCTOR: Noted. The detailed physical exam will be performed during transport.

▾ **Assess the Head**

Student: I am assessing the head. Do I find any DCAP-BTLS? Do I find any evidence of Battle's sign or raccoon eyes?
PROCTOR: No.

▸ **Inspect and Palpate the Head and Ears**

Student: I am assessing the head and ears.
PROCTOR: There are no obvious injuries.

▸ **Assess the Eyes**

Student: I am assessing the eyes. Are the pupils equal, round, and regular in size, and react properly to light (PEARRL)?
PROCTOR: They are PEARRL.

▸ **Assess the Facial Area Including Oral and Nasal Areas**

Student: I am assessing the face, nose, and mouth. Do I see any discharge or hear any obstructions?
PROCTOR: Yes, you hear gurgling.
ALS Proctor: You see blood in the mouth.

Student: I would suction and continue to ventilate per protocol.
PROCTOR: Noted.

Assess the Neck

Inspect and Palpate the Neck

Student: I am assessing the neck for DCAP-BTLS.
PROCTOR: There are small holes.

Assess for Jugular Vein Distention

Student: Do I find any jugular vein distention (JVD)?
PROCTOR: No.

Assess for Tracheal Deviation

Student: Do I see any tracheal deviation?
PROCTOR: No.

Assess the Chest

Student: I am assessing the chest for DCAP-BTLS.
PROCTOR: Noted.

Inspect

Student: What do I see when I look at the chest?
PROCTOR: You see multiple small holes across the chest.
Student: Does the chest appear symmetric?
PROCTOR: Yes.

Palpate

Student: When I touch the chest, do I feel crepitus or a flail segment?
PROCTOR: No. You feel BBs just under the skin.

Auscultate

Student: Are lung sounds present in all fields?
PROCTOR: Yes.
Student: Do I hear any sucking sounds from the chest?
PROCTOR: No (if an occlusive dressing was used).
Student: I would check the occlusive dressing.
PROCTOR: Noted.

Assess the Abdomen/Pelvis

Assess the Abdomen

Student: I am assessing the abdomen for DCAP-BTLS. I am assessing all four quadrants. Do I find any problems?
PROCTOR: No.

Assess the Pelvis

Student: I am assessing the pelvis for DCAP-BTLS. Is the pelvis stable?
PROCTOR: Yes.

Assess the Genitalia/Perineum as Needed (Verbalize in Training)

Student: I am assessing the genitalia/perineum as necessary for DCAP-BTLS.
PROCTOR: The area is unremarkable.

Assess the Extremities

Inspect

Student: I am assessing the lower and upper extremities for DCAP-BTLS. Do I find anything?
PROCTOR: No.

Palpate

Student: Do I feel anything unusual?
PROCTOR: No.

Assess Motor, Sensory, and Circulatory Function

Student: I am checking for DCAP-BTLS, motor and sensory function, and pulses. Right leg?
PROCTOR: Negative DCAP-BTLS. Motor and sensory functions are present. Pulses are weak.
Student: Left leg?
PROCTOR: Negative DCAP-BTLS. Motor and sensory functions are present. Pulses are weak.
Student: Right arm?
PROCTOR: Negative DCAP-BTLS. Motor and sensory functions are present. Pulses are weak.
Student: Left arm?
PROCTOR: Negative DCAP-BTLS. Motor and sensory functions are present. Pulses are weak.

Assess the Posterior

Note: This portion of the detailed physical exam would not be done if the patient were previously backboarded per local protocol.
Student: We will not check the back because it was previously checked and the patient is backboarded.
PROCTOR: Noted.

Manage Secondary Injuries/Wounds

Student: I would direct my partner to monitor the airway, the neck, and the chest.
PROCTOR: Noted.

Reassess Vital Signs

Student: I will reassess vital signs and mental status.
PROCTOR: Blood pressure, 92/66 mm Hg; pulse, 128 beats/min; respirations, per bag-valve device; pulse oximetry reading, 92%; and the patient is tired.
ALS Proctor: *Note:* If RSI was used, the patient will have the following vital signs instead: Blood pressure, 92/66 mm Hg; pulse, 128 beats/min; respirations, per bag-valve device; pulse oximetry reading 96%; and the patient is unresponsive.
Student: The vital signs are deteriorating.
PROCTOR: Noted.

Reassess Interventions

Student: I will reassess my interventions: airway, suction, breathing, bag-valve device, and oxygen; circulation and bleeding control; occlusive dressings; evaluation for tension pneumothorax; immobilization and straps; and treatment for shock.
PROCTOR: Noted.
ALS Student: I will reassess basic life support (BLS) interventions, plus the following: RSI intubation, confirm end tidal CO_2, check lung sounds, monitor the two large-bore IVs, and maintain a systolic blood pressure of 90 mm Hg and cardiac monitor.
ALS Proctor: Noted. The cardiac monitor shows sinus tachycardia. End tidal CO_2 and lung sounds confirm ET tube placement.

Critical Criteria:
- ❑ Did not find or manage problems associated with airway, breathing, hemorrhage or shock (hypoperfusion)

Radio Report

(Provided by the student.)
PROCTOR: Noted.

Ongoing Assessment

Repeat Vital Signs

Student: I will reassess vital signs and mental status.
PROCTOR: Blood pressure, 84/56 mm Hg; pulse, 132 beats/min; respirations, per bag-valve device; pulse oximetry reading, 90%; and the patient is responsive to pain.
ALS Proctor: *Note:* If RSI was used, the patient will have the following vital signs instead: Blood pressure, 84/56 mm Hg; pulse, 132 beats/min; respirations, per bag-valve device; pulse oximetry reading, 97%; and the patient is unresponsive.
Student: The vital signs have deteriorated.
PROCTOR: Noted.

Check Interventions

Student: I will check my interventions: airway, suction, breathing, bag-valve device, and oxygen; circulation and bleeding control; occlusive dressings; evaluation for tension pneumothorax; immobilization and straps; and treatment for shock.

PROCTOR: Noted.

ALS Student: I will check BLS interventions, plus the following: RSI intubation, confirm end tidal CO_2, check lung sounds, monitor the two large-bore IVs, and maintain a systolic blood pressure of 90 mm Hg and cardiac monitor.

ALS Proctor: Noted. The cardiac monitor shows sinus tachycardia. End tidal CO_2 and lung sounds confirm ET tube placement.

Critical Criteria:
- ❑ Did not find or manage problems associated with airway, breathing, hemorrhage or shock (hypoperfusion)

Handoff Report to Emergency Department Staff

Student: The patient's condition deteriorated during transport.

PROCTOR: Noted.

Critical Criteria:
- ❑ Did not transport patient within the (10) minute time limit

Critical Criteria

(Inform the student of items missed, if any.)

❑ Pass ❑ Fail Date: ____________________

Proctor Comments: ____________________

____

____

Dispatch Information

PROCTOR: EMS 10, respond to a 50-year-old male who has been found handcuffed and beaten. He is conscious and breathing. Police are responding to the scene.

Pre-scene Action (BSI)

Student: I am wearing nonlatex gloves and safety glasses.
PROCTOR: Noted.

Critical Criteria:
- ❑ Did not take, or verbalize, body substance isolation (BSI) precautions when necessary

Scene Size-up

Scene Safety

Student: Is the scene safe?
PROCTOR: Yes, police are on scene and you are given clearance to enter.

Mechanism of Injury

Student: What was the mechanism of injury?
PROCTOR: Blunt and penetrating trauma. The patient says he was beaten over his gambling debt.

Number of Patients

Student: How many patients are there?
PROCTOR: One.

Additional Resources

Student: I would call for advanced life support (ALS) assistance.
PROCTOR: Noted.

C-Spine Stabilization

Student: On the basis of the mechanism of injury, I would stabilize the cervical spine (c-spine) in a neutral in-line position.
PROCTOR: Noted.

Critical Criteria:
- ❑ Did not determine scene safety
- ❑ Did not assess for spinal protection
- ❑ Did not provide for spinal protection when indicated

Initial Assessment

Student: As I perform midline c-spine stabilization, I identify myself and ask the patient not to move.
PROCTOR: Noted.

General Impression

Student: My general impression is that the patient's condition is unstable.
PROCTOR: Noted.

Responsiveness/Level of Consciousness

Student: What is the patient's level of consciousness?
PROCTOR: Conscious and alert.

Chief Complaint/Apparent Life Threats

Student: What is the patient's chief complaint?
PROCTOR: The patient is complaining of pain to his head, chest, hands, and shoulders. He had been handcuffed and beaten by his attackers.
Student: I will have the police remove the handcuffs.
PROCTOR: Noted.
Student: There is an apparent life threat; the life threat is the mechanism of injury.
PROCTOR: Noted.

Assess the Airway and Breathing

Student: Is the airway open? Is the patient breathing?
PROCTOR: Yes, the airway is open and the patient is breathing.

Assessment

Student: What are the rate and the quality of breathing?
PROCTOR: Rate: A little fast. Quality: Normal.

Provide Oxygen

Student: I am applying oxygen at 15 L/min via nonrebreathing mask.
PROCTOR: Noted.

Ensure Adequate Ventilation

Student: The patient has adequate ventilations at this time.
PROCTOR: Noted.

Injury Management

Student: I will direct my partner to take over c-spine control as I continue assessment.
PROCTOR: Noted.

Assess Circulation

Student: I am assessing the patient's circulation.
PROCTOR: Noted.

Assess for and Control Major Bleeding

Student: Do I find any major bleeding?
PROCTOR: No.

Assess the Pulse

Student: What are the rate and the quality of pulses?
PROCTOR: Rate: Within normal limits. Quality: Strong.

Assess the Skin

Student: I am assessing the skin. What are the color, temperature, and condition of the skin?
PROCTOR: Color: Flushed. Temperature: Warm. Condition: Moist.

Identify Priority Patients/Make Transport Decision

Student: The patient is a high priority and is a load-and-go. I will begin packaging and transport.
PROCTOR: Noted.

Critical Criteria:
- ❑ Did not provide high concentration of oxygen
- ❑ Did not find or manage problems associated with airway, breathing, hemorrhage or shock (hypoperfusion)
- ❑ Did not differentiate patient's need for transportation versus continued assessment at the scene
- ❑ Did other detailed examination before assessing the airway, breathing and circulation

Focused History and Physical Examination/Rapid Trauma Assessment

Select the Appropriate Assessment (Focused or Rapid)

Student: I am selecting the rapid physical exam to identify and treat life threats.
PROCTOR: Noted.
Student: I am checking for DCAP-BTLS. This acronym stands for deformities, contusions, abrasions, punctures, penetrations, paradoxical motion in the chest, and burns, tenderness, lacerations, and swelling. I am also checking for motor and sensory function and pulses.
PROCTOR: Noted.

Head

Student: I am rapidly assessing the head.
PROCTOR: You find bruises.

▸ Neck

Student: I am rapidly assessing the neck.

PROCTOR: The patient has pain to his neck.

Student: I will apply a cervical collar.

PROCTOR: Noted.

▸ Chest

Student: I am rapidly assessing the chest.

PROCTOR: The patient complains of pain in his ribs.

Student: I will assess the chest for tension pneumothorax by auscultation, and assessment (jugular vein distention [JVD], tracheal deviation, and decreased lung sounds).

PROCTOR: Lung sounds are present, jugular vein distension is not present, and the trachea is midline.

Student: Do I hear any sucking sounds from the chest?

PROCTOR: No.

Student: I will treat the ribs with a bulky dressing.

PROCTOR: Noted.

ALS Student: I will assess the chest for hyperresonance to percussion.

ALS Proctor: Noted. There is no tension noted.

ALS Student: I will monitor the chest.

ALS Proctor: Noted.

▸ Abdomen/Pelvis

Student: I am rapidly assessing the abdomen.

PROCTOR: There is bruising noted.

Student: I am rapidly assessing the pelvis.

PROCTOR: There are no obvious injuries.

▸ Extremities

Student: I am rapidly assessing the extremities.

PROCTOR: There are obvious injuries on the patient's arms and hands. The patient was handcuffed by his attackers.

▸ Assess Motor, Sensory, and Circulatory Function

Student: I am checking for DCAP-BTLS. Right leg?

PROCTOR: Negative DCAP-BTLS. Motor and sensory functions are present. Pulses are present.

Student: Left leg?

PROCTOR: Negative DCAP-BTLS. Motor and sensory functions are present. Pulses are present.

Student: Right arm?

PROCTOR: The shoulder is dislocated and the wrist appears deformed. Motor and sensory functions are present. Pulses are present.

Student: Left arm?

PROCTOR: The shoulder is dislocated and the wrist appears deformed. Motor and sensory functions are present. Pulses are present.

Student: I will apply a sling and swathe the patient's arms, and splint his wrists while en route to the hospital.

PROCTOR: Noted.

▸ Posterior

Student: I will rapidly assess the back. We will now log roll the patient as a unit to check the back. The person at the head will count to three and we will roll the patient.

PROCTOR: You see marks left by a baseball bat.

▸ Assess the Thorax

Student: I am assessing the thorax. Do I find injuries?

PROCTOR: You see marks left by the bat.

▸ Assess the Lumbar Area

Student: I am assessing the flanks and lumbar area. Do I find injuries?

PROCTOR: No.

▸ Assess the Entire Backside

Student: I am assessing the entire backside. Do I find injuries?

PROCTOR: No.

▸ Manage Secondary Injuries/Wounds

Student: We will apply a cervical collar and backboard with full immobilization per local protocol, if not yet done, at this time. I will apply a sling and swathe the patient's arms, and splint his wrists while en route to the hospital.

PROCTOR: Noted.

Student: Are there any changes in motor and sensory functions or pulses?

PROCTOR: No.

ALS Student: I will establish two large-bore IVs en route to the hospital in order to maintain a systolic blood pressure of 90 mm Hg.

ALS Proctor: Noted.

▸ Reevaluate Transport Decision

Student: This patient is a high priority and a load-and-go due to the mechanism of injury. I will transport him to a trauma center.

PROCTOR: Noted.

▾ Baseline Vital Signs

Student: What are the patient's baseline vital signs, including blood pressure, pulse, respirations, pulse oximetry, blood glucose level, and level of consciousness?

PROCTOR: Blood pressure, 160/90 mm Hg; pulse rate, 110 beats/min; respirations, 28 breaths/min; pulse oximetry reading, 100%; blood glucose level, 100 mg/dL; and the patient is alert.

▾ SAMPLE History

Student: At this time I will gather a SAMPLE history from the patient or family. What are the patient's signs and symptoms?

PROCTOR: Pain in the head, neck, chest, arms, and ribs.

Student: Allergies?

PROCTOR: Sulfa medications.

Student: Medications?

PROCTOR: Blood pressure medications.

Student: Pertinent past medical history?

PROCTOR: Heart problems, high blood pressure, and heavy smoking habit.

Student: Last oral intake?

PROCTOR: 4 hours ago.

Student: Events leading up to the incident?

PROCTOR: The patient was at home when some men he owed money to kicked in his door, handcuffed, and beat him with a baseball bat. They struck the handcuff chain several times with the bat.

Critical Criteria:

- ❑ Did not differentiate patient's need for transportation versus continued assessment at the scene
- ❑ Did not provide for spinal protection when indicated

Detailed Physical Examination

Student: I am conducting the detailed physical exam. I am looking for DCAP-BTLS.

PROCTOR: Noted. The detailed physical exam will be performed during transport.

▾ Assess the Head

Student: I am assessing the head. Do I find any DCAP-BTLS? Do I find any evidence of Battle's sign or raccoon eyes?

PROCTOR: Yes, he has a bruise to his forehead.

▸ Inspect and Palpate the Head and Ears

Student: I am assessing the head and ears.

PROCTOR: He has a bruise to his forehead.

▸ Assess the Eyes

Student: I am assessing the eyes. Are the pupils equal, round, and regular in size, and react properly to light (PEARRL)?

PROCTOR: They are PEARRL.

▸ **Assess the Facial Area Including Oral and Nasal Areas**

Student: I am assessing the face, nose, and mouth. Do I see any discharge or hear any obstructions?

PROCTOR: No.

▾ Assess the Neck

▸ **Inspect and Palpate the Neck**

Student: I am assessing the neck for DCAP-BTLS.

PROCTOR: The patient has pain in his neck.

▸ **Assess for Jugular Vein Distention**

Student: Do I find any jugular vein distention (JVD)?

PROCTOR: No.

▸ **Assess for Tracheal Deviation**

Student: Do I see any tracheal deviation?

PROCTOR: No.

▾ Assess the Chest

Student: I am assessing the chest for DCAP-BTLS.

PROCTOR: Noted.

▸ **Inspect**

Student: What do I see when I look at the chest?

PROCTOR: You find impressions from a baseball bat.

Student: Does the chest appear symmetric?

PROCTOR: Yes, but the patient states that he thinks his ribs are cracked. The ribs were treated with a bulky dressing.

▸ **Palpate**

Student: When I touch the chest, do I feel crepitus or a flail segment?

PROCTOR: Yes, you feel crepitus but not a flail segment.

▸ **Auscultate**

Student: Are lung sounds present in all fields?

PROCTOR: Yes.

Student: Do I hear any sucking sounds from the chest?

PROCTOR: No.

Student: I will assess the chest for tension pneumothorax by auscultation, and assessment (jugular vein distention [JVD], tracheal deviation, and decreased lung sounds).

PROCTOR: Lung sounds are present, jugular vein distension is not present, and the trachea is midline.

Student: Do I hear any sucking sounds from the chest?

PROCTOR: No.

ALS Student: I will assess the chest for hyperresonance to percussion.

ALS Proctor: Noted. There is no tension noted.

ALS Student: I will monitor the chest.

ALS Proctor: Noted.

▾ Assess the Abdomen/Pelvis

▸ **Assess the Abdomen**

Student: I am assessing the abdomen for DCAP-BTLS. I am assessing all four quadrants. Do I find any problems?

PROCTOR: Yes, you see bruises from the bat.

▸ **Assess the Pelvis**

Student: I am assessing the pelvis for DCAP-BTLS. Is the pelvis stable?

PROCTOR: Yes.

▾ Assess the Genitalia/Perineum as Needed (Verbalize in Training)

Student: I am assessing the genitalia/perineum as necessary for DCAP-BTLS.

PROCTOR: The area is unremarkable.

▾ Assess the Extremities

▸ **Inspect**

Student: I am assessing the lower and upper extremities for DCAP-BTLS. Do I find anything?

PROCTOR: Yes, the shoulders are painful and the wrists are deformed.

▸ **Palpate**

Student: Do I feel anything unusual?

PROCTOR: Yes, the wrists are deformed.

▸ **Assess Motor, Sensory, and Circulatory Function**

Student: I am checking for DCAP-BTLS, motor and sensory function, and pulses. Right leg?

PROCTOR: Negative DCAP-BTLS. Motor and sensory functions are present. Pulses are present.

Student: Left leg?

PROCTOR: Negative DCAP-BTLS. Motor and sensory functions are present. Pulses are present.

Student: Right arm?

PROCTOR: The shoulder is dislocated and the wrist appears deformed. Motor and sensory functions are present. Pulses are present.

Student: Left arm?

PROCTOR: The shoulder is dislocated and the wrist appears deformed. Motor and sensory functions are present. Pulses are present.

Student: I will apply a sling and swathe the patient's arms and splint his wrists.

PROCTOR: Noted.

▾ Assess the Posterior

Note: This portion of the detailed physical exam would not be done if the patient were previously backboarded per local protocol.

Student: We will not check the back because it was previously checked and the patient is backboarded.

PROCTOR: Noted.

▾ Manage Secondary Injuries/Wounds

Student: I would direct my partner to monitor the airway and to splint both arms if not already done.

PROCTOR: Noted.

▾ Reassess Vital Signs

Student: I will reassess vital signs and mental status.

PROCTOR: Blood pressure, 156/84 mm Hg; pulse rate, 104 beats/min; respirations, 20 breaths/min; pulse oximetry reading, 100%; and the patient is alert.

Student: The vital signs have not changed significantly.

PROCTOR: Noted.

▾ Reassess Interventions

Student: I will reassess my interventions: airway and oxygen; slings, swathes, and splints to both wrists; bulky dressing to the chest; and full immobilization and straps.

PROCTOR: Noted.

ALS Student: I will reassess basic life support (BLS) interventions, plus the following: two large-bore IVs and maintain a systolic blood pressure of 90 mm Hg and a cardiac monitor.

ALS Proctor: Noted. The monitor shows normal sinus rhythm.

Critical Criteria:

❑ Did not find or manage problems associated with airway, breathing, hemorrhage or shock (hypoperfusion)

Radio Report

(Provided by the student.)

PROCTOR: Noted.

Ongoing Assessment

Repeat Vital Signs

Student: I will reassess vital signs and mental status.

PROCTOR: Blood pressure, 150/80 mm Hg; pulse rate, 100 beats/min; respirations, 20 breaths/min; pulse oximetry reading, 100%; and the patient is alert.

Student: The vital signs have not changed significantly.

PROCTOR: Noted.

Check Interventions

Student: I will check my interventions: airway and oxygen; slings, swathes, and splints to both wrists; bulky dressing to the chest; and full immobilization and straps.

PROCTOR: Noted.

ALS Student: I will check BLS interventions, plus the following: monitor the two large-bore IVs and maintain a systolic blood pressure of 90 mm Hg and a cardiac monitor.

ALS Proctor: Noted. The monitor shows normal sinus rhythm.

Critical Criteria:

- ❑ Did not find or manage problems associated with airway, breathing, hemorrhage or shock (hypoperfusion)

Handoff Report to Emergency Department Staff

Student: There was no change in the patient's condition during transport.

PROCTOR: Noted.

Critical Criteria:

- ❑ Did not transport patient within the (10) minute time limit

Critical Criteria

(Inform the student of items missed, if any.)

❑ Pass ❑ Fail Date: ______________________

Proctor Comments: ______________________

____

____

Dispatch Information

PROCTOR: EMS 10, respond to a two-vehicle motor vehicle collision. There are two patients, and one is said to be critical. Police are on the scene.

Pre-scene Action (BSI)

Student: I am wearing nonlatex gloves, safety glasses, mask, and gown.

PROCTOR: Noted.

> **Critical Criteria:**
> - ❑ Did not take, or verbalize, body substance isolation (BSI) precautions when necessary

Scene Size-up

Scene Safety

Student: Is the scene safe?

PROCTOR: Yes, police are on scene and you are given clearance to enter.

Mechanism of Injury

Student: What was the mechanism of injury?

PROCTOR: Puncture wound to the head. The patient was an unrestrained 42-year-old male who was driving a van. The van was struck in the rear driver's side and spun out of control. The driver was impaled through the left temporal region by the gear shifter (on the column). He woke up and pulled his head off of the gear shifter before you could make entry.

Number of Patients

Student: How many patients are there?

PROCTOR: Two, but you are charged with treating only one of them.

Additional Resources

Student: I would call for advanced life support (ALS) assistance and additional resources: fire/rescue.

PROCTOR: Noted.

C-Spine Stabilization

Student: On the basis of the mechanism of injury, I would stabilize the cervical spine (c-spine) in a neutral in-line position.

PROCTOR: Noted.

> **Critical Criteria:**
> - ❑ Did not determine scene safety
> - ❑ Did not assess for spinal protection
> - ❑ Did not provide for spinal protection when indicated

Initial Assessment

Student: As I perform midline c-spine stabilization, I identify myself and ask the patient not to move.

PROCTOR: Noted.

General Impression

Student: My general impression is that the patient's condition is unstable.

PROCTOR: Noted.

Responsiveness/Level of Consciousness

Student: What is the patient's level of consciousness?

PROCTOR: Unresponsive.

Chief Complaint/Apparent Life Threats

Student: What is the patient's chief complaint?

PROCTOR: The patient is now unresponsive.

Student: There is an apparent life threat; the life threat is head trauma.

PROCTOR: Noted.

Assess the Airway and Breathing

Student: Is the airway open? Is the patient breathing?

PROCTOR: Yes, the airway is open and the patient is breathing.

Assessment

Student: What are the rate and the quality of breathing?

PROCTOR: Rate: Bradypneic. Quality: Deep.

Provide Oxygen

Student: I am assisting ventilations with a bag-valve device with 100% oxygen. I will insert an oral/advanced airway.

PROCTOR: Noted.

ALS Student: I will apply basic life support (BLS) interventions, plus the following: intubate, confirm end tidal CO_2, and check lung sounds.

ALS Proctor: Noted. End tidal CO_2 and lung sounds confirm placement of the endotracheal (ET) tube.

Ensure Adequate Ventilation

Student: As noted earlier, I am assisting ventilation with a bag-valve device.

PROCTOR: Noted.

Injury Management

Student: I will direct my partner to take over c-spine control and ventilations as I continue assessment.

PROCTOR: Noted.

Assess Circulation

Student: I am assessing the patient's circulation.

PROCTOR: Noted.

Assess for and Control Major Bleeding

Student: Do I find any major bleeding?

PROCTOR: Yes, from the head wound.

Student: I would apply a dressing per local protocol.

PROCTOR: Noted.

Assess the Pulse

Student: What are the rate and the quality of pulses?

PROCTOR: Rate: Within normal limits. Quality: Bounding.

Assess the Skin

Student: I am assessing the skin. What are the color, temperature, and condition of the skin?

PROCTOR: Color: Ashen. Temperature: Cool. Condition: Moist.

Identify Priority Patients/Make Transport Decision

Student: The patient is a high priority and is a load-and-go. I will begin packaging and transport to a trauma center.

PROCTOR: Noted.

> **Critical Criteria:**
> - ❑ Did not provide high concentration of oxygen
> - ❑ Did not find or manage problems associated with airway, breathing, hemorrhage or shock (hypoperfusion)
> - ❑ Did not differentiate patient's need for transportation versus continued assessment at the scene
> - ❑ Did other detailed examination before assessing the airway, breathing and circulation

Focused History and Physical Examination/Rapid Trauma Assessment

Select the Appropriate Assessment (Focused or Rapid)

Student: I am selecting the rapid physical exam to identify and treat life threats.

PROCTOR: Noted.

Student: I am checking for DCAP-BTLS. This acronym stands for deformities, contusions, abrasions, punctures, penetrations, paradoxical motion in the chest, and burns, tenderness, lacerations, and swelling. I am also checking for motor and sensory function and pulses.

PROCTOR: Noted.

▸ Head

Student: I am rapidly assessing the head.

PROCTOR: There is an open wound to the left temporal region of the head.

Student: I have applied a dressing.

PROCTOR: Noted. Bleeding is controlled.

▸ Neck

Student: I am rapidly assessing the neck.

PROCTOR: There are no obvious injuries.

Student: I will apply a cervical collar.

PROCTOR: Noted.

▸ Chest

Student: I am rapidly assessing the chest.

PROCTOR: There are no obvious injuries.

Student: Are there lung sounds present?

PROCTOR: They are clear bilaterally.

▸ Abdomen/Pelvis

Student: I am rapidly assessing the abdomen.

PROCTOR: There are no obvious injuries.

Student: I am rapidly assessing the pelvis.

PROCTOR: There are no obvious injuries.

▸ Extremities

Student: I am rapidly assessing the extremities.

PROCTOR: There are no obvious injuries.

▸ Assess Motor, Sensory, and Circulatory Function

Student: I am checking for DCAP-BTLS. Right leg?

PROCTOR: Negative DCAP-BTLS. Motor and sensory functions are absent. Pulses are present.

Student: Left leg?

PROCTOR: Negative DCAP-BTLS. Motor and sensory functions are absent. Pulses are present.

Student: Right arm?

PROCTOR: Negative DCAP-BTLS. Motor and sensory functions are absent. Pulses are present.

Student: Left arm?

PROCTOR: Negative DCAP-BTLS. Motor and sensory functions are absent. Pulses are present.

▸ Posterior

Student: I will rapidly assess the back. We will now log roll the patient as a unit to check the back. The person at the head will count to three and we will roll the patient.

PROCTOR: Noted.

▸ Assess the Thorax

Student: I am assessing the thorax. Do I find injuries?

PROCTOR: No.

▸ Assess the Lumbar Area

Student: I am assessing the flanks and lumbar area. Do I find injuries?

PROCTOR: No.

▸ Assess the Entire Backside

Student: I am assessing the entire backside. Do I find injuries?

PROCTOR: No.

▸ Manage Secondary Injuries/Wounds

Student: We will apply a cervical collar and backboard with full immobilization per local protocol, if not yet done, at this time. We will maintain ventilations and suction if necessary.

PROCTOR: Noted.

Student: Are there any changes in motor and sensory functions or pulses?

PROCTOR: No.

ALS Student: I will establish two large-bore IVs en route to the hospital in order to maintain a systolic blood pressure of 90 mm Hg.

ALS Proctor: Noted.

▸ Reevaluate Transport Decision

Student: This patient is a high priority and a load-and-go due to head trauma. He needs transport to a trauma center.

PROCTOR: Noted.

▾ Baseline Vital Signs

Student: What are the patient's baseline vital signs, including blood pressure, pulse, respirations, pulse oximetry, blood glucose level, and level of consciousness?

PROCTOR: Blood pressure, 150/90 mm Hg; pulse rate, 76 beats/min; respirations per bag-valve device; pulse oximetry reading, 95%; blood glucose level, 120 mg/dL; and the patient is unresponsive.

▾ SAMPLE History

Student: At this time I will gather a SAMPLE history from the patient or family. What are the patient's signs and symptoms?

PROCTOR: Unresponsive.

Student: Allergies?

PROCTOR: Unknown.

Student: Medications?

PROCTOR: Unknown.

Student: Pertinent past medical history?

PROCTOR: Unknown.

Student: Last oral intake?

PROCTOR: Unknown.

Student: Events leading up to the incident?

PROCTOR: The driver's van was struck by a car in the front driver's side causing it to spin out of control. The unrestrained driver was impaled by the gearshift from the steering wheel column. The patient removed his head from the gearshift.

Critical Criteria:

- ❑ Did not differentiate patient's need for transportation versus continued assessment at the scene
- ❑ Did not provide for spinal protection when indicated

Detailed Physical Examination

Student: I am conducting the detailed physical exam. I am looking for DCAP-BTLS.

PROCTOR: Noted. The detailed physical exam will be performed during transport.

▾ Assess the Head

Student: I am assessing the head. Do I find any DCAP-BTLS? Do I find any evidence of Battle's sign or raccoon eyes?

PROCTOR: You find an open head wound to the left temporal region. It was treated earlier.

▸ Inspect and Palpate the Head and Ears

Student: I am assessing the head and ears.

PROCTOR: Bleeding and cerebrospinal fluid (CSF) are noted from the wound.

▸ Assess the Eyes

Student: I am assessing the eyes. Are the pupils equal, round, and regular in size, and react properly to light (PEARRL)?

PROCTOR: They are nonreactive.

▸ Assess the Facial Area Including Oral and Nasal Areas

Student: I am assessing the face, nose, and mouth. Do I see any discharge or hear any obstructions?

PROCTOR: No.

ALS Student: I will apply BLS interventions, plus the following: confirm placement of the ET tube with end tidal CO_2 and lung sounds.

ALS Proctor: Noted. End tidal CO_2 and lung sounds confirm placement of the ET tube.

Assess the Neck

Inspect and Palpate the Neck

Student: I am assessing the neck for DCAP-BTLS.
PROCTOR: There are no obvious injuries.

Assess for Jugular Vein Distention

Student: Do I find any jugular vein distention (JVD)?
PROCTOR: No.

Assess for Tracheal Deviation

Student: Do I see any tracheal deviation?
PROCTOR: No.

Assess the Chest

Student: I am assessing the chest for DCAP-BTLS.
PROCTOR: Noted.

Inspect

Student: What do I see when I look at the chest?
PROCTOR: There are no obvious injuries.
Student: Does the chest appear symmetric?
PROCTOR: Yes.

Palpate

Student: When I touch the chest, do I feel crepitus or a flail segment?
PROCTOR: No.

Auscultate

Student: Are lung sounds present in all fields?
PROCTOR: Yes.
Student: Do I hear any sucking sounds from the chest?
PROCTOR: No.

Assess the Abdomen/Pelvis

Assess the Abdomen

Student: I am assessing the abdomen for DCAP-BTLS. I am assessing all four quadrants. Do I find any problems?
PROCTOR: No.

Assess the Pelvis

Student: I am assessing the pelvis for DCAP-BTLS. Is the pelvis stable?
PROCTOR: Yes.

Assess the Genitalia/Perineum as Needed (Verbalize in Training)

Student: I am assessing the genitalia/perineum as necessary for DCAP-BTLS.
PROCTOR: The area is unremarkable.

Assess the Extremities

Inspect

Student: I am assessing the lower and upper extremities for DCAP-BTLS. Do I find anything?
PROCTOR: No.

Palpate

Student: Do I feel anything unusual?
PROCTOR: No.

Assess Motor, Sensory, and Circulatory Function

Student: I am checking for DCAP-BTLS, motor and sensory function, and pulses. Right leg?
PROCTOR: Negative DCAP-BTLS. Motor and sensory functions are absent. Pulses are present.
Student: Left leg?
PROCTOR: Negative DCAP-BTLS. Motor and sensory functions are absent. Pulses are present.
Student: Right arm?
PROCTOR: Negative DCAP-BTLS. Motor and sensory functions are absent. Pulses are present.
Student: Left arm?
PROCTOR: Negative DCAP-BTLS. Motor and sensory functions are absent. Pulses are present.

Assess the Posterior

Note: This portion of the detailed physical exam would not be done if the patient were previously backboarded per local protocol.
Student: We will not check the back because it was previously checked and the patient is backboarded.
PROCTOR: Noted.

Manage Secondary Injuries/Wounds

Student: I would direct my partner to maintain the airway and provide ventilations.
PROCTOR: Noted.

Reassess Vital Signs

Student: I will reassess vital signs and mental status.
PROCTOR: Blood pressure, 154/92 mm Hg; pulse rate, 74 beats/min; respirations per bag-valve device; pulse oximetry reading, 97%; and the patient is unresponsive.
Student: The vital signs have not changed significantly.
PROCTOR: Noted.

Reassess Interventions

Student: I will reassess my interventions: airway, oxygen, oral/advanced airway, suction, and bag-valve device; bleeding control; and immobilization and straps.
PROCTOR: Noted.
ALS Student: I will reassess BLS interventions, plus the following: confirm placement of the ET tube with end tidal CO_2 and lung sounds, establish two large-bore IVs in order to maintain a systolic blood pressure of 90 mm Hg, apply cardiac monitoring, and follow the local protocol.
ALS Proctor: Noted. The cardiac monitor shows normal sinus rhythm and end tidal CO_2 and lung sounds confirm placement of the ET tube.

Critical Criteria:
- ❑ Did not find or manage problems associated with airway, breathing, hemorrhage or shock (hypoperfusion)

Radio Report

(Provided by the student.)
PROCTOR: Noted.

Ongoing Assessment

Repeat Vital Signs

Student: I will reassess vital signs and mental status.
PROCTOR: Blood pressure, 156/86 mm Hg; pulse rate, 72 beats/min; respirations per bag-valve device; pulse oximetry reading, 97%; and the patient is unresponsive.
Student: The vital signs have not changed significantly.
PROCTOR: Noted.

Check Interventions

Student: I will check my interventions: airway, oxygen, oral/advanced airway, suction, and bag-valve device; bleeding control; and immobilization and straps.
PROCTOR: Noted.

ALS Student: I will check BLS interventions, plus the following: confirm placement of the ET tube with end tidal CO_2 and lung sounds, maintain the two large-bore IVs and maintain a systolic blood pressure of 90 mm Hg, cardiac monitoring, and follow the local protocol.

ALS Proctor: Noted. The cardiac monitor shows normal sinus rhythm and end tidal CO_2 and lung sounds confirm placement of the ET tube.

Critical Criteria:
❑ Did not find or manage problems associated with airway, breathing, hemorrhage or shock (hypoperfusion)

Handoff Report to Emergency Department Staff

Student: There was no change in the patient's condition during transport

PROCTOR: Noted.

Critical Criteria:
❑ Did not transport patient within the (10) minute time limit

Critical Criteria

(Inform the student of items missed, if any.)

❑ Pass ❑ Fail Date: ____________________

Proctor Comments: ____________________

____

____

Dispatch Information

PROCTOR: EMS 10, respond to a 23-year-old female who has been sliced across the abdomen with a box cutter. She is conscious and breathing.

Pre-scene Action (BSI)

Student: I am wearing nonlatex gloves, safety glasses, mask, and gown.
PROCTOR: Noted.

Critical Criteria:
- ❑ Did not take, or verbalize, body substance isolation (BSI) precautions when necessary

Scene Size-up

Scene Safety

Student: Is the scene safe?
PROCTOR: Yes.

Mechanism of Injury

Student: What was the mechanism of injury?
PROCTOR: Penetrating trauma. The patient was dancing in a club when she felt a burning sensation across her abdomen. When she looked down, she was bleeding.

Number of Patients

Student: How many patients are there?
PROCTOR: One.

Additional Resources

Student: I would hold off on calling for advanced life support (ALS) assistance.
PROCTOR: Noted.

C-Spine Stabilization

Student: On the basis of the mechanism of injury, I would stabilize the cervical spine (c-spine) in a neutral in-line position.
PROCTOR: Noted.

Critical Criteria:
- ❑ Did not determine scene safety
- ❑ Did not assess for spinal protection
- ❑ Did not provide for spinal protection when indicated

Initial Assessment

Student: As I perform midline c-spine stabilization, I identify myself and ask the patient not to move.
PROCTOR: Noted.

General Impression

Student: My general impression is that the patient's condition is stable.
PROCTOR: Noted.

Responsiveness/Level of Consciousness

Student: What is the patient's level of consciousness?
PROCTOR: Alert and very upset.

Chief Complaint/Apparent Life Threats

Student: What is the patient's chief complaint?
PROCTOR: The patient is complaining of a laceration across her belly. The laceration is not deep.

Assess the Airway and Breathing

Student: Is the airway open? Is the patient breathing?
PROCTOR: Yes, the airway is open and the patient is breathing.
Student: There are no apparent life threats.
PROCTOR: Noted.

Assessment

Student: What are the rate and the quality of breathing?
PROCTOR: Rate: A little fast. Quality: Normal.

Provide Oxygen

Student: I am applying oxygen at 15 L/min via nonrebreathing mask.
PROCTOR: Noted.

Ensure Adequate Ventilation

Student: The patient has adequate ventilations at this time.
PROCTOR: Noted.

Injury Management

Student: I will have my partner control the c-spine as I continue patient assessment.
PROCTOR: Noted.

Assess Circulation

Student: I am assessing the patient's circulation.
PROCTOR: Noted.

Assess for and Control Major Bleeding

Student: Do I find any major bleeding?
PROCTOR: No. Bleeding is minimal. She has a shallow 10- to 12-inch laceration across the abdomen.

Assess the Pulse

Student: What are the rate and the quality of pulses?
PROCTOR: Rate: Within normal limits. Quality: Normal.

Assess the Skin

Student: I am assessing the skin. What are the color, temperature, and condition of the skin?
PROCTOR: Color: Flushed. Temperature: Warm. Condition: Moist.

Identify Priority Patients/Make Transport Decision

Student: The patient is a low priority and does not require immediate transport.
PROCTOR: Noted.

Critical Criteria:
- ❑ Did not provide high concentration of oxygen
- ❑ Did not find or manage problems associated with airway, breathing, hemorrhage or shock (hypoperfusion)
- ❑ Did not differentiate patient's need for transportation versus continued assessment at the scene
- ❑ Did other detailed examination before assessing the airway, breathing and circulation

Focused History and Physical Examination/Rapid Trauma Assessment

Select the Appropriate Assessment (Focused or Rapid)

Student: I am selecting the rapid physical exam to identify and treat life threats.
PROCTOR: Noted.
Student: I am checking for DCAP-BTLS. This acronym stands for deformities, contusions, abrasions, punctures, penetrations, paradoxical motion in the chest, and burns, tenderness, lacerations, and swelling. I am also checking for motor and sensory function and pulses.
PROCTOR: Noted.

Head

Student: I am rapidly assessing the head.
PROCTOR: There are no obvious injuries.

Neck

Student: I am rapidly assessing the neck.
PROCTOR: There are no obvious injuries.
Student: I will apply a cervical collar.
PROCTOR: Noted.

▶ Chest

Student: I am rapidly assessing the chest.
PROCTOR: There are no obvious injuries.
Student: Are there lung sounds present?
PROCTOR: They are clear bilaterally.

▶ Abdomen/Pelvis

Student: I am rapidly assessing the abdomen.
PROCTOR: There is a 10- to 12-inch laceration that is shallow and barely bleeding.
Student: I will apply a dressing.
PROCTOR: Noted. Bleeding is controlled.
Student: I am rapidly assessing the pelvis.
PROCTOR: There are no obvious injuries.

▶ Extremities

Student: I am rapidly assessing the extremities.
PROCTOR: There are no obvious injuries.

▶ Assess Motor, Sensory, and Circulatory Function

Student: I am checking for DCAP-BTLS. Right leg?
PROCTOR: Negative DCAP-BTLS. Motor and sensory functions are present. Pulses are present.
Student: Left leg?
PROCTOR: Negative DCAP-BTLS. Motor and sensory functions are present. Pulses are present.
Student: Right arm?
PROCTOR: Negative DCAP-BTLS. Motor and sensory functions are present. Pulses are present.
Student: Left arm?
PROCTOR: Negative DCAP-BTLS. Motor and sensory functions are present. Pulses are present.

▶ Posterior

Student: I will rapidly assess the back. We will now log roll the patient as a unit to check the back. The person at the head will count to three and we will roll the patient.
PROCTOR: Noted.

▶ Assess the Thorax

Student: I am assessing the thorax. Do I find injuries?
PROCTOR: No.

▶ Assess the Lumbar Area

Student: I am assessing the flanks and lumbar area. Do I find injuries?
PROCTOR: No.

▶ Assess the Entire Backside

Student: I am assessing the entire backside. Do I find injuries?
PROCTOR: No.

▶ Manage Secondary Injuries/Wounds

Student: We will apply a cervical collar and backboard with full immobilization per local protocol, if not yet done, at this time. I will check the dressing.
PROCTOR: Noted.
Student: Are there any changes in motor and sensory functions or pulses?
PROCTOR: No.

▶ Reevaluate Transport Decision

Student: This patient does not require immediate transport.
PROCTOR: Noted.

▼ Baseline Vital Signs

Student: What are the patient's baseline vital signs, including blood pressure, pulse, respirations, pulse oximetry, and level of consciousness?
PROCTOR: Blood pressure, 124/78 mm Hg; pulse, 96 beats/min; respirations, 20 breaths/min; pulse oximetry reading, 98%; and the patient is alert.

▼ SAMPLE History

Student: At this time I will gather a SAMPLE history from the patient or family. What are the patient's signs and symptoms?
PROCTOR: She is very upset and is afraid of disease from the dirty box cutter.
Student: Allergies?
PROCTOR: No allergies.
Student: Medications?
PROCTOR: Inhaler.
Student: Pertinent past medical history?
PROCTOR: Asthma.
Student: Last oral intake?
PROCTOR: 30 minutes ago.
Student: Events leading up to the incident?
PROCTOR: The patient was dancing when she felt a burning sensation across her belly. When she looked down, she saw the blood and her shirt hanging down.

Critical Criteria:
- ❑ Did not differentiate patient's need for transportation versus continued assessment at the scene
- ❑ Did not provide for spinal protection when indicated

Detailed Physical Examination

Student: I am conducting the detailed physical exam. I am looking for DCAP-BTLS.
PROCTOR: Noted. The detailed physical exam will be performed during transport.

▼ Assess the Head

Student: I am assessing the head. Do I find any DCAP-BTLS? Do I find any evidence of Battle's sign or raccoon eyes?
PROCTOR: No.

▶ Inspect and Palpate the Head and Ears

Student: I am assessing the head and ears.
PROCTOR: There are no obvious injuries.

▶ Assess the Eyes

Student: I am assessing the eyes. Are the pupils equal, round, and regular in size, and react properly to light (PEARRL)?
PROCTOR: They are PEARRL.

▶ Assess the Facial Area Including Oral and Nasal Areas

Student: I am assessing the face, nose, and mouth. Do I see any discharge or hear any obstructions?
PROCTOR: No.

▼ Assess the Neck

▶ Inspect and Palpate the Neck

Student: I am assessing the neck for DCAP-BTLS.
PROCTOR: There are no obvious injuries.

▶ Assess for Jugular Vein Distention

Student: Do I find any jugular vein distention (JVD)?
PROCTOR: No.

▶ Assess for Tracheal Deviation

Student: Do I see any tracheal deviation?
PROCTOR: No.

▼ Assess the Chest

Student: I am assessing the chest for DCAP-BTLS.
PROCTOR: Noted.

▶ Inspect

Student: What do I see when I look at the chest?
PROCTOR: There are no obvious injuries.
Student: Does the chest appear symmetric?
PROCTOR: Yes.

▸ Palpate

Student: When I touch the chest, do I feel crepitus or a flail segment?

PROCTOR: No.

▸ Auscultate

Student: Are lung sounds present in all fields?

PROCTOR: Yes.

Student: Do I hear any sucking sounds from the chest?

PROCTOR: No.

▾ Assess the Abdomen/Pelvis

▸ Assess the Abdomen

Student: I am assessing the abdomen for DCAP-BTLS. I am assessing all four quadrants. Do I find any problems?

PROCTOR: You see a 10- to 12-inch-long incision across the top two quadrants. For the most part, blood was oozing from the laceration, with a few spots flowing. You see no spurting blood. Bleeding is controlled.

▸ Assess the Pelvis

Student: I am assessing the pelvis for DCAP-BTLS. Is the pelvis stable?

PROCTOR: Yes.

▾ Assess the Genitalia/Perineum as Needed (Verbalize in Training)

Student: I am assessing the genitalia/perineum as necessary for DCAP-BTLS.

PROCTOR: The area is unremarkable.

▾ Assess the Extremities

▸ Inspect

Student: I am assessing the lower and upper extremities for DCAP-BTLS. Do I find anything?

PROCTOR: No.

▸ Palpate

Student: Do I feel anything unusual?

PROCTOR: No.

▸ Assess Motor, Sensory, and Circulatory Function

Student: I am checking for DCAP-BTLS, motor and sensory functions, and pulses. Right leg?

PROCTOR: Negative DCAP-BTLS. Motor and sensory functions are present. Pulses are present.

Student: Left leg?

PROCTOR: Negative DCAP-BTLS. Motor and sensory functions are present. Pulses are present.

Student: Right arm?

PROCTOR: Negative DCAP-BTLS. Motor and sensory functions are present. Pulses are present.

Student: Left arm?

PROCTOR: Negative DCAP-BTLS. Motor and sensory functions are present. Pulses are present.

▾ Assess the Posterior

Note: This portion of the detailed physical exam would not be done if the patient were previously backboarded per local protocol.

Student: We will not check the back because it was previously checked and the patient is backboarded.

PROCTOR: Noted.

▾ Manage Secondary Injuries/Wounds

Student: I would direct my partner to reassess the abdomen.

PROCTOR: Noted.

▾ Reassess Vital Signs

Student: I will reassess vital signs and mental status.

PROCTOR: Blood pressure, 120/80 mm Hg; pulse, 92 beats/min; respirations, 20 breaths/min; pulse oximetry reading, 99%; and the patient is alert.

Student: The vital signs have not changed significantly.

PROCTOR: Noted.

▾ Reassess Interventions

Student: I will reassess my interventions: airway, breathing, and oxygen; circulation and bleeding control and a dressing; and immobilization and straps.

PROCTOR: Noted.

Critical Criteria:

❑ Did not find or manage problems associated with airway, breathing, hemorrhage or shock (hypoperfusion)

Radio Report

(Provided by the student.)

PROCTOR: Noted.

Ongoing Assessment

▾ Repeat Vital Signs

Student: I will reassess vital signs and mental status.

PROCTOR: Blood pressure, 122/74 mm Hg; pulse, 88 beats/min; respirations, 20 breaths/min; pulse oximetry reading, 99%; and the patient is alert.

Student: The vital signs have not changed significantly.

PROCTOR: Noted.

▾ Check Interventions

Student: I will check my interventions: airway, breathing, and oxygen; circulation and bleeding control; and immobilization and straps.

PROCTOR: Noted.

Critical Criteria:

❑ Did not find or manage problems associated with airway, breathing, hemorrhage or shock (hypoperfusion)

Handoff Report to Emergency Department Staff

Student: There was no change in the patient's condition during transport.

PROCTOR: Noted.

Critical Criteria:

❑ Did not transport patient within the (10) minute time limit

Critical Criteria

(Inform the student of items missed, if any.)

❑ Pass ❑ Fail Date: ______________________

Proctor Comments: ______________________

____

____

CASE 73

Notes

Dispatch Information

PROCTOR: EMS 10, respond to a shooting in front of your station in a blue Mazda pickup. Police are not on scene.

Pre-scene Action (BSI)

Student: I am wearing nonlatex gloves, safety glasses, mask, and gown.
PROCTOR: Noted.

Critical Criteria:
- ❑ Did not take, or verbalize, body substance isolation (BSI) precautions when necessary

Scene Size-up

Scene Safety

Student: Is the scene safe?
PROCTOR: Yes, police are on scene and you are given clearance to enter.

Mechanism of Injury

Student: What was the mechanism of injury?
PROCTOR: Gunshot wound. The 21-year-old patient was buying drugs when he was shot.

Number of Patients

Student: How many patients are there?
PROCTOR: One.

Additional Resources

Student: I would call for advanced life support (ALS) assistance.
PROCTOR: Noted.

C-Spine Stabilization

Student: On the basis of the mechanism of injury, I would stabilize the cervical spine (c-spine) in a neutral in-line position.
PROCTOR: Noted.

Critical Criteria:
- ❑ Did not determine scene safety
- ❑ Did not assess for spinal protection
- ❑ Did not provide for spinal protection when indicated

Initial Assessment

Student: As I perform midline c-spine stabilization, I identify myself and ask the patient not to move.
PROCTOR: Noted.

General Impression

Student: My general impression is that the patient's condition is unstable.
PROCTOR: Noted.

Responsiveness/Level of Consciousness

Student: What is the patient's level of consciousness?
PROCTOR: Conscious and alert.

Chief Complaint/Apparent Life Threats

Student: What is the patient's chief complaint?
PROCTOR: The patient is complaining of multiple gunshot wounds.
Student: There are apparent life threats; the life threats are the multiple gunshot wounds.
PROCTOR: Noted.

Assess the Airway and Breathing

Student: I am opening the airway using the jaw-thrust maneuver. Is the patient breathing?
PROCTOR: Yes.

Assessment

Student: What are the rate and the quality of breathing?
PROCTOR: Rate: Rapid. Quality: Deep.

Provide Oxygen

Student: I am applying oxygen at 15 L/min via nonrebreathing mask.
PROCTOR: Noted.

Ensure Adequate Ventilation

Student: The patient has adequate ventilations at this time.
PROCTOR: Noted.

Injury Management

Student: I will direct my partner to take over c-spine control as I continue assessment.
PROCTOR: Noted.

Assess Circulation

Student: I am assessing the patient's circulation.
PROCTOR: Noted.

Assess for and Control Major Bleeding

Student: Do I find any major bleeding?
PROCTOR: Yes, from the right chest, abdomen, left knee, and left hand.
Student: I would apply an occlusive dressing to the chest and abdomen and direct pressure and dressings to the rest of the wounds.
PROCTOR: Noted.

Assess the Pulse

Student: What are the rate and the quality of pulses?
PROCTOR: Rate: Tachycardic. Quality: Normal.

Assess the Skin

Student: I am assessing the skin. What are the color, temperature, and condition of the skin?
PROCTOR: Color: Pale. Temperature: Cool. Condition: Moist.

Identify Priority Patients/Make Transport Decision

Student: The patient is a high priority and is a load-and-go. I will begin packaging and transport.
PROCTOR: Noted.

Critical Criteria:
- ❑ Did not provide high concentration of oxygen
- ❑ Did not find or manage problems associated with airway, breathing, hemorrhage or shock (hypoperfusion)
- ❑ Did not differentiate patient's need for transportation versus continued assessment at the scene
- ❑ Did other detailed examination before assessing the airway, breathing and circulation

Focused History and Physical Examination/Rapid Trauma Assessment

Select the Appropriate Assessment (Focused or Rapid)

Student: I am selecting the rapid physical exam to identify and treat life threats. I am checking for DCAP-BTLS. This acronym stands for deformities, contusions, abrasions, punctures, penetrations, paradoxical motion in the chest, and burns, tenderness, lacerations, and swelling. I am also checking for motor and sensory function and pulses.
PROCTOR: Noted.

Head

Student: I am rapidly assessing the head.
PROCTOR: There are no obvious injuries.

Neck

Student: I am rapidly assessing the neck.
PROCTOR: There are no obvious injuries.
Student: I will apply a cervical collar.
PROCTOR: Noted.

▶ **Chest**

Student: I am rapidly assessing the chest.

PROCTOR: You see the entrance wound in the right chest. You hear sucking from the chest wound (if not already treated).

Student: I will check the occlusive dressing to the chest.

PROCTOR: Noted.

Student: I will assess the chest for tension pneumothorax by auscultation, and assessment (jugular vein distention [JVD], tracheal deviation, and decreased lung sounds).

PROCTOR: There are decreased lung sounds on the right side, jugular vein distension is present, and the trachea is deviated to the left.

Student: I will burp the occlusive dressing.

PROCTOR: Noted. The treatment was effective.

ALS Student: I will assess the chest for hyperresonance to percussion.

ALS Proctor: Noted. There is a tension pneumothorax on the right side.

ALS Student: I will decompress the chest.

ALS Proctor: Noted. The decompression was effective.

▶ **Abdomen/Pelvis**

Student: I am rapidly assessing the abdomen.

PROCTOR: You see an entrance wound.

Student: I will check the occlusive dressing.

PROCTOR: Noted.

Student: I am rapidly assessing the pelvis.

PROCTOR: There are no obvious injuries.

▶ **Extremities**

Student: I am rapidly assessing the extremities.

PROCTOR: You see an entrance wound in the left hand and left knee.

Student: I will apply dressings.

PROCTOR: Noted.

▶ **Assess Motor, Sensory, and Circulatory Function**

Student: I am checking for DCAP-BTLS. Right leg?

PROCTOR: Negative DCAP-BTLS. Motor and sensory functions are present. Pulses are present.

Student: Left leg?

PROCTOR: Wound noted to the knee. There is some bleeding. Motor and sensory functions are present. Pulses are present.

Student: Right arm?

PROCTOR: Negative DCAP-BTLS. Motor and sensory functions are present. Pulses are present.

Student: Left arm?

PROCTOR: There is a large through-and-through wound to the hand. Motor and sensory functions are present. Pulses are present.

▶ **Posterior**

Student: I will rapidly assess the back. We will now log roll the patient as a unit to check the back. The person at the head will count to three and we will roll the patient.

PROCTOR: Noted.

▶ **Assess the Thorax**

Student: I am assessing the thorax. Do I find injuries?

PROCTOR: No.

▶ **Assess the Lumbar Area**

Student: I am assessing the flanks and lumbar area. Do I find injuries?

PROCTOR: No.

▶ **Assess the Entire Backside**

Student: I am assessing the entire backside. Do I find injuries?

PROCTOR: No.

▶ **Manage Secondary Injuries/Wounds**

Student: We will apply a cervical collar and backboard with full immobilization per local protocol, if not yet done, at this time.

PROCTOR: Noted.

Student: Are there any changes in motor and sensory functions or pulses?

PROCTOR: No.

ALS Student: I will establish two large-bore IVs en route to the hospital and administer a bolus of 20 mL/kg in order to maintain a systolic blood pressure of 90 mm Hg. I will monitor the chest.

ALS Proctor: Noted.

▶ **Reevaluate Transport Decision**

Student: This patient is a load-and-go due to chest and abdominal trauma.

PROCTOR: Noted.

▼ Baseline Vital Signs

Student: What are the patient's baseline vital signs, including blood pressure, pulse, respirations, pulse oximetry, and level of consciousness?

PROCTOR: Blood pressure, 100/66 mm Hg; pulse, 130 beats/min; respirations, 24 breaths/min; pulse oximetry reading, 94%; and the patient is anxious.

▼ SAMPLE History

Student: At this time I will gather a SAMPLE history from the patient or family. What are the patient's signs and symptoms?

PROCTOR: The pain in his chest is killing him.

Student: Allergies?

PROCTOR: No allergies.

Student: Medications?

PROCTOR: Cocaine, methamphetamine, and mushrooms.

Student: Pertinent past medical history?

PROCTOR: No pertinent medical history.

Student: Last oral intake?

PROCTOR: 1 hour ago.

Student: Events leading up to the incident?

PROCTOR: The patient was buying drugs when the dealer shot him.

Critical Criteria:

- ❑ Did not differentiate patient's need for transportation versus continued assessment at the scene
- ❑ Did not provide for spinal protection when indicated

▼ Detailed Physical Examination

Student: I am conducting the detailed physical exam. I am looking for DCAP-BTLS.

PROCTOR: Noted. The detailed physical exam will be performed during transport.

▼ Assess the Head

Student: I am assessing the head. Do I find any DCAP-BTLS? Do I find any evidence of Battle's sign or raccoon eyes?

PROCTOR: No.

▶ **Inspect and Palpate the Head and Ears**

Student: I am assessing the head and ears.

PROCTOR: There are no obvious injuries.

▶ **Assess the Eyes**

Student: I am assessing the eyes. Are the pupils equal, round, and regular in size, and react properly to light (PEARRL)?

PROCTOR: They are PEARRL.

▶ **Assess the Facial Area Including Oral and Nasal Areas**

Student: I am assessing the face, nose, and mouth. Do I see any discharge or hear any obstructions?

PROCTOR: No.

▼ Assess the Neck

▶ **Inspect and Palpate the Neck**

Student: I am assessing the neck for DCAP-BTLS.

PROCTOR: There are no obvious injuries.

▸ **Assess for Jugular Vein Distention**

Student: Do I find any jugular vein distention (JVD)?

PROCTOR: Yes.

▸ **Assess for Tracheal Deviation**

Student: Do I see any tracheal deviation?

PROCTOR: No (if previously treated).

▾ Assess the Chest

Student: I am assessing the chest for DCAP-BTLS.

PROCTOR: Noted.

▸ **Inspect**

Student: What do I see when I look at the chest?

PROCTOR: There is minimal bleeding from the wound.

Student: Does the chest appear symmetric?

PROCTOR: Yes.

▸ **Palpate**

Student: When I touch the chest, do I feel crepitus or a flail segment?

PROCTOR: No.

▸ **Auscultate**

Student: Are lung sounds present in all fields?

PROCTOR: Yes.

Student: Do I hear any sucking sounds from the chest?

PROCTOR: No, if the occlusive dressing is in place.

Student: I will assess the chest for tension pneumothorax by auscultation, and assessment (jugular vein distention [JVD], tracheal deviation, and decreased lung sounds).

PROCTOR: There are equal lung sounds on both sides, jugular vein distension is not present, and the trachea is midline.

ALS Student: I will assess the chest for hyperresonance to percussion.

ALS Proctor: Noted. There is not a tension pneumothorax.

▾ Assess the Abdomen/Pelvis

▸ **Assess the Abdomen**

Student: I am assessing the abdomen for DCAP-BTLS. I am assessing all four quadrants. Do I find any problems?

PROCTOR: Yes, the abdomen is board-like. Bleeding is controlled.

▸ **Assess the Pelvis**

Student: I am assessing the pelvis for DCAP-BTLS. Is the pelvis stable?

PROCTOR: Yes.

▾ Assess the Genitalia/Perineum as Needed (Verbalize in Training)

Student: I am assessing the genitalia/perineum as necessary for DCAP-BTLS.

PROCTOR: The area is unremarkable.

▾ Assess the Extremities

▸ **Inspect**

Student: I am assessing the lower and upper extremities for DCAP-BTLS. Do I find anything?

PROCTOR: No.

▸ **Palpate**

Student: Do I feel anything unusual?

PROCTOR: No.

▸ **Assess Motor, Sensory, and Circulatory Function**

Student: I am checking for DCAP-BTLS, motor and sensory function, and pulses. Right leg?

PROCTOR: Negative DCAP-BTLS. Motor and sensory functions are present. Pulses are present.

Student: Left leg?

PROCTOR: Wound noted to the knee. There is some bleeding. Motor and sensory functions are present. Pulses are present.

Student: Right arm?

PROCTOR: Negative DCAP-BTLS. Motor and sensory functions are present. Pulses are present.

Student: Left arm?

PROCTOR: There is a large through-and-through wound to the hand. Motor and sensory functions are present. Pulses are present.

▾ Assess the Posterior

Note: This portion of the detailed physical exam would not be done if the patient were previously backboarded per local protocol.

Student: We will not check the back because it was previously checked and the patient is backboarded.

PROCTOR: Noted.

▾ Manage Secondary Injuries/Wounds

Student: I would direct my partner to reassess the dressings.

PROCTOR: Noted.

▾ Reassess Vital Signs

Student: I will reassess vital signs and mental status.

PROCTOR: Blood pressure, 94/62 mm Hg; pulse, 134 beats/min; respirations, 20 breaths/min; pulse oximetry reading, 90%; and the patient is anxious.

Student: The vital signs are deteriorating.

PROCTOR: Noted.

▾ Reassess Interventions

Student: I will reassess my interventions: airway, breathing, and oxygen; occlusive dressing (burp as necessary); circulation and bleeding control; immobilization and straps; and treatment for shock.

PROCTOR: Noted.

ALS Student: I will reassess basic life support (BLS) interventions, plus the following: two large-bore IVs to maintain a systolic blood pressure of 90 mm Hg, cardiac monitor, and regional protocol (consider needle decompression if the patient shows signs and symptoms of shock and tracheal deviation).

ALS Proctor: Noted. The cardiac monitor shows sinus tachycardia.

Critical Criteria:

- ☐ Did not find or manage problems associated with airway, breathing, hemorrhage or shock (hypoperfusion)

Radio Report

(Provided by the student.)

PROCTOR: Noted.

Ongoing Assessment

▾ Repeat Vital Signs

Student: I will reassess vital signs and mental status.

PROCTOR: Blood pressure, 92/60 mm Hg; pulse, 136 beats/min; respirations, 20 breaths/min; pulse oximetry reading, 91%; and the patient is anxious.

Student: The vital signs have deteriorated.

PROCTOR: Noted.

▼ Check Interventions

Student: I will check my interventions: airway, breathing, and oxygen; occlusive dressing (burp as necessary); circulation and bleeding control; immobilization and straps; and treatment for shock.

PROCTOR: Noted.

ALS Student: I will check BLS interventions, plus the following: maintain the two large-bore IVs and maintain a systolic blood pressure of 90 mm Hg, cardiac monitor, and regional protocol (consider needle decompression if the patient shows signs and symptoms of shock and tracheal deviation).

ALS Proctor: Noted. The cardiac monitor shows sinus tachycardia.

Critical Criteria:
- ❑ Did not find or manage problems associated with airway, breathing, hemorrhage or shock (hypoperfusion)

▼ Handoff Report to Emergency Department Staff

Student: The patient's condition deteriorated during transport.

PROCTOR: Noted.

Critical Criteria:
- ❑ Did not transport patient within the (10) minute time limit

▼ Critical Criteria

(Inform the student of items missed, if any.)

❑ Pass ❑ Fail Date: ______________________

Proctor Comments: ______________________

____

____

Dispatch Information

PROCTOR: EMS 10, respond to a 34-year-old male who has been shot with a shotgun to the buttocks. He is conscious and breathing. Police are on scene.

Pre-scene Action (BSI)

Student: I am wearing nonlatex gloves, safety glasses, mask, and gown.
PROCTOR: Noted.

> **Critical Criteria:**
> ❑ Did not take, or verbalize, body substance isolation (BSI) precautions when necessary

Scene Size-up

Scene Safety

Student: Is the scene safe?
PROCTOR: Yes, police are on scene and you are given clearance to enter.

Mechanism of Injury

Student: What was the mechanism of injury?
PROCTOR: Gunshot wound. The patient was with his girlfriend when her ex-boyfriend shot him.

Number of Patients

Student: How many patients are there?
PROCTOR: One.

Additional Resources

Student: I would call for advanced life support (ALS) assistance.
PROCTOR: Noted.

C-Spine Stabilization

Student: On the basis of the mechanism of injury, I would stabilize the cervical spine (c-spine) in a neutral in-line position.
PROCTOR: Noted.

> **Critical Criteria:**
> ❑ Did not determine scene safety
> ❑ Did not assess for spinal protection
> ❑ Did not provide for spinal protection when indicated

Initial Assessment

Student: As I perform midline c-spine stabilization, I identify myself and ask the patient not to move.
PROCTOR: Noted.

General Impression

Student: My general impression is that the patient's condition is unstable.
PROCTOR: Noted.

Responsiveness/Level of Consciousness

Student: What is the patient's level of consciousness?
PROCTOR: Alert.

Chief Complaint/Apparent Life Threats

Student: What is the patient's chief complaint?
PROCTOR: The patient is complaining of being shot in the buttocks.
Student: There is an apparent life threat; the life threat is the mechanism of injury.
PROCTOR: Noted.

Assess the Airway and Breathing

Student: I am opening the airway with the jaw-thrust maneuver. Is the patient breathing?
PROCTOR: Yes.

Assessment

Student: What are the rate and the quality of breathing?
PROCTOR: Rate: Within normal limits. Quality: Deep.

Provide Oxygen

Student: I am applying oxygen at 15 L/min via nonrebreathing mask.
PROCTOR: Noted.

Ensure Adequate Ventilation

Student: The patient has adequate ventilations at this time.
PROCTOR: Noted.

Injury Management

Student: I will direct my partner to take over c-spine control as I continue assessment.
PROCTOR: Noted.

Assess Circulation

Student: I am assessing the patient's circulation.
PROCTOR: Noted.

Assess for and Control Major Bleeding

Student: Do I find any major bleeding?
PROCTOR: No.

Assess the Pulse

Student: What are the rate and the quality of pulses?
PROCTOR: Rate: Tachycardic. Quality: Bounding.

Assess the Skin

Student: I am assessing the skin. What are the color, temperature, and condition of the skin?
PROCTOR: Color: Normal. Temperature: Warm. Condition: Moist.

Identify Priority Patients/Make Transport Decision

Student: The patient is a high priority and is a load-and-go. I will begin packaging and transport.
PROCTOR: Noted.

> **Critical Criteria:**
> ❑ Did not provide high concentration of oxygen
> ❑ Did not find or manage problems associated with airway, breathing, hemorrhage or shock (hypoperfusion)
> ❑ Did not differentiate patient's need for transportation versus continued assessment at the scene
> ❑ Did other detailed examination before assessing the airway, breathing and circulation

Focused History and Physical Examination/Rapid Trauma Assessment

Select the Appropriate Assessment (Focused or Rapid)

Student: I am selecting the rapid physical exam to identify and treat life threats. I am checking for DCAP-BTLS. This acronym stands for deformities, contusions, abrasions, punctures, penetrations, paradoxical motion in the chest, and burns, tenderness, lacerations, and swelling.
PROCTOR: Noted.

Head

Student: I am rapidly assessing the head.
PROCTOR: There are no obvious injuries.

Neck

Student: I am rapidly assessing the neck.
PROCTOR: There are no obvious injuries.
Student: I will apply a cervical collar.
PROCTOR: Noted.

Chest

Student: I am rapidly assessing the chest. What are the lung sounds?
PROCTOR: There are no obvious injuries. Lung sounds are clear bilaterally.

▸ **Abdomen/Pelvis**

Student: I am rapidly assessing the abdomen.
PROCTOR: There are no obvious injuries.
Student: I am rapidly assessing the pelvis.
PROCTOR: There are no obvious injuries.

▸ **Extremities**

Student: I am rapidly assessing the extremities.
PROCTOR: There are no obvious injuries.

▸ **Assess Motor, Sensory, and Circulatory Function**

Student: I am checking for DCAP-BTLS. I am also checking for motor and sensory function and pulses. Right leg?
PROCTOR: Negative DCAP-BTLS. Motor and sensory functions are present. Pulses are present.
Student: Left leg?
PROCTOR: Negative DCAP-BTLS. Motor and sensory functions are present. Pulses are present.
Student: Right arm?
PROCTOR: Negative DCAP-BTLS. Motor and sensory functions are present. Pulses are present.
Student: Left arm?
PROCTOR: Negative DCAP-BTLS. Motor and sensory functions are present. Pulses are present.

▸ **Posterior**

Student: I will rapidly assess the back. We will now log roll the patient as a unit to check the back. The person at the head will count to three and we will roll the patient.
PROCTOR: Noted.

▸ **Assess the Thorax**

Student: I am assessing the thorax. Do I find injuries?
PROCTOR: No.

▸ **Assess the Lumbar Area**

Student: I am assessing the flanks and lumbar area. Do I find injuries?
PROCTOR: No.

▸ **Assess the Entire Backside**

Student: I am assessing the entire backside. Do I find injuries?
PROCTOR: Yes, multiple puncture wounds to the buttocks.
Student: I will apply direct pressure with dry, sterile dressings and control bleeding.
PROCTOR: Noted.

▸ **Manage Secondary Injuries/Wounds**

Student: We will apply a cervical collar and backboard with full immobilization per local protocol, if not yet done, at this time.
PROCTOR: Noted.
Student: Are there any changes in motor and sensory functions or pulses?
PROCTOR: No.

▸ **Reevaluate Transport Decision**

Student: This patient is a load-and-go due to the mechanism of injury.
PROCTOR: Noted.

▼ Baseline Vital Signs

Student: What are the patient's baseline vital signs, including blood pressure, pulse, respirations, pulse oximetry, and level of consciousness?
PROCTOR: Blood pressure, 134/85 mm Hg; pulse, 130 beats/min; respirations, 18 breaths/min; pulse oximetry reading, 97%; and the patient is alert.

▼ SAMPLE History

Student: At this time I will gather a SAMPLE history from the patient or family. What are the patient's signs and symptoms?
PROCTOR: Pain in the buttocks.
Student: Allergies?
PROCTOR: No allergies.
Student: Medications?
PROCTOR: No medications.
Student: Pertinent past medical history?
PROCTOR: No pertinent medical history.
Student: Last oral intake?
PROCTOR: 3 hours ago.
Student: Events leading up to the incident?
PROCTOR: The patient was with his girlfriend when he was shot.

Critical Criteria:
- ❑ Did not differentiate patient's need for transportation versus continued assessment at the scene
- ❑ Did not provide for spinal protection when indicated

▼ Detailed Physical Examination

Student: I am conducting the detailed physical exam. I am looking for DCAP-BTLS.
PROCTOR: Noted. The detailed physical exam will be performed during transport.

▼ Assess the Head

Student: I am assessing the head. Do I find any DCAP-BTLS? Do I find any evidence of Battle's sign or raccoon eyes?
PROCTOR: No.

▸ **Inspect and Palpate the Head and Ears**

Student: I am assessing the head and ears.
PROCTOR: There are no obvious injuries.

▸ **Assess the Eyes**

Student: I am assessing the eyes. Are the pupils equal, round, and regular in size, and react properly to light (PEARRL)?
PROCTOR: They are PEARRL.

▸ **Assess the Facial Area Including Oral and Nasal Areas**

Student: I am assessing the face, nose, and mouth. Do I see any discharge or hear any obstructions?
PROCTOR: No.

▼ Assess the Neck

▸ **Inspect and Palpate the Neck**

Student: I am assessing the neck for DCAP-BTLS.
PROCTOR: There are no obvious injuries.

▸ **Assess for Jugular Vein Distention**

Student: Do I find any jugular vein distention (JVD)?
PROCTOR: No.

▸ **Assess for Tracheal Deviation**

Student: Do I see any tracheal deviation?
PROCTOR: No.

▼ Assess the Chest

Student: I am assessing the chest for DCAP-BTLS.
PROCTOR: Noted.

▸ **Inspect**

Student: What do I see when I look at the chest?
PROCTOR: There are no obvious injuries.
Student: Does the chest appear symmetric?
PROCTOR: Yes.

▸ **Palpate**

Student: When I touch the chest, do I feel crepitus or a flail segment?
PROCTOR: No.

▸ **Auscultate**

Student: Are lung sounds present in all fields?
PROCTOR: Yes.
Student: Do I hear any sucking sounds from the chest?
PROCTOR: No.

▼ Assess the Abdomen/Pelvis

▸ **Assess the Abdomen**

Student: I am assessing the abdomen for DCAP-BTLS. I am assessing all four quadrants. Do I find any problems?

PROCTOR: No.

▸ **Assess the Pelvis**

Student: I am assessing the pelvis for DCAP-BTLS. Is the pelvis stable?

PROCTOR: Yes.

▼ Assess the Genitalia/Perineum as Needed (Verbalize in Training)

Student: I am assessing the genitalia/perineum as necessary for DCAP-BTLS.

PROCTOR: The area is unremarkable.

▼ Assess the Extremities

▸ **Inspect**

Student: I am assessing the lower and upper extremities for DCAP-BTLS. Do I find anything?

PROCTOR: No.

▸ **Palpate**

Student: Do I feel anything unusual?

PROCTOR: No.

▸ **Assess Motor, Sensory, and Circulatory Function**

Student: I am checking for DCAP-BTLS, motor and sensory function, and pulses. Right leg?

PROCTOR: Negative DCAP-BTLS. Motor and sensory functions are present. Pulses are present.

Student: Left leg?

PROCTOR: Negative DCAP-BTLS. Motor and sensory functions are present. Pulses are present.

Student: Right arm?

PROCTOR: Negative DCAP-BTLS. Motor and sensory functions are present. Pulses are present.

Student: Left arm?

PROCTOR: Negative DCAP-BTLS. Motor and sensory functions are present. Pulses are present.

▼ Assess the Posterior

Note: This portion of the detailed physical exam would not be done if the patient were previously backboarded per local protocol.

Student: We will not check the back because it was previously checked and the patient is backboarded.

PROCTOR: Noted.

▼ Manage Secondary Injuries/Wounds

Student: I would direct my partner to check the dressing.

PROCTOR: Noted.

▼ Reassess Vital Signs

Student: I will reassess vital signs and mental status.

PROCTOR: Blood pressure, 128/80 mm Hg; pulse, 110 beats/min; respirations, 18 breaths/min; pulse oximetry reading, 98%; and the patient is alert.

Student: The vital signs are improving.

PROCTOR: Noted.

▼ Reassess Interventions

Student: I will reassess my interventions: airway, breathing, and oxygen; circulation and bleeding control; and immobilization and straps.

PROCTOR: Noted.

ALS Student: I will reassess basic life support (BLS) interventions, plus the following: two large-bore IVs and cardiac monitor.

ALS Proctor: Noted. The cardiac monitor shows sinus tachycardia.

Critical Criteria:

❑ Did not find or manage problems associated with airway, breathing, hemorrhage or shock (hypoperfusion)

Radio Report

(Provided by the student.)

PROCTOR: Noted.

Ongoing Assessment

▼ Repeat Vital Signs

Student: I will reassess vital signs and mental status.

PROCTOR: Blood pressure, 122/78 mm Hg; pulse, 100 beats/min; respirations, 18 breaths/min; pulse oximetry reading, 98%; and the patient is alert.

Student: The vital signs have improved.

PROCTOR: Noted.

▼ Check Interventions

Student: I will check my interventions: airway, breathing, and oxygen; circulation and bleeding control; and immobilization and straps.

PROCTOR: Noted.

ALS Student: I will check BLS interventions, plus the following: two large-bore IVs and cardiac monitor.

ALS Proctor: Noted. The cardiac monitor shows sinus tachycardia.

Critical Criteria:

❑ Did not find or manage problems associated with airway, breathing, hemorrhage or shock (hypoperfusion)

Handoff Report to Emergency Department Staff

Student: The patient's condition improved during transport.

PROCTOR: Noted.

Critical Criteria:

❑ Did not transport patient within the (10) minute time limit

Critical Criteria

(Inform the student of items missed, if any.)

❑ Pass ❑ Fail Date: ______________________

Proctor Comments: ______________________

____

____

Notes

Dispatch Information

PROCTOR: EMS 10, respond to a 23-year-old female who has had a seizure. Friends say that she is not acting right. She is conscious and breathing.

Pre-scene Action (BSI)

Student: I am wearing nonlatex gloves and safety glasses.
PROCTOR: Noted.

Critical Criteria:
- ❑ Did not take, or verbalize, body substance isolation (BSI) precautions when necessary

Scene Size-up

Scene Safety

Student: Is the scene safe?
PROCTOR: Yes.

Mechanism of Injury/Nature of Illness

Student: What is the nature of the illness?
PROCTOR: Seizure/possible aspiration. The patient has had a seizure while sitting on a couch and has vomited.

Number of Patients

Student: How many patients are there?
PROCTOR: One.

Additional Resources

Student: I would not call for advanced life support (ALS) assistance.
PROCTOR: Noted.

C-Spine Stabilization

Student: I would not stabilize the cervical spine (c-spine).
PROCTOR: Noted.

Critical Criteria:
- ❑ Did not determine scene safety

Initial Assessment

General Impression

Student: My general impression is that the patient's condition is unstable.
PROCTOR: Noted.

Responsiveness/Level of Consciousness

Student: What is the patient's level of consciousness?
PROCTOR: Drowsy. The patient responds to verbal stimuli.

Chief Complaint/Apparent Life Threats

Student: What is the patient's chief complaint?
PROCTOR: The patient is post seizure.

Assess the Airway and Breathing

Student: Is the airway open?
PROCTOR: Yes.

Assessment

Student: What are the rate and the quality of breathing?
PROCTOR: Rate: Bradypneic. Quality: Shallow.

Provide Oxygen

Student: I will apply suction then oxygen at 15 L/min via nonrebreathing mask.
PROCTOR: Noted.

Ensure Adequate Ventilation

Student: The patient has adequate ventilations at this time.
PROCTOR: Noted.

Assess Circulation

Student: I am assessing the patient's circulation.
PROCTOR: Noted.

Assess for and Control Major Bleeding

Student: Do I find any major bleeding?
PROCTOR: No.

Assess the Pulse

Student: What are the rate and the quality of pulses?
PROCTOR: Rate: Within normal limits. Quality: Bounding.

Assess the Skin

Student: I am assessing the skin. What are the color, temperature, and condition of the skin?
PROCTOR: Color: Pale. Temperature: Cool. Condition: Moist.

Identify Priority Patients/Make Transport Decision

Student: The patient is a low priority and does not require immediate transport.
PROCTOR: Noted.

Critical Criteria:
- ❑ Did not provide high concentration of oxygen
- ❑ Did not find or manage problems associated with airway, breathing, hemorrhage or shock (hypoperfusion)
- ❑ Did not differentiate patient's need for transportation versus continued assessment at the scene
- ❑ Did detailed or focused history/physical examination before assessing the airway, breathing and circulation

Focused History and Physical Examination/Rapid Assessment

Select the Appropriate Assessment (Focused or Rapid)

Student: I am selecting the focused assessment.
PROCTOR: Noted.

SAMPLE History

Student: At this time I will gather a SAMPLE history from the patient or family. What are the patient's signs and symptoms?
PROCTOR: Altered mental status.

> Student: Describe the episode.
> **PROCTOR:** She had a seizure and aspirated vomit.
> Student: When was the onset? What was she doing when this started?
> **PROCTOR:** Visiting with friends.
> Student: What was the duration? How long has this been going on?
> **PROCTOR:** 5 minutes.
> Student: Are there any associated symptoms?
> **PROCTOR:** Yes, you can hear that she has aspirated vomit.
> Student: Is there any evidence of trauma?
> **PROCTOR:** No.
> Student: Have any interventions been tried? Has she done anything to make this better?
> **PROCTOR:** The patient has taken no actions.
> Student: Have there been any seizures?
> **PROCTOR:** Yes.
> Student: Has there been any fever?
> **PROCTOR:** No.

Student: Allergies?
PROCTOR: Unknown.
Student: Medications?
PROCTOR: Seizure medications. Specifics unknown.
Student: Pertinent past medical history?
PROCTOR: Seizures.
Student: Last oral intake?
PROCTOR: Unknown.
Student: Events leading up to the incident?
PROCTOR: The patient was visiting with friends when she had a seizure and vomited.

Perform the Focused Physical Examination

Student: I am performing the focused physical examination.
PROCTOR: Noted.

Student: I am assessing the patient's level of consciousness.
PROCTOR: The patient is drowsy but responds to verbal stimuli (she is in the postictal state).
Student: I will listen to the patient's lung sounds.
PROCTOR: You hear evidence of aspiration.
Student: I will check the patient's blood glucose level.
PROCTOR: The blood glucose level is 110 mg/dL.
Student: I am performing a Cincinnati stroke scale. Does the patient show evidence of facial droop, arm drift, or speech impairment?
PROCTOR: It is negative. There is no facial droop, no arm drift, and no speech impairment.

▼ Baseline Vital Signs

Student: What are the patient's baseline vital signs, including blood pressure, pulse, respirations, pulse oximetry, and level of consciousness?
PROCTOR: Blood pressure, 118/66 mm Hg; pulse, 106 beats/min; respirations, 12 breaths/min; pulse oximetry reading, 96%; and the patient is drowsy.

▼ Interventions

Student: I will continue to suction, apply oxygen, check the blood glucose level, and place the patient in the recovery position.
PROCTOR: Noted. The blood glucose level is 110 mg/dL.
ALS Student: I will apply basic life support (BLS) interventions, plus the following: establish IV access.
ALS Proctor: Noted.

▼ Reevaluate Transport Decision

Student: The patient is a low priority. I will transport her in the recovery position.
PROCTOR: Noted.

▼ Detailed Physical Examination

Possible Answer #1
Student: I would not do a detailed physical exam.
PROCTOR: Noted. (Go to "Radio Report.")

Possible Answer #2
Student: I am conducting the detailed physical exam. I am looking for DCAP-BTLS. This acronym stands for deformities, contusions, abrasions, punctures, penetrations, paradoxical motion in the chest, and burns, tenderness, lacerations, and swelling.
PROCTOR: Noted. The detailed physical exam will be performed during transport.

► Assess the Head

Student: I am assessing the head. Do I find any DCAP-BTLS? Do I find any evidence of Battle's sign or raccoon eyes?
PROCTOR: No.

► Inspect and Palpate the Head and Ears

Student: I am assessing the head and ears.
PROCTOR: There are no obvious injuries.

► Assess the Eyes

Student: I am assessing the eyes. Are the pupils equal, round, and regular in size, and react properly to light (PEARRL)?
PROCTOR: They are sluggish.

► Assess the Facial Area Including Oral and Nasal Areas

Student: I am assessing the face, nose, and mouth. Do I see any discharge or hear any obstructions?
PROCTOR: No.
Student: I will suction the airway as needed.
PROCTOR: Noted.

► Assess the Neck

► Inspect and Palpate the Neck

Student: I am assessing the neck for DCAP-BTLS.
PROCTOR: There are no obvious injuries.

► Assess for Jugular Vein Distention

Student: Do I find any jugular vein distention (JVD)?
PROCTOR: No.

► Assess for Tracheal Deviation

Student: Do I see any tracheal deviation?
PROCTOR: No.

► Assess the Chest

Student: I am assessing the chest for DCAP-BTLS.
PROCTOR: Noted.

► Inspect

Student: What do I see when I look at the chest?
PROCTOR: There are no obvious injuries.
Student: Is the chest symmetric?
PROCTOR: Yes.

► Palpate

Student: When I touch the chest, do I feel crepitus or a flail segment?
PROCTOR: No.

► Auscultate

Student: Are lung sounds present in all fields?
PROCTOR: Yes.
Student: Do I hear any sucking sounds from the chest?
PROCTOR: No.

► Assess the Abdomen/Pelvis

► Assess the Abdomen

Student: I am assessing the abdomen for DCAP-BTLS. I am assessing all four quadrants. Do I find any problems?
PROCTOR: No.

► Assess the Pelvis

Student: I am assessing the pelvis for DCAP-BTLS. Is the pelvis stable?
PROCTOR: Yes.

► Assess the Genitalia/Perineum as Needed (Verbalize in Training)

Student: I am assessing the genitalia/perineum as necessary for DCAP-BTLS.
PROCTOR: The patient is incontinent of urine.

► Assess the Extremities

► Inspect

Student: I am assessing the lower and upper extremities for DCAP-BTLS. Do I find anything?
PROCTOR: No.

► Palpate

Student: Do I feel anything unusual?
PROCTOR: No.

► Assess Motor, Sensory, and Circulatory Function

Student: I am checking for DCAP-BTLS, motor and sensory function, and pulses. Right leg?
PROCTOR: Negative DCAP-BTLS. Motor and sensory functions are present. Pulses are present.
Student: Left leg?
PROCTOR: Negative DCAP-BTLS. Motor and sensory functions are present. Pulses are present.
Student: Right arm?
PROCTOR: Negative DCAP-BTLS. Motor and sensory functions are present. Pulses are present.
Student: Left arm?
PROCTOR: Negative DCAP-BTLS. Motor and sensory functions are present. Pulses are present.

► Assess the Posterior

Student: We will now check the back.
PROCTOR: Noted.

► Assess the Thorax

Student: I am assessing the thorax. Do I find injuries?
PROCTOR: No.

► Assess the Lumbar Area

Student: I am assessing the flanks and lumbar area. Do I find injuries?
PROCTOR: No.

▸ **Assess the Entire Backside**

Student: I am assessing the entire backside. Do I find injuries?

PROCTOR: No.

▸ **Manage Secondary Injuries/Wounds**

Student: I will assess for secondary injuries.

PROCTOR: Noted.

▼ Reassess Interventions

Student: I will reassess my interventions: suction as needed, apply oxygen, and place the patient in the recovery position.

PROCTOR: Noted.

ALS Student: I will reassess BLS interventions, plus the following: IV access.

ALS Proctor: Noted.

Critical Criteria:
- ❑ Did not obtain medical direction or verbalize standing orders for medical interventions
- ❑ Administered a dangerous or inappropriate intervention
- ❑ Did not ask questions about the present illness
- ❑ Did not differentiate patient's need for transportation versus continued assessment at the scene

Radio Report

(Provided by the student.)

PROCTOR: Noted.

Ongoing Assessment

▼ Repeat Vital Signs

Student: I will reassess vital signs and mental status.

PROCTOR: Blood pressure, 122/68 mm Hg; pulse, 102 beats/min; respirations, 16 breaths/min; pulse oximetry reading, 98%; and the patient is drowsy.

Student: The vital signs have not changed significantly.

PROCTOR: Noted.

▼ Check Interventions

Student: I will check my interventions: suction as needed, apply oxygen, and place the patient in the recovery position.

PROCTOR: Noted.

ALS Student: I will check BLS interventions, plus the following: IV access.

ALS Proctor: Noted.

▼ Repeat the Focused Assessment

Student: I will repeat the focused assessment.

PROCTOR: Noted.

Critical Criteria:
- ❑ Did not obtain medical direction or verbalize standing orders for medical interventions
- ❑ Administered a dangerous or inappropriate intervention

Handoff Report to Emergency Department Staff

Student: The patient's condition improved during transport.

PROCTOR: Noted.

Critical Criteria

(Inform the student of items missed, if any.)

❑ Pass ❑ Fail Date: ____________________

Proctor Comments: ____________________

____

____

Notes

Dispatch Information

PROCTOR: EMS 10, respond to a 59-year-old male patient who is conscious but short of breath.

Pre-scene Action (BSI)

Student: I am wearing nonlatex gloves and safety glasses.
PROCTOR: Noted.

Critical Criteria:
❑ Did not take, or verbalize, body substance isolation (BSI) precautions when necessary

Scene Size-up

Scene Safety

Student: Is the scene safe?
PROCTOR: Yes.

Mechanism of Injury/Nature of Illness

Student: What is the nature of the illness?
PROCTOR: The patient is short of breath.

Number of Patients

Student: How many patients are there?
PROCTOR: One.

Additional Resources

Student: I would call for advanced life support (ALS) assistance.
PROCTOR: Noted.

C-Spine Stabilization

Student: I would not stabilize the cervical spine (c-spine).
PROCTOR: Noted.

Critical Criteria:
❑ Did not determine scene safety

Initial Assessment

General Impression

Student: My general impression is that the patient's condition is unstable.
PROCTOR: Noted.

Responsiveness/Level of Consciousness

Student: What is the patient's level of consciousness?
PROCTOR: Alert.

Chief Complaint/Apparent Life Threats

Student: What is the patient's chief complaint?
PROCTOR: The patient is complaining of shortness of breath.

Assess the Airway and Breathing

Student: Is the airway open?
PROCTOR: Yes.

Assessment

Student: What are the rate and the quality of breathing?
PROCTOR: Rate: Tachypneic. Quality: Labored.

Provide Oxygen

Student: I am applying oxygen at 15 L/min via nonrebreathing mask.
PROCTOR: Noted.

Ensure Adequate Ventilation

Student: The patient has adequate ventilations at this time.
PROCTOR: Noted.

Assess Circulation

Student: I am assessing the patient's circulation.
PROCTOR: Noted.

Assess for and Control Major Bleeding

Student: Do I find any major bleeding?
PROCTOR: No.

Assess the Pulse

Student: What are the rate and the quality of pulses?
PROCTOR: Rate: Tachycardic. Quality: Bounding.

Assess the Skin

Student: I am assessing the skin. What are the color, temperature, and condition of the skin?
PROCTOR: Color: Pale. Temperature: Cool. Condition: Diaphoretic.

Identify Priority Patients/Make Transport Decision

Student: The patient is a high priority and is a load-and-go. I will begin packaging and transport.
PROCTOR: Noted.

Critical Criteria:
❑ Did not provide high concentration of oxygen
❑ Did not find or manage problems associated with airway, breathing, hemorrhage or shock (hypoperfusion)
❑ Did not differentiate patient's need for transportation versus continued assessment at the scene
❑ Did detailed or focused history/physical examination before assessing the airway, breathing and circulation

Focused History and Physical Examination/Rapid Assessment

Select the Appropriate Assessment (Focused or Rapid)

Student: I am selecting the focused assessment.
PROCTOR: Noted.

SAMPLE History

Student: At this time I will gather a SAMPLE history from the patient or family. What are the patient's signs and symptoms?
PROCTOR: Respiratory.

Student: Onset: What were you doing when this started?
PROCTOR: Watching TV.
Student: Provokes: What makes your condition worse or better?
PROCTOR: It has not gotten any better.
Student: Quality: Can you describe your pain?
PROCTOR: None.
Student: Radiates: Do you have pain anywhere else?
PROCTOR: No.
Student: Severity: On a scale of 1 to 10 with 10 being the worst possible, how would you rate your distress?
PROCTOR: 7.
Student: Time: How long has this been going on?
PROCTOR: 2 hours.
Student: Interventions: Have you done anything to make this better?
PROCTOR: The patient has taken no actions.

Student: Allergies?
PROCTOR: Penicillin (PCN).
Student: Medications?
PROCTOR: No medications.
Student: Pertinent past medical history?
PROCTOR: No pertinent medical history.
Student: Last oral intake?
PROCTOR: 4 hours ago.
Student: Events leading up to the incident?
PROCTOR: The patient was sitting and watching TV when he experienced sudden onset shortness of breath.

Perform the Focused Physical Examination

Student: I am performing the focused physical examination.
PROCTOR: Noted.
Student: What do I see when I look at the chest?
PROCTOR: There are no obvious injuries.
Student: Is the chest symmetric?
PROCTOR: Yes.

Student: When I touch the chest, do I feel crepitus or a flail segment?
PROCTOR: No.
Student: Are lung sounds present in all fields?
PROCTOR: Yes.

▼ Baseline Vital Signs

Student: What are the patient's baseline vital signs, including blood pressure, pulse, respirations, pulse oximetry, and level of consciousness?
PROCTOR: Blood pressure, 156/90 mm Hg; pulse, 124 beats/min; respirations, 28 breaths/min; pulse oximetry reading, 94%; and the patient is alert.

▼ Interventions

Student: I will continue applying oxygen.
PROCTOR: Noted.
ALS Student: I will apply basic life support (BLS) interventions, plus the following: IV access, cardiac monitoring, 12-lead ECG, and nebulized breathing treatment per protocol.
ALS Proctor: Noted. The cardiac monitor shows sinus tachycardia.

▼ Reevaluate Transport Decision

Student: The patient is a high priority and is a load-and-go.
PROCTOR: Noted.

▼ Detailed Physical Examination

Possible Answer #1
Student: I would not do a detailed physical exam.
PROCTOR: Noted. (Go to "Radio Report.")

Possible Answer #2
Student: I am conducting the detailed physical exam. I am looking for DCAP-BTLS. This acronym stands for deformities, contusions, abrasions, punctures, penetrations, paradoxical motion in the chest, and burns, tenderness, lacerations, and swelling.
PROCTOR: Noted. The detailed physical exam will be performed during transport.

► **Assess the Head**

Student: I am assessing the head. Do I find any DCAP-BTLS? Do I find any evidence of Battle's sign or raccoon eyes?
PROCTOR: No.

► **Inspect and Palpate the Head and Ears**

Student: I am assessing the head and ears.
PROCTOR: There are no obvious injuries.

► **Assess the Eyes**

Student: I am assessing the eyes. Are the pupils equal, round, and regular in size, and react properly to light (PEARRL)?
PROCTOR: They are PEARRL.

► **Assess the Facial Area Including Oral and Nasal Areas**

Student: I am assessing the face, nose, and mouth. Do I see any discharge or hear any obstructions?
PROCTOR: No.

► **Assess the Neck**

► **Inspect and Palpate the Neck**

Student: I am assessing the neck for DCAP-BTLS.
PROCTOR: There are no obvious injuries.

► **Assess for Jugular Vein Distention**

Student: Do I find any jugular vein distention (JVD)?
PROCTOR: No.

► **Assess for Tracheal Deviation**

Student: Do I see any tracheal deviation?
PROCTOR: No.

► **Assess the Chest**

Student: I am assessing the chest for DCAP-BTLS.
PROCTOR: Noted.

► **Inspect**

Student: What do I see when I look at the chest?
PROCTOR: There are no obvious injuries.
Student: Is the chest symmetric?
PROCTOR: Yes.

► **Palpate**

Student: When I touch the chest, do I feel crepitus or a flail segment?
PROCTOR: No.

► **Auscultate**

Student: Are lung sounds present in all fields?
PROCTOR: Yes.
Student: Do I hear any sucking sounds from the chest?
PROCTOR: No.

► **Assess the Abdomen/Pelvis**

► **Assess the Abdomen**

Student: I am assessing the abdomen for DCAP-BTLS. I am assessing all four quadrants. Do I find any problems?
PROCTOR: No.

► **Assess the Pelvis**

Student: I am assessing the pelvis for DCAP-BTLS. Is the pelvis stable?
PROCTOR: Yes.

► **Assess the Genitalia/Perineum as Needed (Verbalize in Training)**

Student: I am assessing the genitalia/perineum as necessary for DCAP-BTLS.
PROCTOR: The area is unremarkable.

► **Assess the Extremities**

► **Inspect**

Student: I am assessing the lower and upper extremities for DCAP-BTLS. Do I find anything?
PROCTOR: No.

► **Palpate**

Student: Do I feel anything unusual?
PROCTOR: No.

► **Assess Motor, Sensory, and Circulatory Function**

Student: I am checking for DCAP-BTLS, motor and sensory function, and pulses. Right leg?
PROCTOR: Negative DCAP-BTLS. Motor and sensory functions are present. Pulses are present.
Student: Left leg?
PROCTOR: Negative DCAP-BTLS. Motor and sensory functions are present. Pulses are present.
Student: Right arm?
PROCTOR: Negative DCAP-BTLS. Motor and sensory functions are present. Pulses are present.
Student: Left arm?
PROCTOR: Negative DCAP-BTLS. Motor and sensory functions are present. Pulses are present.

► **Assess the Posterior**

Student: We will check the back.
PROCTOR: There are no obvious injuries.

► **Manage Secondary Injuries/Wounds**

Student: I would direct my partner to place the patient in the position of comfort.
PROCTOR: Noted.

► **Reassess Interventions**

Student: I will reassess my interventions: oxygen.
PROCTOR: Noted.

ALS Student: I will reassess BLS interventions, plus the following: IV access, cardiac monitoring, 12-lead ECG, and nebulized breathing treatment per protocol.

ALS Proctor: Noted. The cardiac monitor shows sinus tachycardia.

Critical Criteria:
- ❑ Did not obtain medical direction or verbalize standing orders for medical interventions
- ❑ Administered a dangerous or inappropriate intervention
- ❑ Did not ask questions about the present illness
- ❑ Did not differentiate patient's need for transportation versus continued assessment at the scene

Radio Report

(Provided by student.)

PROCTOR: Noted.

Ongoing Assessment

Repeat the Initial Assessment

Student: I will repeat the initial assessment.

PROCTOR: Noted. (Reflected in "Repeat Vital Signs.")

Repeat Vital Signs

Student: I will reassess vital signs and mental status.

PROCTOR: Blood pressure, 148/90 mm Hg; pulse, 112 beats/min; respirations, 22 breaths/min; pulse oximetry reading, 95%; and the patient is alert.

Student: The vital signs have not changed significantly.

PROCTOR: Noted.

Check Interventions

Student: I will check my interventions: oxygen.

PROCTOR: Noted.

ALS Student: I will check BLS interventions, plus the following: IV access, cardiac monitoring, 12-lead ECG, and nebulized breathing treatment per protocol.

ALS Proctor: Noted. The cardiac monitor shows sinus tachycardia.

Repeat the Focused Assessment

Student: I will repeat the focused assessment.

PROCTOR: Noted.

Critical Criteria:
- ❑ Did not obtain medical direction or verbalize standing orders for medical interventions
- ❑ Administered a dangerous or inappropriate intervention

Handoff Report to Emergency Department Staff

Student: There was no change during transport.

PROCTOR: Noted.

Critical Criteria

(Inform the student of items missed, if any.)

❑ Pass ❑ Fail Date: ____________________

Proctor Comments: ____________________

____

____

Notes

Dispatch Information

PROCTOR: EMS 10, respond to a 71-year-old female who is complaining of abdominal pain. She is conscious and breathing.

Pre-scene Action (BSI)

Student: I am wearing nonlatex gloves and safety glasses.
PROCTOR: Noted.

Critical Criteria:
- ❑ Did not take, or verbalize, body substance isolation (BSI) precautions when necessary

Scene Size-up

Scene Safety

Student: Is the scene safe?
PROCTOR: Yes.

Mechanism of Injury/Nature of Illness

Student: What is the nature of the illness?
PROCTOR: The patient has a history of bowel impactions and is complaining of constipation and abdominal pain.

Number of Patients

Student: How many patients are there?
PROCTOR: One.

Additional Resources

Student: I would not call for advanced life support (ALS) assistance.
PROCTOR: Noted.

C-Spine Stabilization

Student: I would not stabilize the cervical spine (c-spine).
PROCTOR: Noted.

Critical Criteria:
- ❑ Did not determine scene safety

Initial Assessment

General Impression

Student: My general impression is that the patient's condition is stable.
PROCTOR: Noted.

Responsiveness/Level of Consciousness

Student: What is the patient's level of consciousness?
PROCTOR: Alert.

Chief Complaint/Apparent Life Threats

Student: What is the patient's chief complaint?
PROCTOR: The patient is complaining of constipation and abdominal pain.

Assess the Airway and Breathing

Student: Is the airway open?
PROCTOR: Yes.

Assessment

Student: What are the rate and the quality of breathing?
PROCTOR: Rate: Within normal limits. Quality: Shallow.

Provide Oxygen

Student: I am applying oxygen at 15 L/min via nonrebreathing mask.
PROCTOR: Noted.

Ensure Adequate Ventilation

Student: The patient has adequate ventilations at this time.
PROCTOR: Noted.

Assess Circulation

Student: I am assessing the patient's circulation.
PROCTOR: Noted.

Assess for and Control Major Bleeding

Student: Do I find any major bleeding?
PROCTOR: No.

Assess the Pulse

Student: What are the rate and the quality of pulses?
PROCTOR: Rate: Within normal limits. Quality: Normal.

Assess the Skin

Student: I am assessing the skin. What are the color, temperature, and condition of the skin?
PROCTOR: Color: Normal. Temperature: Normal. Condition: Moist.

Identify Priority Patients/Make Transport Decision

Student: The patient is a low priority and does not require immediate transport.
PROCTOR: Noted.

Critical Criteria:
- ❑ Did not provide high concentration of oxygen
- ❑ Did not find or manage problems associated with airway, breathing, hemorrhage or shock (hypoperfusion)
- ❑ Did not differentiate patient's need for transportation versus continued assessment at the scene
- ❑ Did detailed or focused history/physical examination before assessing the airway, breathing and circulation

Focused History and Physical Examination/Rapid Assessment

Select the Appropriate Assessment (Focused or Rapid)

Student: I am selecting the focused assessment.
PROCTOR: Noted.

SAMPLE History

Student: At this time I will gather a SAMPLE history from the patient or family. What are the patient's signs and symptoms?
PROCTOR: Abdominal.

> Student: Onset: What were you doing when this started?
> **PROCTOR:** Sleeping; it woke her.
> Student: Provokes: What makes your condition worse or better?
> **PROCTOR:** Going to the hospital and getting "cleaned out" makes it better.
> Student: Quality: Can you describe your pain?
> **PROCTOR:** Cramping.
> Student: Radiates: Do you have pain anywhere else?
> **PROCTOR:** No.
> Student: Severity: On a scale of 1 to 10 with 10 being the worst possible, how would you rate your pain/distress?
> **PROCTOR:** 10.
> Student: Time: How long has this been going on?
> **PROCTOR:** 2 hours.
> Student: Interventions: Have you done anything to make this better?
> **PROCTOR:** The patient has taken no actions.

Student: Allergies?
PROCTOR: No allergies.
Student: Medications?
PROCTOR: Stool softeners.
Student: Pertinent past medical history?
PROCTOR: Bowel impactions.
Student: Last oral intake?
PROCTOR: 12 hours ago.
Student: Events leading up to the incident?
PROCTOR: The patient was sleeping and awoke with the pain.

Perform the Focused Physical Examination

Student: I am performing the focused physical examination.
PROCTOR: Noted.

Student: I am assessing the abdomen for DCAP-BTLS. This acronym stands for deformities, contusions, abrasions, punctures, penetrations, paradoxical motion in the chest, burns, tenderness, lacerations, and swelling. I am assessing all four quadrants. Do I find any problems? Is there any pulsating masses found?
PROCTOR: There is distention and cramping but no pulsating masses noted.
Student: I am assessing the pelvis for DCAP-BTLS. Is the pelvis stable?
PROCTOR: Yes.

▼ Baseline Vital Signs
Student: What are the patient's baseline vital signs, including blood pressure, pulse, respirations, pulse oximetry, and level of consciousness?
PROCTOR: Blood pressure, 140/78 mm Hg; pulse, 96 beats/min; respirations, 16 breaths/min; pulse oximetry reading, 97%; and the patient is alert.

▼ Interventions
Student: I will apply oxygen and transport in the position of comfort.
PROCTOR: Noted.
ALS Student: I will apply basic life support (BLS) interventions plus the following: establish an IV and cardiac monitor.
ALS Proctor: Noted. The cardiac monitor shows normal sinus rhythm.

▼ Reevaluate Transport Decision
Student: The patient does not require immediate transport.
PROCTOR: Noted.

▼ Detailed Physical Examination
Possible Answer #1
Student: I would not do a detailed physical exam.
PROCTOR: Noted. (Go to "Radio Report.")

Possible Answer #2
Student: I am conducting the detailed physical exam. I am looking for DCAP-BTLS.
PROCTOR: Noted. The detailed physical exam will be performed during transport.

► Assess the Head
Student: I am assessing the head. Do I find any DCAP-BTLS? Do I find any evidence of Battle's sign or raccoon eyes?
PROCTOR: No.

► Inspect and Palpate the Head and Ears
Student: I am assessing the head and ears.
PROCTOR: There are no obvious injuries.

► Assess the Eyes
Student: I am assessing the eyes. Are the pupils equal, round, and regular in size, and react properly to light (PEARRL)?
PROCTOR: They are PEARRL.

► Assess the Facial Area Including Oral and Nasal Areas
Student: I am assessing the face, nose, and mouth. Do I see any discharge or hear any obstructions?
PROCTOR: No.

► Assess the Neck

► Inspect and Palpate the Neck
Student: I am assessing the neck for DCAP-BTLS.
PROCTOR: There are no obvious injuries.

► Assess for Jugular Vein Distention
Student: Do I find any jugular vein distention (JVD)?
PROCTOR: No.

► Assess for Tracheal Deviation
Student: Do I see any tracheal deviation?
PROCTOR: No.

► Assess the Chest
Student: I am assessing the chest for DCAP-BTLS.
PROCTOR: Noted.

► Inspect
Student: What do I see when I look at the chest?
PROCTOR: There are no obvious injuries.
Student: Is the chest symmetric?
PROCTOR: Yes.

► Palpate
Student: When I touch the chest, do I feel crepitus or a flail segment?
PROCTOR: No.

► Auscultate
Student: Are lung sounds present in all fields?
PROCTOR: Yes.
Student: Do I hear any sucking sounds from the chest?
PROCTOR: No.

► Assess the Abdomen/Pelvis

► Assess the Abdomen
Student: I am assessing the abdomen for DCAP-BTLS. I am assessing all four quadrants. Do I find any problems? Are there any pulsating masses found?
PROCTOR: There is obvious distention and cramping but no pulsating masses noted.

► Assess the Pelvis
Student: I am assessing the pelvis for DCAP-BTLS. Is the pelvis stable?
PROCTOR: Yes.

► Assess the Genitalia/Perineum as Needed (Verbalize in Training)
Student: I am assessing the genitalia/perineum as necessary for DCAP-BTLS.
PROCTOR: The area is unremarkable.

► Assess the Extremities

► Inspect
Student: I am assessing the lower and upper extremities for DCAP-BTLS. Do I find anything?
PROCTOR: No.

► Palpate
Student: Do I feel anything unusual?
PROCTOR: No.

► Assess Motor, Sensory, and Circulatory Function
Student: I am checking for DCAP-BTLS, motor and sensory function, and pulses. Right leg?
PROCTOR: Negative DCAP-BTLS. Motor and sensory functions are present. Pulses are present.
Student: Left leg?
PROCTOR: Negative DCAP-BTLS. Motor and sensory functions are present. Pulses are present.
Student: Right arm?
PROCTOR: Negative DCAP-BTLS. Motor and sensory functions are present. Pulses are present.
Student: Left arm?
PROCTOR: Negative DCAP-BTLS. Motor and sensory functions are present. Pulses are present.

► Assess the Posterior
Student: We will not check the back.
PROCTOR: Noted.

► Manage Secondary Injuries/Wounds
Student: I would direct my partner to reassure the patient during transport.
PROCTOR: Noted.

Reassess Interventions

Student: I will reassess my interventions: oxygen and transport the patient in the position dictated by local protocol.

PROCTOR: Noted.

ALS Student: I will reassess BLS interventions, plus the following: establish an IV and cardiac monitor.

ALS Proctor: Noted. The cardiac monitor shows normal sinus rhythm.

Critical Criteria:

- ❑ Did not obtain medical direction or verbalize standing orders for medical interventions
- ❑ Administered a dangerous or inappropriate intervention
- ❑ Did not ask questions about the present illness
- ❑ Did not differentiate patient's need for transportation versus continued assessment at the scene

Radio Report

(Provided by the student.)

PROCTOR: Noted.

Ongoing Assessment

Repeat the Initial Assessment

Student: I will repeat the initial assessment.

PROCTOR: Noted. (Reflected in "Repeat Vital Signs.")

Repeat Vital Signs

Student: I will reassess vital signs and mental status.

PROCTOR: Blood pressure, 136/74 mm Hg; pulse, 92 beats/min; respirations, 16 breaths/min; pulse oximetry reading, 98%; and the patient is alert.

Student: The vital signs have not changed significantly.

PROCTOR: Noted.

Check Interventions

Student: I will check my interventions: oxygen and transport the patient in the position dictated by local protocol.

PROCTOR: Noted.

ALS Student: I will check BLS interventions, plus the following: establish an IV and cardiac monitor.

ALS Proctor: Noted. The cardiac monitor shows normal sinus rhythm.

Repeat the Focused Assessment

Student: I will repeat the focused assessment.

PROCTOR: Noted.

Critical Criteria:

- ❑ Did not obtain medical direction or verbalize standing orders for medical interventions
- ❑ Administered a dangerous or inappropriate intervention

Handoff Report to Emergency Department Staff

Student: There was no change during transport.

PROCTOR: Noted.

Critical Criteria

(Inform the student of items missed, if any.)

❑ Pass ❑ Fail Date: ____________________

Proctor Comments: ____________________

____

____

Notes

Dispatch Information

PROCTOR: EMS 10, respond to a 65-year-old male who is complaining of chest pain. He is conscious and breathing.

Pre-scene Action (BSI)

Student: I am wearing nonlatex gloves and safety glasses.
PROCTOR: Noted.

Critical Criteria:
- ❑ Did not take, or verbalize, body substance isolation (BSI) precautions when necessary

Scene Size-up

Scene Safety

Student: Is the scene safe?
PROCTOR: Yes.

Mechanism of Injury/Nature of Illness

Student: What is the nature of the illness?
PROCTOR: The patient has chest pain.

Number of Patients

Student: How many patients are there?
PROCTOR: One.

Additional Resources

Student: I would call for advanced life support (ALS) assistance.
PROCTOR: Noted.

C-Spine Stabilization

Student: I would not stabilize the cervical spine (c-spine).
PROCTOR: Noted.

Critical Criteria:
- ❑ Did not determine scene safety

Initial Assessment

General Impression

Student: My general impression is that the patient's condition is unstable.
PROCTOR: Noted.

Responsiveness/Level of Consciousness

Student: What is the patient's level of consciousness?
PROCTOR: Alert and anxious.

Chief Complaint/Apparent Life Threats

Student: What is the patient's chief complaint?
PROCTOR: The patient is complaining of chest pain.

Assess the Airway and Breathing

Student: Is the airway open?
PROCTOR: Yes.

Assessment

Student: What are the rate and the quality of breathing?
PROCTOR: Rate: Within normal limits. Quality: Normal.

Provide Oxygen

Student: I am applying oxygen at 15 L/min via nonrebreathing mask.
PROCTOR: Noted.

Ensure Adequate Ventilation

Student: The patient has adequate ventilations at this time.
PROCTOR: Noted.

Assess Circulation

Student: I am assessing the patient's circulation.
PROCTOR: Noted.

Assess for and Control Major Bleeding

Student: Do I find any major bleeding?
PROCTOR: No.

Assess the Pulse

Student: What are the rate and the quality of pulses?
PROCTOR: Rate: Within normal limits. Quality: Bounding.

Assess the Skin

Student: I am assessing the skin. What are the color, temperature, and condition of the skin?
PROCTOR: Color: Pale. Temperature: Cool. Condition: Diaphoretic.

Identify Priority Patients/Make Transport Decision

Student: The patient is a high priority and is a load-and-go. I will begin packaging and transport.
PROCTOR: Noted.

Critical Criteria:
- ❑ Did not provide high concentration of oxygen
- ❑ Did not find or manage problems associated with airway, breathing, hemorrhage or shock (hypoperfusion)
- ❑ Did not differentiate patient's need for transportation versus continued assessment at the scene
- ❑ Did detailed or focused history/physical examination before assessing the airway, breathing and circulation

Focused History and Physical Examination/Rapid Assessment

Select the Appropriate Assessment (Focused or Rapid)

Student: I am selecting the focused assessment.
PROCTOR: Noted.

SAMPLE History

Student: At this time I will gather a SAMPLE history from the patient or family. What are the patient's signs and symptoms?
PROCTOR: Cardiac.

> **Student:** Onset: What were you doing when this started?
> **PROCTOR:** Watching TV (the news).
> **Student:** Provokes: What makes your condition worse or better?
> **PROCTOR:** Nothing makes it better.
> **Student:** Quality: Can you describe your pain?
> **PROCTOR:** Crushing chest pain.
> **Student:** Radiates: Do you have pain anywhere else?
> **PROCTOR:** The jaw and left shoulder and arm.
> **Student:** Severity: On a scale of 1 to 10 with 10 being the worst possible, how would you rate your pain/distress?
> **PROCTOR:** 10.
> **Student:** Time: How long has this been going on?
> **PROCTOR:** 1 hour.
> **Student:** Interventions: Have you done anything to make this better?
> **PROCTOR:** The patient took four baby aspirin like the commercial said to do.

Student: Allergies?
PROCTOR: No allergies.
Student: Medications?
PROCTOR: No medications.
Student: Pertinent past medical history?
PROCTOR: No pertinent medical history.
Student: Last oral intake?
PROCTOR: He was eating popcorn when the pain began.
Student: Events leading up to the incident?
PROCTOR: The patient was watching TV (the news) and eating popcorn.

Perform the Focused Physical Examination

Student: I am performing the focused physical examination.
PROCTOR: Noted.

Student: I am assessing the neck for DCAP-BTLS. This acronym stands for deformities, contusions, abrasions, punctures, penetrations, paradoxical motion in the chest, burns, tenderness, lacerations, and swelling.
PROCTOR: There are no obvious injuries.
Student: Do I find any jugular vein distention (JVD)?
PROCTOR: No.
Student: Do I see any tracheal deviation?
PROCTOR: No.
Student: I am assessing the chest for DCAP-BTLS.
PROCTOR: Noted.
Student: What do I see when I look at the chest?
PROCTOR: There are no obvious injuries.
Student: Is the chest symmetric?
PROCTOR: Yes.
Student: When I touch the chest, do I feel crepitus or a flail segment?
PROCTOR: No.
Student: Are lung sounds present in all fields?
PROCTOR: Yes.
Student: Do I hear any sucking sounds from the chest?
PROCTOR: No.
Student: I will assess the extremities for edema.
PROCTOR: There are no obvious injuries.

▼ Baseline Vital Signs

Student: What are the patient's baseline vital signs, including blood pressure, pulse, respirations, pulse oximetry, and level of consciousness?
PROCTOR: Blood pressure, 104/70 mm Hg; pulse, 56 beats/min; respirations, 12 breaths/min; pulse oximetry reading, 96%; and the patient is alert.

▼ Interventions

Student: I will apply oxygen.
PROCTOR: Noted.
ALS Student: I will apply basic life support (BLS) interventions, plus the following: establish IV access, perform cardiac monitoring, 12-lead ECG, and follow advanced cardiac life support (ACLS) (such as nitroglycerin and morphine sulfate) and local protocol.
ALS Proctor: Noted. The cardiac monitor shows sinus bradycardia at 56 beats/min.

▼ Reevaluate Transport Decision

Student: The patient is a high priority and is a load-and-go.
PROCTOR: Noted.

▼ Detailed Physical Examination

Possible Answer #1
Student: I would not do a detailed physical exam.
PROCTOR: Noted. (Go to "Radio Report.")

Possible Answer #2
Student: I am conducting the detailed physical exam. I am looking for DCAP-BTLS.
PROCTOR: Noted. The detailed physical exam will be performed during transport.

► **Assess the Head**

Student: I am assessing the head. Do I find any DCAP-BTLS? Do I find any evidence of Battle's sign or raccoon eyes?
PROCTOR: No.

► **Inspect and Palpate the Head and Ears**

Student: I am assessing the head and ears.
PROCTOR: There are no obvious injuries.

► **Assess the Eyes**

Student: I am assessing the eyes. Are the pupils equal, round, and regular in size, and react properly to light (PEARRL)?
PROCTOR: They are PEARRL.

► **Assess the Facial Area Including Oral and Nasal Areas**

Student: I am assessing the face, nose, and mouth. Do I see any discharge or hear any obstructions?
PROCTOR: No.

► **Assess the Neck**

► **Inspect and Palpate the Neck**

Student: I am assessing the neck for DCAP-BTLS.
PROCTOR: There are no obvious injuries.

► **Assess for Jugular Vein Distention**

Student: Do I find any jugular vein distention (JVD)?
PROCTOR: No.

► **Assess for Tracheal Deviation**

Student: Do I see any tracheal deviation?
PROCTOR: No.

► **Assess the Chest**

Student: I am assessing the chest for DCAP-BTLS.
PROCTOR: Noted.

► **Inspect**

Student: What do I see when I look at the chest?
PROCTOR: There are no obvious injuries.
Student: Is the chest symmetric?
PROCTOR: Yes.

► **Palpate**

Student: When I touch the chest, do I feel crepitus or a flail segment?
PROCTOR: No.

► **Auscultate**

Student: Are lung sounds present in all fields?
PROCTOR: Yes.
Student: Do I hear any sucking sounds from the chest?
PROCTOR: No.

► **Assess the Abdomen/Pelvis**

► **Assess the Abdomen**

Student: I am assessing the abdomen for DCAP-BTLS. I am assessing all four quadrants. Do I find any problems?
PROCTOR: No.

► **Assess the Pelvis**

Student: I am assessing the pelvis for DCAP-BTLS. Is the pelvis stable?
PROCTOR: Yes.

► **Assess the Genitalia/Perineum as Needed (Verbalize in Training)**

Student: I am assessing the genitalia/perineum as necessary for DCAP-BTLS.
PROCTOR: The area is unremarkable.

► **Assess the Extremities**

► **Inspect**

Student: I am assessing the lower and upper extremities for DCAP-BTLS. Do I find anything?
PROCTOR: No.

► **Palpate**

Student: Do I feel anything unusual?
PROCTOR: No.

► **Assess Motor, Sensory, and Circulatory Function**

Student: I am checking for DCAP-BTLS, motor and sensory function, and pulses. Right leg?
PROCTOR: Negative DCAP-BTLS. Motor and sensory functions are present. Pulses are present.

Student: Left leg?

PROCTOR: Negative DCAP-BTLS. Motor and sensory functions are present. Pulses are present.

Student: Right arm?

PROCTOR: Negative DCAP-BTLS. Motor and sensory functions are present. Pulses are present.

Student: Left arm?

PROCTOR: Negative DCAP-BTLS. Motor and sensory functions are present. Pulses are present.

Assess the Posterior

Student: We will not check the back.

PROCTOR: Noted.

Manage Secondary Injuries/Wounds

Student: I would direct my partner to place the patient in the position of comfort.

PROCTOR: Noted.

Reassess Interventions

Student: I will reassess my interventions: oxygen, reassurance, loosen tight-fitting clothing, and transport in the position of comfort.

PROCTOR: Noted.

ALS Student: I will reassess BLS interventions, plus the following: establish IV access, perform cardiac monitoring, 12-lead ECG, and follow ACLS (such as nitroglycerin and morphine sulfate) and local protocol.

ALS Proctor: Noted. The cardiac monitor shows sinus bradycardia at 56 beats/min with an elevated ST segment in leads II, III, and aVF.

Critical Criteria:

- ❑ Did not obtain medical direction or verbalize standing orders for medical interventions
- ❑ Administered a dangerous or inappropriate intervention
- ❑ Did not ask questions about the present illness
- ❑ Did not differentiate patient's need for transportation versus continued assessment at the scene

Radio Report

(Provided by the student.)

PROCTOR: Noted.

Ongoing Assessment

Repeat the Initial Assessment

Student: I will repeat the initial assessment.

PROCTOR: Noted. (Reflected in "Repeat Vital Signs.")

Repeat Vital Signs

Student: I will reassess vital signs and mental status.

PROCTOR: Blood pressure, 106/72 mm Hg; pulse, 62 beats/min; respirations, 16 breaths/min; pulse oximetry reading, 97%; and the patient is alert.

Student: The vital signs have not changed significantly.

PROCTOR: Noted.

Check Interventions

Student: I will check my interventions: oxygen, reassurance, loosen tight-fitting clothing, and transport in the position of comfort.

PROCTOR: Noted.

ALS Student: I will check BLS interventions, plus the following: establish IV access, perform cardiac monitoring, 12-lead ECG, and follow ACLS (such as nitroglycerin and morphine sulfate) and local protocol.

ALS Proctor: Noted. The cardiac monitor shows sinus bradycardia at 56 beats/min with an elevated ST segment in leads II, III, and aVF.

Repeat the Focused Assessment

Student: I will repeat the focused assessment.

PROCTOR: Noted.

Critical Criteria:

- ❑ Did not obtain medical direction or verbalize standing orders for medical interventions
- ❑ Administered a dangerous or inappropriate intervention

Handoff Report to Emergency Department Staff

Student: There was no change during transport.

PROCTOR: Noted.

Critical Criteria

(Inform the student of items missed, if any.)

❑ Pass ❑ Fail Date: ____________________

Proctor Comments: ____________________

____

____

CASE 79

Notes

Dispatch Information

PROCTOR: EMS 10, respond to a 23-year-old female with an altered mental status who is not making sense and is eating raw sausage. She is conscious and breathing.

Pre-scene Action (BSI)

Student: I am wearing nonlatex gloves and safety glasses.
PROCTOR: Noted.

> **Critical Criteria:**
> ❑ Did not take, or verbalize, body substance isolation (BSI) precautions when necessary

Scene Size-up

Scene Safety

Student: Is the scene safe?
PROCTOR: Yes.

Mechanism of Injury/Nature of Illness

Student: What is the nature of the illness?
PROCTOR: The patient is not making any sense when she speaks and she is eating raw sausage. She is a known diabetic.

Number of Patients

Student: How many patients are there?
PROCTOR: One.

Additional Resources

Student: I would not call for advanced life support (ALS) unless she becomes unresponsive.
PROCTOR: Noted.

C-Spine Stabilization

Student: I would not stabilize the cervical spine (c-spine).
PROCTOR: Noted.

> **Critical Criteria:**
> ❑ Did not determine scene safety

Initial Assessment

General Impression

Student: My general impression is that the patient's condition is stable.
PROCTOR: Noted.

Responsiveness/Level of Consciousness

Student: What is the patient's level of consciousness?
PROCTOR: Conscious but confused.

Chief Complaint/Apparent Life Threats

Student: What is the patient's chief complaint?
PROCTOR: The friends are complaining of the patient not making any sense and eating raw sausage.

Assess the Airway and Breathing

Student: Is the airway open?
PROCTOR: Yes.

Assessment

Student: What are the rate and the quality of breathing?
PROCTOR: Rate: Within normal limits. Quality: Normal.

Provide Oxygen

Student: I am applying oxygen at 15 L/min via nonrebreathing mask.
PROCTOR: Noted.

Ensure Adequate Ventilation

Student: The patient has adequate ventilations at this time.
PROCTOR: Noted.

Assess Circulation

Student: I am assessing the patient's circulation.
PROCTOR: Noted.

Assess for and Control Major Bleeding

Student: Do I find any major bleeding?
PROCTOR: No.

Assess the Pulse

Student: What are the rate and the quality of pulses?
PROCTOR: Rate: Within normal limits. Quality: Normal.

Assess the Skin

Student: I am assessing the skin. What are the color, temperature, and condition of the skin?
PROCTOR: Color: Pale. Temperature: Cool. Condition: Clammy.

Identify Priority Patients/Make Transport Decision

Student: The patient is a low priority and does not require immediate transport.
PROCTOR: Noted.

> **Critical Criteria:**
> ❑ Did not provide high concentration of oxygen
> ❑ Did not find or manage problems associated with airway, breathing, hemorrhage or shock (hypoperfusion)
> ❑ Did not differentiate patient's need for transportation versus continued assessment at the scene
> ❑ Did detailed or focused history/physical examination before assessing the airway, breathing and circulation

Focused History and Physical Examination/Rapid Assessment

Select the Appropriate Assessment (Focused or Rapid)

Student: I am selecting the focused assessment.
PROCTOR: Noted.

SAMPLE History

Student: At this time I will gather a SAMPLE history from the patient or family. What are the patient's signs and symptoms?
PROCTOR: Altered mental status.

Student: Describe the episode.
PROCTOR: She has not been acting right. She has been eating raw sausage.
Student: Onset: What was she doing when this started?
PROCTOR: She has been working outside in the yard for four or five hours.
Student: Duration: How long has this been going on?
PROCTOR: 30 minutes.
Student: Are there any associated symptoms?
PROCTOR: Yes, she is very hungry.
Student: Is there any evidence of trauma?
PROCTOR: No.
Student: Interventions: Has she done anything to make this better?
PROCTOR: The patient came in the house and began to eat raw meat.
Student: Have there been any seizures?
PROCTOR: No.
Student: Has there been any fever?
PROCTOR: No.

Student: Allergies?
PROCTOR: Unknown.
Student: Medications?
PROCTOR: Insulin.
Student: Pertinent past medical history?
PROCTOR: Diabetes.
Student: Last oral intake?
PROCTOR: Unknown.
Student: Events leading up to the incident?
PROCTOR: The patient was at a friend's house working in the yard when she began talking "silly" and opened the friend's refrigerator and started eating raw sausage.

▼ Perform the Focused Physical Examination

Student: I am performing the focused physical examination.
PROCTOR: Noted.
Student: I will check the patient's blood glucose level and contact medical control for an oral glucose order.
PROCTOR: Noted. The blood glucose level is 37 mg/dL. The oral glucose order is granted.

▼ Baseline Vital Signs

Student: What are the patient's baseline vital signs, including blood pressure, pulse, respirations, pulse oximetry, and level of consciousness?
PROCTOR: Blood pressure, 132/82 mm Hg; pulse, 88 beats/min; respirations, 12 breaths/min; pulse oximetry reading, 98%; and the patient is alert but confused.

▼ Interventions

Student: I will apply oxygen and administer oral glucose.
PROCTOR: Noted.
ALS Student: I will apply basic life support (BLS) interventions except for the oral glucose. I will establish IV access and administer 25 g of dextrose 50% in water.
ALS Proctor: Noted.

▼ Reevaluate Transport Decision

Student: This patient does not require immediate transport.
PROCTOR: Noted.

▼ Detailed Physical Examination

Possible Answer #1
Student: I would not do a detailed physical exam.
PROCTOR: Noted. (Go to "Radio Report.")

Possible Answer #2
Student: I am conducting the detailed physical exam. I am looking for DCAP-BTLS. This acronym stands for deformities, contusions, abrasions, punctures, penetrations, paradoxical motion in the chest, and burns, tenderness, lacerations, and swelling.
PROCTOR: Noted. The detailed physical exam will be performed during transport.

▸ **Assess the Head**

Student: I am assessing the head. Do I find any DCAP-BTLS? Do I find any evidence of Battle's sign or raccoon eyes?
PROCTOR: No.

▸ **Inspect and Palpate the Head and Ears**

Student: I am assessing the head and ears.
PROCTOR: There are no obvious injuries.

▸ **Assess the Eyes**

Student: I am assessing the eyes. Are the pupils equal, round, and regular in size, and react properly to light (PEARRL)?
PROCTOR: They are PEARRL.

▸ **Assess the Facial Area Including Oral and Nasal Areas**

Student: I am assessing the face, nose, and mouth. Do I see any discharge or hear any obstructions?
PROCTOR: No.

▸ **Assess the Neck**

▸ **Inspect and Palpate the Neck**

Student: I am assessing the neck for DCAP-BTLS.
PROCTOR: There are no obvious injuries.

▸ **Assess for Jugular Vein Distention**

Student: Do I find any jugular vein distention (JVD)?
PROCTOR: No.

▸ **Assess for Tracheal Deviation**

Student: Do I see any tracheal deviation?
PROCTOR: No.

▸ **Assess the Chest**

Student: I am assessing the chest for DCAP-BTLS.
PROCTOR: Noted.

▸ **Inspect**

Student: What do I see when I look at the chest?
PROCTOR: There are no obvious injuries.
Student: Is the chest symmetric?
PROCTOR: Yes.

▸ **Palpate**

Student: When I touch the chest, do I feel crepitus or a flail segment?
PROCTOR: No.

▸ **Auscultate**

Student: Are lung sounds present in all fields?
PROCTOR: Yes.
Student: Do I hear any sucking sounds from the chest?
PROCTOR: No.

▸ **Assess the Abdomen/Pelvis**

▸ **Assess the Abdomen**

Student: I am assessing the abdomen for DCAP-BTLS. I am assessing all four quadrants. Do I find any problems?
PROCTOR: No.

▸ **Assess the Pelvis**

Student: I am assessing the pelvis for DCAP-BTLS. Is the pelvis stable?
PROCTOR: Yes.

▸ **Assess the Genitalia/Perineum as Needed (Verbalize in Training)**

Student: I am assessing the genitalia/perineum as necessary for DCAP-BTLS.
PROCTOR: The area is unremarkable.

▸ **Assess the Extremities**

▸ **Inspect**

Student: I am assessing the lower and upper extremities for DCAP-BTLS. Do I find anything?
PROCTOR: No.

▸ **Palpate**

Student: Do I feel anything unusual?
PROCTOR: No.

▸ **Assess Motor, Sensory, and Circulatory Function**

Student: I am checking for DCAP-BTLS, motor and sensory function, and pulses. Right leg?
PROCTOR: Negative DCAP-BTLS. Motor and sensory functions are present. Pulses are present.
Student: Left leg?
PROCTOR: Negative DCAP-BTLS. Motor and sensory functions are present. Pulses are present.
Student: Right arm?
PROCTOR: Negative DCAP-BTLS. Motor and sensory functions are present. Pulses are present.
Student: Left arm?
PROCTOR: Negative DCAP-BTLS. Motor and sensory functions are present. Pulses are present.

▸ **Assess the Posterior**

Student: We will not check the back.
PROCTOR: Noted.

▸ **Manage Secondary Injuries/Wounds**

Student: I would direct my partner to monitor the airway.
PROCTOR: Noted.

▸ Reassess Interventions

Student: I will reassess my interventions: oxygen, recheck the blood glucose level, and contact medical control with an update.

PROCTOR: Noted. The blood glucose level is now 128 mg/dL.

ALS Student: I will reassess BLS interventions, plus the following: reassess IVs.

ALS Proctor: Noted.

Critical Criteria:

- ❑ Did not obtain medical direction or verbalize standing orders for medical interventions
- ❑ Administered a dangerous or inappropriate intervention
- ❑ Did not ask questions about the present illness
- ❑ Did not differentiate patient's need for transportation versus continued assessment at the scene

Radio Report

(Provided by the student.)

PROCTOR: Noted.

Ongoing Assessment

Repeat the Initial Assessment

Student: I will repeat the initial assessment.

PROCTOR: Noted. (Reflected in "Repeat Vital Signs.")

Repeat Vital Signs

Student: I will reassess vital signs and mental status.

PROCTOR: Blood pressure, 122/74 mm Hg; pulse, 82 beats/min; respirations, 16 breaths/min; pulse oximetry reading, 99%; and the patient is alert.

Student: The vital signs have not changed significantly.

PROCTOR: Noted.

Check Interventions

Student: I will check my interventions: oxygen and recheck the blood glucose level.

PROCTOR: Noted. The blood glucose level is now 128 mg/dL.

ALS Student: I will check BLS interventions, plus the following: IV.

ALS Proctor: Noted.

Repeat the Focused Assessment

Student: I will repeat the focused assessment.

PROCTOR: Noted.

Critical Criteria:

- ❑ Did not obtain medical direction or verbalize standing orders for medical interventions
- ❑ Administered a dangerous or inappropriate intervention

Handoff Report to Emergency Department Staff

Student: There was no change during transport.

PROCTOR: Noted.

Critical Criteria

(Inform the student of items missed, if any.)

❑ Pass ❑ Fail Date: ______________________

Proctor Comments: ______________________

____

____

Notes

Dispatch Information

PROCTOR: EMS 10, respond to the harbor for a 22-year-old sailor who has unusual burns to his chest. He is conscious and breathing. The Hazardous Materials team has cleared the scene of radioactivity and chemicals and a radioactive device has been properly secured.

Pre-scene Action (BSI)

Student: I am wearing nonlatex gloves and safety glasses.
PROCTOR: Noted.

Critical Criteria:
- ❑ Did not take, or verbalize, body substance isolation (BSI) precautions when necessary

Scene Size-up

Scene Safety

Student: Is the scene safe?
PROCTOR: Yes, you are given clearance to enter.

Mechanism of Injury

Student: What was the mechanism of injury?
PROCTOR: Toxic exposure/chest burns. The patient is a sailor on a ship. He was stealing cargo and found an item marked "radioactive source." He broke the seal and stuck the source in his pocket.

Number of Patients

Student: How many patients are there?
PROCTOR: One.

Additional Resources

Student: I would call for advanced life support (ALS) assistance and additional resources: police and fire/rescue.
PROCTOR: Noted.
Student: I will allow the fire/rescue and Hazardous Materials teams to decontaminate the patient. I will call medical control and give a brief radio report to let the receiving facility know that the patient has had a radioactive exposure and has undergone decontamination.
PROCTOR: Noted.

C-Spine Stabilization

Student: I would not stabilize the cervical spine (c-spine).
PROCTOR: Noted.

Critical Criteria:
- ❑ Did not determine scene safety

Initial Assessment

General Impression

Student: My general impression is that the patient's condition is unstable.
PROCTOR: Noted.

Responsiveness/Level of Consciousness

Student: What is the patient's level of consciousness?
PROCTOR: Alert.

Chief Complaint/Apparent Life Threats

Student: What is the patient's chief complaint?
PROCTOR: The patient is complaining of a burn with blistering to the right chest.

Assess the Airway and Breathing

Student: Is the airway open?
PROCTOR: Yes.

Assessment

Student: What are the rate and the quality of breathing?
PROCTOR: Rate: Tachypneic. Quality: Normal.

Provide Oxygen

Student: I am applying oxygen at 15 L/min via nonrebreathing mask.
PROCTOR: Noted.

Ensure Adequate Ventilation

Student: The patient has adequate ventilations at this time.
PROCTOR: Noted.

Assess Circulation

Student: I am assessing the patient's circulation.
PROCTOR: Noted.

Assess for and Control Major Bleeding

Student: Do I find any major bleeding?
PROCTOR: No.

Assess the Pulse

Student: What are the rate and the quality of pulses?
PROCTOR: Rate: Within normal limits. Quality: Bounding.

Assess the Skin

Student: I am assessing the skin. What are the color, temperature, and condition of the skin?
PROCTOR: Color: Flushed. Temperature: Warm. Condition: Moist.

Identify Priority Patients/Make Transport Decision

Student: The patient is a high priority and is a load-and-go. I will begin packaging and transport.
PROCTOR: Noted.

Critical Criteria:
- ❑ Did not provide high concentration of oxygen
- ❑ Did not find or manage problems associated with airway, breathing, hemorrhage or shock (hypoperfusion)
- ❑ Did not differentiate patient's need for transportation versus continued assessment at the scene
- ❑ Did detailed or focused history/physical examination before assessing the airway, breathing and circulation

Focused History and Physical Examination/Rapid Assessment

Select the Appropriate Assessment (Focused or Rapid)

Student: I am selecting the focused assessment.
PROCTOR: Noted.

SAMPLE History

Student: At this time I will gather a SAMPLE history from the patient or family. What are the patient's signs and symptoms?
PROCTOR: Poisoning/overdose.

> **Student:** What was the substance?
> **PROCTOR:** A radioactive source.
> **Student:** When did you ingest or become exposed to the substance?
> **PROCTOR:** 2 hours ago.
> **Student:** How much did you ingest?
> **PROCTOR:** N/A
> **Student:** Over what time period?
> **PROCTOR:** I was around the material for more than 1 hour.
> **Student:** Have you tried any interventions? Have you done anything to make this better?
> **PROCTOR:** No.
> **Student:** What is your weight?
> **PROCTOR:** 150 pounds.

Student: Allergies?
PROCTOR: No allergies.
Student: Medications?
PROCTOR: No medications.
Student: Pertinent past medical history?
PROCTOR: No pertinent medical history.
Student: Last oral intake?
PROCTOR: 4 hours ago.

Student: Events leading up to the incident?
PROCTOR: The patient placed a radioactive source in his shirt pocket.

Perform the Focused Physical Examination

Student: I am performing the focused physical examination.
PROCTOR: Noted.
Student: I am assessing the chest for DCAP-BTLS. This acronym stands for deformities, contusions, abrasions, punctures, penetrations, paradoxical motion in the chest, burns, tenderness, lacerations, and swelling.
PROCTOR: Noted.
Student: What do I see when I look at the chest?
PROCTOR: There is a blistered area in the upper right chest that is about the size of the patient's palm and partial thickness.
Student: I will dress the burn wound per local protocol.
PROCTOR: Noted.

Baseline Vital Signs

Student: What are the patient's baseline vital signs, including blood pressure, pulse, respirations, pulse oximetry, and level of consciousness?
PROCTOR: Blood pressure, 140/76 mm Hg; pulse, 96 beats/min; respirations, 20 breaths/min; pulse oximetry reading, 99%; and the patient is alert.

Interventions

Student: I will apply oxygen and provide reassurance. A dressing has been applied to the burn.
PROCTOR: Noted.
ALS Student: I will apply basic life support (BLS) interventions, plus the following: establish IV access, perform cardiac monitoring, and follow the local protocol.
ALS Proctor: Noted. The cardiac monitor shows normal sinus rhythm.

Reevaluate Transport Decision

Student: The patient is a high priority and is a load-and-go.
PROCTOR: Noted.

Detailed Physical Examination

Possible Answer #1
Student: I would not do a detailed physical exam.
PROCTOR: Noted. (Go to "Radio Report.")

Possible Answer #2
Student: I am conducting the detailed physical exam. I am looking for DCAP-BTLS.
PROCTOR: Noted. The detailed physical exam will be performed during transport.

- **Assess the Head**

Student: I am assessing the head. Do I find any DCAP-BTLS? Do I find any evidence of Battle's sign or raccoon eyes?
PROCTOR: No.

- **Inspect and Palpate the Head and Ears**

Student: I am assessing the head and ears.
PROCTOR: There are no obvious injuries.

- **Assess the Eyes**

Student: I am assessing the eyes. Are the pupils equal, round, and regular in size, and react properly to light (PEARRL)?
PROCTOR: They are PEARRL.

- **Assess the Facial Area Including Oral and Nasal Areas**

Student: I am assessing the face, nose, and mouth. Do I see any discharge or hear any obstructions?
PROCTOR: No.

- **Assess the Neck**
- **Inspect and Palpate the Neck**

Student: I am assessing the neck for DCAP-BTLS.
PROCTOR: There are no obvious injuries.

- **Assess for Jugular Vein Distention**

Student: Do I find any jugular vein distention (JVD)?
PROCTOR: No.

- **Assess for Tracheal Deviation**

Student: Do I see any tracheal deviation?
PROCTOR: No.

- **Assess the Chest**

Student: I am assessing the chest for DCAP-BTLS.
PROCTOR: Noted.

- **Inspect**

Student: What do I see when I look at the chest?
PROCTOR: The burn to the upper right chest has been dressed.
Student: Is the chest symmetric?
PROCTOR: Yes.

- **Palpate**

Student: When I touch the chest, do I feel crepitus or a flail segment?
PROCTOR: No.

- **Auscultate**

Student: Are lung sounds present in all fields?
PROCTOR: Yes.
Student: Do I hear any sucking sounds from the chest?
PROCTOR: No.

- **Assess the Abdomen/Pelvis**
- **Assess the Abdomen**

Student: I am assessing the abdomen for DCAP-BTLS. I am assessing all four quadrants. Do I find any problems?
PROCTOR: No.

- **Assess the Pelvis**

Student: I am assessing the pelvis for DCAP-BTLS. Is the pelvis stable?
PROCTOR: Yes.

- **Assess the Genitalia/Perineum as Needed (Verbalize in Training)**

Student: I am assessing the genitalia/perineum as necessary for DCAP-BTLS.
PROCTOR: The area is unremarkable.

- **Assess the Extremities**
- **Inspect**

Student: I am assessing the lower and upper extremities for DCAP-BTLS. Do I find anything?
PROCTOR: No.

- **Palpate**

Student: Do I feel anything unusual?
PROCTOR: No.

- **Assess Motor, Sensory, and Circulatory Function**

Student: I am checking for DCAP-BTLS, motor and sensory function, and pulses. Right leg?
PROCTOR: Negative DCAP-BTLS. Motor and sensory functions are present. Pulses are present.
Student: Left leg?
PROCTOR: Negative DCAP-BTLS. Motor and sensory functions are present. Pulses are present.
Student: Right arm?
PROCTOR: Negative DCAP-BTLS. Motor and sensory functions are present. Pulses are present.
Student: Left arm?
PROCTOR: Negative DCAP-BTLS. Motor and sensory functions are present. Pulses are present.

- **Assess the Posterior**

Student: We will now check the back.
PROCTOR: Noted.

- **Assess the Thorax**

Student: I am assessing the thorax. Do I find injuries?
PROCTOR: No.

▸ Assess the Lumbar Area

Student: I am assessing the flanks and lumbar area. Do I find injuries?

PROCTOR: No.

▸ Assess the Entire Backside

Student: I am assessing the entire backside. Do I find injuries?

PROCTOR: No.

▸ Manage Secondary Injuries/Wounds

Student: I would reassure the patient.

PROCTOR: Noted.

▸ Reassess Interventions

Student: I will reassess my interventions: reassurance, oxygen, and check the dressing that was applied to the burn.

PROCTOR: Noted.

ALS Student: I will reassess BLS interventions, plus the following: IV access, cardiac monitor, and local protocol.

ALS Proctor: Noted. The cardiac monitor shows normal sinus rhythm.

Critical Criteria:
- ❑ Did not obtain medical direction or verbalize standing orders for medical interventions
- ❑ Administered a dangerous or inappropriate intervention
- ❑ Did not ask questions about the present illness
- ❑ Did not differentiate patient's need for transportation versus continued assessment at the scene

Radio Report

(Provided by the student.)

PROCTOR: Noted.

Ongoing Assessment

Repeat Vital Signs

Student: I will reassess vital signs and mental status.

PROCTOR: Blood pressure, 132/72 mm Hg; pulse, 92 beats/min; respirations, 20 breaths/min; pulse oximetry reading, 99%; and the patient is alert.

Student: The vital signs have not changed significantly.

PROCTOR: Noted.

Check Interventions

Student: I will check my interventions: reassurance, oxygen, and dress the burn per local protocol.

PROCTOR: Noted.

ALS Student: I will check BLS interventions, plus the following: IV access, cardiac monitor, and local protocol.

ALS Proctor: Noted. The cardiac monitor shows normal sinus rhythm.

Repeat the Focused Assessment

Student: I will repeat the focused assessment.

PROCTOR: Noted.

Critical Criteria:
- ❑ Did not obtain medical direction or verbalize standing orders for medical interventions
- ❑ Administered a dangerous or inappropriate intervention

Handoff Report to Emergency Department Staff

Student: There was no change during transport.

PROCTOR: Noted.

Critical Criteria

(Inform the student of items missed, if any.)

❑ Pass ❑ Fail Date: ____________________

Proctor Comments: ____________________

____

____

Notes

Dispatch Information

PROCTOR: EMS 10, respond to a 35-year-old male who is complaining of severe leg pain. He is conscious and breathing.

Pre-scene Action (BSI)

Student: I am wearing nonlatex gloves and safety glasses.
PROCTOR: Noted.

Critical Criteria:
- ❑ Did not take, or verbalize, body substance isolation (BSI) precautions when necessary

Scene Size-up

Scene Safety

Student: Is the scene safe?
PROCTOR: Yes.

Mechanism of Injury/Nature of Illness

Student: What is the nature of the illness?
PROCTOR: The patient was working in a confined space. He felt numbness and tingling to his right leg but continued working. The pain to the leg is now unbearable. The patient is out of the confined space. The patient is in unusually severe pain and you believe this is a life-threatening event. He has a feeling of impending doom.

Number of Patients

Student: How many patients are there?
PROCTOR: One.

Additional Resources

Student: I would call for advanced life support (ALS) assistance due to the patient's distress.
PROCTOR: Noted.

C-Spine Stabilization

Student: I would not stabilize the cervical spine (c-spine).
PROCTOR: Noted.

Critical Criteria:
- ❑ Did not determine scene safety

Initial Assessment

General Impression

Student: My general impression is that the patient's condition is unstable.
PROCTOR: Noted.

Responsiveness/Level of Consciousness

Student: What is the patient's level of consciousness?
PROCTOR: Alert.

Chief Complaint/Apparent Life Threats

Student: What is the patient's chief complaint?
PROCTOR: The patient is complaining of right leg pain.

Assess the Airway and Breathing

Student: Is the airway open?
PROCTOR: Yes.

Assessment

Student: What are the rate and the quality of breathing?
PROCTOR: Rate: Within normal limits. Quality: Deep.

Provide Oxygen

Student: I am applying oxygen at 15 L/min via nonrebreathing mask.
PROCTOR: Noted.

Ensure Adequate Ventilation

Student: The patient has adequate ventilations at this time.
PROCTOR: Noted.

Assess Circulation

Student: I am assessing the patient's circulation.
PROCTOR: Noted.

Assess for and Control Major Bleeding

Student: Do I find any major bleeding?
PROCTOR: No.

Assess the Pulse

Student: What are the rate and the quality of pulses?
PROCTOR: Rate: Tachycardic. Quality: Thready.

Assess the Skin

Student: I am assessing the skin. What are the color, temperature, and condition of the skin?
PROCTOR: Color: Pale. Temperature: Cool. Condition: Diaphoretic.

Identify Priority Patients/Make Transport Decision

Student: The patient is a high priority and is a load-and-go. I will begin packaging and transport.
PROCTOR: Noted.

Critical Criteria:
- ❑ Did not provide high concentration of oxygen
- ❑ Did not find or manage problems associated with airway, breathing, hemorrhage or shock (hypoperfusion)
- ❑ Did not differentiate patient's need for transportation versus continued assessment at the scene
- ❑ Did detailed or focused history/physical examination before assessing the airway, breathing and circulation

Focused History and Physical Examination/Rapid Assessment

Select the Appropriate Assessment (Focused or Rapid)

Student: I am selecting the focused physical exam to identify and treat life threats.
PROCTOR: Noted.

SAMPLE History

Student: At this time I will gather a SAMPLE history from the patient or family. What are the patient's signs and symptoms?
PROCTOR: Unknown leg pain.

> **Student:** Onset: What were you doing when this started?
> **PROCTOR:** He was working in a confined space.
> **Student:** Provokes: What makes your condition worse or better?
> **PROCTOR:** Nothing makes it better.
> **Student:** Quality: Can you describe your pain?
> **PROCTOR:** It is intense pain.
> **Student:** Radiates: Do you have pain anywhere else?
> **PROCTOR:** He also has pain in the groin area.
> **Student:** Severity: On a scale of 1 to 10 with 10 being the worst possible, how would you rate your pain/distress?
> **PROCTOR:** 10.
> **Student:** Time: How long has this been going on?
> **PROCTOR:** 2 hours.
> **Student:** Interventions: Have you done anything to make this better?
> **PROCTOR:** The patient has taken no actions.

Student: Allergies?
PROCTOR: No allergies.
Student: Medications?
PROCTOR: No medications.
Student: Pertinent past medical history?
PROCTOR: No pertinent medical history.
Student: Last oral intake?
PROCTOR: 4 hours ago.
Student: Events leading up to the incident?
PROCTOR: The patient was working in a confined space. He felt numbness and tingling to his right leg but continued working. The pain to the leg is now unbearable.

▼ Perform the Rapid Physical Examination
Student: I am performing the focused physical examination.
PROCTOR: Noted.
Student: I am rapidly assessing the right leg.
PROCTOR: The right leg is cold and cyanotic.

▼ Baseline Vital Signs
Student: What are the patient's baseline vital signs, including blood pressure, pulse, respirations, pulse oximetry, and level of consciousness?
PROCTOR: Blood pressure, 132/88 mm Hg; pulse, 102 beats/min; respiratory rate, 20 breaths/min; pulse oximetry reading, 98%; and the patient is alert.

▼ Interventions
Student: I will apply oxygen and transport the patient in the position of function.
PROCTOR: Noted.

▼ Reevaluate Transport Decision
Student: This patient is a high priority and is a load-and-go.
PROCTOR: Noted.

▼ Detailed Physical Examination
Possible Answer #1
Student: I would not do a detailed physical exam.
PROCTOR: Noted. (Go to "Radio Report.")

Possible Answer #2
Student: I am conducting the detailed physical exam. I am looking for DCAP-BTLS. This acronym stands for deformities, contusions, abrasions, punctures, penetrations, paradoxical motion in the chest, and burns, tenderness, lacerations, and swelling.
PROCTOR: Noted. The detailed physical exam will be performed during transport.

▸ **Assess the Head**
Student: I am assessing the head. Do I find any DCAP-BTLS? Do I find any evidence of Battle's sign or raccoon eyes?
PROCTOR: No.

▸ **Inspect and Palpate the Head and Ears**
Student: I am assessing the head and ears.
PROCTOR: There are no obvious injuries.

▸ **Assess the Eyes**
Student: I am assessing the eyes. Are the pupils equal, round, and regular in size, and react properly to light (PEARRL)?
PROCTOR: They are PEARRL.

▸ **Assess the Facial Area Including Oral and Nasal Areas**
Student: I am assessing the face, nose, and mouth. Do I see any discharge or hear any obstructions?
PROCTOR: No.

▸ **Assess the Neck**

▸ **Inspect and Palpate the Neck**
Student: I am assessing the neck for DCAP-BTLS.
PROCTOR: There are no obvious injuries.

▸ **Assess for Jugular Vein Distention**
Student: Do I find any jugular vein distention (JVD)?
PROCTOR: No.

▸ **Assess for Tracheal Deviation**
Student: Do I see any tracheal deviation?
PROCTOR: No.

▸ **Assess the Chest**
Student: I am assessing the chest for DCAP-BTLS.
PROCTOR: Noted.

▸ **Inspect**
Student: What do I see when I look at the chest?
PROCTOR: There are no obvious injuries.
Student: Is the chest symmetric?
PROCTOR: Yes.

▸ **Palpate**
Student: When I touch the chest, do I feel crepitus or a flail segment?
PROCTOR: No.

▸ **Auscultate**
Student: Are lung sounds present in all fields?
PROCTOR: Yes.
Student: Do I hear any sucking sounds from the chest?
PROCTOR: No.

▸ **Assess the Abdomen/Pelvis**

▸ **Assess the Abdomen**
Student: I am assessing the abdomen for DCAP-BTLS. I am assessing all four quadrants. Do I find any problems?
PROCTOR: No.

▸ **Assess the Pelvis**
Student: I am assessing the pelvis for DCAP-BTLS. Is the pelvis stable?
PROCTOR: Yes.

▸ **Assess the Genitalia/Perineum as Needed (Verbalize in Training)**
Student: I am assessing the genitalia/perineum as necessary for DCAP-BTLS.
PROCTOR: The area is unremarkable.

▸ **Assess the Extremities**

▸ **Inspect**
Student: I am assessing the lower and upper extremities for DCAP-BTLS. Do I find anything?
PROCTOR: Yes, the right leg is cold and cyanotic.

▸ **Palpate**
Student: Do I feel anything unusual?
PROCTOR: Yes.

▸ **Assess Motor, Sensory, and Circulatory Function**
Student: I am checking for DCAP-BTLS, motor and sensory function, and pulses. Right leg?
PROCTOR: Cold and cyanotic. Motor and sensory functions are present. Pulses are absent.
Student: Left leg?
PROCTOR: Negative DCAP-BTLS. Motor and sensory functions are present. Pulses are present.
Student: Right arm?
PROCTOR: Negative DCAP-BTLS. Motor and sensory functions are present. Pulses are present.
Student: Left arm?
PROCTOR: Negative DCAP-BTLS. Motor and sensory functions are present. Pulses are present.

▸ **Assess the Posterior**
Student: We will check the back.
PROCTOR: Noted.

▸ **Assess the Thorax**
Student: I am assessing the thorax. Do I find injuries?
PROCTOR: No.

▸ **Assess the Lumbar Area**
Student: I am assessing the flanks and lumbar area. Do I find injuries?
PROCTOR: No.

▸ **Assess the Entire Backside**
Student: I am assessing the entire backside. Do I find injuries?
PROCTOR: No.

▸ **Manage Secondary Injuries/Wounds**
Student: I would direct my partner to monitor the patient.
PROCTOR: Noted.

▸ **Reassess Interventions**

Student: I will reassess my interventions: breathing, oxygen, and continuously reassess the patient.

PROCTOR: Noted.

Critical Criteria:
- ❑ Did not obtain medical direction or verbalize standing orders for medical interventions
- ❑ Administered a dangerous or inappropriate intervention
- ❑ Did not ask questions about the present illness
- ❑ Did not differentiate patient's need for transportation versus continued assessment at the scene

Radio Report

(Provided by the student.)

PROCTOR: Noted.

Ongoing Assessment

Repeat the Initial Assessment

Student: I will repeat the initial assessment.

PROCTOR: Noted. (Reflected in "Repeat Vital Signs.")

Repeat Vital Signs

Student: I will reassess vital signs and mental status.

PROCTOR: Blood pressure, 0/0 mm Hg; pulse, 0 beats/min; respirations, 0 breaths/min; pulse oximetry reading, N/A; and the patient is unresponsive.

Student: This patient just went into cardiac arrest. I will begin CPR and apply the automated external defibrillator (AED—witnessed arrest).

PROCTOR: Noted. No shock advised.

ALS Student: I will apply basic life support (BLS) interventions, plus the following: intubation, confirm end tidal CO_2, check lung sounds, IV access, cardiac monitor, and advanced cardiac life support (ACLS) or local protocol.

ALS Proctor: Noted. The cardiac monitor shows pulseless electrical activity. End tidal CO_2 and lung sounds confirm placement of the endotracheal (ET) tube.

Check Interventions

Student: I will check my interventions: CPR, oral/advanced airway if permitted to do so, oxygen, bag-valve device, and AED.

PROCTOR: Noted. No shock is advised.

ALS Student: I will check BLS interventions, plus the following: intubation, confirm end tidal CO_2, check lung sounds, IV access, cardiac monitor, and ACLS or local protocol.

ALS Proctor: Noted. The cardiac monitor shows pulseless electrical activity. End tidal CO_2 and lung sounds confirm placement of the ET tube.

Repeat the Focused Assessment

Student: I will repeat the focused assessment.

PROCTOR: Noted.

Critical Criteria:
- ❑ Did not obtain medical direction or verbalize standing orders for medical interventions
- ❑ Administered a dangerous or inappropriate intervention

Handoff Report to Emergency Department Staff

Student: The patient's condition deteriorated during transport.

PROCTOR: Noted.

Critical Criteria

(Inform the student of items missed, if any.)

❑ Pass ❑ Fail Date: ______________________

Proctor Comments: ______________________

____

____

Notes

CASE 83

Dispatch Information

PROCTOR: EMS 10, respond to a 64-year-old male patient with a history of chronic obstructive pulmonary disease (COPD) complaining of difficulty breathing.

Pre-scene Action (BSI)

Student: I am wearing nonlatex gloves and safety glasses.
PROCTOR: Noted.

Critical Criteria:
- ❑ Did not take, or verbalize, body substance isolation (BSI) precautions when necessary

Scene Size-up

Scene Safety

Student: Is the scene safe?
PROCTOR: Yes.

Mechanism of Injury/Nature of Illness

Student: What is the nature of the illness?
PROCTOR: The patient was trying to go to sleep. There is no air conditioning in the home, and the ambient temperature there has reached 94°F (34.4°C). The power went out, and the patient's home oxygen machine stopped working.

Number of Patients

Student: How many patients are there?
PROCTOR: One.

Additional Resources

Student: I would call for advanced life support (ALS) assistance.
PROCTOR: Noted.

C-Spine Stabilization

Student: I would not stabilize the cervical spine (c-spine).
PROCTOR: Noted.

Critical Criteria:
- ❑ Did not determine scene safety

Initial Assessment

General Impression

Student: My general impression is that the patient's condition is unstable.
PROCTOR: Noted.

Responsiveness/Level of Consciousness

Student: What is the patient's level of consciousness?
PROCTOR: Alert.

Chief Complaint/Apparent Life Threats

Student: What is the patient's chief complaint?
PROCTOR: The patient is complaining of shortness of breath.

Assess the Airway and Breathing

Student: Is the airway open?
PROCTOR: Yes.

Assessment

Student: What are the rate and the quality of breathing?
PROCTOR: Rate: Within normal limits. Quality: Labored.

Provide Oxygen

Student: I am applying oxygen with a nonrebreathing mask and 100% oxygen.
PROCTOR: Noted.

Ensure Adequate Ventilation

Student: The patient has adequate ventilations at this time.
PROCTOR: Noted.

Assess Circulation

Student: I am assessing the patient's circulation.
PROCTOR: Noted.

Assess for and Control Major Bleeding

Student: Do I find any major bleeding?
PROCTOR: No.

Assess the Pulse

Student: What are the rate and the quality of pulses?
PROCTOR: Rate: Within normal limits. Quality: Normal.

Assess the Skin

Student: I am assessing the skin. What are the color, temperature, and condition of the skin?
PROCTOR: Color: Pale. Temperature: Hot. Condition: Moist.

Identify Priority Patients/Make Transport Decision

Student: The patient is a high priority and is a load-and-go. I will begin packaging and transport.
PROCTOR: Noted.

Critical Criteria:
- ❑ Did not provide high concentration of oxygen
- ❑ Did not find or manage problems associated with airway, breathing, hemorrhage or shock (hypoperfusion)
- ❑ Did not differentiate patient's need for transportation versus continued assessment at the scene
- ❑ Did detailed or focused history/physical examination before assessing the airway, breathing and circulation

Focused History and Physical Examination/Rapid Assessment

Select the Appropriate Assessment (Focused or Rapid)

Student: I am selecting the focused assessment.
PROCTOR: Noted.

SAMPLE History

Student: At this time I will gather a SAMPLE history from the patient or family. What are the patient's signs and symptoms?
PROCTOR: Respiratory.

> **Student:** Onset: What were you doing when this started?
> **PROCTOR:** It has been going on all day.
> **Student:** Provokes: What makes your condition worse or better?
> **PROCTOR:** Air conditioning and oxygen make the condition better.
> **Student:** Quality: Can you describe your pain?
> **PROCTOR:** None.
> **Student:** Radiates: Do you have pain anywhere else?
> **PROCTOR:** No.
> **Student:** Severity: On a scale of 1 to 10 with 10 being the worst possible, how would you rate your pain/distress?
> **PROCTOR:** 2.
> **Student:** Time: How long has this been going on?
> **PROCTOR:** 12 hours.
> **Student:** Interventions: Have you done anything to make this better?
> **PROCTOR:** The patient has taken no actions.

Student: Allergies?
PROCTOR: No allergies.
Student: Medications?
PROCTOR: Home oxygen, inhaler, and other unknown.
Student: Pertinent past medical history?
PROCTOR: COPD.
Student: Last oral intake?
PROCTOR: 5 hours ago.
Student: Events leading up to the incident?
PROCTOR: The patient was hot in his home and wants to go to the hospital.

Perform Focused Physical Examination

Student: I am performing the focused physical examination.
PROCTOR: Noted.
Student: I am assessing the chest for DCAP-BTLS.
PROCTOR: Noted.
Student: What do I see when I look at the chest?
PROCTOR: There are no obvious injuries.
Student: Is the chest symmetric?
PROCTOR: Yes.
Student: When I touch the chest, do I feel crepitus or a flail segment?
PROCTOR: No.
Student: Are lung sounds present in all fields?
PROCTOR: Lung sounds are diminished due to COPD with wheezing on expiration.
Student: Do I hear any sucking sounds from the chest?
PROCTOR: No.

Baseline Vital Signs

Student: What are the patient's baseline vital signs, including blood pressure, pulse, respirations, pulse oximetry, and level of consciousness?
PROCTOR: Blood pressure, 142/84 mm Hg; pulse rate, 88 beats/min; respirations, 20 breaths/min; pulse oximetry reading, 96%; and the patient is alert.

Interventions

Student: I will apply oxygen and assist the patient with his inhaler.
PROCTOR: Noted.
ALS Student: I will apply basic life support (BLS) interventions, plus the following: establish IV access, perform cardiac monitoring, obtain a 12-lead ECG, and follow local protocol, including bronchodilator treatment if allowed.
ALS Proctor: Noted. The cardiac monitor shows normal sinus rhythm.

Reevaluate Transport Decision

Student: The patient is a load-and-go due to the nature of the illness.
PROCTOR: Noted.

Detailed Physical Examination

Possible Answer #1
Student: I would not do a detailed physical exam.
PROCTOR: Noted. (Go to "Radio Report.")

Possible Answer #2
Student: I am conducting the detailed physical exam. I am looking for DCAP-BTLS. This acronym stands for deformities, contusions, abrasions, punctures, penetrations, paradoxical motion in the chest, and burns, tenderness, lacerations, and swelling.
PROCTOR: Noted. The detailed physical exam will be performed during transport.

Assess the Head

Student: I am assessing the head. Do I find any DCAP-BTLS? Do I find any evidence of Battle's sign or raccoon eyes?
PROCTOR: No.

Inspect and Palpate the Head and Ears

Student: I am assessing the head and ears.
PROCTOR: There are no obvious injuries.

Assess the Eyes

Student: I am assessing the eyes. Are the pupils equal, round, and regular in size, and react properly to light (PEARRL)?
PROCTOR: They are PEARRL.

Assess the Facial Area Including Oral and Nasal Areas

Student: I am assessing the face, nose, and mouth. Do I see any discharge or hear any obstructions?
PROCTOR: No.

Assess the Neck

Inspect and Palpate the Neck

Student: I am assessing the neck for DCAP-BTLS.
PROCTOR: There are no obvious injuries.

Assess for Jugular Vein Distention

Student: Do I find any jugular vein distention (JVD)?
PROCTOR: No.

Assess for Tracheal Deviation

Student: Do I see any tracheal deviation?
PROCTOR: No.

Assess the Chest

Student: I am assessing the chest for DCAP-BTLS.
PROCTOR: Noted.

Inspect

Student: What do I see when I look at the chest?
PROCTOR: There are no obvious injuries.
Student: Is the chest symmetric?
PROCTOR: Yes.

Palpate

Student: When I touch the chest, do I feel crepitus or a flail segment?
PROCTOR: No.

Auscultate

Student: Are lung sounds present in all fields?
PROCTOR: Lung sounds are diminished due to COPD with wheezing on expiration.
Student: Do I hear any sucking sounds from the chest?
PROCTOR: No.

Assess the Abdomen/Pelvis

Assess the Abdomen

Student: I am assessing the abdomen for DCAP-BTLS. I am assessing all four quadrants. Do I find any problems?
PROCTOR: No.

Assess the Pelvis

Student: I am assessing the pelvis for DCAP-BTLS. Is the pelvis stable?
PROCTOR: Yes.

Assess the Genitalia/Perineum as Needed (Verbalize in Training)

Student: I am assessing the genitalia/perineum as necessary for DCAP-BTLS.
PROCTOR: The area is unremarkable.

Assess the Extremities

Inspect

Student: I am assessing the lower and upper extremities for DCAP-BTLS. Do I find anything?
PROCTOR: No.

Palpate

Student: Do I feel anything unusual?
PROCTOR: No.

Assess Motor, Sensory, and Circulatory Function

Student: I am checking for DCAP-BTLS, motor and sensory function, and pulses. Right leg?
PROCTOR: Negative DCAP-BTLS. Motor and sensory functions are present. Pulses are present.
Student: Left leg?
PROCTOR: Negative DCAP-BTLS. Motor and sensory functions are present. Pulses are present.

Student: Right arm?

PROCTOR: Negative DCAP-BTLS. Motor and sensory functions are present. Pulses are present.

Student: Left arm?

PROCTOR: Negative DCAP-BTLS. Motor and sensory functions are present. Pulses are present.

▸ **Assess the Posterior**

Student: We will not check the back.

PROCTOR: Noted.

▸ **Manage Secondary Injuries/Wounds**

Student: I would direct my partner to monitor the airway and pulse oximetry.

PROCTOR: Noted.

▸ **Reassess Interventions**

Student: I will reassess my interventions: airway, breathing, oxygen, and inhaler.

PROCTOR: Noted.

ALS Student: I will reassess BLS interventions, plus the following: IV access, cardiac monitor, 12-lead ECG, and local protocol.

ALS Proctor: Noted. The cardiac monitor shows normal sinus rhythm.

Critical Criteria:
- ❑ Did not obtain medical direction or verbalize standing orders for medical interventions
- ❑ Administered a dangerous or inappropriate intervention
- ❑ Did not ask questions about the present illness
- ❑ Did not differentiate patient's need for transportation versus continued assessment at the scene

Radio Report

(Provided by the student.)

PROCTOR: Noted.

Ongoing Assessment

▾ Repeat the Initial Assessment

Student: I will repeat the initial assessment.

PROCTOR: Noted. (Reflected in "Repeat Vital Signs.")

▾ Repeat Vital Signs

Student: I will reassess vital signs and mental status.

PROCTOR: Blood pressure, 138/80 mm Hg; pulse rate, 82 beats/min; respirations, 16 breaths/min; pulse oximetry reading, 97%; and the patient is alert.

Student: The vital signs have not changed significantly.

PROCTOR: Noted.

▾ Check Interventions

Student: I will check my interventions: oxygen and inhaler.

PROCTOR: Noted.

ALS Student: I will check BLS interventions, plus the following: IV access, cardiac monitor, 12-lead ECG, and local protocol.

ALS Proctor: Noted. The cardiac monitor shows normal sinus rhythm.

▾ Repeat the Focused Assessment

Student: I will repeat the focused assessment.

PROCTOR: Noted.

Critical Criteria:
- ❑ Did not obtain medical direction or verbalize standing orders for medical interventions
- ❑ Administered a dangerous or inappropriate intervention

Handoff Report to Emergency Department Staff

Student: There was no change during transport.

PROCTOR: Noted.

Critical Criteria

(Inform the student of items missed, if any.)

❑ Pass ❑ Fail Date: ______________________

Proctor Comments: ______________________

____

____

CASE 83

Notes

Dispatch Information

PROCTOR: EMS 10, respond to a 65-year-old female who is complaining of diarrhea and vomiting. She is conscious and breathing.

Pre-scene Action (BSI)

Student: I am wearing nonlatex gloves and safety glasses.
PROCTOR: Noted.

Critical Criteria:
- ❑ Did not take, or verbalize, body substance isolation (BSI) precautions when necessary

Scene Size-up

Scene Safety

Student: Is the scene safe?
PROCTOR: Yes.

Mechanism of Injury/Nature of Illness

Student: What is the nature of the illness?
PROCTOR: The patient has been sick with diarrhea and vomiting for two days.

Number of Patients

Student: How many patients are there?
PROCTOR: One.

Additional Resources

Student: I would not call for advanced life support (ALS) assistance.
PROCTOR: Noted.

C-Spine Stabilization

Student: I would not stabilize the cervical spine (c-spine).
PROCTOR: Noted.

Critical Criteria:
- ❑ Did not determine scene safety

Initial Assessment

General Impression

Student: My general impression is that the patient's condition is stable.
PROCTOR: Noted.

Responsiveness/Level of Consciousness

Student: What is the patient's level of consciousness?
PROCTOR: Alert.

Chief Complaint/Apparent Life Threats

Student: What is the patient's chief complaint?
PROCTOR: The patient has been complaining of diarrhea and vomiting for two days.

Assess the Airway and Breathing

Student: Is the airway open?
PROCTOR: Yes.

Assessment

Student: What are the rate and the quality of breathing?
PROCTOR: Rate: Tachypneic. Quality: Deep.

Provide Oxygen

Student: I am applying oxygen at 15 L/min via nonrebreathing mask.
PROCTOR: Noted.

Ensure Adequate Ventilation

Student: The patient has adequate ventilations at this time.
PROCTOR: Noted.

Assess Circulation

Student: I am assessing the patient's circulation.
PROCTOR: Noted.

Assess for and Control Major Bleeding

Student: Do I find any major bleeding?
PROCTOR: No.

Assess the Pulse

Student: What are the rate and the quality of pulses?
PROCTOR: Rate: Tachycardic. Quality: Thready.

Assess the Skin

Student: I am assessing the skin. What are the color, temperature, and condition of the skin?
PROCTOR: Color: Normal. Temperature: Warm. Condition: Dry.

Identify Priority Patients/Make Transport Decision

Student: The patient is a low priority and does not require immediate transport.
PROCTOR: Noted.

Critical Criteria:
- ❑ Did not provide high concentration of oxygen
- ❑ Did not find or manage problems associated with airway, breathing, hemorrhage or shock (hypoperfusion)
- ❑ Did not differentiate patient's need for transportation versus continued assessment at the scene
- ❑ Did detailed or focused history/physical examination before assessing the airway, breathing and circulation

Focused History and Physical Examination/Rapid Assessment

Select the Appropriate Assessment (Focused or Rapid)

Student: I am selecting the focused assessment.
PROCTOR: Noted.

SAMPLE History

Student: At this time I will gather a SAMPLE history from the patient or family. What are the patient's signs and symptoms?
PROCTOR: Sick call.

> **Student:** Onset: What were you doing when this started?
> **PROCTOR:** It has been going on for two days.
> **Student:** Provokes: What makes your condition worse or better?
> **PROCTOR:** Nothing has made it better.
> **Student:** Quality: Can you describe your pain?
> **PROCTOR:** None.
> **Student:** Radiates: Do you have pain anywhere else?
> **PROCTOR:** No.
> **Student:** Severity: On a scale of 1 to 10 with 10 being the worst possible, how would you rate your pain/distress?
> **PROCTOR:** 6.
> **Student:** Time: How long has this been going on?
> **PROCTOR:** 2 days.
> **Student:** Interventions: Have you done anything to make this better?
> **PROCTOR:** The patient has taken over-the-counter medications for diarrhea.

Student: Allergies?
PROCTOR: No allergies.
Student: Medications?
PROCTOR: No medications.
Student: Pertinent past medical history?
PROCTOR: No pertinent medical history.
Student: Last oral intake?
PROCTOR: 16 hours ago.
Student: Events leading up to the incident?
PROCTOR: The patient has had diarrhea and vomiting for two days.

Perform the Focused Physical Examination

Student: I am performing the focused physical examination.
PROCTOR: Noted.

Student: I am assessing the abdomen for DCAP-BTLS. This acronym stands for deformities, contusions, abrasions, punctures, penetrations, paradoxical motion in the chest, burns, tenderness, lacerations, and swelling. I am assessing all four quadrants. Do I find any problems?
PROCTOR: No.
Student: I am assessing the pelvis for DCAP-BTLS. Is the pelvis stable?
PROCTOR: Yes.

▼ Baseline Vital Signs

Student: What are the patient's baseline vital signs, including blood pressure, pulse, respirations, pulse oximetry, blood glucose level, and level of consciousness?
PROCTOR: Blood pressure, 114/70 mm Hg; pulse rate, 120 beats/min; respirations, 28 breaths/min; pulse oximetry reading, 97%; blood glucose level, 74 mg/dL; and the patient is alert.

▼ Interventions

Student: I will apply oxygen and transport the patient in the position of comfort.
PROCTOR: Noted.
ALS Student: I will apply basic life support (BLS) interventions, plus the following: establish IV access, perform cardiac monitoring, 12-lead ECG, and follow the local protocol.
ALS Proctor: Noted. The cardiac monitor shows atrial fibrillation.

▼ Reevaluate Transport Decision

Student: The patient does not require immediate transport.
PROCTOR: Noted.

▼ Detailed Physical Examination

Possible Answer #1
Student: I would not do a detailed physical exam.
PROCTOR: Noted. (Go to "Radio Report.")

Possible Answer #2
Student: I am conducting the detailed physical exam. I am looking for DCAP-BTLS.
PROCTOR: Noted. The detailed physical exam will be performed during transport.

▸ **Assess the Head**

Student: I am assessing the head. Do I find any DCAP-BTLS? Do I find any evidence of Battle's sign or raccoon eyes?
PROCTOR: No.

▸ **Inspect and Palpate the Head and Ears**

Student: I am assessing the head and ears.
PROCTOR: There are no obvious injuries.

▸ **Assess the Eyes**

Student: I am assessing the eyes. Are the pupils equal, round, and regular in size, and react properly to light (PEARRL)?
PROCTOR: They are PEARRL.

▸ **Assess the Facial Area Including Oral and Nasal Areas**

Student: I am assessing the face, nose, and mouth. Do I see any discharge or hear any obstructions?
PROCTOR: No.

▸ **Assess the Neck**

▸ **Inspect and Palpate the Neck**

Student: I am assessing the neck for DCAP-BTLS.
PROCTOR: There are no obvious injuries.

▸ **Assess for Jugular Vein Distention**

Student: Do I find any jugular vein distention (JVD)?
PROCTOR: No.

▸ **Assess for Tracheal Deviation**

Student: Do I see any tracheal deviation?
PROCTOR: No.

▸ **Assess the Chest**

Student: I am assessing the chest for DCAP-BTLS.
PROCTOR: Noted.

▸ **Inspect**

Student: What do I see when I look at the chest?
PROCTOR: There are no obvious injuries.
Student: Is the chest symmetric?
PROCTOR: Yes.

▸ **Palpate**

Student: When I touch the chest, do I feel crepitus or a flail segment?
PROCTOR: No.

▸ **Auscultate**

Student: Are lung sounds present in all fields?
PROCTOR: Yes.
Student: Do I hear any sucking sounds from the chest?
PROCTOR: No.

▸ **Assess the Abdomen/Pelvis**

▸ **Assess the Abdomen**

Student: I am assessing the abdomen for DCAP-BTLS. I am assessing all four quadrants. Do I find any problems?
PROCTOR: No.

▸ **Assess the Pelvis**

Student: I am assessing the pelvis for DCAP-BTLS. Is the pelvis stable?
PROCTOR: Yes.

▸ **Assess the Genitalia/Perineum as Needed (Verbalize in Training)**

Student: I am assessing the genitalia/perineum as necessary for DCAP-BTLS.
PROCTOR: The area is unremarkable.

▸ **Assess the Extremities**

▸ **Inspect**

Student: I am assessing the lower and upper extremities for DCAP-BTLS. Do I find anything?
PROCTOR: No.

▸ **Palpate**

Student: Do I feel anything unusual?
PROCTOR: No.

▸ **Assess Motor, Sensory, and Circulatory Function**

Student: I am checking for DCAP-BTLS, motor and sensory function, and pulses. Right leg?
PROCTOR: Negative DCAP-BTLS. Motor and sensory functions are present. Pulses are present.
Student: Left leg?
PROCTOR: Negative DCAP-BTLS. Motor and sensory functions are present. Pulses are present.
Student: Right arm?
PROCTOR: Negative DCAP-BTLS. Motor and sensory functions are present. Pulses are present.
Student: Left arm?
PROCTOR: Negative DCAP-BTLS. Motor and sensory functions are present. Pulses are present.

▸ **Assess the Posterior**

Student: We will not check the back.
PROCTOR: Noted.

▸ **Manage Secondary Injuries/Wounds**

Student: I would direct my partner to monitor the airway and be prepared for the patient to vomit.

PROCTOR: Noted.

▸ **Reassess Interventions**

Student: I will reassess my interventions: oxygen and transport the patient in the position of comfort.

PROCTOR: Noted.

ALS Student: I will reassess BLS interventions, plus the following: IV access, cardiac monitor, and local protocol.

ALS Proctor: Noted. The cardiac monitor shows atrial fibrillation.

Critical Criteria:

- ❑ Did not obtain medical direction or verbalize standing orders for medical interventions
- ❑ Administered a dangerous or inappropriate intervention
- ❑ Did not ask questions about the present illness
- ❑ Did not differentiate patient's need for transportation versus continued assessment at the scene

Radio Report

(Provided by the student.)

PROCTOR: Noted.

Ongoing Assessment

Repeat the Initial Assessment

Student: I will repeat the initial assessment.

PROCTOR: Noted. (Reflected in "Repeat Vital Signs.")

Repeat Vital Signs

Student: I will reassess vital signs and mental status.

PROCTOR: Blood pressure, 112/72 mm Hg; pulse rate, 118 beats/min; respirations, 24 breaths/min; pulse oximetry reading, 98%; and the patient is alert.

Student: The vital signs have not changed significantly.

PROCTOR: Noted.

Check Interventions

Student: I will check my interventions: oxygen and transport the patient in the position of comfort.

PROCTOR: Noted.

ALS Student: I will check BLS interventions, plus the following: IV access, cardiac monitor, and local protocol.

ALS Proctor: Noted. The cardiac monitor shows atrial fibrillation.

Repeat the Focused Assessment

Student: I will repeat the focused assessment.

PROCTOR: Noted.

Critical Criteria:

- ❑ Did not obtain medical direction or verbalize standing orders for medical interventions
- ❑ Administered a dangerous or inappropriate intervention

Handoff Report to Emergency Department Staff

Student: There was no change during transport.

PROCTOR: Noted.

Critical Criteria

(Inform the student of items missed, if any.)

❑ Pass ❑ Fail Date: ______________________

Proctor Comments: ______________________

____

____

CASE 84

Notes

Dispatch Information

PROCTOR: EMS 10, respond to a 40-year-old male who is complaining of delirium tremens (DTs). He is conscious and breathing.

Pre-scene Action (BSI)

Student: I am wearing nonlatex gloves and safety glasses.
PROCTOR: Noted.

Critical Criteria:
- ❑ Did not take, or verbalize, body substance isolation (BSI) precautions when necessary

Scene Size-up

Scene Safety

Student: Is the scene safe?
PROCTOR: Yes.

Mechanism of Injury/Nature of Illness

Student: What is the nature of the illness?
PROCTOR: The patient has a long history of alcohol abuse. He has not had a drink in a few days and is complaining of tremors.

Number of Patients

Student: How many patients are there?
PROCTOR: One.

Additional Resources

Student: I would not call for advanced life support (ALS) assistance.
PROCTOR: Noted.

C-Spine Stabilization

Student: I would not stabilize the cervical spine (c-spine).
PROCTOR: Noted.

Critical Criteria:
- ❑ Did not determine scene safety

Initial Assessment

General Impression

Student: My general impression is that the patient's condition is stable.
PROCTOR: Noted.

Responsiveness/Level of Consciousness

Student: What is the patient's level of consciousness?
PROCTOR: Alert.

Chief Complaint/Apparent Life Threats

Student: What is the patient's chief complaint?
PROCTOR: The patient is complaining of the DTs and nausea.

Assess the Airway and Breathing

Student: Is the airway open?
PROCTOR: Yes.

Assessment

Student: What are the rate and the quality of breathing?
PROCTOR: Rate: Tachypneic. Quality: Deep.

Provide Oxygen

Student: I am applying oxygen at 15 L/min via nonrebreathing mask.
PROCTOR: Noted.

Ensure Adequate Ventilation

Student: The patient has adequate ventilations at this time.
PROCTOR: Noted.

Assess Circulation

Student: I am assessing the patient's circulation.
PROCTOR: Noted.

Assess for and Control Major Bleeding

Student: Do I find any major bleeding?
PROCTOR: No.

Assess the Pulse

Student: What are the rate and the quality of pulses?
PROCTOR: Rate: Tachycardic. Quality: Bounding.

Assess the Skin

Student: I am assessing the skin. What are the color, temperature, and condition of the skin?
PROCTOR: Color: Jaundice. Temperature: Warm. Condition: Dry.

Identify Priority Patients/Make Transport Decision

Student: The patient is a low priority and does not require immediate transport.
PROCTOR: Noted.

Critical Criteria:
- ❑ Did not provide high concentration of oxygen
- ❑ Did not find or manage problems associated with airway, breathing, hemorrhage or shock (hypoperfusion)
- ❑ Did not differentiate patient's need for transportation versus continued assessment at the scene
- ❑ Did detailed or focused history/physical examination before assessing the airway, breathing and circulation

Focused History and Physical Examination/Rapid Assessment

Select the Appropriate Assessment (Focused or Rapid)

Student: I am selecting the focused assessment.
PROCTOR: Noted.

SAMPLE History

Student: At this time I will gather a SAMPLE history from the patient or family. What are the patient's signs and symptoms?
PROCTOR: DTs.

> Student: Onset: What were you doing when this started?
> **PROCTOR:** Watching TV.
> Student: Provokes: What makes your condition worse or better?
> **PROCTOR:** Drinking makes it better.
> Student: Quality: Can you describe your pain?
> **PROCTOR:** My body will not stop shaking.
> Student: Radiates: Do you have pain anywhere else?
> **PROCTOR:** No.
> Student: Severity: On a scale of 1 to 10 with 10 being the worst possible, how would you rate your distress?
> **PROCTOR:** 8+.
> Student: Time: How long has this been going on?
> **PROCTOR:** 2 days.
> Student: Interventions: Have you done anything to make this better?
> **PROCTOR:** The patient has taken no actions.

Student: Allergies?
PROCTOR: No allergies.
Student: Medications?
PROCTOR: No medications.
Student: Pertinent past medical history?
PROCTOR: Alcohol abuse.
Student: Last oral intake?
PROCTOR: 14 hours ago.
Student: Events leading up to the incident?
PROCTOR: The patient has not had the money to buy alcohol.

Perform the Focused Physical Examination

Student: I am performing the focused physical examination.
PROCTOR: Noted.
Student: I would check his blood glucose level.
PROCTOR: Noted. His blood glucose level is 128 mg/dL.

Baseline Vital Signs

Student: What are the patient's baseline vital signs, including blood pressure, pulse, respirations, pulse oximetry, and level of consciousness?
PROCTOR: Blood pressure, 140/90 mm Hg; pulse rate, 100 beats/min; respirations, 20 breaths/min; pulse oximetry reading, 97%; and the patient is alert.

Interventions

Student: I will apply oxygen.
PROCTOR: Noted.
ALS Student: I will apply basic life support (BLS) interventions, plus the following: establish IV access, perform cardiac monitoring, and follow the local protocol.
ALS Proctor: Noted. The cardiac monitor shows normal sinus rhythm.

Reevaluate Transport Decision

Student: The patient does not require immediate transport.
PROCTOR: Noted.

Detailed Physical Examination

Possible Answer #1
Student: I would not do a detailed physical exam unless there were obvious injuries from falls.
PROCTOR: Noted. (Go to "Radio Report.")

Possible Answer #2
Student: I am conducting the detailed physical exam. I am looking for DCAP-BTLS. This acronym stands for deformities, contusions, abrasions, punctures, penetrations, paradoxical motion in the chest, and burns, tenderness, lacerations, and swelling.
PROCTOR: Noted. The detailed physical exam will be performed during transport.

- **Assess the Head**

Student: I am assessing the head. Do I find any DCAP-BTLS? Do I find any evidence of Battle's sign or raccoon eyes?
PROCTOR: No.

- **Inspect and Palpate the Head and Ears**

Student: I am assessing the head and ears.
PROCTOR: There are no obvious injuries.

- **Assess the Eyes**

Student: I am assessing the eyes. Are the pupils equal, round, and regular in size, and react properly to light (PEARRL)?
PROCTOR: They are PEARRL.

- **Assess the Facial Area Including Oral and Nasal Areas**

Student: I am assessing the face, nose, and mouth. Do I see any discharge or hear any obstructions?
PROCTOR: No.

- **Assess the Neck**
- **Inspect and Palpate the Neck**

Student: I am assessing the neck for DCAP-BTLS.
PROCTOR: There are no obvious injuries.

- **Assess for Jugular Vein Distention**

Student: Do I find any jugular vein distention (JVD)?
PROCTOR: No.

- **Assess for Tracheal Deviation**

Student: Do I see any tracheal deviation?
PROCTOR: No.

- **Assess the Chest**

Student: I am assessing the chest for DCAP-BTLS.
PROCTOR: Noted.

- **Inspect**

Student: What do I see when I look at the chest?
PROCTOR: There are no obvious injuries.
Student: Is the chest symmetric?
PROCTOR: Yes.

- **Palpate**

Student: When I touch the chest, do I feel crepitus or a flail segment?
PROCTOR: No.

- **Auscultate**

Student: Are lung sounds present in all fields?
PROCTOR: Yes.
Student: Do I hear any sucking sounds from the chest?
PROCTOR: No.

- **Assess the Abdomen/Pelvis**
- **Assess the Abdomen**

Student: I am assessing the abdomen for DCAP-BTLS. I am assessing all four quadrants. Do I find any problems?
PROCTOR: No.

- **Assess the Pelvis**

Student: I am assessing the pelvis for DCAP-BTLS. Is the pelvis stable?
PROCTOR: Yes.

- **Assess the Genitalia/Perineum as Needed (Verbalize in Training)**

Student: I am assessing the genitalia/perineum as necessary for DCAP-BTLS.
PROCTOR: The area is unremarkable.

- **Assess the Extremities**
- **Inspect**

Student: I am assessing the lower and upper extremities for DCAP-BTLS. Do I find anything?
PROCTOR: No.

- **Palpate**

Student: Do I feel anything unusual?
PROCTOR: No.

- **Assess Motor, Sensory, and Circulatory Function**

Student: I am checking for DCAP-BTLS, motor and sensory function, and pulses. Right leg?
PROCTOR: Negative DCAP-BTLS. Motor and sensory functions are present. Pulses are present.
Student: Left leg?
PROCTOR: Negative DCAP-BTLS. Motor and sensory functions are present. Pulses are present.
Student: Right arm?
PROCTOR: Negative DCAP-BTLS. Motor and sensory functions are present. Pulses are present.
Student: Left arm?
PROCTOR: Negative DCAP-BTLS. Motor and sensory functions are present. Pulses are present.

- **Assess the Posterior**

Student: We will check the back.
PROCTOR: Noted.

- **Assess the Thorax**

Student: I am assessing the thorax. Do I find injuries?
PROCTOR: No.

- **Assess the Lumbar Area**

Student: I am assessing the flanks and lumbar area. Do I find injuries?
PROCTOR: No.

- **Assess the Entire Backside**

Student: I am assessing the entire backside. Do I find injuries?
PROCTOR: No.

- **Manage Secondary Injuries/Wounds**

Student: I would direct my partner to continue providing oxygen.
PROCTOR: Noted.

▸ **Reassess Interventions**

Student: I will reassess my interventions: oxygen.

PROCTOR: Noted.

ALS Student: I will reassess BLS interventions, plus the following: monitor IVs, perform cardiac monitoring, 12-lead ECG, and local protocol.

ALS Proctor: Noted. The cardiac monitor shows normal sinus rhythm.

Critical Criteria:

- ❑ Did not obtain medical direction or verbalize standing orders for medical interventions
- ❑ Administered a dangerous or inappropriate intervention
- ❑ Did not ask questions about the present illness
- ❑ Did not differentiate patient's need for transportation versus continued assessment at the scene

Radio Report

(Provided by the student.)

PROCTOR: Noted.

Ongoing Assessment

Repeat the Initial Assessment

Student: I will repeat the initial assessment.

PROCTOR: Noted. (Reflected in "Repeat Vital Signs.")

Repeat Vital Signs

Student: I will reassess vital signs and mental status.

PROCTOR: Blood pressure, 148/90 mm Hg; pulse rate, 92 beats/min; respirations, 20 breaths/min; pulse oximetry reading, 98%; and the patient is alert.

Student: The vital signs have not changed significantly.

PROCTOR: Noted.

Check Interventions

Student: I will check my interventions: oxygen.

PROCTOR: Noted.

ALS Student: I will check BLS interventions, plus the following: monitor IVs, cardiac monitor, 12-lead ECG, and local protocol.

ALS Proctor: Noted. The cardiac monitor shows normal sinus rhythm.

Repeat the Focused Assessment

Student: I will repeat the focused assessment.

PROCTOR: Noted.

Critical Criteria:

- ❑ Did not obtain medical direction or verbalize standing orders for medical interventions
- ❑ Administered a dangerous or inappropriate intervention

Handoff Report to Emergency Department Staff

Student: There was no change during transport.

PROCTOR: Noted.

Critical Criteria

(Inform the student of items missed, if any.)

❑ Pass ❑ Fail Date: ____________________

Proctor Comments: ____________________

____

____

CASE 85

Notes

Dispatch Information

PROCTOR: EMS 10, respond to a 55-year-old male who is complaining of difficulty breathing and possible pneumonia. He is conscious and breathing.

Pre-scene Action (BSI)

Student: I am wearing nonlatex gloves, safety glasses, and a mask.
PROCTOR: Noted.

Critical Criteria:
- ❑ Did not take, or verbalize, body substance isolation (BSI) precautions when necessary

Scene Size-up

Scene Safety

Student: Is the scene safe?
PROCTOR: Yes.

Mechanism of Injury/Nature of Illness

Student: What is the nature of the illness?
PROCTOR: The patient is a heavy smoker who has had cold and flu symptoms for the past 4 days.

Number of Patients

Student: How many patients are there?
PROCTOR: One.

Additional Resources

Student: I would call for advanced life support (ALS) assistance if required by local protocol.
PROCTOR: Noted.

C-Spine Stabilization

Student: I would not stabilize the cervical spine (c-spine).
PROCTOR: Noted.

Critical Criteria:
- ❑ Did not determine scene safety

Initial Assessment

General Impression

Student: My general impression is that the patient's condition is stable.
PROCTOR: Noted.

Responsiveness/Level of Consciousness

Student: What is the patient's level of consciousness?
PROCTOR: Alert.

Chief Complaint/Apparent Life Threats

Student: What is the patient's chief complaint?
PROCTOR: The patient is complaining of difficulty breathing, a productive cough, and a high temperature.

Assess the Airway and Breathing

Student: Is the airway open? Is the patient breathing?
PROCTOR: Yes, the airway is open and the patient is breathing.

Assessment

Student: What are the rate and the quality of breathing?
PROCTOR: Rate: Tachypneic. Quality: Labored.

Provide Oxygen

Student: I am applying oxygen at 15 L/min via nonrebreathing mask.
PROCTOR: Noted.

Ensure Adequate Ventilation

Student: The patient has adequate ventilations at this time.
PROCTOR: Noted.

Assess Circulation

Student: I am assessing the patient's circulation.
PROCTOR: Noted.

Assess for and Control Major Bleeding

Student: Do I find any major bleeding?
PROCTOR: No.

Assess the Pulse

Student: What are the rate and the quality of pulses?
PROCTOR: Rate: Tachycardic. Quality: Bounding.

Assess the Skin

Student: I am assessing the skin. What are the color, temperature, and condition of the skin?
PROCTOR: Color: Flushed. Temperature: Hot (101°F if taken). Condition: Dry.

Identify Priority Patients/Make Transport Decision

Student: The patient is a low priority and does not require immediate transport.
PROCTOR: Noted.

Critical Criteria:
- ❑ Did not provide high concentration of oxygen
- ❑ Did not find or manage problems associated with airway, breathing, hemorrhage or shock (hypoperfusion)
- ❑ Did not differentiate patient's need for transportation versus continued assessment at the scene
- ❑ Did detailed or focused history/physical examination before assessing the airway, breathing and circulation

Focused History and Physical Examination/Rapid Assessment

Select the Appropriate Assessment (Focused or Rapid)

Student: I am selecting the focused assessment.
PROCTOR: Noted.

SAMPLE History

Student: At this time I will gather a SAMPLE history from the patient or family. What are the patient's signs and symptoms?
PROCTOR: Respiratory.

Student: Onset: What were you doing when this started?
PROCTOR: He started getting sick 4 days ago.
Student: Provokes: What makes your condition worse or better?
PROCTOR: Sitting up makes it easier to breathe.
Student: Quality: Can you describe your pain?
PROCTOR: Dull chest pain when he coughs. The cough is productive.
Student: Radiates: Do you have pain anywhere else?
PROCTOR: No.
Student: Severity: On a scale of 1 to 10 with 10 being the worst possible, how would you rate your pain/distress?
PROCTOR: 3.
Student: Time: How long has this been going on?
PROCTOR: 1 day.
Student: Interventions: Have you done anything to make this better?
PROCTOR: Hot soup and cough medicine.

Student: Allergies?
PROCTOR: No allergies.
Student: Medications?
PROCTOR: Over-the-counter cough and cold medications.
Student: Pertinent past medical history?
PROCTOR: Has smoked 2½ packs of cigarettes per day for 35 years.
Student: Last oral intake?
PROCTOR: 2 hours ago.
Student: Events leading up to the incident?
PROCTOR: The patient started getting sick 4 days ago.

▼ Perform Focused Physical Examination

Student: I am performing the focused physical examination.

PROCTOR: Noted.

Student: I am assessing the chest for DCAP-BTLS. This acronym stands for deformities, contusions, abrasions, punctures, penetrations, paradoxical motion in the chest, and burns, tenderness, lacerations, and swelling.

PROCTOR: Noted.

Student: Are lung sounds present in all fields?

PROCTOR: Yes, with wheezing noted.

Student: Is there any edema in the extremities?

PROCTOR: No.

Student: Do I hear any sucking sounds from the chest?

PROCTOR: No.

▼ Baseline Vital Signs

Student: What are the patient's baseline vital signs, including blood pressure, pulse, respirations, pulse oximetry, blood glucose level, and level of consciousness?

PROCTOR: Blood pressure, 140/84 mm Hg; pulse, 122 beats/min; respirations, 28 breaths/min; pulse oximetry reading, 96%; blood glucose level, 108 mg/dL; and the patient is alert.

▼ Interventions

Student: I will check the effectiveness of the oxygen via nonrebreathing mask.

PROCTOR: Noted.

ALS Student: I will apply basic life support (BLS) interventions, plus the following: establish IV access, perform cardiac monitoring, and follow the local protocol.

ALS Proctor: Noted. The cardiac monitor shows sinus tachycardia.

▼ Reevaluate Transport Decision

Student: The patient is a low priority and does not require immediate transport.

PROCTOR: Noted.

▼ Detailed Physical Examination

Possible Answer #1

Student: I would not do a detailed physical exam.

PROCTOR: Noted. (Go to "Radio Report.")

Possible Answer #2

Student: I am conducting the detailed physical exam. I am looking for DCAP-BTLS.

PROCTOR: Noted. The detailed physical exam will be performed during transport.

▸ **Assess the Head**

Student: I am assessing the head. Do I find any DCAP-BTLS? Do I find any evidence of Battle's sign or raccoon eyes?

PROCTOR: No.

▸ **Inspect and Palpate the Head and Ears**

Student: I am assessing the head and ears.

PROCTOR: There are no obvious injuries.

▸ **Assess the Eyes**

Student: I am assessing the eyes. Are the pupils equal, round, and regular in size, and react properly to light (PEARRL)?

PROCTOR: They are PEARRL.

▸ **Assess the Facial Area Including Oral and Nasal Areas**

Student: I am assessing the face, nose, and mouth. Do I see any discharge or hear any obstructions?

PROCTOR: No.

▸ **Assess the Neck**

▸ **Inspect and Palpate the Neck**

Student: I am assessing the neck for DCAP-BTLS.

PROCTOR: There are no obvious injuries.

▸ **Assess for Jugular Vein Distention**

Student: Do I find any jugular vein distention (JVD)?

PROCTOR: No.

▸ **Assess for Tracheal Deviation**

Student: Do I see any tracheal deviation?

PROCTOR: No.

▸ **Assess the Chest**

Student: I am assessing the chest for DCAP-BTLS.

PROCTOR: Noted.

▸ **Inspect**

Student: What do I see when I look at the chest?

PROCTOR: There are no obvious injuries.

Student: Is the chest symmetric?

PROCTOR: Yes.

▸ **Palpate**

Student: When I touch the chest, do I feel crepitus or a flail segment?

PROCTOR: No.

▸ **Auscultate**

Student: Are lung sounds present in all fields?

PROCTOR: Yes, with some wheezing noted.

Student: Do I hear any sucking sounds from the chest?

PROCTOR: No.

▸ **Assess the Abdomen/Pelvis**

▸ **Assess the Abdomen**

Student: I am assessing the abdomen for DCAP-BTLS. I am assessing all four quadrants. Do I find any problems?

PROCTOR: No.

▸ **Assess the Pelvis**

Student: I am assessing the pelvis for DCAP-BTLS. Is the pelvis stable?

PROCTOR: Yes.

▸ **Assess the Genitalia/Perineum as Needed (Verbalize in Training)**

Student: I am assessing the genitalia/perineum as necessary for DCAP-BTLS.

PROCTOR: The area is unremarkable.

▸ **Assess the Extremities**

▸ **Inspect**

Student: I am assessing the lower and upper extremities for DCAP-BTLS. Do I find anything?

PROCTOR: No.

▸ **Palpate**

Student: Do I feel anything unusual?

PROCTOR: No.

▸ **Assess Motor, Sensory, and Circulatory Function**

Student: I am checking for DCAP-BTLS, motor and sensory function, and pulses. Right leg?

PROCTOR: Negative DCAP-BTLS. Motor and sensory functions are present. Pulses are present.

Student: Left leg?

PROCTOR: Negative DCAP-BTLS. Motor and sensory functions are present. Pulses are present.

Student: Right arm?

PROCTOR: Negative DCAP-BTLS. Motor and sensory functions are present. Pulses are present.

Student: Left arm?

PROCTOR: Negative DCAP-BTLS. Motor and sensory functions are present. Pulses are present.

▸ **Assess the Posterior**

Student: We will check the back.

PROCTOR: Noted.

▸ Assess the Thorax

Student: I am assessing the thorax. Do I find injuries?

PROCTOR: No.

▸ Assess the Lumbar Area

Student: I am assessing the flanks and lumbar area. Do I find injuries?

PROCTOR: No.

▸ Assess the Entire Backside

Student: I am assessing the entire backside. Do I find injuries?

PROCTOR: No.

▸ Manage Secondary Injuries/Wounds

Student: I would direct my partner to continue providing oxygen.

PROCTOR: Noted.

▸ Reassess Interventions

Student: I will reassess my interventions: oxygen.

PROCTOR: Noted.

ALS Student: I will reassess BLS interventions, plus the following: IV access, cardiac monitoring, 12-lead ECG, and local protocol.

ALS Proctor: Noted. The cardiac monitor shows sinus tachycardia.

Critical Criteria:
- ❑ Did not obtain medical direction or verbalize standing orders for medical interventions
- ❑ Administered a dangerous or inappropriate intervention
- ❑ Did not ask questions about the present illness
- ❑ Did not differentiate patient's need for transportation versus continued assessment at the scene

Radio Report

(Provided by the student.)

PROCTOR: Noted.

Ongoing Assessment

Repeat the Initial Assessment

Student: I will repeat the initial assessment.

PROCTOR: Noted. (Reflected in "Repeat Vital Signs.")

Repeat Vital Signs

Student: I will reassess vital signs and mental status.

PROCTOR: Blood pressure, 142/82 mm Hg; pulse, 118 beats/min; respirations, 24 breaths/min; pulse oximetry reading, 99%; and the patient is alert.

Student: The vital signs have not changed significantly.

PROCTOR: Noted.

Check Interventions

Student: I will check my interventions: oxygen.

PROCTOR: Noted.

ALS Student: I will check BLS interventions, plus the following: IV access, cardiac monitoring, 12-lead ECG, and local protocol.

ALS Proctor: Noted. The cardiac monitor shows sinus tachycardia.

Repeat the Focused Assessment

Student: I will repeat the focused assessment.

PROCTOR: Noted.

Critical Criteria:
- ❑ Did not obtain medical direction or verbalize standing orders for medical interventions
- ❑ Administered a dangerous or inappropriate intervention

Handoff Report to Emergency Department Staff

Student: There was no change during transport.

PROCTOR: Noted.

Critical Criteria

(Inform the student of items missed, if any.)

❑ Pass ❑ Fail Date: ______________________________

Proctor Comments: ______________________________

____

____

Notes

Dispatch Information

PROCTOR: EMS 10, respond to a 74-year-old male who is complaining of chest pain. He is conscious and breathing.

Pre-scene Action (BSI)

Student: I am wearing nonlatex gloves and safety glasses.
PROCTOR: Noted.

Critical Criteria:
- ❑ Did not take, or verbalize, body substance isolation (BSI) precautions when necessary

Scene Size-up

Scene Safety

Student: Is the scene safe?
PROCTOR: Yes.

Mechanism of Injury/Nature of Illness

Student: What is the nature of the illness?
PROCTOR: The patient has chest pain. He said that it is the worst pain he could imagine.

Number of Patients

Student: How many patients are there?
PROCTOR: One.

Additional Resources

Student: I would call for advanced life support (ALS) assistance.
PROCTOR: Noted.

C-Spine Stabilization

Student: I would not stabilize the cervical spine (c-spine).
PROCTOR: Noted.

Critical Criteria:
- ❑ Did not determine scene safety

Initial Assessment

General Impression

Student: My general impression is that the patient's condition is unstable.
PROCTOR: Noted.

Responsiveness/Level of Consciousness

Student: What is the patient's level of consciousness?
PROCTOR: Alert.

Chief Complaint/Apparent Life Threats

Student: What is the patient's chief complaint?
PROCTOR: The patient is complaining of chest pain.

Assess the Airway and Breathing

Student: Is the airway open? Is the patient breathing?
PROCTOR: Yes, the airway is open and the patient is breathing.

Assessment

Student: What are the rate and the quality of breathing?
PROCTOR: Rate: Within normal limits. Quality: Normal.

Provide Oxygen

Student: I am applying oxygen at 15 L/min via nonrebreathing mask.
PROCTOR: Noted.

Ensure Adequate Ventilation

Student: The patient has adequate ventilations at this time.
PROCTOR: Noted.

Assess Circulation

Student: I am assessing the patient's circulation.
PROCTOR: Noted.

Assess for and Control Major Bleeding

Student: Do I find any major bleeding?
PROCTOR: No.

Assess the Pulse

Student: What are the rate and the quality of pulses?
PROCTOR: Rate: A little slow. Quality: Thready.

Assess the Skin

Student: I am assessing the skin. What are the color, temperature, and condition of the skin?
PROCTOR: Color: Pale. Temperature: Cool. Condition: Diaphoretic.

Identify Priority Patients/Make Transport Decision

Student: The patient is a high priority and is a load-and-go. I will begin packaging and transport.
PROCTOR: Noted.

Critical Criteria:
- ❑ Did not provide high concentration of oxygen
- ❑ Did not find or manage problems associated with airway, breathing, hemorrhage or shock (hypoperfusion)
- ❑ Did not differentiate patient's need for transportation versus continued assessment at the scene
- ❑ Did detailed or focused history/physical examination before assessing the airway, breathing and circulation

Focused History and Physical Examination/Rapid Assessment

Select the Appropriate Assessment (Focused or Rapid)

Student: I am selecting the focused assessment.
PROCTOR: Noted.

SAMPLE History

Student: At this time I will gather a SAMPLE history from the patient or family. What are the patient's signs and symptoms?
PROCTOR: Cardiac.

> **Student:** Onset: What were you doing when this started?
> **PROCTOR:** Sleeping and woke up with the chest pain.
> **Student:** Provokes: What makes your condition worse or better?
> **PROCTOR:** Nothing makes it better.
> **Student:** Quality: Can you describe your pain?
> **PROCTOR:** An elephant is sitting on my chest.
> **Student:** Radiates: Do you have pain anywhere else?
> **PROCTOR:** In the jaw.
> **Student:** Severity: On a scale of 1 to 10 with 10 being the worst possible, how would you rate your pain/distress?
> **PROCTOR:** 10.
> **Student:** Time: How long has this been going on?
> **PROCTOR:** 3 hours.
> **Student:** Interventions: Have you done anything to make this better?
> **PROCTOR:** The patient has taken no actions.

Student: Allergies?
PROCTOR: No allergies.
Student: Medications? Has the patient used any erectile dysfunction medication?
PROCTOR: No medications, and no erectile dysfunction medication.
Student: Pertinent past medical history?
PROCTOR: No pertinent medical history.
Student: Last oral intake?
PROCTOR: 14 hours ago.
Student: Events leading up to the incident?
PROCTOR: The patient was sleeping and awoke with this pain.

Perform the Focused Physical Examination

Student: I am performing the focused physical examination.
PROCTOR: Noted.

Student: I am assessing the neck for DCAP-BTLS. This acronym stands for deformities, contusions, abrasions, punctures, penetrations, paradoxical motion in the chest, and burns, tenderness, lacerations, and swelling.
PROCTOR: There are no obvious injuries.
Student: Are lung sounds present in all fields?
PROCTOR: Yes, they are clear bilaterally.
Student: Do I hear any sucking sounds from the chest?
PROCTOR: No.
Student: Is there any pedal edema?
PROCTOR: None noted.

▼ Baseline Vital Signs

Student: What are the patient's baseline vital signs, including blood pressure, pulse, respirations, pulse oximetry, blood glucose level, and level of consciousness?
PROCTOR: Blood pressure, 90/60 mm Hg; pulse, 54 beats/min; respirations, 12 breaths/min; pulse oximetry reading, 95%; blood glucose level, 99 mg/dL; and the patient is alert.

▼ Interventions

Student: I will apply oxygen, loosen tight-fitting clothing, and transport the patient in the position of comfort.
PROCTOR: Noted.
ALS Student: I will apply basic life support (BLS) interventions, plus the following: establish IV access, perform cardiac monitoring, 12-lead ECG, and follow advanced cardiac life support (ACLS) or local protocol.
ALS Proctor: Noted. The cardiac monitor shows sinus bradycardia. 12-lead ECG shows ST elevation in leads V_3 and V_4.

▼ Reevaluate Transport Decision

Student: The patient is a load-and-go.
PROCTOR: Noted.

▼ Detailed Physical Examination

Possible Answer #1
Student: I would not do a detailed physical exam.
PROCTOR: Noted. (Go to "Radio Report.")

Possible Answer #2
Student: I am conducting the detailed physical exam. I am looking for DCAP-BTLS.
PROCTOR: Noted. The detailed physical exam will be performed during transport.

▸ **Assess the Head**

Student: I am assessing the head. Do I find any DCAP-BTLS? Do I find any evidence of Battle's sign or raccoon eyes?
PROCTOR: No.

▸ **Inspect and Palpate the Head and Ears**

Student: I am assessing the head and ears.
PROCTOR: There are no obvious injuries.

▸ **Assess the Eyes**

Student: I am assessing the eyes. Are the pupils equal, round, and regular in size, and react properly to light (PEARRL)?
PROCTOR: They are PEARRL.

▸ **Assess the Facial Area Including Oral and Nasal Areas**

Student: I am assessing the face, nose, and mouth. Do I see any discharge or hear any obstructions?
PROCTOR: No.

▸ **Assess the Neck**

▸ **Inspect and Palpate the Neck**

Student: I am assessing the neck for DCAP-BTLS.
PROCTOR: There are no obvious injuries.

▸ **Assess for Jugular Vein Distention**

Student: Do I find any jugular vein distention (JVD)?
PROCTOR: No.

▸ **Assess for Tracheal Deviation**

Student: Do I see any tracheal deviation?
PROCTOR: No.

▸ **Assess the Chest**

Student: I am assessing the chest for DCAP-BTLS.
PROCTOR: Noted.

▸ **Inspect**

Student: What do I see when I look at the chest?
PROCTOR: There are no obvious injuries.
Student: Is the chest symmetric?
PROCTOR: Yes.

▸ **Palpate**

Student: When I touch the chest, do I feel crepitus or a flail segment?
PROCTOR: No.

▸ **Auscultate**

Student: Are lung sounds present in all fields?
PROCTOR: Yes.
Student: Do I hear any sucking sounds from the chest?
PROCTOR: No.

▸ **Assess the Abdomen/Pelvis**

▸ **Assess the Abdomen**

Student: I am assessing the abdomen for DCAP-BTLS. I am assessing all four quadrants. Do I find any problems?
PROCTOR: No.

▸ **Assess the Pelvis**

Student: I am assessing the pelvis for DCAP-BTLS. Is the pelvis stable?
PROCTOR: Yes.

▸ **Assess the Genitalia/Perineum as Needed (Verbalize in Training)**

Student: I am assessing the genitalia/perineum as necessary for DCAP-BTLS.
PROCTOR: The area is unremarkable.

▸ **Assess the Extremities**

▸ **Inspect**

Student: I am assessing the lower and upper extremities for DCAP-BTLS. Do I find anything?
PROCTOR: No.

▸ **Palpate**

Student: Do I feel anything unusual?
PROCTOR: No.

▸ **Assess Motor, Sensory, and Circulatory Function**

Student: I am checking for DCAP-BTLS, motor and sensory function, and pulses. Right leg?
PROCTOR: Negative DCAP-BTLS. Motor and sensory functions are present. Pulses are present.
Student: Left leg?
PROCTOR: Negative DCAP-BTLS. Motor and sensory functions are present. Pulses are present.
Student: Right arm?
PROCTOR: Negative DCAP-BTLS. Motor and sensory functions are present. Pulses are present.
Student: Left arm?
PROCTOR: Negative DCAP-BTLS. Motor and sensory functions are present. Pulses are present.

▸ **Assess the Posterior**

Student: We will check the back.
PROCTOR: Noted.

▸ Assess the Thorax

Student: I am assessing the thorax. Do I find injuries?

PROCTOR: No.

▸ Assess the Lumbar Area

Student: I am assessing the flanks and lumbar area. Do I find injuries?

PROCTOR: No.

▸ Assess the Entire Backside

Student: I am assessing the entire backside. Do I find injuries?

PROCTOR: No.

▸ Manage Secondary Injuries/Wounds

Student: I would reassure the patient.

PROCTOR: Noted.

▸ Reassess Interventions

Student: I will reassess my interventions: airway, breathing, and oxygen; circulation; and reassurance.

PROCTOR: Noted.

Critical Criteria:

- ❑ Did not obtain medical direction or verbalize standing orders for medical interventions
- ❑ Administered a dangerous or inappropriate intervention
- ❑ Did not ask questions about the present illness
- ❑ Did not differentiate patient's need for transportation versus continued assessment at the scene

Radio Report

(Provided by the student.)

PROCTOR: Noted.

Ongoing Assessment

Repeat the Initial Assessment

Student: I will repeat initial assessment.

PROCTOR: Noted. (Reflected in "Repeat Vital Signs.")

Repeat Vital Signs

Student: I will reassess vital signs and mental status.

PROCTOR: Blood pressure, 96/62 mm Hg; pulse, 62 beats/min; respirations, 16 breaths/min; pulse oximetry reading, 97%; and the patient is alert.

Student: The vital signs have improved.

PROCTOR: Noted.

Check Interventions

Student: I will check my interventions: oxygen, loosen tight-fitting clothing, and transport in the position of comfort.

PROCTOR: Noted.

ALS Student: I will check BLS interventions, plus the following: IV access, cardiac monitoring, 12-lead ECG, and ACLS or local protocol (morphine per local protocol, aspirin 325 mg, nitroglycerin spray or sublingual after blood pressure is within local protocol range and no recent history of erectile dysfunction medication usage).

ALS Proctor: Noted. The cardiac monitor shows normal sinus rhythm with a rate of 62 beats/min. 12-lead ECG shows ST elevation in leads V_3 and V_4.

Repeat the Focused Assessment

Student: I will repeat the focused assessment.

PROCTOR: Noted.

Critical Criteria:

- ❑ Did not obtain medical direction or verbalize standing orders for medical interventions
- ❑ Administered a dangerous or inappropriate intervention

Handoff Report to Emergency Department Staff

Student: The patient's condition improved during transport.

PROCTOR: Noted.

Critical Criteria

(Inform the student of items missed, if any.)

❑ Pass ❑ Fail Date: ____________________

Proctor Comments: ____________________

____

____

Notes

Dispatch Information

PROCTOR: EMS 10, respond to a 23-year-old female who is possibly having an allergic reaction. She is conscious and breathing.

Pre-scene Action (BSI)

Student: I am wearing nonlatex gloves and safety glasses.
PROCTOR: Noted.

Critical Criteria:
- ❑ Did not take, or verbalize, body substance isolation (BSI) precautions when necessary

Scene Size-up

Scene Safety

Student: Is the scene safe?
PROCTOR: Yes.

Mechanism of Injury/Nature of Illness

Student: What is the nature of the illness?
PROCTOR: The patient was eating seafood when she tried some crab meat and immediately felt tightness in her chest, swelling in her throat, voice changes, and fear.

Number of Patients

Student: How many patients are there?
PROCTOR: One.

Additional Resources

Student: I would call for advanced life support (ALS) assistance.
PROCTOR: Noted.

C-Spine Stabilization

Student: I would not stabilize the cervical spine (c-spine).
PROCTOR: Noted.

Critical Criteria:
- ❑ Did not determine scene safety

Initial Assessment

General Impression

Student: My general impression is that the patient's condition is unstable.
PROCTOR: Noted.

Responsiveness/Level of Consciousness

Student: What is the patient's level of consciousness?
PROCTOR: Alert.

Chief Complaint/Apparent Life Threats

Student: What is the patient's chief complaint?
PROCTOR: The patient is complaining of tightness in her chest, swelling in her throat, voice changes, and fear.

Assess the Airway and Breathing

Student: Is the airway open?
PROCTOR: Yes.

Assessment

Student: What are the rate and the quality of breathing?
PROCTOR: Rate: Tachypneic. Quality: Labored.

Provide Oxygen

Student: I am applying oxygen at 15 L/min via nonrebreathing mask.
PROCTOR: Noted.

Ensure Adequate Ventilation

Student: The patient has adequate ventilations at this time.
PROCTOR: Noted.

Assess Circulation

Student: I am assessing the patient's circulation.
PROCTOR: Noted.

Assess for and Control Major Bleeding

Student: Do I find any major bleeding?
PROCTOR: No.

Assess the Pulse

Student: What are the rate and the quality of pulses?
PROCTOR: Rate: Tachycardic. Quality: Thready.

Assess the Skin

Student: I am assessing the skin. What are the color, temperature, and condition of the skin?
PROCTOR: Color: Pale. Temperature: Cool. Condition: Diaphoretic.

Identify Priority Patients/Make Transport Decision

Student: The patient is a high priority and is a load-and-go. I will begin packaging and transport.
PROCTOR: Noted.

Critical Criteria:
- ❑ Did not provide high concentration of oxygen
- ❑ Did not find or manage problems associated with airway, breathing, hemorrhage or shock (hypoperfusion)
- ❑ Did not differentiate patient's need for transportation versus continued assessment at the scene
- ❑ Did detailed or focused history/physical examination before assessing the airway, breathing and circulation

Focused History and Physical Examination/Rapid Assessment

Select the Appropriate Assessment (Focused or Rapid)

Student: I am selecting the focused assessment.
PROCTOR: Noted.

SAMPLE History

Student: At this time I will gather a SAMPLE history from the patient or family. What are the patient's signs and symptoms?
PROCTOR: Allergic reaction.

> **Student:** Is there a history of allergies?
> **PROCTOR:** No.
> **Student:** What were you exposed to?
> **PROCTOR:** The patient ate seafood and the problem began when she ate crab meat.
> **Student:** How were you exposed?
> **PROCTOR:** During a meal.
> **Student:** What were the effects?
> **PROCTOR:** Tightness in her chest, swelling in her throat, voice changes, and fear.
> **Student:** Has the condition progressed?
> **PROCTOR:** Yes, it has progressed to difficulty breathing.
> **Student:** Interventions: Have you done anything to make this better?
> **PROCTOR:** The patient has taken no actions.

Student: Allergies?
PROCTOR: No known allergies.
Student: Medications?
PROCTOR: No medications.
Student: Pertinent past medical history?
PROCTOR: No pertinent medical history.
Student: Last oral intake?
PROCTOR: 15 minutes ago.
Student: Events leading up to the incident?
PROCTOR: The patient was eating seafood and the symptoms started after she ate the crab meat.

▼ Perform the Focused Physical Examination

Student: I will perform the focused physical examination while en route to the hospital.
PROCTOR: Noted.

▼ Baseline Vital Signs

Student: What are the patient's baseline vital signs, including blood pressure, pulse, respirations, pulse oximetry, and level of consciousness?
PROCTOR: Blood pressure, 112/64 mm Hg; pulse, 128 beats/min; respirations, 24 breaths/min; pulse oximetry reading, 96%; and the patient is alert.

▼ Interventions

Student: I will apply oxygen 15 L/min via nonrebreathing mask and administer an epinephrine auto injector (EpiPen) 0.3 mg if carried and allowed per protocol.
PROCTOR: Noted.
ALS Student: I will apply basic life support (BLS) interventions, plus the following: establish IV access, perform cardiac monitoring, administer epinephrine 1:1,000, 0.3 mg IM, and administer Benadryl 50 mg IV.
ALS Proctor: Noted. The cardiac monitor shows sinus tachycardia.

▼ Reevaluate Transport Decision

Student: The patient is a high priority and is a load-and-go.
PROCTOR: Noted.

▼ Detailed Physical Examination

Possible Answer #1
Student: I would not do a detailed physical exam.
PROCTOR: Noted. (Go to "Radio Report.")

Possible Answer #2
Student: I am conducting the detailed physical exam. I am looking for DCAP-BTLS. This acronym stands for deformities, contusions, abrasions, punctures, penetrations, paradoxical motion in the chest, and burns, tenderness, lacerations, and swelling.
PROCTOR: Noted. The detailed physical exam will be performed during transport.

► **Assess the Head**

Student: I am assessing the head. Do I find any DCAP-BTLS? Do I find any evidence of Battle's sign or raccoon eyes?
PROCTOR: No.

► **Inspect and Palpate the Head and Ears**

Student: I am assessing the head and ears.
PROCTOR: There are no obvious injuries.

► **Assess the Eyes**

Student: I am assessing the eyes. Are the pupils equal, round, and regular in size, and react properly to light (PEARRL)?
PROCTOR: They are sluggish.

► **Assess the Facial Area Including Oral and Nasal Areas**

Student: I am assessing the face, nose, and mouth. Do I see any discharge or hear any obstructions?
PROCTOR: Yes, when the patient speaks, she sounds hoarse or raspy.

► **Assess the Neck**

► **Inspect and Palpate the Neck**

Student: I am assessing the neck for DCAP-BTLS.
PROCTOR: You see hives on the upper chest at the base of the neck.

► **Assess for Jugular Vein Distention**

Student: Do I find any jugular vein distention (JVD)?
PROCTOR: No.

► **Assess for Tracheal Deviation**

Student: Do I see any tracheal deviation?
PROCTOR: No.

► **Assess the Chest**

Student: I am assessing the chest for DCAP-BTLS.
PROCTOR: Noted.

► **Inspect**

Student: What do I see when I look at the chest?
PROCTOR: You see hives on the upper chest at the base of the neck.
Student: Is the chest symmetric?
PROCTOR: Yes.

► **Palpate**

Student: When I touch the chest, do I feel crepitus or a flail segment?
PROCTOR: No.

► **Auscultate**

Student: Are lung sounds present in all fields? Any wheezing?
PROCTOR: Yes.
Student: Do I hear any sucking sounds from the chest?
PROCTOR: No.

► **Assess the Abdomen/Pelvis**

► **Assess the Abdomen**

Student: I am assessing the abdomen for DCAP-BTLS. I am assessing all four quadrants. Do I find any problems?
PROCTOR: No.

► **Assess the Pelvis**

Student: I am assessing the pelvis for DCAP-BTLS. Is the pelvis stable?
PROCTOR: Yes.

► **Assess the Genitalia/Perineum as Needed (Verbalize in Training)**

Student: I am assessing the genitalia/perineum as necessary for DCAP-BTLS.
PROCTOR: The area is unremarkable.

► **Assess the Extremities**

► **Inspect**

Student: I am assessing the lower and upper extremities for DCAP-BTLS. Do I find anything?
PROCTOR: No.

► **Palpate**

Student: Do I feel anything unusual?
PROCTOR: No.

► **Assess Motor, Sensory, and Circulatory Function**

Student: I am checking for DCAP-BTLS, motor and sensory function, and pulses. Right leg?
PROCTOR: Negative DCAP-BTLS. Motor and sensory functions are present. Pulses are present.
Student: Left leg?
PROCTOR: Negative DCAP-BTLS. Motor and sensory functions are present. Pulses are present.
Student: Right arm?
PROCTOR: Negative DCAP-BTLS. Motor and sensory functions are present. Pulses are present.
Student: Left arm?
PROCTOR: Negative DCAP-BTLS. Motor and sensory functions are present. Pulses are present.

► **Assess the Posterior**

Student: We will check the back.
PROCTOR: Noted.

► **Assess the Thorax**

Student: I am assessing the thorax. Do I find injuries?
PROCTOR: No.

► **Assess the Lumbar Area**

Student: I am assessing the flanks and lumbar area. Do I find injuries?
PROCTOR: No.

► **Assess the Entire Backside**

Student: I am assessing the entire backside. Do I find injuries?
PROCTOR: No.

▸ Manage Secondary Injuries/Wounds

Student: I would monitor the airway oxygen and administer an epinephrine auto injector (EpiPen) 0.3 mg if carried and allowed per protocol, if not done previously.

PROCTOR: Noted.

▸ Reassess Interventions

Student: I will check my interventions: oxygen.

PROCTOR: Noted.

ALS Student: I will check BLS interventions, plus the following: check IV flow, perform cardiac monitoring, check for improvement from medications, and follow local protocol.

ALS Proctor: Noted. The cardiac monitor shows sinus tachycardia.

Critical Criteria:
- ❑ Did not obtain medical direction or verbalize standing orders for medical interventions
- ❑ Administered a dangerous or inappropriate intervention
- ❑ Did not ask questions about the present illness
- ❑ Did not differentiate patient's need for transportation versus continued assessment at the scene

Radio Report

(Provided by the student.)

PROCTOR: Noted.

Ongoing Assessment

Repeat the Initial Assessment

Student: I will repeat the initial assessment.

PROCTOR: Noted. (Reflected in "Repeat Vital Signs.")

Repeat Vital Signs

Student: I will reassess vital signs.

PROCTOR: Blood pressure, 114/62 mm Hg; pulse, 120 beats/min; respirations, 20 breaths/min; pulse oximetry reading, 97%; and the patient is alert.

Student: The vital signs have not changed significantly.

PROCTOR: Noted.

Check Interventions

Student: I will check my interventions: oxygen.

PROCTOR: Noted.

ALS Student: I will check BLS interventions, plus the following: check IV flow, perform cardiac monitoring, check for improvement from medications, and follow local protocol.

ALS Proctor: Noted. The cardiac monitor shows sinus tachycardia.

Repeat the Focused Assessment

Student: I will repeat the focused assessment.

PROCTOR: Noted.

Critical Criteria:
- ❑ Did not obtain medical direction or verbalize standing orders for medical interventions
- ❑ Administered a dangerous or inappropriate intervention

Handoff Report to Emergency Department Staff

Student: There was no change during transport.

PROCTOR: Noted.

Critical Criteria

(Inform the student of items missed, if any.)

❑ Pass ❑ Fail Date: ______________________

Proctor Comments: ______________________

____

____

Notes

Dispatch Information

PROCTOR: EMS 10, respond to a 73-year-old female who is complaining of shortness of breath. She is conscious and breathing.

Pre-scene Action (BSI)

Student: I am wearing nonlatex gloves and safety glasses.
PROCTOR: Noted.

Critical Criteria:
- ❑ Did not take, or verbalize, body substance isolation (BSI) precautions when necessary

Scene Size-up

Scene Safety

Student: Is the scene safe?
PROCTOR: Yes.

Mechanism of Injury/Nature of Illness

Student: What is the nature of the illness?
PROCTOR: The patient has a history of emphysema and is complaining of shortness of breath. She received bad news tonight of her sister's death. She is visibly shaken over the news.

Number of Patients

Student: How many patients are there?
PROCTOR: One.

Additional Resources

Student: I would hold off on calling advanced life support (ALS).
PROCTOR: Noted.

C-Spine Stabilization

Student: I would not stabilize the cervical spine (c-spine).
PROCTOR: Noted.

Critical Criteria:
- ❑ Did not determine scene safety

Initial Assessment

General Impression

Student: My general impression is that the patient's condition is stable.
PROCTOR: Noted.

Responsiveness/Level of Consciousness

Student: What is the patient's level of consciousness?
PROCTOR: Alert.

Chief Complaint/Apparent Life Threats

Student: What is the patient's chief complaint?
PROCTOR: The patient is complaining of shortness of breath.

Assess the Airway and Breathing

Student: Is the airway open?
PROCTOR: Yes.

Assessment

Student: What are the rate and the quality of breathing?
PROCTOR: Rate: A little fast. Quality: Crying.

Provide Oxygen

Student: I am applying oxygen at 15 L/min via nonrebreathing mask.
PROCTOR: Noted.

Ensure Adequate Ventilation

Student: The patient has adequate ventilations at this time.
PROCTOR: Noted.

Assess Circulation

Student: I am assessing the patient's circulation.
PROCTOR: Noted.

Assess for and Control Major Bleeding

Student: Do I find any major bleeding?
PROCTOR: No.

Assess the Pulse

Student: What are the rate and the quality of pulses?
PROCTOR: Rate: Within normal limits. Quality: Strong.

Assess the Skin

Student: I am assessing the skin. What are the color, temperature, and condition of the skin?
PROCTOR: Color: Flushed. Temperature: Normal. Condition: Normal.

Identify Priority Patients/Make Transport Decision

Student: The patient is a low priority and does not require immediate transport.
PROCTOR: Noted.

Critical Criteria:
- ❑ Did not provide high concentration of oxygen
- ❑ Did not find or manage problems associated with airway, breathing, hemorrhage or shock (hypoperfusion)
- ❑ Did not differentiate patient's need for transportation versus continued assessment at the scene
- ❑ Did detailed or focused history/physical examination before assessing the airway, breathing and circulation

Focused History and Physical Examination/Rapid Assessment

Select the Appropriate Assessment (Focused or Rapid)

Student: I am selecting the focused assessment.
PROCTOR: Noted.

SAMPLE History

Student: At this time I will gather a SAMPLE history from the patient or family. What are the patient's signs and symptoms?
PROCTOR: Respiratory.

> **Student:** Onset: What were you doing when this started?
> **PROCTOR:** On the phone receiving word of her sister's death.
> **Student:** Provokes: What makes your condition worse or better?
> **PROCTOR:** She is just upset.
> **Student:** Quality: Can you describe your pain?
> **PROCTOR:** None.
> **Student:** Radiates: Do you have pain anywhere else?
> **PROCTOR:** No.
> **Student:** Severity: On a scale of 1 to 10 with 10 being the worst possible, how would you rate your distress?
> **PROCTOR:** 3.
> **Student:** Time: How long has this been going on?
> **PROCTOR:** 30 minutes.
> **Student:** Interventions: Have you done anything to make this better?
> **PROCTOR:** The patient has taken no actions.

Student: Allergies?
PROCTOR: No allergies.
Student: Medications?
PROCTOR: Respiratory medications, home oxygen, and an inhaler.
Student: Pertinent past medical history?
PROCTOR: Emphysema.
Student: Last oral intake?
PROCTOR: 2 hours ago.
Student: Events leading up to the incident?
PROCTOR: The patient received word of her sister's death.

Perform Focused Physical Examination

Student: I am performing the focused physical examination.
PROCTOR: Noted.
Student: Are lung sounds present in all fields?
PROCTOR: Yes, you can hear wheezes.
Student: Does she have a cough? If so, is it productive?
PROCTOR: Yes, she has a cough and it is productive.

Baseline Vital Signs

Student: What are the patient's baseline vital signs, including blood pressure, pulse, respirations, pulse oximetry, and level of consciousness?
PROCTOR: Blood pressure, 148/82 mm Hg; pulse, 88 beats/min; respirations, 20 breaths/min; pulse oximetry reading, 96%; and the patient is alert.

Interventions

Student: I will apply oxygen, assist the patient with her inhaler if available, and transport the patient.
PROCTOR: Noted.
ALS Student: I will apply basic life support (BLS) interventions, plus the following: IV access, cardiac monitoring and 12-lead ECG and breathing treatment per protocol.
ALS Proctor: Noted. The monitor shows normal sinus rhythm.

Reevaluate Transport Decision

Student: The patient is a low priority and does not require immediate transport.
PROCTOR: Noted.

Detailed Physical Examination

Possible Answer #1
Student: I would not do a detailed physical exam.
PROCTOR: Noted. (Go to "Radio Report.")

Possible Answer #2
Student: I am conducting the detailed physical exam. I am checking for DCAP-BTLS. This acronym stands for deformities, contusions, abrasions, punctures, penetrations, and paradoxical motion in the chest, and burns, tenderness, lacerations, and swelling.
PROCTOR: Noted. The detailed physical exam will be performed during transport.

Assess the Head

Student: I am assessing the head. Do I find any DCAP-BTLS? Do I find any evidence of Battle's sign or raccoon eyes?
PROCTOR: No.

Inspect and Palpate the Head and Ears

Student: I am assessing the head and ears.
PROCTOR: There are no obvious injuries.

Assess the Eyes

Student: I am assessing the eyes. Are the pupils equal, round, and regular in size, and react properly to light (PEARRL)?
PROCTOR: They are PEARRL.

Assess the Facial Area Including Oral and Nasal Areas

Student: I am assessing the face, nose, and mouth. Do I see any discharge or hear any obstructions?
PROCTOR: No.

Assess the Neck

Inspect and Palpate the Neck

Student: I am assessing the neck for DCAP-BTLS.
PROCTOR: There are no obvious injuries.

Assess for Jugular Vein Distention

Student: Do I find any jugular vein distention (JVD)?
PROCTOR: No.

Assess for Tracheal Deviation

Student: Do I see any tracheal deviation?
PROCTOR: No.

Assess the Chest

Student: I am assessing the chest for DCAP-BTLS.
PROCTOR: Noted.

Inspect

Student: What do I see when I look at the chest?
PROCTOR: There are no obvious injuries.
Student: Is the chest symmetric?
PROCTOR: Yes.

Palpate

Student: When I touch the chest, do I feel crepitus or a flail segment?
PROCTOR: No.

Auscultate

Student: Are lung sounds present in all fields?
PROCTOR: Yes.
Student: Do I hear any sucking sounds from the chest?
PROCTOR: No.

Assess the Abdomen/Pelvis

Assess the Abdomen

Student: I am assessing the abdomen for DCAP-BTLS. I am assessing all four quadrants. Do I find any problems?
PROCTOR: No.

Assess the Pelvis

Student: I am assessing the pelvis for DCAP-BTLS. Is the pelvis stable?
PROCTOR: Yes.

Assess the Genitalia/Perineum as Needed (Verbalize in Training)

Student: I am assessing the genitalia/perineum as necessary for DCAP-BTLS.
PROCTOR: The area is unremarkable.

Assess the Extremities

Inspect

Student: I am assessing the lower and upper extremities for DCAP-BTLS. Do I find anything?
PROCTOR: No.

Palpate

Student: Do I feel anything unusual?
PROCTOR: No.

Assess Motor, Sensory, and Circulatory Function

Student: I am checking for DCAP-BTLS, motor and sensory function, and pulses. Right leg?
PROCTOR: Negative DCAP-BTLS. Motor and sensory functions are present. Pulses are present.
Student: Left leg?
PROCTOR: Negative DCAP-BTLS. Motor and sensory functions are present. Pulses are present.
Student: Right arm?
PROCTOR: Negative DCAP-BTLS. Motor and sensory functions are present. Pulses are present.
Student: Left arm?
PROCTOR: Negative DCAP-BTLS. Motor and sensory functions are present. Pulses are present.

Assess the Posterior

Student: We will not check the back.
PROCTOR: Noted.

▸ Manage Secondary Injuries/Wounds

Student: I would reassure the patient.

PROCTOR: Noted.

▸ Reassess Interventions

Student: I will reassess my interventions: airway, breathing, oxygen, and inhaler assistance; and circulation.

PROCTOR: Noted.

ALS Student: I will reassess BLS interventions, plus the following: breathing treatment, check that the IV is flowing, and check cardiac monitor and 12-lead ECG.

ALS Proctor: Noted.

Critical Criteria:
- ❑ Did not obtain medical direction or verbalize standing orders for medical interventions
- ❑ Administered a dangerous or inappropriate intervention
- ❑ Did not ask questions about the present illness
- ❑ Did not differentiate patient's need for transportation versus continued assessment at the scene

Radio Report

(Provided by the student.)

PROCTOR: Noted.

Ongoing Assessment

Repeat the Initial Assessment

Student: I will repeat the initial assessment.

PROCTOR: Noted. (Reflected in "Repeat Vital Signs.")

Repeat Vital Signs

Student: I will reassess vital signs and mental status.

PROCTOR: Blood pressure, 138/78 mm Hg; pulse, 84 beats/min; respirations, 16 breaths/min; pulse oximetry reading, 97%; and the patient is alert.

Student: The vital signs have not changed significantly.

PROCTOR: Noted.

Check Interventions

Student: I will check my interventions: oxygen, inhaler assistance, reassurance, and transport.

PROCTOR: Noted.

ALS Student: I will check BLS interventions, plus the following: breathing treatment, check that the IV is flowing, and check cardiac monitor and 12-lead ECG.

ALS Proctor: Noted. The monitor shows normal sinus rhythm.

Repeat the Focused Assessment

Student: I will repeat the focused assessment.

PROCTOR: Noted.

Critical Criteria:
- ❑ Did not obtain medical direction or verbalize standing orders for medical interventions
- ❑ Administered a dangerous or inappropriate intervention

Handoff Report to Emergency Department Staff

Student: There was no change during transport.

PROCTOR: Noted.

Critical Criteria

(Inform the student of items missed, if any.)

❑ Pass ❑ Fail Date: ______________________

Proctor Comments: ______________________

Notes

Dispatch Information

PROCTOR: EMS 10, respond to 40-year-old male who was laying blacktop asphalt and became overheated. He is conscious and breathing.

Pre-scene Action (BSI)

Student: I am wearing nonlatex gloves and safety glasses.
PROCTOR: Noted.

Critical Criteria:
- ❑ Did not take, or verbalize, body substance isolation (BSI) precautions when necessary

Scene Size-up

Scene Safety

Student: Is the scene safe?
PROCTOR: Yes.

Mechanism of Injury/Nature of Illness

Student: What is the nature of the illness?
PROCTOR: The patient was laying blacktop asphalt and became overheated.

Number of Patients

Student: How many patients are there?
PROCTOR: One.

Additional Resources

Student: I would call for advanced life support (ALS) assistance.
PROCTOR: Noted.

C-Spine Stabilization

Student: I would not stabilize the cervical spine (c-spine).
PROCTOR: Noted.

Critical Criteria:
- ❑ Did not determine scene safety

Initial Assessment

General Impression

Student: My general impression is that the patient's condition is unstable.
PROCTOR: Noted.

Responsiveness/Level of Consciousness

Student: What is the patient's level of consciousness?
PROCTOR: Alert.

Chief Complaint/Apparent Life Threats

Student: What is the patient's chief complaint?
PROCTOR: The patient is complaining of a being hot and feeling weak.

Assess the Airway and Breathing

Student: Is the airway open?
PROCTOR: Yes.

Assessment

Student: What are the rate and the quality of breathing?
PROCTOR: Rate: Rapid. Quality: Shallow.

Provide Oxygen

Student: I am applying oxygen at 15 L/min via nonrebreathing mask.
PROCTOR: Noted.

Ensure Adequate Ventilation

Student: The patient has adequate ventilations at this time.
PROCTOR: Noted.

Assess Circulation

Student: I am assessing the patient's circulation.
PROCTOR: Noted.

Assess for and Control Major Bleeding

Student: Do I find any major bleeding?
PROCTOR: No.

Assess the Pulse

Student: What are the rate and the quality of pulses?
PROCTOR: Rate: Tachycardic. Quality: Bounding.

Assess the Skin

Student: I am assessing the skin. What are the color, temperature, and condition of the skin?
PROCTOR: Color: Flushed. Temperature: Hot. Condition: Dry.

Identify Priority Patients/Make Transport Decision

Student: The patient is a high priority and is a load-and-go. I will move him to a cooler environment and begin cooling measures. I will begin packaging and transport.
PROCTOR: Noted.

Critical Criteria:
- ❑ Did not provide high concentration of oxygen
- ❑ Did not find or manage problems associated with airway, breathing, hemorrhage or shock (hypoperfusion)
- ❑ Did not differentiate patient's need for transportation versus continued assessment at the scene
- ❑ Did detailed or focused history/physical examination before assessing the airway, breathing and circulation

Focused History and Physical Examination/Rapid Assessment

Select the Appropriate Assessment (Focused or Rapid)

Student: I am selecting the focused assessment.
PROCTOR: Noted.

SAMPLE History

Student: At this time I will gather a SAMPLE history from the patient or family. What are the patient's signs and symptoms?
PROCTOR: Environmental emergency.
Student: What was the source?
PROCTOR: Outdoor heat while laying blacktop.
Student: What was the environment?
PROCTOR: The temperature outdoors was 101°F.
Student: What was the duration?
PROCTOR: More than 6 hours.
Student: Was there any loss of consciousness?
PROCTOR: Yes, for 30 seconds (he did not fall).
Student: What were the effects—local or general?
PROCTOR: The whole body.
Student: Allergies?
PROCTOR: No allergies.
Student: Medications?
PROCTOR: No medications.
Student: Pertinent past medical history?
PROCTOR: No pertinent medical history.
Student: Last oral intake?
PROCTOR: 2 hours ago.
Student: Events leading up to the incident?
PROCTOR: The patient was laying blacktop in 101°F conditions.

Perform the Focused Physical Examination

Student: I am performing the focused physical examination.
PROCTOR: Noted.

Baseline Vital Signs

Student: What are the patient's baseline vital signs, including blood pressure, pulse, respirations, pulse oximetry, blood glucose level, and level of consciousness?
PROCTOR: Blood pressure, 150/88 mm Hg; pulse, 130 beats/min; respirations, 28 breaths/min; pulse oximetry reading, 97%; blood glucose level, 129 mg/dL; and the patient is alert.

▼ Interventions

Student: I will apply oxygen, continuously reassess and monitor the patient, remove the patient from the hot environment into a cool one (air conditioning on cold in the ambulance), remove the patient's clothing, and place a cold pack or ice wraps (to the neck, underarms, and groin).

PROCTOR: Noted.

ALS Student: I will apply basic life support (BLS) interventions, plus the following: establish IV access, perform cardiac monitoring, 12-lead ECG, and follow the local protocol.

ALS Proctor: Noted. The cardiac monitor shows sinus tachycardia.

▼ Reevaluate Transport Decision

Student: The patient is a high priority and is a load-and-go.

PROCTOR: Noted.

▼ Detailed Physical Examination

Possible Answer #1

Student: I would not do a detailed physical exam.

PROCTOR: Noted. (Go to "Radio Report.")

Possible Answer #2

Student: I am conducting the detailed physical exam. I am looking for DCAP-BTLS. This acronym stands for deformities, contusions, abrasions, punctures, penetrations, paradoxical motion in the chest, and burns, tenderness, lacerations, and swelling.

PROCTOR: Noted. The detailed physical exam will be performed during transport.

▸ **Assess the Head**

Student: I am assessing the head. Do I find any DCAP-BTLS? Do I find any evidence of Battle's sign or raccoon eyes?

PROCTOR: No.

▸ **Inspect and Palpate the Head and Ears**

Student: I am assessing the head and ears.

PROCTOR: There are no obvious injuries.

▸ **Assess the Eyes**

Student: I am assessing the eyes. Are the pupils equal, round, and regular in size, and react properly to light (PEARRL)?

PROCTOR: They are dilated but reactive.

▸ **Assess the Facial Area Including Oral and Nasal Areas**

Student: I am assessing the face, nose, and mouth. Do I see any discharge or hear any obstructions?

PROCTOR: No.

▸ **Assess the Neck**

▸ **Inspect and Palpate the Neck**

Student: I am assessing the neck for DCAP-BTLS.

PROCTOR: There are no obvious injuries.

▸ **Assess for Jugular Vein Distention**

Student: Do I find any jugular vein distention (JVD)?

PROCTOR: No.

▸ **Assess for Tracheal Deviation**

Student: Do I see any tracheal deviation?

PROCTOR: No.

▸ **Assess the Chest**

Student: I am assessing the chest for DCAP-BTLS.

PROCTOR: Noted.

▸ **Inspect**

Student: What do I see when I look at the chest?

PROCTOR: There are no obvious injuries.

Student: Is the chest symmetric?

PROCTOR: Yes.

▸ **Palpate**

Student: When I touch the chest, do I feel crepitus or a flail segment?

PROCTOR: No.

▸ **Auscultate**

Student: Are lung sounds present in all fields?

PROCTOR: Yes.

Student: Do I hear any sucking sounds from the chest?

PROCTOR: No.

▸ **Assess the Abdomen/Pelvis**

▸ **Assess the Abdomen**

Student: I am assessing the abdomen for DCAP-BTLS. I am assessing all four quadrants. Do I find any problems?

PROCTOR: No.

▸ **Assess the Pelvis**

Student: I am assessing the pelvis for DCAP-BTLS. Is the pelvis stable?

PROCTOR: Yes.

▸ **Assess the Genitalia/Perineum as Needed (Verbalize in Training)**

Student: I am assessing the genitalia/perineum as necessary for DCAP-BTLS.

PROCTOR: The area is unremarkable.

▸ **Assess the Extremities**

▸ **Inspect**

Student: I am assessing the lower and upper extremities for DCAP-BTLS. Do I find anything?

PROCTOR: No.

▸ **Palpate**

Student: Do I feel anything unusual?

PROCTOR: No.

▸ **Assess Motor, Sensory, and Circulatory Function**

Student: I am checking for DCAP-BTLS, motor and sensory function, and pulses. Right leg?

PROCTOR: Negative DCAP-BTLS. Motor and sensory functions are present. Pulses are present.

Student: Left leg?

PROCTOR: Negative DCAP-BTLS. Motor and sensory functions are present. Pulses are present.

Student: Right arm?

PROCTOR: Negative DCAP-BTLS. Motor and sensory functions are present. Pulses are present.

Student: Left arm?

PROCTOR: Negative DCAP-BTLS. Motor and sensory functions are present. Pulses are present.

▸ **Assess the Posterior**

Student: We will check the back.

PROCTOR: Noted.

▸ **Assess the Thorax**

Student: I am assessing the thorax. Do I find injuries?

PROCTOR: No.

▸ **Assess the Lumbar Area**

Student: I am assessing the flanks and lumbar area. Do I find injuries?

PROCTOR: No.

▸ **Assess the Entire Backside**

Student: I am assessing the entire backside. Do I find injuries?

PROCTOR: No.

▸ **Manage Secondary Injuries/Wounds**

Student: I would continuously monitor vital signs.

PROCTOR: Noted.

▸ **Reassess Interventions**

Student: I will reassess my interventions: airway, breathing, and oxygen; circulation and cooling measures.

PROCTOR: Noted.

Critical Criteria:
- ❑ Did not obtain medical direction or verbalize standing orders for medical interventions
- ❑ Administered a dangerous or inappropriate intervention
- ❑ Did not ask questions about the present illness
- ❑ Did not differentiate patient's need for transportation versus continued assessment at the scene

Radio Report

(Provided by the student.)

PROCTOR: Noted.

Ongoing Assessment

Repeat the Initial Assessment

Student: I will repeat the initial assessment.

PROCTOR: Noted. (Reflected in "Repeat Vital Signs.")

Repeat Vital Signs

Student: I will reassess vital signs.

PROCTOR: Blood pressure, 144/86 mm Hg; pulse, 122 beats/min; respirations, 24 breaths/min; pulse oximetry reading, 98%; and the patient is alert. Patient temperature, if taken, is 99.7°F.

Student: The vital signs have not changed significantly.

PROCTOR: Noted.

Check Interventions

Student: I will check my interventions: oxygen, continuously reassess and monitor the patient, remove patient from the hot environment into a cool one (air conditioning on cold in the ambulance), remove the patient's clothing, and place cold pack or ice wraps (to the neck, underarms, and groin).

PROCTOR: Noted.

ALS Student: I will check BLS interventions, plus the following: establish IV access, perform cardiac monitoring, 12-lead ECG, and follow the local protocol.

ALS Proctor: Noted. The cardiac monitor shows sinus tachycardia.

Repeat the Focused Assessment

Student: I will repeat the focused assessment.

PROCTOR: Noted.

Critical Criteria:
- ❑ Did not obtain medical direction or verbalize standing orders for medical interventions
- ❑ Administered a dangerous or inappropriate intervention

Handoff Report to Emergency Department Staff

Student: There was no change during transport.

PROCTOR: Noted.

Critical Criteria

(Inform the student of items missed, if any.)

❑ Pass ❑ Fail Date: ______________________

Proctor Comments: ______________________

____

____

Notes

Dispatch Information

PROCTOR: EMS 10, respond to a 65-year-old female who is complaining of a clogged tracheostomy tube. She is conscious and breathing.

Pre-scene Action (BSI)

Student: I am wearing nonlatex gloves and safety glasses.
PROCTOR: Noted.

Critical Criteria:
- ❑ Did not take, or verbalize, body substance isolation (BSI) precautions when necessary

Scene Size-up

Scene Safety

Student: Is the scene safe?
PROCTOR: Yes.

Mechanism of Injury/Nature of Illness

Student: What is the nature of the illness?
PROCTOR: The patient has had recent throat surgery for the removal of cancer. She now has a tracheostomy tube. She is hesitant in its care and maintenance. The tube is partially obstructed, making it difficult to breathe. She is conscious and breathing.

Number of Patients

Student: How many patients are there?
PROCTOR: One.

Additional Resources

Student: I would not call for advanced life support (ALS) assistance.
PROCTOR: Noted.

C-Spine Stabilization

Student: I would not stabilize the cervical spine (c-spine).
PROCTOR: Noted.

Critical Criteria:
- ❑ Did not determine scene safety

Initial Assessment

General Impression

Student: My general impression is that the patient's condition is stable.
PROCTOR: Noted.

Responsiveness/Level of Consciousness

Student: What is the patient's level of consciousness?
PROCTOR: Alert.

Chief Complaint/Apparent Life Threats

Student: What is the patient's chief complaint?
PROCTOR: The patient is complaining of a partially obstructed tracheostomy tube.

Assess the Airway and Breathing

Student: Is the airway open?
PROCTOR: Yes.

Assessment

Student: What are the rate and the quality of breathing?
PROCTOR: Rate: Tachypneic. Quality: Gurgling.
Student: I would either suction the tube with a French catheter or remove and clean the inner tube and then reinsert it (per local protocol).
PROCTOR: Noted.

Provide Oxygen

Student: I am applying oxygen at 15 L/min via nonrebreathing or tracheostomy mask.
PROCTOR: Noted.

Ensure Adequate Ventilation

Student: The patient has adequate ventilations at this time.
PROCTOR: Noted.

Assess Circulation

Student: I am assessing the patient's circulation.
PROCTOR: Noted.

Assess for and Control Major Bleeding

Student: Do I find any major bleeding?
PROCTOR: No.

Assess the Pulse

Student: What are the rate and the quality of pulses?
PROCTOR: Rate: Tachycardic. Quality: Strong.

Assess the Skin

Student: I am assessing the skin. What are the color, temperature, and condition of the skin?
PROCTOR: Color: Pale. Temperature: Warm. Condition: Moist.

Identify Priority Patients/Make Transport Decision

Student: The patient is a low priority and does not require immediate transport.
PROCTOR: Noted.

Critical Criteria:
- ❑ Did not provide high concentration of oxygen
- ❑ Did not find or manage problems associated with airway, breathing, hemorrhage or shock (hypoperfusion)
- ❑ Did not differentiate patient's need for transportation versus continued assessment at the scene
- ❑ Did detailed or focused history/physical examination before assessing the airway, breathing and circulation

Focused History and Physical Examination/Rapid Assessment

Select the Appropriate Assessment (Focused or Rapid)

Student: I am selecting the focused assessment.
PROCTOR: Noted.

SAMPLE History

Student: At this time I will gather a SAMPLE history from the patient or family. What are the patient's signs and symptoms?
PROCTOR: Respiratory.

> **Student:** Onset: What were you doing when this started?
> **PROCTOR:** Watching TV.
> **Student:** Provokes: What makes your condition worse or better?
> **PROCTOR:** Coughing makes her condition worse.
> **Student:** Quality: Can you describe your pain?
> **PROCTOR:** None.
> **Student:** Radiates: Do you have pain anywhere else?
> **PROCTOR:** No.
> **Student:** Severity: On a scale of 1 to 10 with 10 being the worst possible, how would you rate your distress?
> **PROCTOR:** 4.
> **Student:** Time: How long has this been going on?
> **PROCTOR:** 30 minutes.
> **Student:** Interventions: Have you done anything to make this better?
> **PROCTOR:** The patient has taken no actions.

Student: Allergies?
PROCTOR: No allergies.

Student: Medications?
PROCTOR: Asthma medications.
Student: Pertinent past medical history?
PROCTOR: She has a history of 30 years of smoking, asthma, and throat cancer.
Student: Last oral intake?
PROCTOR: 3 hours ago.
Student: Events leading up to the incident?
PROCTOR: The patient was watching TV. She began to cough and felt restriction through her tracheostomy tube.

▼ Perform the Focused Physical Examination

Student: I am performing the focused physical examination.
PROCTOR: Noted.
Student: I am assessing the face, nose, and mouth. Do I see any discharge or hear any obstructions?
PROCTOR: No.
Student: I am assessing the neck for DCAP-BTLS. This acronym stands for deformities, contusions, abrasions, punctures, penetrations, paradoxical motion in the chest, and burns, tenderness, lacerations, and swelling.
PROCTOR: There is a tracheostomy tube in place. It consists of an outer tube which is sewn to the skin. The inner tube is removable for cleaning.
Student: I will clean the inner tube per protocol.
PROCTOR: Noted.
Student: Are lung sounds present in all fields?
PROCTOR: Yes, lung sounds are clear bilaterally.
Student: Do I hear any sucking sounds from the chest?
PROCTOR: No.

▼ Baseline Vital Signs

Student: What are the patient's baseline vital signs, including blood pressure, pulse, respirations, pulse oximetry, and level of consciousness?
PROCTOR: Blood pressure, 140/84 mm Hg; pulse, 112 beats/min; respirations, 24 breaths/min; pulse oximetry reading, 95%; and the patient is alert.

▼ Interventions

Student: I will apply suction as needed during transport, continue applying oxygen, provide reassurance, and transport in the position of function.
PROCTOR: Noted.

▼ Reevaluate Transport Decision

Student: The patient is a low priority and does not require immediate transport.
PROCTOR: Noted.

▼ Detailed Physical Examination

Possible Answer #1
Student: I would not do a detailed physical exam.
PROCTOR: Noted. (Go to "Radio Report.")

Possible Answer #2
Student: I am conducting the detailed physical exam. I am looking for DCAP-BTLS.
PROCTOR: Noted.

▸ **Assess the Head**

Student: I am assessing the head. Do I find any DCAP-BTLS? Do I find any evidence of Battle's sign or raccoon eyes?
PROCTOR: No.

▸ **Inspect and Palpate the Head and Ears**

Student: I am assessing the head and ears.
PROCTOR: There are no obvious injuries.

▸ **Assess the Eyes**

Student: I am assessing the eyes. Are the pupils equal, round, and regular in size, and react properly to light (PEARRL)?
PROCTOR: They are PEARRL.

▸ **Assess the Facial Area Including Oral and Nasal Areas**

Student: I am assessing the face, nose, and mouth. Do I see any discharge or hear any obstructions?
PROCTOR: No.

▸ **Assess the Neck**

▸ **Inspect and Palpate the Neck**

Student: I am assessing the neck for DCAP-BTLS.
PROCTOR: There are no obvious injuries.

▸ **Assess for Jugular Vein Distention**

Student: Do I find any jugular vein distention (JVD)?
PROCTOR: No.

▸ **Assess for Tracheal Deviation**

Student: Do I see any tracheal deviation?
PROCTOR: No.

▸ **Assess the Chest**

Student: I am assessing the chest for DCAP-BTLS.
PROCTOR: Noted.

▸ **Inspect**

Student: What do I see when I look at the chest?
PROCTOR: There are no obvious injuries.
Student: Is the chest symmetric?
PROCTOR: Yes.

▸ **Palpate**

Student: When I touch the chest, do I feel crepitus or a flail segment?
PROCTOR: No.

▸ **Auscultate**

Student: Are lung sounds present in all fields?
PROCTOR: Yes, lung sounds are clear bilaterally.
Student: Do I hear any sucking sounds from the chest?
PROCTOR: No.

▸ **Assess the Abdomen/Pelvis**

▸ **Assess the Abdomen**

Student: I am assessing the abdomen for DCAP-BTLS. I am assessing all four quadrants. Do I find any problems?
PROCTOR: No.

▸ **Assess the Pelvis**

Student: I am assessing the pelvis for DCAP-BTLS. Is the pelvis stable?
PROCTOR: Yes.

▸ **Assess the Genitalia/Perineum as Needed (Verbalize in Training)**

Student: I am assessing the genitalia/perineum as necessary for DCAP-BTLS.
PROCTOR: The area is unremarkable.

▸ **Assess the Extremities**

▸ **Inspect**

Student: I am assessing the lower and upper extremities for DCAP-BTLS. Do I find anything?
PROCTOR: No.

▸ **Palpate**

Student: Do I feel anything unusual?
PROCTOR: No.

▸ **Assess Motor, Sensory, and Circulatory Function**

Student: I am checking for DCAP-BTLS, motor and sensory function, and pulses. Right leg?
PROCTOR: Negative DCAP-BTLS. Motor and sensory functions are present. Pulses are present.

Student: Left leg?
PROCTOR: Negative DCAP-BTLS. Motor and sensory functions are present. Pulses are present.
Student: Right arm?
PROCTOR: Negative DCAP-BTLS. Motor and sensory functions are present. Pulses are present.
Student: Left arm?
PROCTOR: Negative DCAP-BTLS. Motor and sensory functions are present. Pulses are present.

▸ **Assess the Posterior**

Student: We will now check the back.
PROCTOR: Noted.

▸ **Assess the Thorax**

Student: I am assessing the thorax. Do I find injuries?
PROCTOR: No.

▸ **Assess the Lumbar Area**

Student: I am assessing the flanks and lumbar area. Do I find injuries?
PROCTOR: No.

▸ **Assess the Entire Backside**

Student: I am assessing the entire backside. Do I find injuries?
PROCTOR: No.

▸ **Manage Secondary Injuries/Wounds**

Student: I would suction as necessary during transport.
PROCTOR: Noted.

▸ **Reassess Interventions**

Student: I will reassess my interventions: suction, oxygen, reassurance, and transport in the position of comfort.
PROCTOR: Noted.

Critical Criteria:
- ❑ Did not obtain medical direction or verbalize standing orders for medical interventions
- ❑ Administered a dangerous or inappropriate intervention
- ❑ Did not ask questions about the present illness
- ❑ Did not differentiate patient's need for transportation versus continued assessment at the scene

Radio Report

(Provided by the student.)
PROCTOR: Noted.

Ongoing Assessment

Repeat the Initial Assessment

Student: I will repeat the initial assessment.
PROCTOR: Noted. (Reflected in "Repeat Vital Signs.")

Repeat Vital Signs

Student: I will reassess vital signs and mental status.
PROCTOR: Blood pressure, 136/82 mm Hg; pulse, 108 beats/min; respirations, 22 breaths/min; pulse oximetry reading, 97%; and the patient is alert.
Student: The vital signs have not changed significantly.
PROCTOR: Noted.

Check Interventions

Student: I will check my interventions: suction, oxygen, reassurance, and transport in the position of comfort.
PROCTOR: Noted.

Repeat the Focused Assessment

Student: I will repeat the focused assessment.
PROCTOR: Noted.

Critical Criteria:
- ❑ Did not obtain medical direction or verbalize standing orders for medical interventions
- ❑ Administered a dangerous or inappropriate intervention

Handoff Report to Emergency Department Staff

Student: There was no change during transport.
PROCTOR: Noted.

Critical Criteria

(Inform the student of items missed, if any.)

❑ Pass ❑ Fail Date: ______________________

Proctor Comments: ______________________

Notes

Dispatch Information

PROCTOR: EMS 10, respond to a 61-year-old male who is complaining of chest pain. He is conscious and breathing.

Pre-scene Action (BSI)

Student: I am wearing nonlatex gloves and safety glasses.
PROCTOR: Noted.

Critical Criteria:
- ❑ Did not take, or verbalize, body substance isolation (BSI) precautions when necessary

Scene Size-up

Scene Safety

Student: Is the scene safe?
PROCTOR: Yes.

Mechanism of Injury/Nature of Illness

Student: What is the nature of the illness?
PROCTOR: The patient has pain in the chest and neck.

Number of Patients

Student: How many patients are there?
PROCTOR: One.

Additional Resources

Student: I would call for advanced life support (ALS) assistance.
PROCTOR: Noted.

C-Spine Stabilization

Student: I would not stabilize the cervical spine (c-spine).
PROCTOR: Noted.

Critical Criteria:
- ❑ Did not determine scene safety

Initial Assessment

General Impression

Student: My general impression is that the patient's condition is unstable.
PROCTOR: Noted.

Responsiveness/Level of Consciousness

Student: What is the patient's level of consciousness?
PROCTOR: Alert.

Chief Complaint/Apparent Life Threats

Student: What is the patient's chief complaint?
PROCTOR: The patient is complaining of pain in the chest and the neck.

Assess the Airway and Breathing

Student: Is the airway open?
PROCTOR: Yes.

Assessment

Student: What are the rate and the quality of breathing?
PROCTOR: Rate: Tachypneic. Quality: Deep.

Provide Oxygen

Student: I am applying oxygen at 15 L/min via nonrebreathing mask.
PROCTOR: Noted.

Ensure Adequate Ventilation

Student: The patient has adequate ventilations at this time.
PROCTOR: Noted.

Assess Circulation

Student: I am assessing the patient's circulation.
PROCTOR: Noted.

Assess for and Control Major Bleeding

Student: Do I find any major bleeding?
PROCTOR: No.

Assess the Pulse

Student: What are the rate and the quality of pulses?
PROCTOR: Rate: Bradycardic. Quality: Thready.

Assess the Skin

Student: I am assessing the skin. What are the color, temperature, and condition of the skin?
PROCTOR: Color: Pale. Temperature: Cool. Condition: Diaphoretic.

Identify Priority Patients/Make Transport Decision

Student: The patient is a high priority and is a load-and-go. I will begin packaging and transport.
PROCTOR: Noted.

Critical Criteria:
- ❑ Did not provide high concentration of oxygen
- ❑ Did not find or manage problems associated with airway, breathing, hemorrhage or shock (hypoperfusion)
- ❑ Did not differentiate patient's need for transportation versus continued assessment at the scene
- ❑ Did detailed or focused history/physical examination before assessing the airway, breathing and circulation

Focused History and Physical Examination/Rapid Assessment

Select the Appropriate Assessment (Focused or Rapid)

Student: I am selecting the focused assessment.
PROCTOR: Noted.

SAMPLE History

Student: At this time I will gather a SAMPLE history from the patient or family. What are the patient's signs and symptoms?
PROCTOR: Cardiac.

> **Student:** Onset: What were you doing when this started?
> **PROCTOR:** Eating dinner.
> **Student:** Provokes: What makes your condition worse or better?
> **PROCTOR:** Nothing makes it better.
> **Student:** Quality: Can you describe your pain?
> **PROCTOR:** Heaviness and tightness in the chest.
> **Student:** Radiates: Do you have pain anywhere else?
> **PROCTOR:** In the neck.
> **Student:** Severity: On a scale of 1 to 10 with 10 being the worst possible, how would you rate your pain/distress?
> **PROCTOR:** 10.
> **Student:** Time: How long has this been going on?
> **PROCTOR:** 30 minutes.
> **Student:** Interventions: Have you done anything to make this better?
> **PROCTOR:** The patient has taken three nitroglycerin tablets with no pain relief. He now has a headache as well.

Student: Allergies?
PROCTOR: Penicillin (PCN).
Student: Medications? Has the patient used any erectile dysfunction medication?
PROCTOR: Nitroglycerin. No, the patient has not used any erectile dysfunction medication.
Student: Pertinent past medical history?
PROCTOR: Angina.
Student: Last oral intake?
PROCTOR: 30 minutes ago.
Student: Events leading up to the incident?
PROCTOR: The patient was eating dinner about 30 minutes ago when the pain began.

▼ **Perform the Focused Physical Examination**

Student: I am performing the focused physical examination.
PROCTOR: Noted.
Student: Are lung sounds present in all fields?
PROCTOR: Yes.
Student: Is there any edema to the extremities?
PROCTOR: No.

▼ **Baseline Vital Signs**

Student: What are the patient's baseline vital signs, including blood pressure, pulse, respirations, pulse oximetry, and level of consciousness?
PROCTOR: Blood pressure, 124/60 mm Hg; pulse rate, 68 beats/min; respirations, 12 breaths/min; pulse oximetry reading, 95%; and the patient is alert.

▼ **Interventions**

Student: I will apply oxygen, loosen tight-fitting clothing, and treat for shock.
PROCTOR: Noted.
ALS Student: I will apply basic life support (BLS) interventions, plus the following: IV access, cardiac monitor, 12-lead ECG, advanced cardiac life support (ACLS) or local protocol, 325 mg baby aspirin, and morphine.
ALS Proctor: Noted. The cardiac monitor shows normal sinus rhythm. 12-lead ECG shows ST elevation in V_1 and V_2.

▼ **Reevaluate Transport Decision**

Student: The patient is a load-and-go due to the nature of the illness.
PROCTOR: Noted.

▼ **Detailed Physical Examination**

Possible Answer #1
Student: I would not do a detailed physical exam.
PROCTOR: Noted. (Go to "Radio Report.")

Possible Answer #2
Student: I am conducting the detailed physical exam. I am checking for DCAP-BTLS. This acronym stands for deformities, contusions, abrasions, punctures, penetrations, and paradoxical motion in the chest, and burns, tenderness, lacerations, and swelling.
PROCTOR: Noted. The detailed physical exam will be performed during transport.

► **Assess the Head**

Student: I am assessing the head. Do I find any DCAP-BTLS? Do I find any evidence of Battle's sign or raccoon eyes?
PROCTOR: No.

► **Inspect and Palpate the Head and Ears**

Student: I am assessing the head and ears.
PROCTOR: There are no obvious injuries.

► **Assess the Eyes**

Student: I am assessing the eyes. Are the pupils equal, round, and regular in size, and react properly to light (PEARRL)?
PROCTOR: They are PEARRL.

► **Assess the Facial Area Including Oral and Nasal Areas**

Student: I am assessing the face, nose, and mouth. Do I see any discharge or hear any obstructions?
PROCTOR: No.

► **Assess the Neck**

► **Inspect and Palpate the Neck**

Student: I am assessing the neck for DCAP-BTLS.
PROCTOR: There are no obvious injuries.

► **Assess for Jugular Vein Distention**

Student: Do I find any JVD?
PROCTOR: No.

► **Assess for Tracheal Deviation**

Student: Do I see any tracheal deviation?
PROCTOR: No.

► **Assess the Chest**

Student: I am assessing the chest for DCAP-BTLS.
PROCTOR: Noted.

► **Inspect**

Student: What do I see when I look at the chest?
PROCTOR: There are no obvious injuries.
Student: Is the chest symmetric?
PROCTOR: Yes.

► **Palpate**

Student: When I touch the chest, do I feel crepitus or a flail segment?
PROCTOR: No.

► **Auscultate**

Student: Are lung sounds present in all fields?
PROCTOR: Yes.
Student: Do I hear any sucking sounds from the chest?
PROCTOR: No.

► **Assess the Abdomen/Pelvis**

► **Assess the Abdomen**

Student: I am assessing the abdomen for DCAP-BTLS. I am assessing all four quadrants. Do I find any problems?
PROCTOR: No.

► **Assess the Pelvis**

Student: I am assessing the pelvis for DCAP-BTLS. Is the pelvis stable?
PROCTOR: Yes.

► **Assess the Genitalia/Perineum as Needed (Verbalize in Training)**

Student: I am assessing the genitalia/perineum as necessary for DCAP-BTLS.
PROCTOR: The area is unremarkable.

► **Assess the Extremities**

► **Inspect**

Student: I am assessing the lower and upper extremities for DCAP-BTLS. Do I find anything?
PROCTOR: No.

► **Palpate**

Student: Do I feel anything unusual?
PROCTOR: No.

► **Assess Motor, Sensory, and Circulatory Function**

Student: I am checking for DCAP-BTLS, motor and sensory function, and pulses. Right leg?
PROCTOR: Negative DCAP-BTLS. Motor and sensory functions are present. Pulses are present.
Student: Left leg?
PROCTOR: Negative DCAP-BTLS. Motor and sensory functions are present. Pulses are present.

Student: Right arm?

PROCTOR: Negative DCAP-BTLS. Motor and sensory functions are present. Pulses are present.

Student: Left arm?

PROCTOR: Negative DCAP-BTLS. Motor and sensory functions are present. Pulses are present.

▸ **Assess the Posterior**

Student: We will check the back.

PROCTOR: Noted.

▸ **Assess the Thorax**

Student: I am assessing the thorax. Do I find injuries?

PROCTOR: No.

▸ **Assess the Lumbar Area**

Student: I am assessing the flanks and lumbar area. Do I find injuries?

PROCTOR: No.

▸ **Assess the Entire Backside**

Student: I am assessing the entire backside. Do I find injuries?

PROCTOR: No.

▸ **Manage Secondary Injuries/Wounds**

Student: I would direct my partner to monitor the airway.

PROCTOR: Noted.

▸ **Reassess Interventions**

Student: I will reassess my interventions: apply oxygen, loosen tight-fitting clothing, and transport the patient in the position of comfort.

PROCTOR: Noted.

ALS Student: I will reassess BLS interventions, plus the following: IV access, cardiac monitor, 12-lead ECG, ACLS or local protocol, and check for pain relief from baby aspirin.

ALS Proctor: Noted. The cardiac monitor shows normal sinus rhythm. 12-lead ECG shows ST elevation in V_1 and V_2.

Critical Criteria:
- ❑ Did not obtain medical direction or verbalize standing orders for medical interventions
- ❑ Administered a dangerous or inappropriate intervention
- ❑ Did not ask questions about the present illness
- ❑ Did not differentiate patient's need for transportation versus continued assessment at the scene

Radio Report

(Provided by the student.)

PROCTOR: Noted.

Ongoing Assessment

Repeat the Initial Assessment

Student: I will repeat the initial assessment.

PROCTOR: Noted. (Reflected in "Repeat Vital Signs.")

Repeat Vital Signs

Student: I will reassess vital signs and mental status.

PROCTOR: Blood pressure, 116/62 mm Hg; pulse rate, 72 beats/min; respirations, 16 breaths/min; pulse oximetry reading, 97%; and the patient is alert.

Student: The vital signs have improved.

PROCTOR: Noted.

Check Interventions

Student: I will check my interventions: apply oxygen, loosen tight-fitting clothing, and transport the patient in the position of comfort.

PROCTOR: Noted.

ALS Student: I will check BLS interventions, plus the following: IV access, cardiac monitor, ACLS or local protocol, and check for pain relief from baby aspirin and morphine.

ALS Proctor: Noted. The cardiac monitor shows sinus bradycardia.

Repeat the Focused Assessment

Student: I will repeat the focused assessment.

PROCTOR: Noted.

Critical Criteria:
- ❑ Did not obtain medical direction or verbalize standing orders for medical interventions
- ❑ Administered a dangerous or inappropriate intervention

Handoff Report to Emergency Department Staff

Student: The patient's condition improved during transport.

PROCTOR: Noted.

Critical Criteria

(Inform the student of items missed, if any.)

❑ Pass ❑ Fail Date: ______________________

Proctor Comments: ______________________

____

____

CASE 92

Notes

Dispatch Information

PROCTOR: EMS 10, respond to 29-year-old male who attempted suicide by eating d-CON mouse poison.

Pre-scene Action (BSI)

Student: I am wearing nonlatex gloves and safety glasses.
PROCTOR: Noted.

Critical Criteria:
- ❑ Did not take, or verbalize, body substance isolation (BSI) precautions when necessary

Scene Size-up

Scene Safety

Student: Is the scene safe?
PROCTOR: Yes.

Mechanism of Injury/Nature of Illness

Student: What is the nature of the illness?
PROCTOR: The patient was trying to kill himself by eating d-CON mouse poison.

Number of Patients

Student: How many patients are there?
PROCTOR: One.

Additional Resources

Student: I would call for advanced life support (ALS) assistance.
PROCTOR: Noted.

C-Spine Stabilization

Student: I would not stabilize the cervical spine (c-spine).
PROCTOR: Noted.

Critical Criteria:
- ❑ Did not determine scene safety

Initial Assessment

General Impression

Student: My general impression is that the patient's condition is stable.
PROCTOR: Noted.

Responsiveness/Level of Consciousness

Student: What is the patient's level of consciousness?
PROCTOR: Alert.

Chief Complaint/Apparent Life Threats

Student: What is the patient's chief complaint?
PROCTOR: The patient is complaining of vomiting and stomach upset. He believes that he has vomited all of the d-CON up.

Assess the Airway and Breathing

Student: Is the airway open?
PROCTOR: Yes.

Assessment

Student: What are the rate and the quality of breathing?
PROCTOR: Rate: Within normal limits. Quality: Normal.

Provide Oxygen

Student: I am applying oxygen at 15 L/min via nonrebreathing mask.
PROCTOR: Noted.

Ensure Adequate Ventilation

Student: The patient has adequate ventilations at this time.
PROCTOR: Noted.

Assess Circulation

Student: I am assessing the patient's circulation.
PROCTOR: Noted.

Assess for and Control Major Bleeding

Student: Do I find any major bleeding?
PROCTOR: No.

Assess the Pulse

Student: What are the rate and the quality of pulses?
PROCTOR: Rate: Within normal limits. Quality: Normal.

Assess the Skin

Student: I am assessing the skin. What are the color, temperature, and condition of the skin?
PROCTOR: Color: Pale. Temperature: Warm. Condition: Moist.

Identify Priority Patients/Make Transport Decision

Student: The patient is a low priority and does not require immediate transport.
PROCTOR: Noted.

Critical Criteria:
- ❑ Did not provide high concentration of oxygen
- ❑ Did not find or manage problems associated with airway, breathing, hemorrhage or shock (hypoperfusion)
- ❑ Did not differentiate patient's need for transportation versus continued assessment at the scene
- ❑ Did detailed or focused history/physical examination before assessing the airway, breathing and circulation

Focused History and Physical Examination/Rapid Assessment

Select the Appropriate Assessment (Focused or Rapid)

Student: I am selecting the focused assessment.
PROCTOR: Noted.

SAMPLE History

Student: At this time I will gather a SAMPLE history from the patient or family. What are the patient's signs and symptoms?
PROCTOR: Behavioral and poisoning/overdose.

> Student: I will ask behavioral questions first. How do you feel?
> **PROCTOR:** He is sick to his stomach and has vomited.
> Student: Do you want to hurt or kill yourself?
> **PROCTOR:** Yes.
> Student: Is the patient a threat to self or others? What do you think?
> **PROCTOR:** Yes.
> Student: Is there a medical problem?
> **PROCTOR:** No.
> Student: Interventions: Have you done anything to make this better?
> **PROCTOR:** No.
> Student: I will now ask poisoning/overdose questions. What was the substance?
> **PROCTOR:** d-CON.
> Student: When did you ingest/become exposed?
> **PROCTOR:** It was 20 minutes ago.
> Student: How much did you ingest?
> **PROCTOR:** The whole box.
> Student: Over what time period?
> **PROCTOR:** Over 10 minutes.
> Student: Interventions? Have you done anything to make this better?
> **PROCTOR:** Yes, I vomited.
> Student: What is your weight?
> **PROCTOR:** 210 pounds.

Student: Allergies?
PROCTOR: No allergies.
Student: Medications?
PROCTOR: No medications.
Student: Pertinent past medical history?
PROCTOR: No pertinent medical history.

Student: Last oral intake?
PROCTOR: 1 hour.
Student: Events leading up to the incident?
PROCTOR: The patient was upset about the economy and decided to eat mouse poison. It did not taste good, so he made it into a tea. He got sick to his stomach and called for help.

▼ Perform the Focused Physical Examination

Student: I am performing the focused physical examination.
PROCTOR: Noted.
Student: I am assessing the abdomen for DCAP-BTLS. This acronym stands for deformities, contusions, abrasions, punctures, penetrations, paradoxical motion in the chest, and burns, tenderness, lacerations, and swelling. I am assessing all four quadrants. Do I find any problems?
PROCTOR: No.
Student: I am assessing the pelvis for DCAP-BTLS. Is the pelvis stable?
PROCTOR: Yes.

▼ Baseline Vital Signs

Student: What are the patient's baseline vital signs, including blood pressure, pulse, respirations, pulse oximetry, and level of consciousness?
PROCTOR: Blood pressure, 136/88 mm Hg; pulse, 78; respirations, 16 breaths/min; pulse oximetry reading, 98%; and the patient is alert.

▼ Interventions

Student: I will apply oxygen and call medical control for a poison control consult, and the possibility of using activated charcoal.
PROCTOR: Noted.
ALS Student: I will apply basic life support (BLS) interventions, plus the following: establish IV access, perform cardiac monitoring, and follow the local protocol.
ALS Proctor: Noted. The cardiac monitor shows normal sinus rhythm.

▼ Reevaluate Transport Decision

Student: This patient does not require immediate transport.
PROCTOR: Noted.

▼ Detailed Physical Examination

Possible Answer #1
Student: I would not do a detailed physical exam.
PROCTOR: Noted. (Go to "Radio Report.")

Possible Answer #2
Student: I am conducting the detailed physical exam. I am looking for DCAP-BTLS.
PROCTOR: Noted. The detailed physical exam will be performed during transport.

► Assess the Head

Student: I am assessing the head. Do I find any DCAP-BTLS? Do I find any evidence of Battle's sign or raccoon eyes?
PROCTOR: No.

► Inspect and Palpate the Head and Ears

Student: I am assessing the head and ears.
PROCTOR: There are no obvious injuries.

► Assess the Eyes

Student: I am assessing the eyes. Are the pupils equal, round, and regular in size, and react properly to light (PEARRL)?
PROCTOR: They are PEARRL.

► Assess the Facial Area Including Oral and Nasal Areas

Student: I am assessing the face, nose, and mouth. Do I see any discharge or hear any obstructions?
PROCTOR: No.

► Assess the Neck

► Inspect and Palpate the Neck

Student: I am assessing the neck for DCAP-BTLS.
PROCTOR: There are no obvious injuries.

► Assess for Jugular Vein Distention

Student: Do I find any jugular vein distention (JVD)?
PROCTOR: No.

► Assess for Tracheal Deviation

Student: Do I see any tracheal deviation?
PROCTOR: No.

► Assess the Chest

Student: I am assessing the chest for DCAP-BTLS.
PROCTOR: Noted.

► Inspect

Student: What do I see when I look at the chest?
PROCTOR: There are no obvious injuries.
Student: Is the chest symmetric?
PROCTOR: Yes.

► Palpate

Student: When I touch the chest, do I feel crepitus or a flail segment?
PROCTOR: No.

► Auscultate

Student: Are lung sounds present in all fields?
PROCTOR: Yes.
Student: Do I hear any sucking sounds from the chest?
PROCTOR: No.

► Assess the Abdomen/Pelvis

► Assess the Abdomen

Student: I am assessing the abdomen for DCAP-BTLS. I am assessing all four quadrants. Do I find any problems?
PROCTOR: No.

► Assess the Pelvis

Student: I am assessing the pelvis for DCAP-BTLS. Is the pelvis stable?
PROCTOR: Yes.

► Assess the Genitalia/Perineum as Needed (Verbalize in Training)

Student: I am assessing the genitalia/perineum as necessary for DCAP-BTLS.
PROCTOR: The area is unremarkable.

► Assess the Extremities

► Inspect

Student: I am assessing the lower and upper extremities for DCAP-BTLS. Do I find anything?
PROCTOR: No.

► Palpate

Student: Do I feel anything unusual?
PROCTOR: No.

► Assess Motor, Sensory, and Circulatory Function

Student: I am checking for DCAP-BTLS, motor and sensory function, and pulses. Right leg?
PROCTOR: Negative DCAP-BTLS. Motor and sensory functions are present. Pulses are present.
Student: Left leg?
PROCTOR: Negative DCAP-BTLS. Motor and sensory functions are present. Pulses are present.
Student: Right arm?
PROCTOR: Negative DCAP-BTLS. Motor and sensory functions are present. Pulses are present.
Student: Left arm?
PROCTOR: Negative DCAP-BTLS. Motor and sensory functions are present. Pulses are present.

▸ Assess the Posterior

Student: We will not check the back.

PROCTOR: Noted.

▸ Manage Secondary Injuries/Wounds

Student: I would reassure the patient.

PROCTOR: Noted.

▸ Reassess Interventions

Student: I will reassess my interventions: oxygen and call medical control. Monitor patient for continued vomiting and airway maintenance.

PROCTOR: Noted.

ALS Student: I will reassess BLS interventions, plus the following: IV access, cardiac monitoring, and local protocol.

ALS Proctor: Noted. The cardiac monitor shows normal sinus rhythm.

Critical Criteria:

- ❑ Did not obtain medical direction or verbalize standing orders for medical interventions
- ❑ Administered a dangerous or inappropriate intervention
- ❑ Did not ask questions about the present illness
- ❑ Did not differentiate patient's need for transportation versus continued assessment at the scene

Radio Report

(Provided by the student.)

PROCTOR: Noted.

Ongoing Assessment

Repeat the Initial Assessment

Student: I will repeat the initial assessment.

PROCTOR: Noted. (Reflected in "Repeat Vital Signs.")

Repeat Vital Signs

Student: I will reassess vital signs and mental status.

PROCTOR: Blood pressure, 132/84 mm Hg; pulse, 76 beats/min; respirations, 16 breaths/min; pulse oximetry reading, 99%; and the patient is alert.

Student: The vital signs have not changed significantly.

PROCTOR: Noted.

Check Interventions

Student: I will check my interventions: oxygen.

PROCTOR: Noted.

ALS Student: I will check BLS interventions, plus the following: IV access, cardiac monitoring, and local protocol.

ALS Proctor: Noted. The cardiac monitor shows normal sinus rhythm.

Repeat the Focused Assessment

Student: I will repeat the focused assessment.

PROCTOR: Noted.

Critical Criteria:

- ❑ Did not obtain medical direction or verbalize standing orders for medical interventions
- ❑ Administered a dangerous or inappropriate intervention

Handoff Report to Emergency Department Staff

Student: There was no change during transport.

PROCTOR: Noted.

Critical Criteria

(Inform the student of items missed, if any.)

❑ Pass ❑ Fail Date: ____________________

Proctor Comments: ____________________

Notes

Dispatch Information

PROCTOR: EMS 10, respond to a 17-year-old female complaining of abdominal pain. She is conscious and breathing.

Pre-scene Action (BSI)

Student: I am wearing nonlatex gloves and safety glasses.
PROCTOR: Noted.

Critical Criteria:
- ❑ Did not take, or verbalize, body substance isolation (BSI) precautions when necessary

Scene Size-up

Scene Safety

Student: Is the scene safe?
PROCTOR: Yes.

Mechanism of Injury/Nature of Illness

Student: What is the nature of the illness?
PROCTOR: The patient is complaining of abdominal pain.

Number of Patients

Student: How many patients are there?
PROCTOR: One.

Additional Resources

Student: I would call for advanced life support (ALS) assistance.
PROCTOR: Noted.

C-Spine Stabilization

Student: I would not stabilize the cervical spine (c-spine).
PROCTOR: Noted.

Critical Criteria:
- ❑ Did not determine scene safety

Initial Assessment

General Impression

Student: My general impression is that the patient's condition is unstable.
PROCTOR: Noted.

Responsiveness/Level of Consciousness

Student: What is the patient's level of consciousness?
PROCTOR: Alert.

Chief Complaint/Apparent Life Threats

Student: What is the patient's chief complaint?
PROCTOR: The patient is complaining of abdominal pain.

Assess the Airway and Breathing

Student: Is the airway open?
PROCTOR: Yes.

Assessment

Student: What are the rate and the quality of breathing?
PROCTOR: Rate: Tachypneic. Quality: Crying.

Provide Oxygen

Student: I am applying oxygen at 15 L/min via nonrebreathing mask.
PROCTOR: Noted.

Ensure Adequate Ventilation

Student: The patient has adequate ventilations at this time.
PROCTOR: Noted.

Assess Circulation

Student: I am assessing the patient's circulation.
PROCTOR: Noted.

Assess for and Control Major Bleeding

Student: Do I find any major bleeding?
PROCTOR: No.

Assess the Pulse

Student: What are the rate and the quality of pulses?
PROCTOR: Rate: Tachycardic. Quality: Thready.

Assess the Skin

Student: I am assessing the skin. What are the color, temperature, and condition of the skin?
PROCTOR: Color: Pale. Temperature: Cool. Condition: Diaphoretic.

Identify Priority Patients/Make Transport Decision

Student: The patient is a high priority and is a load-and-go. I will begin packaging and transport.
PROCTOR: Noted.

Critical Criteria:
- ❑ Did not provide high concentration of oxygen
- ❑ Did not find or manage problems associated with airway, breathing, hemorrhage or shock (hypoperfusion)
- ❑ Did not differentiate patient's need for transportation versus continued assessment at the scene
- ❑ Did detailed or focused history/physical examination before assessing the airway, breathing and circulation

Focused History and Physical Examination/Rapid Assessment

Select the Appropriate Assessment (Focused or Rapid)

Student: I am selecting the focused assessment.
PROCTOR: Noted.

SAMPLE History

Student: At this time I will gather a SAMPLE history from the patient or family. What are the patient's signs and symptoms?
PROCTOR: Obstetrics.
> **Student:** Are you pregnant?
> **PROCTOR:** Maybe.
> **Student:** How long have you been pregnant?
> **PROCTOR:** I am not sure.
> **Student:** Are you having pain or contractions?
> **PROCTOR:** No.
> **Student:** Are you having any bleeding or discharge?
> **PROCTOR:** Yes, it is heavy.
> **Student:** Do you feel the need to push?
> **PROCTOR:** No.
> **Student:** When was your last menstrual period?
> **PROCTOR:** 2 or 3 months ago.

Student: Allergies?
PROCTOR: No allergies.
Student: Medications?
PROCTOR: No medications.
Student: Pertinent past medical history?
PROCTOR: No pertinent medical history.
Student: Last oral intake?
PROCTOR: 3 hours ago.
Student: Events leading up to the incident?
PROCTOR: The patient was shopping with friends at the mall when the abdominal pain and vaginal bleeding started.

Perform the Focused Physical Examination

Student: I am performing the focused physical examination.
PROCTOR: Noted.
Student: I am assessing the abdomen for DCAP-BTLS. This acronym stands for deformities, contusions, abrasions, punctures, penetrations, paradoxical motion in the chest, and burns, tenderness, lacerations, and swelling. I am assessing all four quadrants. Do I find any problems?
PROCTOR: She has point tenderness in the lower middle abdomen.
Student: Is there any miscarriage tissue?
PROCTOR: No.

▼ Baseline Vital Signs

Student: What are the patient's baseline vital signs, including blood pressure, pulse, respirations, pulse oximetry, and level of consciousness?

PROCTOR: Blood pressure, 102/68 mm Hg; pulse, 132 beats/min; respirations, 28 breaths/min; pulse oximetry reading, 97%; and the patient is alert.

▼ Interventions

Student: I will apply oxygen, and treat for shock.

PROCTOR: Noted.

ALS Student: I will apply basic life support (BLS) interventions, plus the following: establish two large-bore IVs.

ALS Proctor: Noted.

▼ Reevaluate Transport Decision

Student: The patient is a load-and-go.

PROCTOR: Noted.

▼ Detailed Physical Examination

Possible Answer #1

Student: I would not do a detailed physical exam.

PROCTOR: Noted. (Go to "Radio Report.")

Possible Answer #2

Student: I am conducting the detailed physical exam. I am looking for DCAP-BTLS.

PROCTOR: Noted. The detailed physical exam will be performed during transport.

▸ **Assess the Head**

Student: I am assessing the head. Do I find any DCAP-BTLS? Do I find any evidence of Battle's sign or raccoon eyes?

PROCTOR: No.

▸ **Inspect and Palpate the Head and Ears**

Student: I am assessing the head and ears.

PROCTOR: There are no obvious injuries.

▸ **Assess the Eyes**

Student: I am assessing the eyes. Are the pupils equal, round, and regular in size, and react properly to light (PEARRL)?

PROCTOR: They are PEARRL.

▸ **Assess the Facial Area Including Oral and Nasal Areas**

Student: I am assessing the face, nose, and mouth. Do I see any discharge or hear any obstructions?

PROCTOR: No.

▸ **Assess the Neck**

▸ **Inspect and Palpate the Neck**

Student: I am assessing the neck for DCAP-BTLS.

PROCTOR: There are no obvious injuries.

▸ **Assess for Jugular Vein Distention**

Student: Do I find any jugular vein distention (JVD)?

PROCTOR: No.

▸ **Assess for Tracheal Deviation**

Student: Do I see any tracheal deviation?

PROCTOR: No.

▸ **Assess the Chest**

Student: I am assessing the chest for DCAP-BTLS.

PROCTOR: Noted.

▸ **Inspect**

Student: What do I see when I look at the chest?

PROCTOR: There are no obvious injuries.

Student: Is the chest symmetric?

PROCTOR: Yes.

▸ **Palpate**

Student: When I touch the chest, do I feel crepitus or a flail segment?

PROCTOR: No.

▸ **Auscultate**

Student: Are lung sounds present in all fields?

PROCTOR: Yes.

Student: Do I hear any sucking sounds from the chest?

PROCTOR: No.

▸ **Assess the Abdomen/Pelvis**

▸ **Assess the Abdomen**

Student: I am assessing the abdomen for DCAP-BTLS. I am assessing all four quadrants. Do I find any problems?

PROCTOR: She has point tenderness in the lower middle abdomen.

▸ **Assess the Pelvis**

Student: I am assessing the pelvis for DCAP-BTLS. Is the pelvis stable?

PROCTOR: Yes.

▸ **Assess the Genitalia/Perineum as Needed (Verbalize in Training)**

Student: I am assessing the genitalia/perineum as necessary for DCAP-BTLS.

PROCTOR: There is heavy bleeding. She has used three pads.

▸ **Assess the Extremities**

▸ **Inspect**

Student: I am assessing the lower and upper extremities for DCAP-BTLS. Do I find anything?

PROCTOR: No.

▸ **Palpate**

Student: Do I feel anything unusual?

PROCTOR: No.

▸ **Assess Motor, Sensory, and Circulatory Function**

Student: I am checking for DCAP-BTLS, motor and sensory function, and pulses. Right leg?

PROCTOR: Negative DCAP-BTLS. Motor and sensory functions are present. Pulses are present.

Student: Left leg?

PROCTOR: Negative DCAP-BTLS. Motor and sensory functions are present. Pulses are present.

Student: Right arm?

PROCTOR: Negative DCAP-BTLS. Motor and sensory functions are present. Pulses are present.

Student: Left arm?

PROCTOR: Negative DCAP-BTLS. Motor and sensory functions are present. Pulses are present.

▸ **Assess the Posterior**

Student: We will not check the back.

PROCTOR: Noted.

▸ **Manage Secondary Injuries/Wounds**

Student: I would reassure the patient and continue oxygen therapy.

PROCTOR: Noted.

▸ **Reassess Interventions**

Student: I will reassess my interventions: oxygen, and transport in the position of comfort or shock position.

PROCTOR: Noted.

Critical Criteria:

- ❑ Did not obtain medical direction or verbalize standing orders for medical interventions
- ❑ Administered a dangerous or inappropriate intervention
- ❑ Did not ask questions about the present illness
- ❑ Did not differentiate patient's need for transportation versus continued assessment at the scene

▼ Radio Report

(Provided by the student.)

PROCTOR: Noted.

Ongoing Assessment

Repeat the Initial Assessment

Student: I will repeat the initial assessment.

PROCTOR: Noted. (Reflected in "Repeat Vital Signs.")

Repeat Vital Signs

Student: I will reassess vital signs and mental status.

PROCTOR: Blood pressure, 98/64 mm Hg; pulse, 130 beats/min; respirations, 24 breaths/min; pulse oximetry reading, 98%; and the patient is alert.

Student: The vital signs have not changed significantly.

PROCTOR: Noted.

Check Interventions

Student: I will check my interventions: oxygen, and transport in the shock position.

PROCTOR: Noted.

ALS Student: I will check BLS interventions, plus the following: two large-bore IVs.

ALS Proctor: Noted.

Repeat the Focused Assessment

Student: I will repeat the focused assessment.

PROCTOR: Noted.

Critical Criteria:
- ❑ Did not obtain medical direction or verbalize standing orders for medical interventions
- ❑ Administered a dangerous or inappropriate intervention

Handoff Report to Emergency Department Staff

Student: There was no change during transport.

PROCTOR: Noted.

Critical Criteria

(Inform the student of items missed, if any.)

❑ Pass ❑ Fail Date: ____________________

Proctor Comments: ____________________

____

____

Notes

Dispatch Information

PROCTOR: EMS 10, respond to an 85-year-old female who has wandered away from a nursing home. She is conscious and breathing.

Pre-scene Action (BSI)

Student: I am wearing nonlatex gloves and safety glasses.
PROCTOR: Noted.

> **Critical Criteria:**
> ❑ Did not take, or verbalize, body substance isolation (BSI) precautions when necessary

Scene Size-up

Scene Safety

Student: Is the scene safe?
PROCTOR: Yes.

Mechanism of Injury/Nature of Illness

Student: What is the nature of the illness?
PROCTOR: The patient was found lying next to a creek a mile from the nursing home. It is 40°F (4.4°C) with high winds. It is raining and the patient is wearing only a nightgown. She has multiple small cuts and abrasions on her extremities.

Number of Patients

Student: How many patients are there?
PROCTOR: One.

Additional Resources

Student: I would call for advanced life support (ALS) assistance.
PROCTOR: Noted.

C-Spine Stabilization

Student: On the basis of the mechanism of injury, I would stabilize the cervical spine (c-spine) in a neutral in-line position.
PROCTOR: Noted.

> **Critical Criteria:**
> ❑ Did not determine scene safety

Initial Assessment

General Impression

Student: My general impression is that the patient's condition is unstable.
PROCTOR: Noted.

Responsiveness/Level of Consciousness

Student: What is the patient's level of consciousness?
PROCTOR: Alert but confused.

Chief Complaint/Apparent Life Threats

Student: What is the patient's chief complaint?
PROCTOR: The patient is complaining of being cold.

Assess the Airway and Breathing

Student: Is the airway open?
PROCTOR: Yes.

Assessment

Student: What are the rate and the quality of breathing?
PROCTOR: Rate: Within normal limits. Quality: Deep.

Provide Oxygen

Student: I am applying oxygen at 15 L/min via nonrebreathing mask.
PROCTOR: Noted.

Ensure Adequate Ventilation

Student: The patient has adequate ventilations at this time.
PROCTOR: Noted.

Assess Circulation

Student: I am assessing the patient's circulation.
PROCTOR: Noted.

Assess for and Control Major Bleeding

Student: Do I find any major bleeding?
PROCTOR: No. Just small cuts and abrasions.

Assess the Pulse

Student: What are the rate and the quality of pulses?
PROCTOR: Rate: Tachycardic. Quality: Thready.

Assess the Skin

Student: I am assessing the skin. What are the color, temperature, and condition of the skin?
PROCTOR: Color: Pale. Temperature: Cold. Condition: Moist.

Identify Priority Patients/Make Transport Decision

Student: The patient is a high priority and is a load-and-go. I will remove wet clothes, cover her with blankets to prevent any further heat loss, and move her out of the cold environment to the back of the heated ambulance. I will begin packaging with a backboard and cervical collar and transport gently to prevent ventricular fibrillation.
PROCTOR: Noted.

> **Critical Criteria:**
> ❑ Did not provide high concentration of oxygen
> ❑ Did not find or manage problems associated with airway, breathing, hemorrhage or shock (hypoperfusion)
> ❑ Did not differentiate patient's need for transportation versus continued assessment at the scene
> ❑ Did detailed or focused history/physical examination before assessing the airway, breathing and circulation

Focused History and Physical Examination/Rapid Assessment

Select the Appropriate Assessment (Focused or Rapid)

Student: I am selecting the rapid physical exam to identify and treat life threats. I am checking for DCAP-BTLS. This acronym stands for deformities, contusions, abrasions, punctures, penetrations, and paradoxical motion in the chest, and burns, tenderness, lacerations, and swelling.
PROCTOR: Noted.

Head

Student: I am rapidly assessing the head.
PROCTOR: There are no obvious injuries.

Neck

Student: I am rapidly assessing the neck.
PROCTOR: There are no obvious injuries.
Student: I will apply a cervical collar.
PROCTOR: Noted.

Chest

Student: I am rapidly assessing the chest.
PROCTOR: There are no obvious injuries.

Abdomen/Pelvis

Student: I am rapidly assessing the abdomen.
PROCTOR: There are no obvious injuries.
Student: I am rapidly assessing the pelvis.
PROCTOR: There are no obvious injuries.

Extremities

Student: I am rapidly assessing the extremities.
PROCTOR: There are small cuts and abrasions noted.

Assess Motor, Sensory, and Circulatory Function

Student: I am checking for DCAP-BTLS. I am also checking pulses, and motor and sensory function. Right leg?
PROCTOR: Negative DCAP-BTLS. Motor and sensory functions are present. Pulses are present.

Student: Left leg?

PROCTOR: Negative DCAP-BTLS. Motor and sensory functions are present. Pulses are present.

Student: Right arm?

PROCTOR: Negative DCAP-BTLS. Motor and sensory functions are present. Pulses are present.

Student: Left arm?

PROCTOR: Negative DCAP-BTLS. Motor and sensory functions are present. Pulses are present.

▸ **Posterior**

Student: I am rapidly assessing the back. We will now log roll the patient as a unit to check the back. The person at the head will count to three and we will roll the patient.

PROCTOR: Noted.

▸ **Assess the Thorax**

Student: I am assessing the thorax. Do I find injuries?

PROCTOR: No.

▸ **Assess the Lumbar Area**

Student: I am assessing the flanks and lumbar area. Do I find injuries?

PROCTOR: No.

▸ **Assess the Entire Backside**

Student: I am assessing the entire backside. Do I find injuries?

PROCTOR: No.

▸ **Manage Secondary Injuries/Wounds**

Student: We will apply a cervical collar and backboard with full immobilization per local protocol, if not yet done, at this time.

PROCTOR: Noted.

Student: Are there any changes in motor and sensory functions or pulses?

PROCTOR: No.

▾ SAMPLE History

Student: At this time I will gather a SAMPLE history from the patient or family. What are the patient's signs and symptoms?

PROCTOR: Environmental emergency.

Student: What was the source?

PROCTOR: Cold air and rain.

Student: What was the environment?

PROCTOR: It was 40°F (4.4°C).

Student: What was the duration?

PROCTOR: More than 45 minutes.

Student: Was there any loss of consciousness?

PROCTOR: No.

Student: What were the effects—local or general?

PROCTOR: The whole body.

Student: Allergies?

PROCTOR: Unknown.

Student: Medications?

PROCTOR: Unknown.

Student: Pertinent past medical history?

PROCTOR: Unknown.

Student: Last oral intake?

PROCTOR: Unknown.

Student: Events leading up to the incident?

PROCTOR: The patient walked away from a nursing home 45 minutes ago.

▾ Baseline Vital Signs

Student: What are the patient's baseline vital signs, including blood pressure, pulse, respirations, pulse oximetry, and level of consciousness?

PROCTOR: Blood pressure, 110/68 mm Hg; pulse, 110 beats/min; respirations, 26 breaths/min; pulse oximetry reading, N/A; and the patient is alert but confused.

▾ Interventions

Student: I will replace the patient's wet clothing, administer oxygen, and check her blood glucose level. She is fully immobilized.

PROCTOR: Noted. Her blood glucose level is 90 mg/dL.

Student: I will perform a Cincinnati stroke scale on this patient.

PROCTOR: It is negative.

ALS Student: I will apply basic life support (BLS) interventions, plus the following: establish IV access, perform cardiac monitoring, and follow the local protocol.

ALS Proctor: Noted. The cardiac monitor shows sinus tachycardia.

▾ Reevaluate Transport Decision

Student: This patient is a high priority and is a load-and-go due to altered mental status and hypothermia.

PROCTOR: Noted.

▾ Detailed Physical Examination

Student: I am conducting the detailed physical exam. I am looking for DCAP-BTLS.

PROCTOR: Noted. The detailed physical exam will be performed during transport.

▸ **Assess the Head**

Student: I am assessing the head. Do I find any DCAP-BTLS? Do I find any evidence of Battle's sign or raccoon eyes?

PROCTOR: No.

▸ **Inspect and Palpate the Head and Ears**

Student: I am assessing the head and ears.

PROCTOR: There are no obvious injuries.

▸ **Assess the Eyes**

Student: I am assessing the eyes. Are the pupils equal, round, and regular in size, and react properly to light (PEARRL)?

PROCTOR: They are sluggish.

▸ **Assess the Facial Area Including Oral and Nasal Areas**

Student: I am assessing the face, nose, and mouth. Do I see any discharge or hear any obstructions?

PROCTOR: No.

▸ **Assess the Neck**

▸ **Inspect and Palpate the Neck**

Student: I am assessing the neck for DCAP-BTLS.

PROCTOR: There are no obvious injuries.

▸ **Assess for Jugular Vein Distention**

Student: Do I find any jugular vein distention (JVD)?

PROCTOR: No.

▸ **Assess for Tracheal Deviation**

Student: Do I see any tracheal deviation?

PROCTOR: No.

▸ **Assess the Chest**

Student: I am assessing the chest for DCAP-BTLS.

PROCTOR: Noted.

▸ **Inspect**

Student: What do I see when I look at the chest?

PROCTOR: There are no obvious injuries.

Student: Is the chest symmetric?

PROCTOR: Yes.

▸ **Palpate**

Student: When I touch the chest, do I feel crepitus or a flail segment?

PROCTOR: No.

▸ **Auscultate**

Student: Are lung sounds present in all fields?

PROCTOR: Yes.

Student: Do I hear any sucking sounds from the chest?

PROCTOR: No.

▸ Assess the Abdomen/Pelvis

▸ Assess the Abdomen

Student: I am assessing the abdomen for DCAP-BTLS. I am assessing all four quadrants. Do I find any problems?

PROCTOR: No.

▸ Assess the Pelvis

Student: I am assessing the pelvis for DCAP-BTLS. Is the pelvis stable?

PROCTOR: Yes.

▸ Assess the Genitalia/Perineum as Needed (Verbalize in Training)

Student: I am assessing the genitalia/perineum as necessary for DCAP-BTLS.

PROCTOR: The area is unremarkable.

▸ Assess the Extremities

▸ Inspect

Student: I am assessing the lower and upper extremities for DCAP-BTLS. Do I find anything?

PROCTOR: No.

▸ Palpate

Student: Do I feel anything unusual?

PROCTOR: No.

▸ Assess Motor, Sensory, and Circulatory Function

Student: I am checking for DCAP-BTLS, motor and sensory function, and pulses. Right leg?

PROCTOR: Negative DCAP-BTLS. Motor and sensory functions are present. Pulses are present.

Student: Left leg?

PROCTOR: Negative DCAP-BTLS. Motor and sensory functions are present. Pulses are present.

Student: Right arm?

PROCTOR: Negative DCAP-BTLS. Motor and sensory functions are present. Pulses are present.

Student: Left arm?

PROCTOR: Negative DCAP-BTLS. Motor and sensory functions are present. Pulses are present.

▸ Assess the Posterior

Note: This portion of the detailed physical exam would not be done if the patient were previously backboarded per local protocol.

Student: We will not check the back since it was previously checked and the patient is backboarded.

PROCTOR: Noted.

▸ Manage Secondary Injuries/Wounds

Student: I would direct my partner to continue providing oxygen and warming measures.

PROCTOR: Noted.

▸ Reassess Interventions

Student: I will reassess my interventions: airway, breathing, and oxygen; and immobilization, straps, and warm blankets.

PROCTOR: Noted.

ALS Student: I will reassess BLS interventions, plus the following: IV access with warm fluids, cardiac monitor, and local protocol.

ALS Proctor: Noted. The cardiac monitor shows sinus tachycardia.

Critical Criteria:

- ❑ Did not obtain medical direction or verbalize standing orders for medical interventions
- ❑ Administered a dangerous or inappropriate intervention
- ❑ Did not ask questions about the present illness
- ❑ Did not differentiate patient's need for transportation versus continued assessment at the scene

Radio Report

(Provided by the student.)

PROCTOR: Noted.

Ongoing Assessment

Repeat the Initial Assessment

Student: I will repeat the initial assessment.

PROCTOR: Noted. (Reflected in "Repeat Vital Signs.")

Repeat Vital Signs

Student: I will reassess vital signs and mental status.

PROCTOR: Blood pressure, 114/66 mm Hg; pulse, 112 beats/min; respirations, 24 breaths/min; pulse oximetry reading, N/A; and the patient is alert.

Student: The vital signs have not changed significantly.

PROCTOR: Noted.

Check Interventions

Student: I will check my interventions: oxygen, immobilization, and drying.

PROCTOR: Noted.

ALS Student: I will check BLS interventions, plus the following: IV access, cardiac monitor, and local protocol.

ALS Proctor: Noted. The cardiac monitor shows sinus tachycardia.

Repeat the Focused Assessment

Student: I will repeat the focused assessment.

PROCTOR: Noted.

Critical Criteria:

- ❑ Did not obtain medical direction or verbalize standing orders for medical interventions
- ❑ Administered a dangerous or inappropriate intervention

Handoff Report to Emergency Department Staff

Student: There was no change during transport.

PROCTOR: Noted.

Critical Criteria

(Inform the student of items missed, if any.)

❑ Pass ❑ Fail Date: ____________________

Proctor Comments: ____________________

____

____

Notes

Dispatch Information

PROCTOR: EMS 10, respond to a 56-year-old female who is complaining of shortness of breath. She weighs 700 pounds. She is conscious and breathing.

Pre-scene Action (BSI)

Student: I am wearing nonlatex gloves and safety glasses.
PROCTOR: Noted.

> **Critical Criteria:**
> - ❑ Did not take, or verbalize, body substance isolation (BSI) precautions when necessary

Scene Size-up

Scene Safety

Student: Is the scene safe?
PROCTOR: Yes.

Mechanism of Injury/Nature of Illness

Student: What is the nature of the illness?
PROCTOR: The patient does not have air conditioning and is complaining of shortness of breath during a regional heat wave.

Number of Patients

Student: How many patients are there?
PROCTOR: One.

Additional Resources

Student: I would call for advanced life support (ALS) assistance and additional resources: fire/rescue for assistance lifting and a specially equipped ambulance to handle her weight if available.
PROCTOR: Noted.

C-Spine Stabilization

Student: I would not stabilize the cervical spine (c-spine).
PROCTOR: Noted.

> **Critical Criteria:**
> - ❑ Did not determine scene safety

Initial Assessment

General Impression

Student: My general impression is that the patient's condition is unstable.
PROCTOR: Noted.

Responsiveness/Level of Consciousness

Student: What is the patient's level of consciousness?
PROCTOR: Alert.

Chief Complaint/Apparent Life Threats

Student: What is the patient's chief complaint?
PROCTOR: The patient is complaining of shortness of breath.

Assess the Airway and Breathing

Student: Is the airway open?
PROCTOR: Yes.

Assessment

Student: What are the rate and the quality of breathing?
PROCTOR: Rate: Tachypneic. Quality: Shallow.

Provide Oxygen

Student: I am applying oxygen at 15 L/min via nonrebreathing mask.
PROCTOR: Noted.

Ensure Adequate Ventilation

Student: The patient has adequate ventilations at this time.
PROCTOR: Noted.

Assess Circulation

Student: I am assessing the patient's circulation.
PROCTOR: Noted.

Assess for and Control Major Bleeding

Student: Do I find any major bleeding?
PROCTOR: No.

Assess the Pulse

Student: What are the rate and the quality of pulses?
PROCTOR: Rate: Within normal limits. Quality: Normal.

Assess the Skin

Student: I am assessing the skin. What are the color, temperature, and condition of the skin?
PROCTOR: Color: Flushed. Temperature: Hot. Condition: Moist.

Identify Priority Patients/Make Transport Decision

Student: The patient is a high priority and is a load-and-go. I will begin packaging and transport.
PROCTOR: Noted.

> **Critical Criteria:**
> - ❑ Did not provide high concentration of oxygen
> - ❑ Did not find or manage problems associated with airway, breathing, hemorrhage or shock (hypoperfusion)
> - ❑ Did not differentiate patient's need for transportation versus continued assessment at the scene
> - ❑ Did detailed or focused history/physical examination before assessing the airway, breathing and circulation

Focused History and Physical Examination/Rapid Assessment

Select the Appropriate Assessment (Focused or Rapid)

Student: I am selecting the focused assessment.
PROCTOR: Noted.

SAMPLE History

Student: At this time I will gather a SAMPLE history from the patient or family. What are the patient's signs and symptoms?
PROCTOR: Respiratory, cardiac, and environmental emergency.

> **Student:** Onset: What were you doing when this started?
> **PROCTOR:** Trying to go to sleep.
> **Student:** Provokes: What makes your condition worse or better?
> **PROCTOR:** Not having air conditioning makes it worse.
> **Student:** Quality: Can you describe your pain?
> **PROCTOR:** None.
> **Student:** Radiates: Do you have pain anywhere else?
> **PROCTOR:** No.
> **Student:** Severity: On a scale of 1 to 10 with 10 being the worst possible, how would you rate your distress?
> **PROCTOR:** 6.
> **Student:** Time: How long has this been going on?
> **PROCTOR:** 3 hours.
> **Student:** Interventions: Have you done anything to make this better?
> **PROCTOR:** The patient has taken no actions.
> **Student:** I will now ask the patient questions about the environmental emergency. What was the source?
> **PROCTOR:** There is a regional heat wave and the patient does not have air conditioning.
> **Student:** What was the environment?
> **PROCTOR:** It was 96°F.
> **Student:** What was the duration?
> **PROCTOR:** Over 22 hours.
> **Student:** Was there any loss of consciousness?
> **PROCTOR:** No.
> **Student:** What were the effects—local or general?
> **PROCTOR:** Her whole body is hot and sweaty.

Student: Allergies?
PROCTOR: No allergies.
Student: Medications?
PROCTOR: Insulin.

Student: Pertinent past medical history?
PROCTOR: Diabetes.
Student: Last oral intake?
PROCTOR: 7 hours ago.
Student: Events leading up to the incident?
PROCTOR: The patient was trying to sleep in a hot house.

▼ Perform the Focused Physical Examination

Student: I am performing the focused physical examination.
PROCTOR: Noted.
Student: Are lung sounds present in all fields?
PROCTOR: Yes.
Student: I am assessing for pedal edema. Is there any?
PROCTOR: No.

▼ Baseline Vital Signs

Student: What are the patient's baseline vital signs, including blood pressure, pulse, respirations, pulse oximetry, and level of consciousness?
PROCTOR: Blood pressure, N/A due to the size of her arm; pulse rate, 96 beats/min; respirations, 28 breaths/min; pulse oximetry reading, 97%; and the patient is alert.

▼ Interventions

Student: I will apply high-flow oxygen, loosen tight-fitting clothing, cool with moistened cloths, and transport in an air conditioned ambulance at a comfortable setting. I would allow her to drink if permitted by protocol.
PROCTOR: Noted.
ALS Student: I will apply basic life support (BLS) interventions, plus the following: establish IV access, perform cardiac monitoring and a 12-lead ECG, and follow the local protocol.
ALS Proctor: Noted. The cardiac monitor shows normal sinus rhythm.

▼ Reevaluate Transport Decision

Student: The patient is a high priority and is a load-and-go.
PROCTOR: Noted.

▼ Detailed Physical Examination

Possible Answer #1
Student: I would not do a detailed physical exam.
PROCTOR: Noted. (Go to "Radio Report.")

Possible Answer #2
Student: I am conducting the detailed physical exam. I am looking for DCAP-BTLS. This acronym stands for deformities, contusions, abrasions, punctures, penetrations, paradoxical motion in the chest, and burns, tenderness, lacerations, and swelling.
PROCTOR: Noted. The detailed physical exam will be performed during transport.

▸ Assess the Head

Student: I am assessing the head. Do I find any DCAP-BTLS? Do I find any evidence of Battle's sign or raccoon eyes?
PROCTOR: No.

▸ Inspect and Palpate the Head and Ears

Student: I am assessing the head and ears.
PROCTOR: There are no obvious injuries.

▸ Assess the Eyes

Student: I am assessing the eyes. Are the pupils equal, round, and regular in size, and react properly to light (PEARRL)?
PROCTOR: They are PEARRL.

▸ Assess the Facial Area Including Oral and Nasal Areas

Student: I am assessing the face, nose, and mouth. Do I see any discharge or hear any obstructions?
PROCTOR: No.

▸ Assess the Neck

▸ Inspect and Palpate the Neck

Student: I am assessing the neck for DCAP-BTLS.
PROCTOR: There are no obvious injuries.

▸ Assess for Jugular Vein Distention

Student: Do I find any jugular vein distention (JVD)?
PROCTOR: No.

▸ Assess for Tracheal Deviation

Student: Do I see any tracheal deviation?
PROCTOR: No.

▸ Assess the Chest

Student: I am assessing the chest for DCAP-BTLS.
PROCTOR: Noted.

▸ Inspect

Student: What do I see when I look at the chest?
PROCTOR: There are no obvious injuries.
Student: Is the chest symmetric?
PROCTOR: Yes.

▸ Palpate

Student: When I touch the chest, do I feel crepitus or a flail segment?
PROCTOR: No.

▸ Auscultate

Student: Are lung sounds present in all fields?
PROCTOR: Yes.
Student: Do I hear any sucking sounds from the chest?
PROCTOR: No.

▸ Assess the Abdomen/Pelvis

▸ Assess the Abdomen

Student: I am assessing the abdomen for DCAP-BTLS. I am assessing all four quadrants. Do I find any problems?
PROCTOR: No.

▸ Assess the Pelvis

Student: I am assessing the pelvis for DCAP-BTLS. Is the pelvis stable?
PROCTOR: Yes.

▸ Assess the Genitalia/Perineum as Needed (Verbalize in Training)

Student: I am assessing the genitalia/perineum as necessary for DCAP-BTLS.
PROCTOR: The area is unremarkable.

▸ Assess the Extremities

▸ Inspect

Student: I am assessing the lower and upper extremities for DCAP-BTLS. Do I find anything?
PROCTOR: No.

▸ Palpate

Student: Do I feel anything unusual?
PROCTOR: No.

▸ Assess Motor, Sensory, and Circulatory Function

Student: I am checking for DCAP-BTLS, motor and sensory function, and pulses. Right leg?
PROCTOR: Negative DCAP-BTLS. Motor and sensory functions are present. Pulses are present.
Student: Left leg?
PROCTOR: Negative DCAP-BTLS. Motor and sensory functions are present. Pulses are present.
Student: Right arm?
PROCTOR: Negative DCAP-BTLS. Motor and sensory functions are present. Pulses are present.
Student: Left arm?
PROCTOR: Negative DCAP-BTLS. Motor and sensory functions are present. Pulses are present.

▸ Assess the Posterior

Student: We will check the back.

PROCTOR: Noted.

▸ Assess the Thorax

Student: I am assessing the thorax. Do I find injuries?

PROCTOR: No.

▸ Assess the Lumbar Area

Student: I am assessing the flanks and lumbar area. Do I find injuries?

PROCTOR: No.

▸ Assess the Entire Backside

Student: I am assessing the entire backside. Do I find injuries?

PROCTOR: No.

▸ Manage Secondary Injuries/Wounds

Student: I would reassure the patient and transport her in the most appropriate ambulance.

PROCTOR: Noted.

▸ Reassess Interventions

Student: I will reassess my interventions: high-flow oxygen, loosen tight-fitting clothing, cool with moistened cloths, and transport in an air conditioned ambulance at a comfortable setting. I would allow her to drink if permitted by protocol.

PROCTOR: Noted.

ALS Student: I will reassess BLS interventions, plus the following: monitor IV fluids, cardiac monitor, and local protocols.

ALS Proctor: Noted. The cardiac monitor shows normal sinus rhythm.

Critical Criteria:
- ❑ Did not obtain medical direction or verbalize standing orders for medical interventions
- ❑ Administered a dangerous or inappropriate intervention
- ❑ Did not ask questions about the present illness
- ❑ Did not differentiate patient's need for transportation versus continued assessment at the scene

▼ Radio Report

(Provided by the student.)

PROCTOR: Noted.

▼ Ongoing Assessment

▼ Repeat the Initial Assessment

Student: I will repeat the initial assessment.

PROCTOR: Noted. (Reflected in "Repeat Vital Signs.")

▼ Repeat Vital Signs

Student: I will reassess vital signs and mental status.

PROCTOR: Blood pressure, N/A; pulse rate, 92 beats/min; respirations, 24 breaths/min; pulse oximetry reading, 99%; and the patient is alert.

Student: The vital signs have not changed significantly.

PROCTOR: Noted.

▼ Check Interventions

Student: I will check my interventions: high-flow oxygen, loosen tight-fitting clothing, cool with moistened cloths, and transport in an air conditioned ambulance at a comfortable setting. I would allow her to drink if permitted by protocol.

PROCTOR: Noted.

ALS Student: I will check BLS interventions, plus the following: monitor IV, cardiac monitor, and local protocols.

ALS Proctor: Noted. The cardiac monitor shows normal sinus rhythm.

▼ Repeat the Focused Assessment

Student: I will repeat the focused assessment.

PROCTOR: Noted.

Critical Criteria:
- ❑ Did not obtain medical direction or verbalize standing orders for medical interventions
- ❑ Administered a dangerous or inappropriate intervention

▼ Handoff Report to Emergency Department Staff

Student: There was no change during transport.

PROCTOR: Noted.

▼ Critical Criteria

(Inform the student of items missed, if any.)

❑ Pass ❑ Fail Date: ____________________

Proctor Comments: ____________________

____

____

Notes

Dispatch Information

PROCTOR: EMS 10, respond to a 24-year-old female who is pregnant and having a seizure.

Pre-scene Action (BSI)

Student: I am wearing nonlatex gloves and safety glasses.
PROCTOR: Noted.

Critical Criteria:
- ❑ Did not take, or verbalize, body substance isolation (BSI) precautions when necessary

Scene Size-up

Scene Safety

Student: Is the scene safe?
PROCTOR: Yes.

Mechanism of Injury/Nature of Illness

Student: What is the nature of the illness?
PROCTOR: The patient was watching TV and complained of a headache and ringing in the ears before having a seizure.

Number of Patients

Student: How many patients are there?
PROCTOR: One.

Additional Resources

Student: I would call for advanced life support (ALS) assistance.
PROCTOR: Noted.

C-Spine Stabilization

Student: I would not stabilize the cervical spine (c-spine).
PROCTOR: Noted.

Critical Criteria:
- ❑ Did not determine scene safety

Initial Assessment

General Impression

Student: My general impression is that the patient's condition is unstable.
PROCTOR: Noted.

Responsiveness/Level of Consciousness

Student: What is the patient's level of consciousness?
PROCTOR: Unresponsive.

Chief Complaint/Apparent Life Threats

Student: What is the patient's chief complaint?
PROCTOR: The patient is just coming out of a seizure.

Assess the Airway and Breathing

Student: Is the airway open?
PROCTOR: Yes.

▸ Assessment

Student: What are the rate and the quality of breathing?
PROCTOR: Rate: Slow. Quality: Shallow.

▸ Provide Oxygen

Student: I am assisting ventilations with a bag-valve device with 100% oxygen.
PROCTOR: Noted.

▸ Ensure Adequate Ventilation

Student: As noted, I will assist ventilation with the bag-valve device.
PROCTOR: Noted.

Assess Circulation

Student: I am assessing the patient's circulation.
PROCTOR: Noted.

▸ Assess for and Control Major Bleeding

Student: Do I find any major bleeding?
PROCTOR: No.

▸ Assess the Pulse

Student: What are the rate and the quality of pulses?
PROCTOR: Rate: Tachycardic. Quality: Bounding.

▸ Assess the Skin

Student: I am assessing the skin. What are the color, temperature, and condition of the skin?
PROCTOR: Color: Cyanotic. Temperature: Warm. Condition: Moist.

Identify Priority Patients/Make Transport Decision

Student: The patient is a high priority and is a load-and-go. I will begin packaging and transport.
PROCTOR: Noted.

Critical Criteria:
- ❑ Did not provide high concentration of oxygen
- ❑ Did not find or manage problems associated with airway, breathing, hemorrhage or shock (hypoperfusion)
- ❑ Did not differentiate patient's need for transportation versus continued assessment at the scene
- ❑ Did detailed or focused history/physical examination before assessing the airway, breathing and circulation

Focused History and Physical Examination/Rapid Assessment

Select the Appropriate Assessment (Focused or Rapid)

Student: I am selecting the focused assessment.
PROCTOR: Noted.

SAMPLE History

Student: At this time I will gather a SAMPLE history from the patient or family. What are the patient's signs and symptoms?
PROCTOR: Altered mental status.
- **Student:** Describe the episode.
- **PROCTOR:** She has been having a seizure for 5 minutes.
- **Student:** Onset: What was she doing when this started?
- **PROCTOR:** Watching TV.
- **Student:** Duration: How long has this been going on?
- **PROCTOR:** 5 minutes.
- **Student:** Are there any associated symptoms?
- **PROCTOR:** Yes, she has had a headache with ringing in the ears and swollen feet.
- **Student:** Is there any evidence of trauma?
- **PROCTOR:** No.
- **Student:** Interventions: Has she done anything to make this better?
- **PROCTOR:** The patient has taken no actions.
- **Student:** Have there been any seizures?
- **PROCTOR:** Yes.
- **Student:** Has there been any fever?
- **PROCTOR:** No.
- **Student:** I will now ask questions related to obstetrics. Is she pregnant?
- **PROCTOR:** Yes.
- **Student:** How long has she been pregnant?
- **PROCTOR:** 8 months.
- **Student:** Has she had pain or contractions?
- **PROCTOR:** No.
- **Student:** Has she had bleeding or discharge?
- **PROCTOR:** No.
- **Student:** Does she feel the need to push?
- **PROCTOR:** No.
- **Student:** When was her last menstrual period?
- **PROCTOR:** 9 months ago.

Student: Allergies?
PROCTOR: No allergies.

Student: Medications?
PROCTOR: Vitamins.
Student: Pertinent past medical history?
PROCTOR: She is 8 months pregnant.
Student: Last oral intake?
PROCTOR: 4 hours ago.
Student: Events leading up to the incident?
PROCTOR: The patient was watching TV and complained of a headache with ringing in the ears and swollen feet. The seizure came on suddenly.

▼ Perform the Focused Physical Examination

Student: I am performing the focused physical examination.
PROCTOR: Noted.
Student: Has she received any injuries during the seizure?
PROCTOR: No.
Student: Is she having contractions?
PROCTOR: No.
Student: I will check her blood glucose level.
PROCTOR: Her blood glucose level is 118 mg/dL.

▼ Baseline Vital Signs

Student: What are the patient's baseline vital signs, including blood pressure, pulse, respirations, pulse oximetry, and level of consciousness?
PROCTOR: Blood pressure, 180/110 mm Hg; pulse, 112 beats/min; respirations, 12 breaths/min; pulse oximetry reading, 95%; and the patient is unresponsive.

▼ Interventions

Student: I will assess the effectiveness of the oxygen as I watch her recover from the postictal state.
PROCTOR: Noted.
ALS Student: I will apply basic life support (BLS) interventions, plus the following: establish IV access, perform cardiac monitoring, and follow the local protocol (magnesium sulfate per local protocol if seizures continue).
ALS Proctor: Noted. The cardiac monitor shows sinus tachycardia.

▼ Reevaluate Transport Decision

Student: The patient is a high priority and is a load-and-go.
PROCTOR: Noted.

▼ Detailed Physical Examination

Possible Answer #1
Student: I would not do a detailed physical exam.
PROCTOR: Noted. (Go to "Radio Report.")

Possible Answer #2
Student: I am conducting the detailed physical exam. I am looking for DCAP-BTLS. This acronym stands for deformities, contusions, abrasions, punctures, penetrations, paradoxical motion in the chest, and burns, tenderness, lacerations, and swelling.
PROCTOR: Noted. The detailed physical exam will be performed during transport.

► Assess the Head

Student: I am assessing the head. Do I find any DCAP-BTLS? Do I find any evidence of Battle's sign or raccoon eyes?
PROCTOR: No.

► Inspect and Palpate the Head and Ears

Student: I am assessing the head and ears.
PROCTOR: There are no obvious injuries.

► Assess the Eyes

Student: I am assessing the eyes. Are the pupils equal, round, and regular in size, and react properly to light (PEARRL)?
PROCTOR: They are PEARRL.

► Assess the Facial Area Including Oral and Nasal Areas

Student: I am assessing the face, nose, and mouth. Do I see any discharge or hear any obstructions?
PROCTOR: Yes, the teeth are clenched.

► Assess the Neck

► Inspect and Palpate the Neck

Student: I am assessing the neck for DCAP-BTLS.
PROCTOR: There are no obvious injuries.

► Assess for Jugular Vein Distention

Student: Do I find any jugular vein distention (JVD)?
PROCTOR: No.

► Assess for Tracheal Deviation

Student: Do I see any tracheal deviation?
PROCTOR: No.

► Assess the Chest

Student: I am assessing the chest for DCAP-BTLS.
PROCTOR: Noted.

► Inspect

Student: What do I see when I look at the chest?
PROCTOR: There are no obvious injuries.
Student: Is the chest symmetric?
PROCTOR: Yes.

► Palpate

Student: When I touch the chest, do I feel crepitus or a flail segment?
PROCTOR: No.

► Auscultate

Student: Are lung sounds present in all fields?
PROCTOR: Yes, and her rate is increasing to normal.
Student: I would switch over to a nonrebreathing mask with 100% oxygen.
PROCTOR: Noted.
Student: Do I hear any sucking sounds from the chest?
PROCTOR: No.

► Assess the Abdomen/Pelvis

► Assess the Abdomen

Student: I am assessing the abdomen for DCAP-BTLS. I am assessing all four quadrants. Do I find any problems?
PROCTOR: The abdomen is obviously distended due to pregnancy.

► Assess the Pelvis

Student: I am assessing the pelvis for DCAP-BTLS. Is the pelvis stable?
PROCTOR: Yes.

► Assess the Genitalia/Perineum as Needed (Verbalize in Training)

Student: I am assessing the genitalia/perineum as necessary for DCAP-BTLS.
PROCTOR: The area is unremarkable.

► Assess the Extremities

► Inspect

Student: I am assessing the lower and upper extremities for DCAP-BTLS. Do I find anything?
PROCTOR: No.

► Palpate

Student: Do I feel anything unusual?
PROCTOR: No.

► Assess Motor, Sensory, and Circulatory Function

Student: I am checking for DCAP-BTLS, motor and sensory function, and pulses. Right leg?
PROCTOR: Foot is notably swollen. Motor and sensory functions are absent. Pulses are present.
Student: Left leg?
PROCTOR: Foot is notably swollen. Motor and sensory functions are absent. Pulses are present.

Student: Right arm?
PROCTOR: Negative DCAP-BTLS. Motor and sensory functions are absent. Pulses are present.
Student: Left arm?
PROCTOR: Negative DCAP-BTLS. Motor and sensory functions are absent. Pulses are present.

▸ Assess the Posterior

Student: We will check the back.
PROCTOR: Noted.

▸ Assess the Thorax

Student: I am assessing the thorax. Do I find injuries?
PROCTOR: No.

▸ Assess the Lumbar Area

Student: I am assessing the flanks and lumbar area. Do I find injuries?
PROCTOR: No.

▸ Assess the Entire Backside

Student: I am assessing the entire backside. Do I find injuries?
PROCTOR: No.

▸ Manage Secondary Injuries/Wounds

Student: I would transport the patient on her left side in the recovery position.
PROCTOR: Noted.

▸ Reassess Vital Signs

Student: I will reassess vital signs and mental status.
PROCTOR: Blood pressure, 170/100 mm Hg; pulse rate, 100 beats/min; respirations, 16 breaths/min; pulse oximetry reading, 96%; and the patient is becoming more responsive.
Student: The vital signs have not significantly changed.
PROCTOR: Noted.

▾ Reassess Interventions

Student: I will reassess my interventions: oxygen.
PROCTOR: Noted.
ALS Student: I will reassess basic life support (BLS) interventions, plus the following: IV access, cardiac monitoring, and local protocol (magnesium sulfate per local protocol).
ALS Proctor: Noted. The cardiac monitor shows sinus tachycardia.

Critical Criteria:
- ❑ Did not obtain medical direction or verbalize standing orders for medical interventions
- ❑ Administered a dangerous or inappropriate intervention
- ❑ Did not ask questions about the present illness
- ❑ Did not differentiate patient's need for transportation versus continued assessment at the scene

▼ Radio Report

(Provided by the student.)
PROCTOR: Noted.

▼ Ongoing Assessment

▾ Repeat the Initial Assessment

Student: I will repeat the initial assessment.
PROCTOR: Noted. (Reflected in "Repeat Vital Signs.")

▾ Repeat Vital Signs

Student: I will reassess vital signs and mental status.
PROCTOR: Blood pressure, 162/94 mm Hg; pulse, 110 beats/min; respirations, 16 breaths/min; pulse oximetry reading, 96%; and the patient is responsive.
Student: The vital signs have not significantly changed.
PROCTOR: Noted.

▾ Check Interventions

Student: I will check my interventions: oxygen.
PROCTOR: Noted.
ALS Student: I will check BLS interventions, plus the following: IV access, cardiac monitoring, and local protocol (magnesium sulfate per local protocol).
ALS Proctor: Noted. The cardiac monitor shows sinus tachycardia.

▾ Repeat the Focused Assessment

Student: I will repeat the focused assessment.
PROCTOR: Noted.

Critical Criteria:
- ❑ Did not obtain medical direction or verbalize standing orders for medical interventions
- ❑ Administered a dangerous or inappropriate intervention

▼ Handoff Report to Emergency Department Staff

Student: The patient's condition improved during transport.
PROCTOR: Noted.

▼ Critical Criteria

(Inform the student of items missed, if any.)

❑ Pass ❑ Fail Date: ______________________

Proctor Comments: ______________________

____

____

Notes

CASE 98

Dispatch Information

PROCTOR: EMS 10, respond to a 50 year-old-female who is complaining of chest pain. She is conscious and breathing.

Pre-scene Action (BSI)

Student: I am wearing nonlatex gloves and safety glasses.
PROCTOR: Noted.

Critical Criteria:
- ❑ Did not take, or verbalize, body substance isolation (BSI) precautions when necessary

Scene Size-up

Scene Safety

Student: Is the scene safe?
PROCTOR: Yes.

Mechanism of Injury/Nature of Illness

Student: What is the nature of the illness?
PROCTOR: The patient was making dinner when the sudden onset of pain began.

Number of Patients

Student: How many patients are there?
PROCTOR: One.

Additional Resources

Student: I would call for advanced life support (ALS) assistance.
PROCTOR: Noted.

C-Spine Stabilization

Student: I would not stabilize the cervical spine (c-spine).
PROCTOR: Noted.

Critical Criteria:
- ❑ Did not determine scene safety

Initial Assessment

General Impression

Student: My general impression is that the patient's condition is unstable.
PROCTOR: Noted.

Responsiveness/Level of Consciousness

Student: What is the patient's level of consciousness?
PROCTOR: Alert.

Chief Complaint/Apparent Life Threats

Student: What is the patient's chief complaint?
PROCTOR: The patient is complaining of chest pain on the right side.

Assess the Airway and Breathing

Student: Is the airway open?
PROCTOR: Yes.

Assessment

Student: What are the rate and the quality of breathing?
PROCTOR: Rate: Rapid. Quality: Shallow.

Provide Oxygen

Student: I am applying oxygen at 15 L/min via nonrebreathing mask.
PROCTOR: Noted.

Ensure Adequate Ventilation

Student: The patient has adequate ventilations at this time.
PROCTOR: Noted.

Assess Circulation

Student: I am assessing the patient's circulation.
PROCTOR: Noted.

Assess for and Control Major Bleeding

Student: Do I find any major bleeding?
PROCTOR: No.

Assess the Pulse

Student: What are the rate and the quality of pulses?
PROCTOR: Rate: Tachycardic. Quality: Bounding.

Assess the Skin

Student: I am assessing the skin. What are the color, temperature, and condition of the skin?
PROCTOR: Color: Cyanotic. Temperature: Cool. Condition: Diaphoretic.

Identify Priority Patients/Make Transport Decision

Student: The patient is a high priority and is a load-and-go. I will begin packaging and transport.
PROCTOR: Noted.

Critical Criteria:
- ❑ Did not provide high concentration of oxygen
- ❑ Did not find or manage problems associated with airway, breathing, hemorrhage or shock (hypoperfusion)
- ❑ Did not differentiate patient's need for transportation versus continued assessment at the scene
- ❑ Did detailed or focused history/physical examination before assessing the airway, breathing and circulation

Focused History and Physical Examination/Rapid Assessment

Select the Appropriate Assessment (Focused or Rapid)

Student: I am selecting the focused assessment.
PROCTOR: Noted.

SAMPLE History

Student: At this time I will gather a SAMPLE history from the patient or family. What are the patient's signs and symptoms?
PROCTOR: Respiratory.

> **Student:** Onset: What were you doing when this started?
> **PROCTOR:** The patient was cooking dinner.
> **Student:** Provokes: What makes your condition worse or better?
> **PROCTOR:** Nothing makes it better.
> **Student:** Quality: Can you describe your pain?
> **PROCTOR:** Stabbing.
> **Student:** Radiates: Do you have pain anywhere else?
> **PROCTOR:** No.
> **Student:** Severity: On a scale of 1 to 10 with 10 being the worst possible, how would you rate your pain/distress?
> **PROCTOR:** 10.
> **Student:** Time: How long has this been going on?
> **PROCTOR:** 15 minutes.
> **Student:** Interventions: Have you done anything to make this better?
> **PROCTOR:** The patient has taken no actions.

Student: Allergies?
PROCTOR: Penicillin (PCN).
Student: Medications?
PROCTOR: Aspirin.
Student: Pertinent past medical history?
PROCTOR: Pulmonary embolism.
Student: Last oral intake?
PROCTOR: 4 hours ago.
Student: Events leading up to the incident?
PROCTOR: The patient was cooking dinner.

Perform the Focused Physical Examination

Student: I am performing the focused physical examination.
PROCTOR: Noted.

Student: Are lung sounds present in all fields?
PROCTOR: They are diminished on the right side.
Student: Do I see any tracheal deviation?
PROCTOR: No.

▼ Baseline Vital Signs

Student: What are the patient's baseline vital signs, including blood pressure, pulse, respirations, pulse oximetry, and level of consciousness?
PROCTOR: Blood pressure, 140/86 mm Hg; pulse rate, 120 beats/min; respirations, 28 breaths/min; pulse oximetry reading, 84%; and the patient is alert.

▼ Interventions

Student: I will apply oxygen, loosen tight-fitting clothing, and transport the patient in the position of comfort.
PROCTOR: Noted.
ALS Student: I will apply basic life support (BLS) interventions, plus the following: IV access, cardiac monitor, 12-lead ECG, advanced cardiac life support (ACLS) or local protocol, and apply continuous positive airway pressure (CPAP) per local protocol.
ALS Proctor: Noted. The cardiac monitor shows sinus tachycardia.

▼ Reevaluate Transport Decision

Student: The patient is a high priority and is a load-and-go.
PROCTOR: Noted.

▼ Detailed Physical Examination

Possible Answer #1
Student: I would not do a detailed physical exam.
PROCTOR: Noted. (Go to "Radio Report.")

Possible Answer #2
Student: I am conducting the detailed physical exam. I am looking for DCAP-BTLS. This acronym stands for deformities, contusions, abrasions, punctures, penetrations, paradoxical motion in the chest, and burns, tenderness, lacerations, and swelling.
PROCTOR: Noted. The detailed physical exam will be performed during transport.

► **Assess the Head**

Student: I am assessing the head. Do I find any DCAP-BTLS? Do I find any evidence of Battle's sign or raccoon eyes?
PROCTOR: No.

► **Inspect and Palpate the Head and Ears**

Student: I am assessing the head and ears.
PROCTOR: There are no obvious injuries.

► **Assess the Eyes**

Student: I am assessing the eyes. Are the pupils equal, round, and regular in size, and react properly to light (PEARRL)?
PROCTOR: They are PEARRL.

► **Assess the Facial Area Including Oral and Nasal Areas**

Student: I am assessing the face, nose, and mouth. Do I see any discharge or hear any obstructions?
PROCTOR: No.

► **Assess the Neck**

► **Inspect and Palpate the Neck**

Student: I am assessing the neck for DCAP-BTLS.
PROCTOR: There are no obvious injuries.

► **Assess for Jugular Vein Distention**

Student: Do I find any jugular vein distention (JVD)?
PROCTOR: No.

► **Assess for Tracheal Deviation**

Student: Do I see any tracheal deviation?
PROCTOR: No.

► **Assess the Chest**

Student: I am assessing the chest for DCAP-BTLS.
PROCTOR: Noted.

► **Inspect**

Student: What do I see when I look at the chest?
PROCTOR: There are no obvious injuries.
Student: Is the chest symmetric?
PROCTOR: Yes.

► **Palpate**

Student: When I touch the chest, do I feel crepitus or a flail segment?
PROCTOR: No.

► **Auscultate**

Student: Are lung sounds present in all fields?
PROCTOR: They are diminished on the right side.
Student: Do I hear any sucking sounds from the chest?
PROCTOR: No.

► **Assess the Abdomen/Pelvis**

► **Assess the Abdomen**

Student: I am assessing the abdomen for DCAP-BTLS. I am assessing all four quadrants. Do I find any problems?
PROCTOR: No.

► **Assess the Pelvis**

Student: I am assessing the pelvis for DCAP-BTLS. Is the pelvis stable?
PROCTOR: Yes.

► **Assess the Genitalia/Perineum as Needed (Verbalize in Training)**

Student: I am assessing the genitalia/perineum as necessary for DCAP-BTLS.
PROCTOR: The area is unremarkable.

► **Assess the Extremities**

► **Inspect**

Student: I am assessing the lower and upper extremities for DCAP-BTLS. Do I find anything?
PROCTOR: No.

► **Palpate**

Student: Do I feel anything unusual?
PROCTOR: No.

► **Assess Motor, Sensory, and Circulatory Function**

Student: I am checking for DCAP-BTLS, motor and sensory function, and pulses. Right leg?
PROCTOR: Negative DCAP-BTLS. Motor and sensory functions are present. Pulses are present.
Student: Left leg?
PROCTOR: Negative DCAP-BTLS. Motor and sensory functions are present. Pulses are present.
Student: Right arm?
PROCTOR: Negative DCAP-BTLS. Motor and sensory functions are present. Pulses are present.
Student: Left arm?
PROCTOR: Negative DCAP-BTLS. Motor and sensory functions are present. Pulses are present.

► **Assess the Posterior**

Student: We will not check the back.
PROCTOR: Noted.

► **Manage Secondary Injuries/Wounds**

Student: I would direct my partner to monitor the airway.
PROCTOR: Noted.

► **Reassess Interventions**

Student: I will reassess my interventions: airway, breathing, oxygen, and local protocol.
PROCTOR: Noted.

ALS Student: I will reassess BLS interventions, plus the following: IV access, cardiac monitoring, 12-lead ECG, ACLS or local protocol, and monitor CPAP per local protocol.

ALS Proctor: Noted. The cardiac monitor shows sinus tachycardia.

Critical Criteria:
- ❑ Did not obtain medical direction or verbalize standing orders for medical interventions
- ❑ Administered a dangerous or inappropriate intervention
- ❑ Did not ask questions about the present illness
- ❑ Did not differentiate patient's need for transportation versus continued assessment at the scene

Radio Report

(Provided by the student.)

PROCTOR: Noted.

Ongoing Assessment

Repeat the Initial Assessment

Student: I will repeat the initial assessment.

PROCTOR: Noted. (Reflected in "Repeat Vital Signs.")

Repeat Vital Signs

Student: I will reassess vital signs and mental status.

PROCTOR: Blood pressure, 136/68 mm Hg; pulse rate, 118 beats/min; respirations, 24 breaths/min; pulse oximetry reading, 89%; and the patient is alert.

Student: The vital signs have not significantly changed.

PROCTOR: Noted.

Check Interventions

Student: I will check my interventions: oxygen, loosen tight-fitting clothing, transport the patient in the position of comfort, and local protocol.

PROCTOR: Noted.

ALS Student: I will check BLS interventions, plus the following: IV access, cardiac monitoring, 12-lead ECG, and ACLS or local protocol, and monitor CPAP per local protocol.

ALS Proctor: Noted. The cardiac monitor shows sinus tachycardia.

Repeat the Focused Assessment

Student: I will repeat the focused assessment.

PROCTOR: Noted.

Critical Criteria:
- ❑ Did not obtain medical direction or verbalize standing orders for medical interventions
- ❑ Administered a dangerous or inappropriate intervention

Handoff Report to Emergency Department Staff

Student: There was no change during transport.

PROCTOR: Noted.

Critical Criteria

(Inform the student of items missed, if any.)

❑ Pass ❑ Fail Date: ______________________

Proctor Comments: ______________________

____

____

Notes

Dispatch Information

PROCTOR: EMS 10, respond to a 17-year-old male who is unresponsive. He is breathing but his lips are cyanotic.

Pre-scene Action (BSI)

Student: I am wearing nonlatex gloves and safety glasses.
PROCTOR: Noted.

Critical Criteria:
- ❑ Did not take, or verbalize, body substance isolation (BSI) precautions when necessary

Scene Size-up

Scene Safety

Student: Is the scene safe?
PROCTOR: Yes.

Mechanism of Injury/Nature of Illness

Student: What is the nature of the illness?
PROCTOR: The patient was drinking a slushy drink (blue in color) when he passed out and his face went forward into his drink.

Number of Patients

Student: How many patients are there?
PROCTOR: One.

Additional Resources

Student: I would call for advanced life support (ALS) assistance.
PROCTOR: Noted.

C-Spine Stabilization

Student: I would not stabilize the cervical spine (c-spine).
PROCTOR: Noted.

Critical Criteria:
- ❑ Did not determine scene safety

Initial Assessment

General Impression

Student: My general impression is that the patient's condition is unstable.
PROCTOR: Noted.

Responsiveness/Level of Consciousness

Student: What is the patient's level of consciousness?
PROCTOR: Alert.

Chief Complaint/Apparent Life Threats

Student: What is the patient's chief complaint?
PROCTOR: The patient is complaining of having passed out, but is now conscious and alert.

Assess the Airway and Breathing

Student: Is the airway open?
PROCTOR: Yes.

Assessment

Student: What are the rate and the quality of breathing?
PROCTOR: Rate: Within normal limits. Quality: Normal.

Provide Oxygen

Student: I am applying oxygen at 15 L/min via nonrebreathing mask.
PROCTOR: Noted.

Ensure Adequate Ventilation

Student: The patient has adequate ventilations at this time.
PROCTOR: Noted.

Assess Circulation

Student: I am assessing the patient's circulation.
PROCTOR: Noted.

Assess for and Control Major Bleeding

Student: Do I find any major bleeding?
PROCTOR: No.

Assess the Pulse

Student: What are the rate and the quality of pulses?
PROCTOR: Rate: Within normal limits. Quality: Strong.

Assess the Skin

Student: I am assessing the skin. What are the color, temperature, and condition of the skin?
PROCTOR: Color: Normal. Temperature: Warm. Condition: Moist.

Identify Priority Patients/Make Transport Decision

Student: The patient is a low priority and does not require immediate transport.
PROCTOR: Noted.

Critical Criteria:
- ❑ Did not provide high concentration of oxygen
- ❑ Did not find or manage problems associated with airway, breathing, hemorrhage or shock (hypoperfusion)
- ❑ Did not differentiate patient's need for transportation versus continued assessment at the scene
- ❑ Did detailed or focused history/physical examination before assessing the airway, breathing and circulation

Focused History and Physical Examination/Rapid Assessment

Select the Appropriate Assessment (Focused or Rapid)

Student: I am selecting the focused assessment.
PROCTOR: Noted.

SAMPLE History

Student: At this time I will gather a SAMPLE history from the patient or family. What are the patient's signs and symptoms?
PROCTOR: Respiratory/cardiac.

> Student: Onset: What were you doing when this started?
> **PROCTOR:** Drinking a slushy with friends.
> Student: Provokes: What makes your condition worse or better?
> **PROCTOR:** Lying down for a while makes the condition better.
> Student: Quality: Can you describe your pain?
> **PROCTOR:** None.
> Student: Radiates: Do you have pain anywhere else?
> **PROCTOR:** No.
> Student: Severity: On a scale of 1 to 10 with 10 being the worst possible, how would you rate your distress?
> **PROCTOR:** 0.
> Student: Time: How long has this been going on?
> **PROCTOR:** 1 minute.
> Student: Interventions: Have you done anything to make this better?
> **PROCTOR:** The patient has taken no actions.

Student: Allergies?
PROCTOR: No allergies.
Student: Medications?
PROCTOR: No medications.
Student: Pertinent past medical history?
PROCTOR: Passing out for unknown reasons.
Student: Last oral intake?
PROCTOR: 5 minutes ago.
Student: Events leading up to the incident?
PROCTOR: The patient was drinking a slushy with friends when he passed out.

Perform the Focused Physical Examination

Student: I am performing the focused physical examination. I will check the patient's blood glucose level.
PROCTOR: Noted. His blood glucose level is 128 mg/dL.

▼ Baseline Vital Signs

Student: What are the patient's baseline vital signs, including blood pressure, pulse, respirations, pulse oximetry, and level of consciousness?

PROCTOR: Blood pressure, 118/72 mm Hg; pulse, 90 beats/min; respirations, 16 breaths/min; pulse oximetry reading, 98%; and the patient is alert.

▼ Interventions

Student: I will apply oxygen.

PROCTOR: Noted.

ALS Student: I will apply basic life support (BLS) interventions, plus the following: establish IV access, perform cardiac monitoring, a 12-lead ECG, and follow the local protocol.

ALS Proctor: Noted. The cardiac monitor shows normal sinus rhythm.

▼ Reevaluate Transport Decision

Student: This patient does not require immediate transport.

PROCTOR: Noted.

▼ Detailed Physical Examination

Possible Answer #1

Student: I would not do a detailed physical exam.

PROCTOR: Noted. (Go to "Radio Report.")

Possible Answer #2

Student: I am conducting the detailed physical exam. I am looking for DCAP-BTLS. This acronym stands for deformities, contusions, abrasions, punctures, penetrations, paradoxical motion in the chest, and burns, tenderness, lacerations, and swelling.

PROCTOR: Noted. The detailed physical exam will be performed during transport.

► **Assess the Head**

Student: I am assessing the head. Do I find any DCAP-BTLS? Do I find any evidence of Battle's sign or raccoon eyes?

PROCTOR: No.

► **Inspect and Palpate the Head and Ears**

Student: I am assessing the head and ears.

PROCTOR: There are no obvious injuries.

► **Assess the Eyes**

Student: I am assessing the eyes. Are the pupils equal, round, and regular in size, and react properly to light (PEARRL)?

PROCTOR: They are PEARRL.

► **Assess the Facial Area Including Oral and Nasal Areas**

Student: I am assessing the face, nose, and mouth. Do I see any discharge or hear any obstructions?

PROCTOR: No.

► **Assess the Neck**

► **Inspect and Palpate the Neck**

Student: I am assessing the neck for DCAP-BTLS.

PROCTOR: There are no obvious injuries.

► **Assess for Jugular Vein Distention**

Student: Do I find any jugular vein distention (JVD)?

PROCTOR: No.

► **Assess for Tracheal Deviation**

Student: Do I see any tracheal deviation?

PROCTOR: No.

► **Assess the Chest**

Student: I am assessing the chest for DCAP-BTLS.

PROCTOR: Noted.

► **Inspect**

Student: What do I see when I look at the chest?

PROCTOR: There are no obvious injuries.

Student: Is the chest symmetric?

PROCTOR: Yes.

► **Palpate**

Student: When I touch the chest, do I feel crepitus or a flail segment?

PROCTOR: No.

► **Auscultate**

Student: Are lung sounds present in all fields?

PROCTOR: Yes.

Student: Do I hear any sucking sounds from the chest?

PROCTOR: No.

► **Assess the Abdomen/Pelvis**

► **Assess the Abdomen**

Student: I am assessing the abdomen for DCAP-BTLS. I am assessing all four quadrants. Do I find any problems?

PROCTOR: No.

► **Assess the Pelvis**

Student: I am assessing the pelvis for DCAP-BTLS. Is the pelvis stable?

PROCTOR: Yes.

► **Assess the Genitalia/Perineum as Needed (Verbalize in Training)**

Student: I am assessing the genitalia/perineum as necessary for DCAP-BTLS.

PROCTOR: The area is unremarkable.

► **Assess the Extremities**

► **Inspect**

Student: I am assessing the lower and upper extremities for DCAP-BTLS. Do I find anything?

PROCTOR: No.

► **Palpate**

Student: Do I feel anything unusual?

PROCTOR: No.

► **Assess Motor, Sensory, and Circulatory Function**

Student: I am checking for DCAP-BTLS, motor and sensory function, and pulses. Right leg?

PROCTOR: Negative DCAP-BTLS. Motor and sensory functions are present. Pulses are present.

Student: Left leg?

PROCTOR: Negative DCAP-BTLS. Motor and sensory functions are present. Pulses are present.

Student: Right arm?

PROCTOR: Negative DCAP-BTLS. Motor and sensory functions are present. Pulses are present.

Student: Left arm?

PROCTOR: Negative DCAP-BTLS. Motor and sensory functions are present. Pulses are present.

► **Assess the Posterior**

Student: We will check the back.

PROCTOR: Noted.

► **Assess the Thorax**

Student: I am assessing the thorax. Do I find injuries?

PROCTOR: No.

► **Assess the Lumbar Area**

Student: I am assessing the flanks and lumbar area. Do I find injuries?

PROCTOR: No.

► **Assess the Entire Backside**

Student: I am assessing the entire backside. Do I find injuries?

PROCTOR: No.

► **Manage Secondary Injuries/Wounds**

Student: I would direct my partner to monitor the airway.

PROCTOR: Noted.

▸ Reassess Interventions

Student: I will reassess my interventions: oxygen.

PROCTOR: Noted.

ALS Student: I will reassess BLS interventions, plus the following: IV access, cardiac monitor, a 12-lead ECG, and local protocol.

ALS Proctor: Noted. The cardiac monitor shows normal sinus rhythm.

Critical Criteria:
- ❑ Did not obtain medical direction or verbalize standing orders for medical interventions
- ❑ Administered a dangerous or inappropriate intervention
- ❑ Did not ask questions about the present illness
- ❑ Did not differentiate patient's need for transportation versus continued assessment at the scene

Radio Report

(Provided by the student.)

PROCTOR: Noted.

Ongoing Assessment

Repeat the Initial Assessment

Student: I will repeat the initial assessment.

PROCTOR: Noted. (Reflected in "Repeat Vital Signs.")

Repeat Vital Signs

Student: I will reassess vital signs and mental status.

PROCTOR: Blood pressure, 120/72 mm Hg; pulse, 88 beats/min; respirations, 16 breaths/min; pulse oximetry reading, 99%; and the patient is alert.

Student: The vital signs have not significantly changed.

PROCTOR: Noted.

Check Interventions

Student: I will check my interventions: oxygen.

PROCTOR: Noted.

ALS Student: I will check BLS interventions, plus the following: monitor IV, cardiac monitor, a 12-lead ECG, and local protocol.

ALS Proctor: Noted. The cardiac monitor shows normal sinus rhythm.

Repeat the Focused Assessment

Student: I will repeat the focused assessment.

PROCTOR: Noted.

Critical Criteria:
- ❑ Did not obtain medical direction or verbalize standing orders for medical interventions
- ❑ Administered a dangerous or inappropriate intervention

Handoff Report to Emergency Department Staff

Student: There was no change during transport.

PROCTOR: Noted.

Critical Criteria

(Inform the student of items missed, if any.)

❑ Pass ❑ Fail Date: ______________________

Proctor Comments: ______________________

____

____

Notes

CASE 100

Dispatch Information

PROCTOR: EMS 10, respond to a 21-year-old college student who was running in a cross-country event and was stung by a bee. She is having an allergic reaction and does not have her EpiPen. She is conscious and breathing but in respiratory distress.

Pre-scene Action (BSI)

Student: I am wearing nonlatex gloves and safety glasses.
PROCTOR: Noted.

Critical Criteria:
- ❑ Did not take, or verbalize, body substance isolation (BSI) precautions when necessary

Scene Size-up

Scene Safety

Student: Is the scene safe?
PROCTOR: Yes.

Mechanism of Injury/Nature of Illness

Student: What is the nature of the illness?
PROCTOR: The patient was stung by a bee and she is allergic to bee venom.

Number of Patients

Student: How many patients are there?
PROCTOR: One.

Additional Resources

Student: I would call for advanced life support (ALS) assistance.
PROCTOR: Noted.

C-Spine Stabilization

Student: I would not stabilize the cervical spine (c-spine).
PROCTOR: Noted.

Critical Criteria:
- ❑ Did not determine scene safety

Initial Assessment

General Impression

Student: My general impression is that the patient's condition is unstable.
PROCTOR: Noted.

Responsiveness/Level of Consciousness

Student: What is the patient's level of consciousness?
PROCTOR: Alert.

Chief Complaint/Apparent Life Threats

Student: What is the patient's chief complaint?
PROCTOR: The patient is complaining of shortness of breath and chest pain, her tongue is swelling, and she has a rash.

Assess the Airway and Breathing

Student: Is the airway open?
PROCTOR: Yes.

Assessment

Student: What are the rate and the quality of breathing?
PROCTOR: Rate: Tachypneic. Quality: Labored.

Provide Oxygen

Student: I am applying oxygen at 15 L/min via nonrebreathing mask.
PROCTOR: Noted.

Ensure Adequate Ventilation

Student: Ventilations are adequate right now. I will monitor her ventilations and continue with assessment.
PROCTOR: Noted.

Assess Circulation

Student: I am assessing the patient's circulation.
PROCTOR: Noted.

Assess for and Control Major Bleeding

Student: Do I find any major bleeding?
PROCTOR: No.

Assess the Pulse

Student: What are the rate and the quality of pulses?
PROCTOR: Rate: Tachycardic. Quality: Thready.

Assess the Skin

Student: I am assessing the skin. What are the color, temperature, and condition of the skin?
PROCTOR: Color: Pale with hives noted across the neck, chest, and arms. Temperature: Cool. Condition: Diaphoretic.

Identify Priority Patients/Make Transport Decision

Student: The patient is a high priority and is a load-and-go. I will begin packaging and transport. I will request an onboard EpiPen administration if permitted per local protocol.
PROCTOR: Noted. Granted.

Critical Criteria:
- ❑ Did not provide high concentration of oxygen
- ❑ Did not find or manage problems associated with airway, breathing, hemorrhage or shock (hypoperfusion)
- ❑ Did not differentiate patient's need for transportation versus continued assessment at the scene
- ❑ Did detailed or focused history/physical examination before assessing the airway, breathing and circulation

Focused History and Physical Examination/Rapid Assessment

Select the Appropriate Assessment (Focused or Rapid)

Student: I am selecting the focused assessment.
PROCTOR: Noted.

SAMPLE History

Student: At this time I will gather a SAMPLE history from the patient or family. What are the patient's signs and symptoms?
PROCTOR: Allergic reaction.
> **Student:** Is there a history of allergies?
> **PROCTOR:** Yes, to bees.
> **Student:** What were you exposed to?
> **PROCTOR:** A bee sting.
> **Student:** How were you exposed?
> **PROCTOR:** Stinger. The stinger was removed by the bee.
> **Student:** What were the effects?
> **PROCTOR:** Shortness of breath, chest pain, swelling of the tongue, and a rash.
> **Student:** Has the condition progressed?
> **PROCTOR:** Yes, breathing is becoming more difficult.
> **Student:** Interventions: Have you done anything to make this better?
> **PROCTOR:** The patient has taken no actions.

Student: Allergies?
PROCTOR: To yellow jackets, hornets, and bees.
Student: Medications?
PROCTOR: She has a prescribed EpiPen but does not have it with her.
Student: Pertinent past medical history?
PROCTOR: Allergic reactions to yellow jackets, hornets, and bees.
Student: Last oral intake?
PROCTOR: 3 hours ago.
Student: Events leading up to the incident?
PROCTOR: The patient was running in a cross-country foot race and was stung by a bee.

▼ Perform the Focused Physical Examination

Student: I am performing the focused physical examination.
PROCTOR: Noted.
Student: What are her lung sounds?
PROCTOR: She has wheezing noted bilaterally.

▼ Baseline Vital Signs

Student: What are the patient's baseline vital signs, including blood pressure, pulse, respirations, pulse oximetry, and level of consciousness?
PROCTOR: Blood pressure, 108/60 mm Hg; pulse, 134 beats/min; respirations, 28 breaths/min; pulse oximetry reading, 97%; and the patient is alert.

▼ Interventions

Student: I will apply oxygen and begin rapid transport. I will request an order for an EpiPen if permitted per local protocol. I will monitor her vital signs every five minutes or less during transport.
PROCTOR: Noted. Granted.
ALS Student: I will apply basic life support (BLS) interventions, plus the following: establish IV access, perform cardiac monitoring, and follow the local protocol.
ALS Proctor: Noted. The cardiac monitor shows sinus tachycardia with occasional premature ventricular complexes.

▼ Reevaluate Transport Decision

Student: The patient is a high priority and is a load-and-go.
PROCTOR: Noted.

▼ Detailed Physical Examination

Possible Answer #1
Student: I would not do a detailed physical exam.
PROCTOR: Noted. (Go to "Radio Report.")

Possible Answer #2
Student: I am conducting the detailed physical exam. I am looking for DCAP-BTLS. This acronym stands for deformities, contusions, abrasions, punctures, penetrations, paradoxical motion in the chest, and burns, tenderness, lacerations, and swelling.
PROCTOR: Noted. The detailed physical exam will be performed during transport.

▸ **Assess the Head**

Student: I am assessing the head. Do I find any DCAP-BTLS? Do I find any evidence of Battle's sign or raccoon eyes?
PROCTOR: No.

▸ **Inspect and Palpate the Head and Ears**

Student: I am assessing the head and ears.
PROCTOR: There are no obvious injuries.

▸ **Assess the Eyes**

Student: I am assessing the eyes. Are the pupils equal, round, and regular in size, and react properly to light (PEARRL)?
PROCTOR: They are PEARRL.

▸ **Assess the Facial Area Including Oral and Nasal Areas**

Student: I am assessing the face, nose, and mouth. Do I see any discharge or hear any obstructions?
PROCTOR: No.

▸ **Assess the Neck**

▸ **Inspect and Palpate the Neck**

Student: I am assessing the neck for DCAP-BTLS.
PROCTOR: There are no obvious injuries.

▸ **Assess for Jugular Vein Distention**

Student: Do I find any jugular vein distention (JVD)?
PROCTOR: No.

▸ **Assess for Tracheal Deviation**

Student: Do I see any tracheal deviation?
PROCTOR: No.

▸ **Assess the Chest**

Student: I am assessing the chest for DCAP-BTLS.
PROCTOR: Noted.

▸ **Inspect**

Student: What do I see when I look at the chest?
PROCTOR: There are no obvious injuries.
Student: Is the chest symmetric?
PROCTOR: Yes.

▸ **Palpate**

Student: When I touch the chest, do I feel crepitus or a flail segment?
PROCTOR: No.

▸ **Auscultate**

Student: Are lung sounds present in all fields?
PROCTOR: Yes, with improvement noted following the EpiPen injection.
Student: Do I hear any sucking sounds from the chest?
PROCTOR: No.

▸ **Assess the Abdomen/Pelvis**

▸ **Assess the Abdomen**

Student: I am assessing the abdomen for DCAP-BTLS. I am assessing all four quadrants. Do I find any problems?
PROCTOR: No.

▸ **Assess the Pelvis**

Student: I am assessing the pelvis for DCAP-BTLS. Is the pelvis stable?
PROCTOR: Yes.

▸ **Assess the Genitalia/Perineum as Needed (Verbalize in Training)**

Student: I am assessing the genitalia/perineum as necessary for DCAP-BTLS.
PROCTOR: The area is unremarkable.

▸ **Assess the Extremities**

▸ **Inspect**

Student: I am assessing the lower and upper extremities for DCAP-BTLS. Do I find anything?
PROCTOR: No.

▸ **Palpate**

Student: Do I feel anything unusual?
PROCTOR: No.

▸ **Assess Motor, Sensory, and Circulatory Function**

Student: I am checking for DCAP-BTLS, motor and sensory function, and pulses. Right leg?
PROCTOR: Negative DCAP-BTLS. Motor and sensory functions are present. Pulses are present.
Student: Left leg?
PROCTOR: Negative DCAP-BTLS. Motor and sensory functions are present. Pulses are present.
Student: Right arm?
PROCTOR: Negative DCAP-BTLS. Motor and sensory functions are present. Pulses are present.
Student: Left arm?
PROCTOR: Negative DCAP-BTLS. Motor and sensory functions are present. Pulses are present.

▸ **Assess the Posterior**

Student: We will check the back.
PROCTOR: Noted.

▸ **Assess the Thorax**

Student: I am assessing the thorax. Do I find injuries?
PROCTOR: No.

▸ **Assess the Lumbar Area**

Student: I am assessing the flanks and lumbar area. Do I find injuries?
PROCTOR: No.

▸ **Assess the Entire Backside**

Student: I am assessing the entire backside. Do I find injuries?
PROCTOR: No.

▸ **Manage Secondary Injuries/Wounds**

Student: I would direct my partner to monitor the airway.

PROCTOR: Noted.

▸ **Reassess Interventions**

Student: I will reassess my interventions: oxygen, EpiPen, and rapid transport.

PROCTOR: Noted.

ALS Student: I will reassess BLS interventions, plus the following: IV access, cardiac monitor, and local protocol.

ALS Proctor: Noted. The cardiac monitor shows sinus tachycardia with occasional premature ventricular complexes.

Critical Criteria:

- ❑ Did not obtain medical direction or verbalize standing orders for medical interventions
- ❑ Administered a dangerous or inappropriate intervention
- ❑ Did not ask questions about the present illness
- ❑ Did not differentiate patient's need for transportation versus continued assessment at the scene

Radio Report

(Provided by the student.)

PROCTOR: Noted.

Ongoing Assessment

Repeat the Initial Assessment

Student: I will repeat the initial assessment.

PROCTOR: Noted. (Reflected in "Repeat Vital Signs.")

Repeat Vital Signs

Student: I will reassess vital signs and mental status.

PROCTOR: Blood pressure, 110/62 mm Hg; pulse, 138 beats/min; respirations, 24 breaths/min; pulse oximetry reading, 98%; and the patient is alert.

Student: The vital signs have improved with the EpiPen.

PROCTOR: Noted.

Check Interventions

Student: I will check my interventions: oxygen and EpiPen.

PROCTOR: Noted.

ALS Student: I will check BLS interventions, plus the following: IV access, cardiac monitor, and local protocol.

ALS Proctor: Noted. The cardiac monitor shows sinus tachycardia with occasional premature ventricular complexes.

Repeat the Focused Assessment

Student: I will repeat the focused assessment.

PROCTOR: Noted.

Critical Criteria:

- ❑ Did not obtain medical direction or verbalize standing orders for medical interventions
- ❑ Administered a dangerous or inappropriate intervention

Handoff Report to Emergency Department Staff

Student: The patient's condition improved during transport.

PROCTOR: Noted.

Critical Criteria

(Inform the student of items missed, if any.)

❑ Pass ❑ Fail Date: ______________________

Proctor Comments: ______________________

____

____

CASE 100

Notes

Dispatch Information

PROCTOR: EMS 10, respond to a 32-year-old pregnant female complaining of contractions that are 5 minutes apart. This is her first child. She is conscious and breathing.

Pre-scene Action (BSI)

Student: I am wearing nonlatex gloves and safety glasses.
PROCTOR: Noted.

Critical Criteria:
- ❑ Did not take, or verbalize, body substance isolation (BSI) precautions when necessary

Scene Size-up

Scene Safety

Student: Is the scene safe?
PROCTOR: Yes.

Mechanism of Injury/Nature of Illness

Student: What is the nature of the illness?
PROCTOR: The patient is pregnant and complaining of contractions 5 minutes apart.

Number of Patients

Student: How many patients are there?
PROCTOR: One.

Additional Resources

Student: I would call for advanced life support (ALS) assistance.
PROCTOR: Noted.

C-Spine Stabilization

Student: I would not stabilize the cervical spine (c-spine).
PROCTOR: Noted.

Critical Criteria:
- ❑ Did not determine scene safety

Initial Assessment

General Impression

Student: My general impression is that the patient's condition is stable.
PROCTOR: Noted.

Responsiveness/Level of Consciousness

Student: What is the patient's level of consciousness?
PROCTOR: Alert.

Chief Complaint/Apparent Life Threats

Student: What is the patient's chief complaint?
PROCTOR: The patient is complaining of contractions 5 minutes apart.

Assess the Airway and Breathing

Student: Is the airway open?
PROCTOR: Yes.

Assessment

Student: What are the rate and the quality of breathing?
PROCTOR: Rate: Tachypneic. Quality: Shallow.

Provide Oxygen

Student: I am applying oxygen at 15 L/min via nonrebreathing mask.
PROCTOR: Noted.

Ensure Adequate Ventilation

Student: The patient has adequate ventilations at this time.
PROCTOR: Noted.

Assess Circulation

Student: I am assessing the patient's circulation.
PROCTOR: Noted.

Assess for and Control Major Bleeding

Student: Do I find any major bleeding?
PROCTOR: No.

Assess the Pulse

Student: What are the rate and the quality of pulses?
PROCTOR: Rate: Tachycardic. Quality: Bounding.

Assess the Skin

Student: I am assessing the skin. What are the color, temperature, and condition of the skin?
PROCTOR: Color: Normal. Temperature: Warm. Condition: Moist.

Identify Priority Patients/Make Transport Decision

Student: The patient is a low priority and does not require immediate transport.
PROCTOR: Noted.

Critical Criteria:
- ❑ Did not provide high concentration of oxygen
- ❑ Did not find or manage problems associated with airway, breathing, hemorrhage or shock (hypoperfusion)
- ❑ Did not differentiate patient's need for transportation versus continued assessment at the scene
- ❑ Did detailed or focused history/physical examination before assessing the airway, breathing and circulation

Focused History and Physical Examination/Rapid Assessment

Select the Appropriate Assessment (Focused or Rapid)

Student: I am selecting the focused assessment.
PROCTOR: Noted.

SAMPLE History

Student: At this time I will gather a SAMPLE history from the patient or family. What are the patient's signs and symptoms?
PROCTOR: Obstetrics.

> Student: Are you pregnant? Have you received prenatal care?
> **PROCTOR:** Yes. She has been under the care of an OB/GYN without known complications.
> Student: How long have you been pregnant? When are you due?
> **PROCTOR:** 9 months. She is due to deliver in 2 days.
> Student: Are you having pain or contractions?
> **PROCTOR:** Yes, the contractions are 5 minutes apart.
> Student: Are you having any bleeding or discharge?
> **PROCTOR:** No.
> Student: Do you feel the need to push?
> **PROCTOR:** Sometimes.
> Student: When was your last menstrual period?
> **PROCTOR:** 10 months ago.

Student: Allergies?
PROCTOR: No allergies.
Student: Medications?
PROCTOR: Prenatal vitamins.
Student: Pertinent past medical history?
PROCTOR: No pertinent medical history.
Student: Last oral intake?
PROCTOR: 3 hours ago.
Student: Events leading up to the incident?
PROCTOR: The patient was at home in bed when the contractions began.

Perform the Focused Physical Examination

Student: I am performing the focused physical examination.
PROCTOR: Noted.
Student: I am assessing the abdomen for DCAP-BTLS. This acronym stands for deformities, contusions, abrasions, punctures, penetrations, paradoxical motion in the chest, and burns, tenderness, lacerations, and swelling. I am assessing all four quadrants. What do I see and feel?
PROCTOR: She has an obviously pregnant, distended abdomen, with contractions every 5 minutes that last about 1 minute.
Student: I am assessing the pelvis for DCAP-BTLS. Is the pelvis stable?
PROCTOR: Yes.
Student: I will check for crowning.
PROCTOR: There are no signs of crowning.

Baseline Vital Signs

Student: What are the patient's baseline vital signs, including blood pressure, pulse, respirations, pulse oximetry, and level of consciousness?
PROCTOR: Blood pressure, 138/78 mm Hg; pulse, 112 beats/min; respirations, 24 breaths/min; pulse oximetry reading, 99%; and the patient is alert.

Interventions

Student: I will apply oxygen and transport the patient on her left side.
PROCTOR: Noted.
ALS Student: I will apply basic life support (BLS) interventions, plus the following: IV access.
ALS Proctor: Noted.

Reevaluate Transport Decision

Student: This patient does not require immediate transport.
PROCTOR: Noted.

Detailed Physical Examination

Possible Answer #1
Student: I would not do a detailed physical exam.
PROCTOR: Noted. (Go to "Radio Report.")

Possible Answer #2
Student: I am conducting the detailed physical exam. I am looking for DCAP-BTLS.
PROCTOR: Noted. The detailed physical exam will be performed during transport.

Assess the Head

Student: I am assessing the head. Do I find any DCAP-BTLS? Do I find any evidence of Battle's sign or raccoon eyes?
PROCTOR: No.

Inspect and Palpate the Head and Ears

Student: I am assessing the head and ears.
PROCTOR: There are no obvious injuries.

Assess the Eyes

Student: I am assessing the eyes. Are the pupils equal, round, and regular in size, and react properly to light (PEARRL)?
PROCTOR: They are PEARRL.

Assess the Facial Area Including Oral and Nasal Areas

Student: I am assessing the face, nose, and mouth. Do I see any discharge or hear any obstructions?
PROCTOR: No.

Assess the Neck

Inspect and Palpate the Neck

Student: I am assessing the neck for DCAP-BTLS.
PROCTOR: There are no obvious injuries.

Assess for Jugular Vein Distention

Student: Do I find any jugular vein distention (JVD)?
PROCTOR: No.

Assess for Tracheal Deviation

Student: Do I see any tracheal deviation?
PROCTOR: No.

Assess the Chest

Student: I am assessing the chest for DCAP-BTLS.
PROCTOR: Noted.

Inspect

Student: What do I see when I look at the chest?
PROCTOR: There are no obvious injuries.
Student: Is the chest symmetric?
PROCTOR: Yes.

Palpate

Student: When I touch the chest, do I feel crepitus or a flail segment?
PROCTOR: No.

Auscultate

Student: Are lung sounds present in all fields?
PROCTOR: Yes.
Student: Do I hear any sucking sounds from the chest?
PROCTOR: No.

Assess the Abdomen/Pelvis

Assess the Abdomen

Student: I am assessing the abdomen for DCAP-BTLS. I am assessing all four quadrants. Do I find any problems?
PROCTOR: She has an obviously distended abdomen, with contractions every 5 minutes and lasting about 1 minute.

Assess the Pelvis

Student: I am assessing the pelvis for DCAP-BTLS. Is the pelvis stable?
PROCTOR: Yes.

Assess the Genitalia/Perineum as Needed (Verbalize in Training)

Student: I am assessing the genitalia/perineum as necessary for DCAP-BTLS.
PROCTOR: There are no signs of crowning and her bag of water has not ruptured.

Assess the Extremities

Inspect

Student: I am assessing the lower and upper extremities for DCAP-BTLS. Do I find anything?
PROCTOR: No.

Palpate

Student: Do I feel anything unusual?
PROCTOR: No.

Assess Motor, Sensory, and Circulatory Function

Student: I am checking for DCAP-BTLS, motor and sensory function, and pulses. Right leg?
PROCTOR: Negative DCAP-BTLS. Motor and sensory functions are present. Pulses are present.
Student: Left leg?
PROCTOR: Negative DCAP-BTLS. Motor and sensory functions are present. Pulses are present.
Student: Right arm?
PROCTOR: Negative DCAP-BTLS. Motor and sensory functions are present. Pulses are present.
Student: Left arm?
PROCTOR: Negative DCAP-BTLS. Motor and sensory functions are present. Pulses are present.

Assess the Posterior

Student: We will not check the back.
PROCTOR: Noted.

Manage Secondary Injuries/Wounds

Student: I would reassure the patient and transport.
PROCTOR: Noted.

▸ Reassess Interventions

Student: I will reassess my interventions: oxygen, reassurance, and left-sided transport.

PROCTOR: Noted.

ALS Student: I will reassess BLS interventions, plus the following: IV access.

ALS Proctor: Noted.

Critical Criteria:
- ❑ Did not obtain medical direction or verbalize standing orders for medical interventions
- ❑ Administered a dangerous or inappropriate intervention
- ❑ Did not ask questions about the present illness
- ❑ Did not differentiate patient's need for transportation versus continued assessment at the scene

Radio Report

(Provided by the student.)

PROCTOR: Noted.

Ongoing Assessment

Repeat the Initial Assessment

Student: I will repeat the initial assessment.

PROCTOR: Noted. (Reflected in "Repeat Vital Signs.")

Repeat Vital Signs

Student: I will reassess vital signs and mental status.

PROCTOR: Blood pressure, 132/70 mm Hg; pulse, 110 beats/min; respirations, 20 breaths/min; pulse oximetry reading, 99%; and the patient is alert.

Student: The vital signs have not significantly changed.

PROCTOR: Noted.

Check Interventions

Student: I will check my interventions: oxygen and transport the patient on her left side.

PROCTOR: Noted.

ALS Student: I will check BLS interventions, plus the following: IV access.

ALS Proctor: Noted.

Repeat the Focused Assessment

Student: I will repeat the focused assessment.

PROCTOR: Noted.

Critical Criteria:
- ❑ Did not obtain medical direction or verbalize standing orders for medical interventions
- ❑ Administered a dangerous or inappropriate intervention

Handoff Report to Emergency Department Staff

Student: There was no change during transport.

PROCTOR: Noted.

Critical Criteria

(Inform the student of items missed, if any.)

❑ Pass ❑ Fail Date: ______________________________

Proctor Comments: ______________________________

____

____

CASE 101

Notes

Dispatch Information

PROCTOR: EMS 10, respond to a possible diabetic emergency. The 46-year-old male patient is in a car and is conscious and breathing.

Pre-scene Action (BSI)

Student: I am wearing nonlatex gloves and safety glasses.
PROCTOR: Noted.

Critical Criteria:
- ❑ Did not take, or verbalize, body substance isolation (BSI) precautions when necessary

Scene Size-up

Scene Safety

Student: Is the scene safe?
PROCTOR: Yes.

Mechanism of Injury/Nature of Illness

Student: What is the nature of the illness?
PROCTOR: The patient was stopped by the police for speeding. He then said he was having a diabetic emergency.

Number of Patients

Student: How many patients are there?
PROCTOR: One.

Additional Resources

Student: I would call for advanced life support (ALS) assistance.
PROCTOR: Noted.

C-Spine Stabilization

Student: I would not stabilize the cervical spine (c-spine).
PROCTOR: Noted.

Critical Criteria:
- ❑ Did not determine scene safety

Initial Assessment

General Impression

Student: My general impression is that the patient's condition is stable.
PROCTOR: Noted.

Responsiveness/Level of Consciousness

Student: What is the patient's level of consciousness?
PROCTOR: Alert.

Chief Complaint/Apparent Life Threats

Student: What is the patient's chief complaint?
PROCTOR: The patient says that he thinks his blood sugar is low.

Assess the Airway and Breathing

Student: Is the airway open?
PROCTOR: Yes.

Assessment

Student: What are the rate and the quality of breathing?
PROCTOR: Rate: Within normal limits. Quality: Normal.

Provide Oxygen

Student: I am applying oxygen at 15 L/min via nonrebreathing mask.
PROCTOR: Noted.

Ensure Adequate Ventilation

Student: The patient has adequate ventilations at this time.
PROCTOR: Noted.

Assess Circulation

Student: I am assessing the patient's circulation.
PROCTOR: Noted.

Assess for and Control Major Bleeding

Student: Do I find any major bleeding?
PROCTOR: No.

Assess the Pulse

Student: What are the rate and the quality of pulses?
PROCTOR: Rate: Within normal limits. Quality: Normal.

Assess the Skin

Student: I am assessing the skin. What are the color, temperature, and condition of the skin?
PROCTOR: Color: Normal. Temperature: Warm. Condition: Moist.

Identify Priority Patients/Make Transport Decision

Student: The patient is a low priority and does not require immediate transport.
PROCTOR: Noted.

Critical Criteria:
- ❑ Did not provide high concentration of oxygen
- ❑ Did not find or manage problems associated with airway, breathing, hemorrhage or shock (hypoperfusion)
- ❑ Did not differentiate patient's need for transportation versus continued assessment at the scene
- ❑ Did detailed or focused history/physical examination before assessing the airway, breathing and circulation

Focused History and Physical Examination/Rapid Assessment

Select the Appropriate Assessment (Focused or Rapid)

Student: I am selecting the focused assessment.
PROCTOR: Noted.

SAMPLE History

Student: At this time I will gather a SAMPLE history from the patient or family. What are the patient's signs and symptoms?
PROCTOR: Altered mental status.

> Student: Describe the episode.
> **PROCTOR:** He was stopped by the police and said he thinks his blood sugar is low.
> Student: Onset: What was he doing when this started?
> **PROCTOR:** Driving.
> Student: Duration: How long has this been going on?
> **PROCTOR:** 20 minutes (per the patient).
> Student: Are there any associated symptoms?
> **PROCTOR:** No.
> Student: Is there any evidence of trauma?
> **PROCTOR:** No.
> Student: Interventions: Has he done anything to make this better?
> **PROCTOR:** The patient has taken no actions.
> Student: Have there been any seizures?
> **PROCTOR:** No.
> Student: Has there been any fever?
> **PROCTOR:** No.

Student: Allergies?
PROCTOR: No allergies.
Student: Medications?
PROCTOR: Insulin.
Student: Pertinent past medical history?
PROCTOR: Diabetes.
Student: Last oral intake?
PROCTOR: 3 hours ago.
Student: Events leading up to the incident?
PROCTOR: The patient was stopped by the police and said he was having a diabetic emergency.

Perform the Focused Physical Examination

Student: I am performing the focused physical examination.
PROCTOR: Noted.
Student: I will check the patient's blood glucose level.
PROCTOR: Noted. The blood glucose level is 118 mg/dL.

Baseline Vital Signs

Student: What are the patient's baseline vital signs, including blood pressure, pulse, respirations, pulse oximetry, and level of consciousness?
PROCTOR: Blood pressure, 136/82 mm Hg; pulse rate, 90 beats/min; respirations, 16 breaths/min; pulse oximetry reading, 99%; and the patient is alert and oriented.

Interventions

Student: I will perform a Cincinnati Stroke Scale assessment, call medical control, and transport the patient, canceling the request for ALS assistance.
PROCTOR: The Cincinnati Stroke Scale is negative.

Reevaluate Transport Decision

Student: The patient does not require immediate transport.
PROCTOR: Noted.

Detailed Physical Examination

Possible Answer #1
Student: I would not do a detailed physical exam.
PROCTOR: Noted. (Go to "Radio Report.")

Possible Answer #2
Student: I am conducting the detailed physical exam. I am looking for DCAP-BTLS. This acronym stands for deformities, contusions, abrasions, punctures, penetrations, paradoxical motion in the chest, and burns, tenderness, lacerations, and swelling.
PROCTOR: Noted. The detailed physical exam will be performed during transport.

- **Assess the Head**

Student: I am assessing the head. Do I find any DCAP-BTLS? Do I find any evidence of Battle's sign or raccoon eyes?
PROCTOR: No.

  - **Inspect and Palpate the Head and Ears**

Student: I am assessing the head and ears.
PROCTOR: There are no obvious injuries.

  - **Assess the Eyes**

Student: I am assessing the eyes. Are the pupils equal, round, and regular in size, and react properly to light (PEARRL)?
PROCTOR: They are PEARRL.

  - **Assess the Facial Area Including Oral and Nasal Areas**

Student: I am assessing the face, nose, and mouth. Do I see any discharge or hear any obstructions?
PROCTOR: No.

- **Assess the Neck**
  - **Inspect and Palpate the Neck**

Student: I am assessing the neck for DCAP-BTLS.
PROCTOR: There are no obvious injuries.

  - **Assess for Jugular Vein Distention**

Student: Do I find any jugular vein distention (JVD)?
PROCTOR: No.

  - **Assess for Tracheal Deviation**

Student: Do I see any tracheal deviation?
PROCTOR: No.

- **Assess the Chest**

Student: I am assessing the chest for DCAP-BTLS.
PROCTOR: Noted.

  - **Inspect**

Student: What do I see when I look at the chest?
PROCTOR: There are no obvious injuries.
Student: Is the chest symmetric?
PROCTOR: Yes.

  - **Palpate**

Student: When I touch the chest, do I feel crepitus or a flail segment?
PROCTOR: No.

  - **Auscultate**

Student: Are lung sounds present in all fields?
PROCTOR: Yes.
Student: Do I hear any sucking sounds from the chest?
PROCTOR: No.

- **Assess the Abdomen/Pelvis**
  - **Assess the Abdomen**

Student: I am assessing the abdomen for DCAP-BTLS. I am assessing all four quadrants. Do I find any problems?
PROCTOR: No.

  - **Assess the Pelvis**

Student: I am assessing the pelvis for DCAP-BTLS. Is the pelvis stable?
PROCTOR: Yes.

  - **Assess the Genitalia/Perineum as Needed (Verbalize in Training)**

Student: I am assessing the genitalia/perineum as necessary for DCAP-BTLS.
PROCTOR: The area is unremarkable.

- **Assess the Extremities**
  - **Inspect**

Student: I am assessing the lower and upper extremities for DCAP-BTLS. Do I find anything?
PROCTOR: No.

  - **Palpate**

Student: Do I feel anything unusual?
PROCTOR: No.

  - **Assess Motor, Sensory, and Circulatory Function**

Student: I am checking for DCAP-BTLS, motor and sensory function, and pulses. Right leg?
PROCTOR: Negative DCAP-BTLS. Motor and sensory functions are present. Pulses are present.
Student: Left leg?
PROCTOR: Negative DCAP-BTLS. Motor and sensory functions are present. Pulses are present.
Student: Right arm?
PROCTOR: Negative DCAP-BTLS. Motor and sensory functions are present. Pulses are present.
Student: Left arm?
PROCTOR: Negative DCAP-BTLS. Motor and sensory functions are present. Pulses are present.

- **Assess the Posterior**

Student: We will not check the back.
PROCTOR: Noted.

- **Manage Secondary Injuries/Wounds**

Student: I would direct my partner to monitor the patient.
PROCTOR: Noted.

- **Reassess Interventions**

Student: I will reassess my interventions: check the blood glucose level, call medical control, and transport the patient.
PROCTOR: Noted. The blood glucose level is 118 mg/dL.

Critical Criteria:
- ❑ Did not obtain medical direction or verbalize standing orders for medical interventions
- ❑ Administered a dangerous or inappropriate intervention
- ❑ Did not ask questions about the present illness
- ❑ Did not differentiate patient's need for transportation versus continued assessment at the scene

Radio Report

(Provided by the student.)

PROCTOR: Noted.

Ongoing Assessment

Repeat the Initial Assessment

Student: I will repeat the initial assessment.

PROCTOR: Noted. (Reflected in "Repeat Vital Signs.")

Repeat Vital Signs

Student: I will reassess vital signs and mental status.

PROCTOR: Blood pressure, 132/76 mm Hg; pulse rate, 84 beats/min; respirations, 16 breaths/min; pulse oximetry reading, 99%; and the patient is alert.

Trend Vital Signs

Student: The vital signs have not significantly changed.

PROCTOR: Noted.

Check Interventions

Student: I will check my interventions: blood glucose level, call medical control, and transport the patient.

PROCTOR: Noted. The blood glucose level is 118 mg/dL.

Repeat the Focused Assessment

Student: I will repeat the focused assessment.

PROCTOR: Noted.

Critical Criteria:

- ❑ Did not obtain medical direction or verbalize standing orders for medical interventions
- ❑ Administered a dangerous or inappropriate intervention

Handoff Report to Emergency Department Staff

Student: There was no change during transport.

PROCTOR: Noted.

Critical Criteria

(Inform the student of items missed, if any.)

❑ Pass ❑ Fail Date: ______________________________

Proctor Comments: ______________________________

____

____

Notes

Dispatch Information

PROCTOR: EMS 10, respond to a 50-year-old male who is complaining of difficulty breathing. He is conscious and breathing.

Pre-scene Action (BSI)

Student: I am wearing nonlatex gloves and safety glasses.
PROCTOR: Noted.

Critical Criteria:
- ❑ Did not take, or verbalize, body substance isolation (BSI) precautions when necessary

Scene Size-up

Scene Safety

Student: Is the scene safe?
PROCTOR: Yes.

Mechanism of Injury/Nature of Illness

Student: What is the nature of the illness?
PROCTOR: The patient was sitting on the toilet bearing down when he had a sudden onset of difficulty breathing and right-sided chest pain.

Number of Patients

Student: How many patients are there?
PROCTOR: One.

Additional Resources

Student: I would call for advanced life support (ALS) assistance.
PROCTOR: Noted.

C-Spine Stabilization

Student: I would not stabilize the cervical spine (c-spine).
PROCTOR: Noted.

Critical Criteria:
- ❑ Did not determine scene safety

Initial Assessment

General Impression

Student: My general impression is that the patient's condition is unstable.
PROCTOR: Noted.

Responsiveness/Level of Consciousness

Student: What is the patient's level of consciousness?
PROCTOR: Alert.

Chief Complaint/Apparent Life Threats

Student: What is the patient's chief complaint?
PROCTOR: He is complaining of shortness of breath and right-sided chest pain.

Assess the Airway and Breathing

Student: Is the airway open?
PROCTOR: Yes.

Assessment

Student: What are the rate and the quality of breathing?
PROCTOR: Rate: Within normal limits. Quality: Labored.

Provide Oxygen

Student: I am applying oxygen at 15 L/min via nonrebreathing mask.
PROCTOR: Noted.

Ensure Adequate Ventilation

Student: The patient has adequate ventilations at this time.
PROCTOR: Noted.

Assess Circulation

Student: I am assessing the patient's circulation.
PROCTOR: Noted.

Assess for and Control Major Bleeding

Student: Do I find any major bleeding?
PROCTOR: No.

Assess the Pulse

Student: What are the rate and the quality of pulses?
PROCTOR: Rate: Tachycardic. Quality: Bounding.

Assess the Skin

Student: I am assessing the skin. What are the color, temperature, and condition of the skin?
PROCTOR: Color: Cyanotic. Temperature: Cool. Condition: Diaphoretic.

Identify Priority Patients/Make Transport Decision

Student: The patient is a high priority and is a load-and-go. I will begin packaging and transport.
PROCTOR: Noted.

Critical Criteria:
- ❑ Did not provide high concentration of oxygen
- ❑ Did not find or manage problems associated with airway, breathing, hemorrhage or shock (hypoperfusion)
- ❑ Did not differentiate patient's need for transportation versus continued assessment at the scene
- ❑ Did detailed or focused history/physical examination before assessing the airway, breathing and circulation

Focused History and Physical Examination/Rapid Assessment

Select the Appropriate Assessment (Focused or Rapid)

Student: I am selecting the focused assessment.
PROCTOR: Noted.

SAMPLE History

Student: At this time I will gather a SAMPLE history from the patient or family. What are the patient's signs and symptoms?
PROCTOR: Respiratory.

> **Student:** Onset: What were you doing when this started?
> **PROCTOR:** The patient was sitting on the toilet bearing down when he had a sudden onset of difficulty breathing and right-sided chest pain.
> **Student:** Provokes: What makes your condition worse or better?
> **PROCTOR:** Nothing makes it better.
> **Student:** Quality: Can you describe your pain?
> **PROCTOR:** Stabbing on the right side of the chest.
> **Student:** Radiates: Do you have pain anywhere else?
> **PROCTOR:** No.
> **Student:** Severity: On a scale of 1 to 10 with 10 being the worst possible, how would you rate your pain/distress?
> **PROCTOR:** 9.
> **Student:** Time: How long has this been going on?
> **PROCTOR:** 20 minutes.
> **Student:** Interventions: Have you done anything to make this better?
> **PROCTOR:** The patient has taken no actions.

Student: Allergies?
PROCTOR: No allergies.
Student: Medications?
PROCTOR: No medications.
Student: Pertinent past medical history?
PROCTOR: Hypertension and the patient smokes 1½ packs of cigarettes per day.
Student: Last oral intake?
PROCTOR: 3 hours ago.

Student: Events leading up to the incident?
PROCTOR: The patient was sitting on the toilet bearing down when he had a sudden onset of difficulty breathing and right-sided chest pain.

Perform the Focused Physical Examination

Student: I am performing the focused physical examination.
PROCTOR: Noted.
Student: I am assessing the neck for DCAP-BTLS. This acronym stands for deformities, contusions, abrasions, punctures, penetrations, paradoxical motion in the chest, and burns, tenderness, lacerations, and swelling.
PROCTOR: He has tracheal deviation to the left.
Student: I am assessing the chest for DCAP-BTLS.
PROCTOR: Noted.
Student: What do I see when I look at the chest?
PROCTOR: There are no obvious injuries.
Student: Is the chest symmetric?
PROCTOR: Yes.
Student: When I touch the chest, do I feel crepitus or a flail segment?
PROCTOR: No.
Student: Are lung sounds present in all fields?
PROCTOR: They are diminished on the right side.
Student: Do I hear any sucking sounds from the chest?
PROCTOR: No.

Baseline Vital Signs

Student: What are the patient's baseline vital signs, including blood pressure, pulse, respirations, pulse oximetry, and level of consciousness?
PROCTOR: Blood pressure, 100/60 mm Hg; pulse rate, 140 beats/min; respirations, 20 breaths/min; pulse oximetry reading, 94%; and the patient is alert but very anxious.

Interventions

Student: I will apply 100% oxygen via nonrebreathing mask.
PROCTOR: Noted.
ALS Student: I will apply basic life support (BLS) interventions, plus the following: establish IV access, perform cardiac monitoring, and assess for a tension pneumothorax (jugular vein distention [JVD], tracheal deviation), percuss the chest, and decompress the right chest.
ALS Proctor: Noted. The cardiac monitor shows sinus tachycardia. There is tracheal deviation present to the left side. Hyperresonance is present. Lung sounds are diminished on the right. Chest decompression is effective.

Reevaluate Transport Decision

Student: The patient is a high priority and is a load-and-go.
PROCTOR: Noted.

Detailed Physical Examination

Possible Answer #1
Student: I would not do a detailed physical exam.
PROCTOR: Noted. (Go to "Radio Report.")

Possible Answer #2
Student: I am conducting the detailed physical exam. I am looking for DCAP-BTLS.
PROCTOR: Noted. The detailed physical exam will be performed during transport.

Assess the Head

Student: I am assessing the head. Do I find any DCAP-BTLS? Do I find any evidence of Battle's sign or raccoon eyes?
PROCTOR: No.

Inspect and Palpate the Head and Ears

Student: I am assessing the head and ears.
PROCTOR: There are no obvious injuries.

Assess the Eyes

Student: I am assessing the eyes. Are the pupils equal, round, and regular in size, and react properly to light (PEARRL)?
PROCTOR: They are PEARRL.

Assess the Facial Area Including Oral and Nasal Areas

Student: I am assessing the face, nose, and mouth. Do I see any discharge or hear any obstructions?
PROCTOR: No.

Assess the Neck

Inspect and Palpate the Neck

Student: I am assessing the neck for DCAP-BTLS.
PROCTOR: There are no obvious injuries.

Assess for Jugular Vein Distention

Student: Do I find any JVD?
PROCTOR: No (if treated).

Assess for Tracheal Deviation

Student: Do I see any tracheal deviation?
PROCTOR: No (if treated with a needle decompression).

Assess the Chest

Student: I am assessing the chest for DCAP-BTLS.
PROCTOR: Noted.

Inspect

Student: What do I see when I look at the chest?
PROCTOR: There are no obvious injuries.
Student: Is the chest symmetric?
PROCTOR: Yes.

Palpate

Student: When I touch the chest, do I feel crepitus or a flail segment?
PROCTOR: No.

Auscultate

Student: Are lung sounds present in all fields?
PROCTOR: Yes (if treated with a needle decompression).
Student: Do I hear any sucking sounds from the chest?
PROCTOR: No.

Assess the Abdomen/Pelvis

Assess the Abdomen

Student: I am assessing the abdomen for DCAP-BTLS. I am assessing all four quadrants. Do I find any problems?
PROCTOR: No.

Assess the Pelvis

Student: I am assessing the pelvis for DCAP-BTLS. Is the pelvis stable?
PROCTOR: Yes.

Assess the Genitalia/Perineum as Needed (Verbalize in Training)

Student: I am assessing the genitalia/perineum as necessary for DCAP-BTLS.
PROCTOR: The area is unremarkable.

Assess the Extremities

Inspect

Student: I am assessing the lower and upper extremities for DCAP-BTLS. Do I find anything?
PROCTOR: No.

Palpate

Student: Do I feel anything unusual?
PROCTOR: No.

Assess Motor, Sensory, and Circulatory Function

Student: I am checking for DCAP-BTLS, motor and sensory function, and pulses. Right leg?
PROCTOR: Negative DCAP-BTLS. Motor and sensory functions are present. Pulses are present.
Student: Left leg?
PROCTOR: Negative DCAP-BTLS. Motor and sensory functions are present. Pulses are present.

Student: Right arm?
PROCTOR: Negative DCAP-BTLS. Motor and sensory functions are present. Pulses are present.
Student: Left arm?
PROCTOR: Negative DCAP-BTLS. Motor and sensory functions are present. Pulses are present.

▸ **Assess the Posterior**

Student: We will not check the back.
PROCTOR: Noted.

▸ **Manage Secondary Injuries/Wounds**

Student: I would direct my partner to monitor the airway.
PROCTOR: Noted.

▸ **Reassess Interventions**

Student: I will reassess my interventions: airway, breathing, and oxygen.
PROCTOR: Noted.
ALS Student: I will reassess BLS interventions, plus the following: assess the decompression, IV access, cardiac monitor, and 12-lead ECG.
ALS Proctor: Noted. The cardiac monitor shows sinus tachycardia.

Critical Criteria:
- ❑ Did not obtain medical direction or verbalize standing orders for medical interventions
- ❑ Administered a dangerous or inappropriate intervention
- ❑ Did not ask questions about the present illness
- ❑ Did not differentiate patient's need for transportation versus continued assessment at the scene

Radio Report

(Provided by the student.)
PROCTOR: Noted.

Ongoing Assessment

Repeat the Initial Assessment

Student: I will repeat the initial assessment.
PROCTOR: (Reflected in "Repeat Vital Signs.")

Repeat Vital Signs

Student: I will reassess vital signs and mental status.
PROCTOR: Blood pressure, 110/66 mm Hg; pulse rate, 136 beats/min; respirations, 20 breaths/min; pulse oximetry reading, 95%; and the patient is alert but very anxious.
Student: The vital signs have not significantly changed.
PROCTOR: Noted.

Check Interventions

Student: I will check my interventions: oxygen.
PROCTOR: Noted.
ALS Student: I will check BLS interventions, plus the following: IV access, cardiac monitor, assess for a tension pneumothorax, and percuss the chest.
ALS Proctor: Noted. The cardiac monitor shows sinus tachycardia. Tracheal deviation is absent if treated previously. Hyperresonance is absent if treated previously.

Repeat the Focused Assessment

Student: I will repeat the focused assessment.
PROCTOR: Noted.

Critical Criteria:
- ❑ Did not obtain medical direction or verbalize standing orders for medical interventions
- ❑ Administered a dangerous or inappropriate intervention

Handoff Report to Emergency Department Staff

Student: The patient's condition improved during transport.
PROCTOR: Noted.

Critical Criteria

(Inform the student of items missed, if any.)

❑ Pass ❑ Fail Date: __________

Proctor Comments: __________

CASE 103

Notes

Dispatch Information

PROCTOR: EMS 10, respond to a 50-year-old male who has had an unidentified powder fall on him. His skin has a burning sensation. He is conscious and breathing.

Pre-scene Action (BSI)

Student: I am wearing nonlatex gloves and safety glasses.
PROCTOR: Noted.

> **Critical Criteria:**
> ❑ Did not take, or verbalize, body substance isolation (BSI) precautions when necessary

Scene Size-up

Scene Safety

Student: Is the scene safe?
PROCTOR: Yes.

Mechanism of Injury/Nature of Illness

Student: What is the nature of the illness?
PROCTOR: The patient was working in a barn when a bag of an unknown powder opened and spilled on him.

Number of Patients

Student: How many patients are there?
PROCTOR: One.

Additional Resources

Student: I would call for advanced life support (ALS) assistance and additional resources: fire/rescue and hazardous materials responders. I will direct the patient to brush off any powder and remove contaminated clothing. I will have the hazardous materials team decontaminate the patient prior to making patient contact.
PROCTOR: Noted.

C-Spine Stabilization

Student: I would not stabilize the cervical spine (c-spine).
PROCTOR: Noted.

> **Critical Criteria:**
> ❑ Did not determine scene safety

Initial Assessment

General Impression

Student: My general impression is that the patient's condition is unstable.
PROCTOR: Noted.

Responsiveness/Level of Consciousness

Student: What is the patient's level of consciousness?
PROCTOR: Alert.

Chief Complaint/Apparent Life Threats

Student: What is the patient's chief complaint?
PROCTOR: The patient is complaining of his skin having a burning sensation.

Assess the Airway and Breathing

Student: Is the airway open?
PROCTOR: Yes.

Assessment

Student: What are the rate and the quality of breathing?
PROCTOR: Rate: Tachypneic. Quality: Labored.

Provide Oxygen

Student: I am applying oxygen at 15 L/min via nonrebreathing mask.
PROCTOR: Noted.

Ensure Adequate Ventilation

Student: Ventilations are adequate at this time.
PROCTOR: Noted.

Assess Circulation

Student: I am assessing the patient's circulation.
PROCTOR: Noted.

Assess for and Control Major Bleeding

Student: Do I find any major bleeding?
PROCTOR: No.

Assess the Pulse

Student: What are the rate and the quality of pulses?
PROCTOR: Rate: Tachycardic. Quality: Bounding.

Assess the Skin

Student: I am assessing the skin. What are the color, temperature, and condition of the skin?
PROCTOR: Color: Flushed. Temperature: Warm. Condition: Moist.

Identify Priority Patients/Make Transport Decision

Student: The patient is a high priority and is a load-and-go. I will begin packaging and transport.
PROCTOR: Noted.

> **Critical Criteria:**
> ❑ Did not provide high concentration of oxygen
> ❑ Did not find or manage problems associated with airway, breathing, hemorrhage or shock (hypoperfusion)
> ❑ Did not differentiate patient's need for transportation versus continued assessment at the scene
> ❑ Did detailed or focused history/physical examination before assessing the airway, breathing and circulation

Focused History and Physical Examination/Rapid Assessment

Select the Appropriate Assessment (Focused or Rapid)

Student: I am selecting the rapid assessment. I will make sure that he is completely decontaminated prior to assessment and treatment.
PROCTOR: Noted.

Head

Student: I am rapidly assessing the head.
PROCTOR: There are no obvious injuries.

Neck

Student: I am rapidly assessing the neck.
PROCTOR: There are no obvious injuries.

Chest

Student: I am rapidly assessing the chest.
PROCTOR: He has redness present at the top of his chest. The powder entered the front of his open shirt.

Abdomen/Pelvis

Student: I am rapidly assessing the abdomen. Do I find any problems?
PROCTOR: You see redness over all four quadrants of the abdomen.
Student: I am rapidly assessing the pelvis.
PROCTOR: The powder did not make it past the patient's belt.

Extremities

Student: I am rapidly assessing the lower and upper extremities.
PROCTOR: He has redness noted to both arms.

Assess Motor, Sensory, and Circulatory Function

Student: I am checking for DCAP-BTLS. This acronym stands for deformities, contusions, abrasions, punctures, penetrations, paradoxical motion in the chest, and burns, tenderness, lacerations, and swelling. I am also checking motor and sensory function, and pulses. Right leg?
PROCTOR: Negative DCAP-BTLS. Motor and sensory functions are present. Pulses are present.

Student: Left leg?
PROCTOR: Negative DCAP-BTLS. Motor and sensory functions are present. Pulses are present.
Student: Right arm?
PROCTOR: Negative DCAP-BTLS. Motor and sensory functions are present. Pulses are present.
Student: Left arm?
PROCTOR: Negative DCAP-BTLS. Motor and sensory functions are present. Pulses are present.

▸ **Posterior**

Student: We will rapidly check the back.
PROCTOR: Noted. There is no redness noted to his back.

▸ **Assess the Thorax**

Student: I am rapidly assessing the thorax. Do I find injuries?
PROCTOR: No.

▸ **Assess the Lumbar Area**

Student: I am rapidly assessing the flanks and lumbar area. Do I find injuries?
PROCTOR: No.

▸ **Assess the Entire Backside**

Student: I am rapidly assessing the entire backside. Do I find injuries?
PROCTOR: No.

▸ **Manage Secondary Injuries/Wounds**

Student: I would direct my partner to irrigate per local protocol.
PROCTOR: Noted.

▾ SAMPLE History

Student: At this time I will gather a SAMPLE history from the patient or family. What are the patient's signs and symptoms?
PROCTOR: Poisoning/overdose.
Student: What was the substance?
PROCTOR: The patient does not know. It was not labeled. It was a white powder in a milk container that had its top cut off.
Student: Did you ingest any of the substance?
PROCTOR: No.
Student: When did you become exposed?
PROCTOR: It was 15 minutes ago.
Student: Over what time period?
PROCTOR: Over a few minutes.
Student: Interventions: Have you done anything to make this better?
PROCTOR: Yes, the patient tried to brush some of the powder off.
Student: What is your weight?
PROCTOR: 195 pounds.
Student: Allergies?
PROCTOR: No allergies.
Student: Medications?
PROCTOR: No medications.
Student: Pertinent past medical history?
PROCTOR: No pertinent medical history.
Student: Last oral intake?
PROCTOR: 3 hours ago.
Student: Events leading up to the incident?
PROCTOR: The patient was working in a barn when the powder spilled on him.

▾ Baseline Vital Signs

Student: What are the patient's baseline vital signs, including blood pressure, pulse, respirations, pulse oximetry, and level of consciousness?
PROCTOR: Blood pressure, 150/84 mm Hg; pulse rate, 124 beats/min; respirations, 24 breaths/min; pulse oximetry reading, 98%; and the patient is alert.

▾ Interventions

Student: I had the hazardous materials team decontaminate the patient by first dry-brushing him and then decontaminating him per local protocol. I will administer 100% oxygen via nonrebreathing mask. I will continue irrigation throughout transport, being careful to stay out of the runoff water.
PROCTOR: Noted.
ALS Student: I will apply basic life support (BLS) interventions, plus the following: IV access, cardiac monitor, and local protocol.
ALS Proctor: Noted. The cardiac monitor shows sinus tachycardia.

▾ Reevaluate Transport Decision

Student: The patient is a high priority and is a load-and-go.
PROCTOR: Noted.

▾ Detailed Physical Examination

Possible Answer #1
Student: I would not do a detailed physical exam.
PROCTOR: Noted. (Go to "Radio Report.")

Possible Answer #2
Student: I am conducting the detailed physical exam. I am looking for DCAP-BTLS.
PROCTOR: Noted. The detailed physical exam will be performed during transport.

▸ **Assess the Head**

Student: I am assessing the head. Do I find any DCAP-BTLS? Do I find any evidence of Battle's sign or raccoon eyes?
PROCTOR: No.

▸ **Inspect and Palpate the Head and Ears**

Student: I am assessing the head and ears.
PROCTOR: There are no obvious injuries.

▸ **Assess the Eyes**

Student: I am assessing the eyes. Are the pupils equal, round, and regular in size, and react properly to light (PEARRL)?
PROCTOR: They are PEARRL.

▸ **Assess the Facial Area Including Oral and Nasal Areas**

Student: I am assessing the face, nose, and mouth. Do I see any discharge or hear any obstructions?
PROCTOR: No.

▸ **Assess the Neck**

▸ **Inspect and Palpate the Neck**

Student: I am assessing the neck for DCAP-BTLS.
PROCTOR: There are no obvious injuries.

▸ **Assess for Jugular Vein Distention**

Student: Do I find any jugular vein distention (JVD)?
PROCTOR: No.

▸ **Assess for Tracheal Deviation**

Student: Do I see any tracheal deviation?
PROCTOR: No.

▸ **Assess the Chest**

Student: I am assessing the chest for DCAP-BTLS.
PROCTOR: Noted.

▸ **Inspect**

Student: What do I see when I look at the chest?
PROCTOR: He has redness present at the top of his chest. The powder entered the front of his open shirt.
Student: Is the chest symmetric?
PROCTOR: Yes.

▸ **Palpate**

Student: When I touch the chest, do I feel crepitus or a flail segment?
PROCTOR: No.

▸ **Auscultate**

Student: Are lung sounds present in all fields?

PROCTOR: Yes.

Student: Do I hear any sucking sounds from the chest?

PROCTOR: No.

▸ **Assess the Abdomen/Pelvis**

▸ **Assess the Abdomen**

Student: I am assessing the abdomen for DCAP-BTLS. I am assessing all four quadrants. Do I find any problems?

PROCTOR: You see redness over all four quadrants of the abdomen.

▸ **Assess the Pelvis**

Student: I am assessing the pelvis for DCAP-BTLS. Is the pelvis stable?

PROCTOR: Yes. The powder did not make it past the patient's belt.

▸ **Assess the Genitalia/Perineum as Needed (Verbalize in Training)**

Student: I am assessing the genitalia/perineum as necessary for DCAP-BTLS.

PROCTOR: The area is unremarkable.

▸ **Assess the Extremities**

▸ **Inspect**

Student: I am assessing the lower and upper extremities for DCAP-BTLS. Do I find anything?

PROCTOR: Yes, he has redness noted to both arms.

▸ **Palpate**

Student: Do I feel anything unusual?

PROCTOR: No.

▸ **Assess Motor, Sensory, and Circulatory Function**

Student: I am checking for DCAP-BTLS, motor and sensory function, and pulses. Right leg?

PROCTOR: Negative DCAP-BTLS. Motor and sensory functions are present. Pulses are present.

Student: Left leg?

PROCTOR: Negative DCAP-BTLS. Motor and sensory functions are present. Pulses are present.

Student: Right arm?

PROCTOR: Negative DCAP-BTLS. Motor and sensory functions are present. Pulses are present.

Student: Left arm?

PROCTOR: Negative DCAP-BTLS. Motor and sensory functions are present. Pulses are present.

▸ **Assess the Posterior**

Student: We will check the back.

PROCTOR: Noted. There is no redness noted to his back.

▸ **Assess the Thorax**

Student: I am assessing the thorax. Do I find injuries?

PROCTOR: No.

▸ **Assess the Lumbar Area**

Student: I am assessing the flanks and lumbar area. Do I find injuries?

PROCTOR: No.

▸ **Assess the Entire Backside**

Student: I am assessing the entire backside. Do I find injuries?

PROCTOR: No.

▸ **Manage Secondary Injuries/Wounds**

Student: I would direct my partner to dress the burns per local protocol.

PROCTOR: Noted.

▸ **Reassess Interventions**

Student: I will reassess my interventions: apply oxygen and ask the patient about areas that still feel as though they are burning. If burning is still felt, we will continue to irrigate until it subsides.

PROCTOR: Noted. The burning is being relieved.

ALS Student: I will reassess BLS interventions, plus the following: IV access, cardiac monitor, local protocol, and pain management.

ALS Proctor: Noted. The cardiac monitor shows sinus tachycardia. The blood glucose level is now 136 mg/dL.

Critical Criteria:
- ❑ Did not obtain medical direction or verbalize standing orders for medical interventions
- ❑ Administered a dangerous or inappropriate intervention
- ❑ Did not ask questions about the present illness
- ❑ Did not differentiate patient's need for transportation versus continued assessment at the scene

Radio Report

(Provided by the student.)

PROCTOR: Noted.

Ongoing Assessment

Repeat the Initial Assessment

Student: I will repeat the initial assessment.

PROCTOR: Noted. (Reflected in "Repeat Vital Signs.")

Repeat Vital Signs

Student: I will reassess vital signs and mental status.

PROCTOR: Blood pressure, 144/80 mm Hg; pulse rate, 114 beats/min; respirations, 20 breaths/min; pulse oximetry reading, 99%; and the patient is alert.

Student: The vital signs have not significantly changed.

PROCTOR: Noted.

Check Interventions

Student: I will check my interventions: oxygen.

PROCTOR: Noted.

ALS Student: I will check BLS interventions, plus the following: IV access, cardiac monitor, local protocol, and pain management.

ALS Proctor: Noted. The cardiac monitor shows sinus tachycardia.

Repeat the Focused Assessment

Student: I will repeat the focused assessment.

PROCTOR: Noted.

Critical Criteria:
- ❑ Did not obtain medical direction or verbalize standing orders for medical interventions
- ❑ Administered a dangerous or inappropriate intervention

Handoff Report to Emergency Department Staff

Student: There was no change during transport.

PROCTOR: Noted.

Critical Criteria

(Inform the student of items missed, if any.)

❑ Pass ❑ Fail Date: ____________________

Proctor Comments: ____________________

Notes

Dispatch Information

PROCTOR: EMS 10, respond to a 30-year-old female with possible alcohol intoxication. She is unresponsive and not breathing.

Pre-scene Action (BSI)

Student: I am wearing nonlatex gloves and safety glasses.

Critical Criteria:
- ❑ Did not take, or verbalize, body substance isolation (BSI) precautions when necessary

Scene Size-up

Scene Safety

Student: Is the scene safe?
PROCTOR: Yes.

Mechanism of Injury/Nature of Illness

Student: What is the nature of the illness?
PROCTOR: The patient has been drinking at a business convention. She is unresponsive and not breathing.

Number of Patients

Student: How many patients are there?
PROCTOR: One.

Additional Resources

Student: I would call for advanced life support (ALS) assistance.
PROCTOR: Noted.

C-Spine Stabilization

Student: On the basis of the mechanism of injury, I would stabilize the cervical spine (c-spine) in a neutral in-line position.
PROCTOR: Noted.

Critical Criteria:
- ❑ Did not determine scene safety

Initial Assessment

Student: As I perform midline c-spine stabilization, I identify myself and ask the patient not to move.
PROCTOR: Noted.

General Impression

Student: My general impression is that the patient's condition is unstable.
PROCTOR: Noted.

Responsiveness/Level of Consciousness

Student: What is the patient's level of consciousness?
PROCTOR: Unresponsive.

Chief Complaint/Apparent Life Threats

Student: What is the patient's chief complaint?
PROCTOR: The patient is unresponsive.

Assess the Airway and Breathing

Student: I will open the airway using the jaw-thrust maneuver.
PROCTOR: Noted.

Assessment

Student: What are the rate and the quality of breathing?
PROCTOR: Rate: Slow. Quality: Shallow.

Provide Oxygen

Student: I am assisting ventilations with a bag-valve device with 100% oxygen. I will insert an oral or advanced airway.
PROCTOR: Noted.

Ensure Adequate Ventilation

Student: I will assist ventilation with the bag-valve device and oral or advanced airway.
PROCTOR: Noted.

Assess Circulation

Student: I am assessing the patient's circulation.
PROCTOR: Noted.

Assess for and Control Major Bleeding

Student: Do I find any major bleeding?
PROCTOR: No.

Assess the Pulse

Student: What are the rate and the quality of pulses?
PROCTOR: Rate: Tachycardic. Quality: Thready.

Assess the Skin

Student: I am assessing the skin. What are the color, temperature, and condition of the skin?
PROCTOR: Color: Pale. Temperature: Cool. Condition: Diaphoretic.

Identify Priority Patients/Make Transport Decision

Student: The patient is a high priority and is a load-and-go. I will begin packaging and transport.
PROCTOR: Noted.

Critical Criteria:
- ❑ Did not provide high concentration of oxygen
- ❑ Did not find or manage problems associated with airway, breathing, hemorrhage or shock (hypoperfusion)
- ❑ Did not differentiate patient's need for transportation versus continued assessment at the scene
- ❑ Did detailed or focused history/physical examination before assessing the airway, breathing and circulation

Focused History and Physical Examination/Rapid Assessment

Select the Appropriate Assessment (Focused or Rapid)

Student: I am selecting the rapid assessment.
PROCTOR: Noted.

Head

Student: I am rapidly assessing the head.
PROCTOR: There are no obvious injuries.

Neck

Inspect and Palpate the Neck

Student: I am rapidly assessing the neck.
PROCTOR: There are no obvious injuries.
Student: I will apply a cervical collar.
PROCTOR: Noted.

Chest

Student: I am rapidly assessing the chest.
PROCTOR: There are no obvious injuries.

Abdomen/Pelvis

Student: I am rapidly assessing the abdomen.
PROCTOR: There are no obvious injuries.
Student: I am rapidly assessing the pelvis.
PROCTOR: There are no obvious injuries.

Extremities

Student: I am rapidly assessing the extremities.
PROCTOR: There are no obvious injuries.

Assess Motor, Sensory, and Circulatory Function

Student: I am checking for DCAP-BTLS. This acronym stands for deformities, contusions, abrasions, punctures, penetrations, paradoxical motion in the chest, and burns, tenderness, lacerations, and swelling. I am also checking motor and sensory function, and pulses. Right leg?
PROCTOR: Negative DCAP-BTLS. Motor and sensory functions are absent. Pulses are present.
Student: Left leg?
PROCTOR: Negative DCAP-BTLS. Motor and sensory functions are absent. Pulses are present.

Student: Right arm?
PROCTOR: Negative DCAP-BTLS. Motor and sensory functions are absent. Pulses are present.
Student: Left arm?
PROCTOR: Negative DCAP-BTLS. Motor and sensory functions are absent. Pulses are present.

▸ **Posterior**

Student: I will rapidly assess the back.
PROCTOR: Noted.

▸ **Assess the Thorax**

Student: I am rapidly assessing the thorax. Do I find injuries?
PROCTOR: No.

▸ **Assess the Lumbar Area**

Student: I am rapidly assessing the flanks and lumbar area. Do I find injuries?
PROCTOR: No.

▸ **Assess the Entire Backside**

Student: I am rapidly assessing the entire backside. Do I find injuries?
PROCTOR: No.

▸ **Manage Secondary Injuries/Wounds**

Student: We will apply a cervical collar and backboard with full immobilization per local protocol, if not yet done, at this time.
PROCTOR: Noted.
Student: Are there any changes in motor and sensory functions or pulses?
PROCTOR: No.

▾ SAMPLE History

Student: At this time I will gather a SAMPLE history from the patient or bystanders. What are the signs and symptoms?
PROCTOR: Poisoning/overdose.
  Student: What was the substance?
  PROCTOR: Beer and mixed drinks.
  Student: When did the patient consume these substances?
  PROCTOR: It was 45 minutes ago.
  Student: Over what time period?
  PROCTOR: Continuous ingestion over 6 hours.
  Student: Interventions? Has anyone done anything to make this better?
  PROCTOR: No actions have been taken.
  Student: What is the patient's weight?
  PROCTOR: 120 to 130 pounds.
Student: Allergies?
PROCTOR: Unknown.
Student: Medications?
PROCTOR: Unknown.
Student: Pertinent past medical history?
PROCTOR: Unknown.
Student: Last oral intake?
PROCTOR: The patient has been drinking all evening.
Student: Events leading up to the incident?
PROCTOR: The patient was drinking all evening and then passed out.

▾ Baseline Vital Signs

Student: What are the patient's baseline vital signs, including blood pressure, pulse, respirations, pulse oximetry, blood glucose level, and level of consciousness?
PROCTOR: Blood pressure, 122/72 mm Hg; pulse, 124 beats/min; respirations, per bag-valve device; pulse oximetry reading, 90%, blood glucose level, 42 mg/dL; and the patient is unresponsive.

▾ Interventions

Student: I have applied oxygen via bag-valve device and an oral or advanced airway.
PROCTOR: Noted.
ALS Student: I will apply basic life support (BLS) interventions, plus the following: intubate, confirm with end tidal CO_2 and lung sounds, establish IV access, perform cardiac monitoring, administer IV, a bolus of 25 grams of D_{50}, and medications per local protocol.
ALS Proctor: Noted. The cardiac monitor shows sinus tachycardia. End tidal CO_2 confirms endotracheal (ET) tube placement.

▾ Reevaluate Transport Decision

Student: The patient is a high priority and is a load-and-go.
PROCTOR: Noted.

▾ Detailed Physical Examination

Possible Answer #1
Student: I would not do a detailed physical exam.
PROCTOR: Noted. (Go to "Radio Report.")

Possible Answer #2
Student: I am conducting the detailed physical exam. I am looking for DCAP-BTLS.
PROCTOR: Noted. The detailed physical exam will be performed during transport.

▸ **Assess the Head**

Student: I am assessing the head. Do I find any DCAP-BTLS? Do I find any evidence of Battle's sign or raccoon eyes?
PROCTOR: No.

▸ **Inspect and Palpate the Head and Ears**

Student: I am assessing the head and ears.
PROCTOR: There are no obvious injuries.

▸ **Assess the Eyes**

Student: I am assessing the eyes. Are the pupils equal, round, and regular in size, and react properly to light (PEARRL)?
PROCTOR: They are equal but nonreactive.

▸ **Assess the Facial Area Including Oral and Nasal Areas**

Student: I am assessing the face, nose, and mouth. Do I see any discharge or hear any obstructions?
PROCTOR: No.

▸ **Assess the Neck**

▸ **Inspect and Palpate the Neck**

Student: I am assessing the neck for DCAP-BTLS.
PROCTOR: There are no obvious injuries.

▸ **Assess for Jugular Vein Distention**

Student: Do I find any jugular vein distention (JVD)?
PROCTOR: No.

▸ **Assess for Tracheal Deviation**

Student: Do I see any tracheal deviation?
PROCTOR: No.

▸ **Assess the Chest**

Student: I am assessing the chest for DCAP-BTLS.
PROCTOR: Noted.

▸ **Inspect**

Student: What do I see when I look at the chest?
PROCTOR: There are no obvious injuries.
Student: Is the chest symmetric?
PROCTOR: Yes.

▸ **Palpate**

Student: When I touch the chest, do I feel crepitus or a flail segment?
PROCTOR: No.

▸ **Auscultate**

Student: Are lung sounds present in all fields?
PROCTOR: Yes.
Student: Do I hear any sucking sounds from the chest?
PROCTOR: No.

▸ **Assess the Abdomen/Pelvis**

▸ **Assess the Abdomen**

Student: I am assessing the abdomen for DCAP-BTLS. I am assessing all four quadrants. Do I find any problems?

PROCTOR: No.

▸ **Assess the Pelvis**

Student: I am assessing the pelvis for DCAP-BTLS. Is the pelvis stable?

PROCTOR: Yes.

▸ **Assess the Genitalia/Perineum as Needed (Verbalize in Training)**

Student: I am assessing the genitalia/perineum as necessary for DCAP-BTLS.

PROCTOR: The area is unremarkable.

▸ **Assess the Extremities**

▸ **Inspect**

Student: I am assessing the lower and upper extremities for DCAP-BTLS. Do I find anything?

PROCTOR: No.

▸ **Palpate**

Student: Do I feel anything unusual?

PROCTOR: No.

▸ **Assess Motor, Sensory, and Circulatory Function**

Student: I am checking for DCAP-BTLS, motor and sensory function, and pulses. Right leg?

PROCTOR: Negative DCAP-BTLS. Motor and sensory functions are absent. Pulses are present.

Student: Left leg?

PROCTOR: Negative DCAP-BTLS. Motor and sensory functions are absent. Pulses are present.

Student: Right arm?

PROCTOR: Negative DCAP-BTLS. Motor and sensory functions are absent. Pulses are present.

Student: Left arm?

PROCTOR: Negative DCAP-BTLS. Motor and sensory functions are absent. Pulses are present.

▸ **Assess the Posterior**

Note: This portion of the detailed physical exam would not be done if the patient were previously backboarded per local protocol.

Student: We will not check the back since it was previously checked and the patient is backboarded.

PROCTOR: Noted.

▸ **Manage Secondary Injuries/Wounds**

Student: I would direct my partner to continue providing ventilations.

PROCTOR: Noted.

▸ **Reassess Interventions**

Student: I will reassess my interventions: bag-valve ventilation, oxygen, and an oral or advanced airway.

PROCTOR: Noted.

ALS Student: I will reassess BLS interventions, plus the following: intubate, confirm end tidal CO_2 and lung sounds, establish IV access, perform cardiac monitoring, monitor blood glucose levels, and follow the local protocol.

ALS Proctor: Noted. The cardiac monitor shows sinus tachycardia. End tidal CO_2 confirms ET tube placement.

Critical Criteria:

- ❑ Did not obtain medical direction or verbalize standing orders for medical interventions
- ❑ Administered a dangerous or inappropriate intervention
- ❑ Did not ask questions about the present illness
- ❑ Did not differentiate patient's need for transportation versus continued assessment at the scene

Radio Report

(Provided by the student.)

PROCTOR: Noted.

Ongoing Assessment

Repeat the Initial Assessment

Student: I will repeat the initial assessment. (Reflected in "Repeat Vital Signs.")

Repeat Vital Signs

Student: I will reassess vital signs and mental status.

PROCTOR: Blood pressure, 120/70 mm Hg; pulse, 120 beats/min; respirations, per bag-valve device; pulse oximetry reading, N/A; blood glucose level, 136 mg/dL; and the patient is unresponsive.

Student: The vital signs have not significantly changed.

PROCTOR: Noted.

Check Interventions

Student: I will check my interventions: oxygen and an oral/advanced airway.

PROCTOR: Noted.

ALS Student: I will check BLS interventions, plus the following: intubate, confirm end tidal CO_2 and lung sounds, monitor IV, perform cardiac monitoring, and follow the local protocol.

ALS Proctor: Noted. The cardiac monitor shows sinus tachycardia. End tidal CO_2 confirms ET tube placement.

Repeat the Focused Assessment

Student: I will repeat the focused assessment.

PROCTOR: Noted.

Critical Criteria:

- ❑ Did not obtain medical direction or verbalize standing orders for medical interventions
- ❑ Administered a dangerous or inappropriate intervention

Handoff Report to Emergency Department Staff

Student: There was no change during transport.

PROCTOR: Noted.

Critical Criteria

(Inform the student of items missed, if any.)

❑ Pass ❑ Fail Date: ____________________

Proctor Comments: ____________________

Notes

CASE 106

Dispatch Information

PROCTOR: EMS 10, respond to a 15-year-old male who is complaining of difficulty breathing. He is conscious and breathing.

Pre-scene Action (BSI)

Student: I am wearing nonlatex gloves and safety glasses.
PROCTOR: Noted.

Critical Criteria:
- ❑ Did not take, or verbalize, body substance isolation (BSI) precautions when necessary

Scene Size-up

Scene Safety

Student: Is the scene safe?
PROCTOR: Yes.

Mechanism of Injury/Nature of Illness

Student: What is the nature of the illness?
PROCTOR: The patient had been seeing how long he could hold his breath under water when he coughed and inhaled some chlorinated water. He has been coughing and crying.

Number of Patients

Student: How many patients are there?
PROCTOR: One.

Additional Resources

Student: I would call for advanced life support (ALS) assistance.
PROCTOR: Noted.

C-Spine Stabilization

Student: I would not stabilize the cervical spine (c-spine).
PROCTOR: Noted.

Critical Criteria:
- ❑ Did not determine scene safety

Initial Assessment

General Impression

Student: My general impression is that the patient's condition is unstable.
PROCTOR: Noted.

Responsiveness/Level of Consciousness

Student: What is the patient's level of consciousness?
PROCTOR: Alert and anxious.

Chief Complaint/Apparent Life Threats

Student: What is the patient's chief complaint?
PROCTOR: The patient is complaining of difficulty breathing and coughing. He inhaled pool water while trying to hold his breath under water.

Assess the Airway and Breathing

Student: Is the airway open? Is the patient breathing?
PROCTOR: Yes, the airway is open and the patient is breathing.

► Assessment

Student: What are the rate and the quality of breathing?
PROCTOR: Rate: Rapid. Quality: Crying.

► Provide Oxygen

Student: I am applying oxygen at 15 L/min via nonrebreathing mask.
PROCTOR: Noted.

► Ensure Adequate Ventilation

Student: The patient has adequate ventilations at this time.
PROCTOR: Noted.

Assess Circulation

Student: I am assessing the patient's circulation.
PROCTOR: Noted.

► Assess for and Control Major Bleeding

Student: Do I find any major bleeding?
PROCTOR: No.

► Assess the Pulse

Student: What are the rate and the quality of pulses?
PROCTOR: Rate: Tachycardic. Quality: Bounding.

► Assess the Skin

Student: I am assessing the skin. What are the color, temperature, and condition of the skin?
PROCTOR: Color: Flushed. Temperature: Warm. Condition: Moist.

Identify Priority Patients/Make Transport Decision

Student: The patient is a high priority and is a load-and-go. I will begin packaging and transport.
PROCTOR: Noted.

Critical Criteria:
- ❑ Did not provide high concentration of oxygen
- ❑ Did not find or manage problems associated with airway, breathing, hemorrhage or shock (hypoperfusion)
- ❑ Did not differentiate patient's need for transportation versus continued assessment at the scene
- ❑ Did detailed or focused history/physical examination before assessing the airway, breathing and circulation

Focused History and Physical Examination/Rapid Assessment

Select the Appropriate Assessment (Focused or Rapid)

Student: I am selecting the focused assessment.
PROCTOR: Noted.

SAMPLE History

Student: At this time I will gather a SAMPLE history from the patient or family. What are the patient's signs and symptoms?
PROCTOR: Respiratory.

> **Student:** Onset: What were you doing when this started?
> **PROCTOR:** He was swimming and seeing how long he could hold his breath while under water when he coughed and inhaled pool water.
> **Student:** Provokes: What makes your condition worse or better?
> **PROCTOR:** Nothing.
> **Student:** Quality: Can you describe your pain?
> **PROCTOR:** Irritation in his lungs.
> **Student:** Radiates: Do you have pain anywhere else?
> **PROCTOR:** No.
> **Student:** Severity: On a scale of 1 to 10 with 10 being the worst possible, how would you rate your pain/distress?
> **PROCTOR:** 10.
> **Student:** Time: How long has this been going on?
> **PROCTOR:** 30 minutes. He was under water for a minute or two.
> **Student:** Interventions: Have you done anything to make this better?
> **PROCTOR:** The patient has taken no actions.

Student: Allergies?
PROCTOR: No allergies.
Student: Medications?
PROCTOR: No medications.
Student: Pertinent past medical history?
PROCTOR: No pertinent medical history.
Student: Last oral intake?
PROCTOR: 3 hours ago.

Student: Events leading up to the incident?
PROCTOR: The patient was seeing how long he could hold his breath when he coughed and inhaled pool water.

▼ Perform Focused Physical Examination
Student: I am performing the focused physical examination.
PROCTOR: Noted.
Student: What are the patient's lung sounds?
PROCTOR: The lung sounds are rales bilaterally.
Student: Does he have any pain in his joints?
PROCTOR: No. He coughs forcibly.

▼ Baseline Vital Signs
Student: What are the patient's baseline vital signs, including blood pressure, pulse, respirations, pulse oximetry, and level of consciousness?
PROCTOR: Blood pressure, 124/80 mm Hg; pulse, 124 beats/min; respirations, 28 breaths/min; pulse oximetry reading, 95%; and the patient is alert.

▼ Interventions
Student: I will continue applying oxygen and reassure the patient.
PROCTOR: Noted.
ALS Student: I will apply basic life support (BLS) interventions, plus the following: establish IV access, perform cardiac monitoring, and follow the local protocol.
ALS Proctor: Noted. The cardiac monitor shows sinus tachycardia.

▼ Reevaluate Transport Decision
Student: The patient is a high priority and is a load-and-go.
PROCTOR: Noted.

▼ Detailed Physical Examination
Possible Answer #1
Student: I would not do a detailed physical exam.
PROCTOR: Noted. (Go to "Radio Report.")

Possible Answer #2
Student: I am conducting the detailed physical exam. I am looking for DCAP-BTLS. This acronym stands for deformities, contusions, abrasions, punctures, penetrations, paradoxical motion in the chest, and burns, tenderness, lacerations, and swelling.
PROCTOR: Noted. The detailed physical exam will be performed during transport.

► Assess the Head
Student: I am assessing the head. Do I find any DCAP-BTLS? Do I find any evidence of Battle's sign or raccoon eyes?
PROCTOR: No.

► Inspect and Palpate the Head and Ears
Student: I am assessing the head and ears.
PROCTOR: There are no obvious injuries.

► Assess the Eyes
Student: I am assessing the eyes. Are the pupils equal, round, and regular in size, and react properly to light (PEARRL)?
PROCTOR: They are PEARRL.

► Assess the Facial Area Including Oral and Nasal Areas
Student: I am assessing the face, nose, and mouth. Do I see any discharge or hear any obstructions?
PROCTOR: No.

► Assess the Neck

► Inspect and Palpate the Neck
Student: I am assessing the neck for DCAP-BTLS.
PROCTOR: There are no obvious injuries.

► Assess for Jugular Vein Distention
Student: Do I find any jugular vein distention?
PROCTOR: No.

► Assess for Tracheal Deviation
Student: Do I see any tracheal deviation?
PROCTOR: No.

► Assess the Chest
Student: I am assessing the chest for DCAP-BTLS.
PROCTOR: Noted.

► Inspect
Student: What do I see when I look at the chest?
PROCTOR: There are no obvious injuries.
Student: Is the chest symmetric?
PROCTOR: Yes.

► Palpate
Student: When I touch the chest, do I feel crepitus or a flail segment?
PROCTOR: No.

► Auscultate
Student: Are lung sounds present in all fields?
PROCTOR: Yes, you hear rales.
Student: Do I hear any sucking sounds from the chest?
PROCTOR: No.

► Assess the Abdomen/Pelvis

► Assess the Abdomen
Student: I am assessing the abdomen for DCAP-BTLS. I am assessing all four quadrants. Do I find any problems?
PROCTOR: No.

► Assess the Pelvis
Student: I am assessing the pelvis for DCAP-BTLS. Is the pelvis stable?
PROCTOR: Yes.

► Assess the Genitalia/Perineum as Needed (Verbalize in Training)
Student: I am assessing the genitalia/perineum as necessary for DCAP-BTLS.
PROCTOR: The area is unremarkable.

► Assess the Extremities

► Inspect
Student: I am assessing the lower and upper extremities for DCAP-BTLS. Do I find anything?
PROCTOR: No.

► Palpate
Student: Do I feel anything unusual?
PROCTOR: No.

► Assess Motor, Sensory, and Circulatory Function
Student: I am checking for DCAP-BTLS, motor and sensory function, and pulses. Right leg?
PROCTOR: Negative DCAP-BTLS. Motor and sensory functions are present. Pulses are present.
Student: Left leg?
PROCTOR: Negative DCAP-BTLS. Motor and sensory functions are present. Pulses are present.
Student: Right arm?
PROCTOR: Negative DCAP-BTLS. Motor and sensory functions are present. Pulses are present.
Student: Left arm?
PROCTOR: Negative DCAP-BTLS. Motor and sensory functions are present. Pulses are present.

► Assess the Posterior
Student: We will check the back.
PROCTOR: Noted.

► Assess the Thorax
Student: I am assessing the thorax. Do I find injuries?
PROCTOR: No.

► Assess the Lumbar Area
Student: I am assessing the flanks and lumbar area. Do I find injuries?
PROCTOR: No.

► Assess the Entire Backside
Student: I am assessing the entire backside. Do I find injuries?
PROCTOR: No.

▸ Manage Secondary Injuries/Wounds

Student: I would direct my partner to monitor the airway.

PROCTOR: Noted.

▸ Reassess Interventions

Student: I will reassess my interventions: oxygen and reassurance.

PROCTOR: Noted.

ALS Student: I will reassess BLS interventions, plus the following: oxygen, IV access, cardiac monitor, and local protocol.

ALS Proctor: Noted. The cardiac monitor shows sinus tachycardia.

Critical Criteria:

- ❑ Did not obtain medical direction or verbalize standing orders for medical interventions
- ❑ Administered a dangerous or inappropriate intervention
- ❑ Did not ask questions about the present illness
- ❑ Did not differentiate patient's need for transportation versus continued assessment at the scene

Radio Report

(Provided by the student.)

PROCTOR: Noted.

Ongoing Assessment

Repeat the Initial Assessment

Student: I will repeat the initial assessment.

PROCTOR: Noted. (Reflected in "Repeat Vital Signs.")

Repeat Vital Signs

Student: I will reassess vital signs and mental status.

PROCTOR: Blood pressure, 124/80 mm Hg; pulse, 124 beats/min; respirations, 28 breaths/min; pulse oximetry reading, 95%; and the patient is alert.

Student: The vital signs have not changed significantly.

PROCTOR: Noted.

Check Interventions

Student: I will check my interventions: oxygen.

PROCTOR: Noted.

ALS Student: I will check BLS interventions, plus the following: oxygen, IV access, cardiac monitor, and local protocol.

ALS Proctor: Noted. The cardiac monitor shows sinus tachycardia.

Repeat the Focused Assessment

Student: I will repeat the focused assessment.

PROCTOR: Noted.

Critical Criteria:

- ❑ Did not obtain medical direction or verbalize standing orders for medical interventions
- ❑ Administered a dangerous or inappropriate intervention

Handoff Report to Emergency Department Staff

Student: There was no change in the patient's condition during transport.

PROCTOR: Noted.

Critical Criteria

(Inform the student of items missed, if any.)

❑ Pass ❑ Fail Date: ____________________

Proctor Comments: ____________________

____

____

Notes

Dispatch Information

PROCTOR: EMS 10, respond to a 3-year-old male who is having a seizure.

Pre-scene Action (BSI)

Student: I am wearing nonlatex gloves and safety glasses.
PROCTOR: Noted.

Critical Criteria:
- ❑ Did not take, or verbalize, body substance isolation (BSI) precautions when necessary

Scene Size-up

Scene Safety

Student: Is the scene safe?
PROCTOR: Yes.

Mechanism of Injury/Nature of Illness

Student: What is the nature of the illness?
PROCTOR: The patient had a seizure and has gone limp.

Number of Patients

Student: How many patients are there?
PROCTOR: One.

Additional Resources

Student: I would call for advanced life support (ALS) assistance.
PROCTOR: Noted.

C-Spine Stabilization

Student: I would not stabilize the cervical spine (c-spine) if there was no trauma.
PROCTOR: Noted.

Critical Criteria:
- ❑ Did not determine scene safety

Initial Assessment

General Impression

Student: My general impression is that the patient's condition is stable.
PROCTOR: Noted.

Responsiveness/Level of Consciousness

Student: What is the patient's level of consciousness?
PROCTOR: Sleepy with snoring respirations.
Student: I will open the airway with a head-tilt chin-lift or recovery position per protocol.
PROCTOR: Noted.

Chief Complaint/Apparent Life Threats

Student: What is the patient's chief complaint?
PROCTOR: The patient is sleepy.

Assess the Airway and Breathing

Student: I will open the child's airway. Is the child breathing?
PROCTOR: Noted. The child is breathing.

▸ Assessment

Student: What are the rate and the quality of breathing?
PROCTOR: Rate: Bradypneic (normal once opened by the responder). Quality: Snoring (clear once opened by the responder).
Student: I will position the airway.
PROCTOR: Noted.

▸ Provide Oxygen

Student: I am applying oxygen at 15 L/min via pediatric nonrebreathing mask.
PROCTOR: Noted.

▸ Ensure Adequate Ventilation

Student: The patient has adequate ventilations at this time.
PROCTOR: Noted.

Assess Circulation

Student: I am assessing the patient's circulation.
PROCTOR: Noted.

▸ Assess for and Control Major Bleeding

Student: Do I find any major bleeding?
PROCTOR: No.

▸ Assess the Pulse

Student: What are the rate and the quality of pulses?
PROCTOR: Rate: Within normal limits. Quality: Bounding.

▸ Assess the Skin

Student: I am assessing the skin. What are the color, temperature, and condition of the skin?
PROCTOR: Color: Flushed. Temperature: Hot. Condition: Dry.

Identify Priority Patients/Make Transport Decision

Student: The patient is no longer having a seizure, so he is a low priority and does not require immediate transport.
PROCTOR: Noted.

Critical Criteria:
- ❑ Did not provide high concentration of oxygen
- ❑ Did not find or manage problems associated with airway, breathing, hemorrhage or shock (hypoperfusion)
- ❑ Did not differentiate patient's need for transportation versus continued assessment at the scene
- ❑ Did detailed or focused history/physical examination before assessing the airway, breathing and circulation

Focused History and Physical Examination/Rapid Assessment

Select the Appropriate Assessment (Focused or Rapid)

Student: I am selecting the focused assessment.
PROCTOR: Noted.

SAMPLE History

Student: At this time I will gather a SAMPLE history from the patient or family. What are the patient's signs and symptoms?
PROCTOR: Altered mental status.

> **Student:** Describe the episode.
> **PROCTOR:** The patient has had the flu for a few days.
> **Student:** Onset: What was he doing when this started?
> **PROCTOR:** Watching TV.
> **Student:** Duration: How long has this been going on?
> **PROCTOR:** 2 minutes.
> **Student:** Are there any associated symptoms?
> **PROCTOR:** Yes, he is worn out.
> **Student:** Is there any evidence of trauma?
> **PROCTOR:** No.
> **Student:** Interventions: Has the patient or his parents done anything to make this better?
> **PROCTOR:** The patient and his parents have taken no actions.
> **Student:** Have there been any seizures?
> **PROCTOR:** Yes, just this one.
> **Student:** Has there been any fever?
> **PROCTOR:** Yes, 102.5°F (39.2°C).

Student: Allergies?
PROCTOR: No allergies.
Student: Medications?
PROCTOR: Children's Tylenol about 20 minutes ago.
Student: Pertinent past medical history?
PROCTOR: No pertinent medical history.

Student: Last oral intake?
PROCTOR: The patient has been drinking Kool-Aid.
Student: Events leading up to the incident?
PROCTOR: The patient was watching TV.

▾ Perform the Focused Physical Examination

Student: I am performing the focused physical examination.
PROCTOR: Noted.
Student: What is the patient's level of consciousness, at this time?
PROCTOR: He is tired but responds to verbal stimuli.
Student: Are there any injuries from the seizure?
PROCTOR: There are no obvious injuries.
Student: What is the patient's blood glucose level?
PROCTOR: It is 94 mg/dL.

▾ Baseline Vital Signs

Student: What are the patient's baseline vital signs, including blood pressure, pulse, respirations, pulse oximetry, blood glucose level, and level of consciousness?
PROCTOR: Blood pressure, N/A; pulse, 132 beats/min; respirations, 32 breaths/min; pulse oximetry reading, N/A; blood glucose level, 94 mg/dL; and the patient is tired.

▾ Interventions

Student: I will apply oxygen, monitor the airway, and cool per local protocol.
PROCTOR: Noted.
ALS Student: I will apply basic life support (BLS) interventions, plus the following: establish IV access.
ALS Proctor: Noted.

▾ Reevaluate Transport Decision

Student: This patient does not require immediate transport.
PROCTOR: Noted.

▾ Detailed Physical Examination

Possible Answer #1
Student: I would not do a detailed physical exam.
PROCTOR: Noted. (Go to "Radio Report.")

Possible Answer #2
Student: I am conducting the detailed physical exam. I am looking for DCAP-BTLS. This acronym stands for deformities, contusions, abrasions, punctures, penetrations, paradoxical motion in the chest, and burns, tenderness, lacerations, and swelling.
PROCTOR: Noted. The detailed physical exam will be performed during transport.

▸ Assess the Head

Student: I am assessing the head. Do I find any DCAP-BTLS? Do I find any evidence of Battle's sign or raccoon eyes?
PROCTOR: No.

▸ Inspect and Palpate the Head and Ears

Student: I am assessing the head and ears.
PROCTOR: There are no obvious injuries.

▸ Assess the Eyes

Student: I am assessing the eyes. Are the pupils equal, round, and regular in size, and react properly to light (PEARRL)?
PROCTOR: They are slow to react.

▸ Assess the Facial Area Including Oral and Nasal Areas

Student: I am assessing the face, nose, and mouth. Do I see any discharge or hear any obstructions?
PROCTOR: The airway is clear once it is opened by the responder.

▸ Assess the Neck

▸ Inspect and Palpate the Neck

Student: I am assessing the neck for DCAP-BTLS.
PROCTOR: There are no obvious injuries.

▸ Assess for Jugular Vein Distention

Student: Do I find any jugular vein distention (JVD)?
PROCTOR: No.

▸ Assess for Tracheal Deviation

Student: Do I see any tracheal deviation?
PROCTOR: No.

▸ Assess the Chest

Student: I am assessing the chest for DCAP-BTLS.
PROCTOR: Noted.

▸ Inspect

Student: What do I see when I look at the chest?
PROCTOR: There are no obvious injuries.
Student: Is the chest symmetric?
PROCTOR: Yes.

▸ Palpate

Student: When I touch the chest, do I feel crepitus or a flail segment?
PROCTOR: No.

▸ Auscultate

Student: Are lung sounds present in all fields?
PROCTOR: Yes.
Student: Do I hear any sucking sounds from the chest?
PROCTOR: No.

▸ Assess the Abdomen/Pelvis

▸ Assess the Abdomen

Student: I am assessing the abdomen for DCAP-BTLS. I am assessing all four quadrants. Do I find any problems?
PROCTOR: No.

▸ Assess the Pelvis

Student: I am assessing the pelvis for DCAP-BTLS. Is the pelvis stable?
PROCTOR: Yes.

▸ Assess the Genitalia/Perineum as Needed (Verbalize in Training)

Student: I am assessing the genitalia/perineum as necessary for DCAP BTLS.
PROCTOR: The area is unremarkable.

▸ Assess the Extremities

▸ Inspect

Student: I am assessing the lower and upper extremities for DCAP-BTLS. Do I find anything?
PROCTOR: No.

▸ Palpate

Student: Do I feel anything unusual?
PROCTOR: No.

▸ Assess Motor, Sensory, and Circulatory Function

Student: I am checking for DCAP-BTLS, motor and sensory function, and pulses. Right leg?
PROCTOR: Negative DCAP-BTLS. Motor and sensory functions are present. Pulses are present.
Student: Left leg?
PROCTOR: Negative DCAP-BTLS. Motor and sensory functions are present. Pulses are present.
Student: Right arm?
PROCTOR: Negative DCAP-BTLS. Motor and sensory functions are present. Pulses are present.
Student: Left arm?
PROCTOR: Negative DCAP-BTLS. Motor and sensory functions are present. Pulses are present.

▸ Assess the Posterior

Student: We will check the back.
PROCTOR: Noted.

▸ Assess the Thorax

Student: I am assessing the thorax. Do I find injuries?
PROCTOR: No.

▸ Assess the Lumbar Area

Student: I am assessing the flanks and lumbar area. Do I find injuries?
PROCTOR: No.

▸ Assess the Entire Backside

Student: I am assessing the entire backside. Do I find injuries?

PROCTOR: No.

▸ Manage Secondary Injuries/Wounds

Student: I would direct my partner to maintain the airway.

PROCTOR: Noted.

▸ Reassess Interventions

Student: I will reassess my interventions: airway, breathing, oxygen, and cool per local protocol.

PROCTOR: Noted.

ALS Student: I will reassess BLS interventions, plus the following: IV access.

ALS Proctor: Noted.

Critical Criteria:

- ❑ Did not obtain medical direction or verbalize standing orders for medical interventions
- ❑ Administered a dangerous or inappropriate intervention
- ❑ Did not ask questions about the present illness
- ❑ Did not differentiate patient's need for transportation versus continued assessment at the scene

Radio Report

(Provided by the student.)

PROCTOR: Noted.

Ongoing Assessment

Repeat the Initial Assessment

Student: I will repeat the initial assessment.

PROCTOR: Noted. (Reflected in "Repeat Vital Signs.")

Repeat Vital Signs

Student: I will reassess vital signs and mental status.

PROCTOR: Blood pressure, N/A; pulse, 128 beats/min; respirations, 28 breaths/min; pulse oximetry reading, N/A; and the patient is tired.

Student: The vital signs have not changed significantly.

PROCTOR: Noted.

Check Interventions

Student: I will check my interventions: airway, breathing, oxygen, and cool per local protocol.

PROCTOR: Noted.

ALS Student: I will check BLS interventions, plus the following: IV access.

ALS Proctor: Noted.

Repeat the Focused Assessment

Student: I will repeat the focused assessment.

PROCTOR: Noted.

Critical Criteria:

- ❑ Did not obtain medical direction or verbalize standing orders for medical interventions
- ❑ Administered a dangerous or inappropriate intervention

Handoff Report to Emergency Department Staff

Student: There was no change during transport.

PROCTOR: Noted.

Critical Criteria

(Inform the student of items missed, if any.)

❑ Pass ❑ Fail Date: ____________________

Proctor Comments: ____________________

____

____

Notes

CASE 108

Dispatch Information

PROCTOR: EMS 10, respond to a 23-year-old pregnant female complaining of feeling light-headed, like she could pass out. She is conscious and breathing.

Pre-scene Action (BSI)

Student: I am wearing nonlatex gloves and safety glasses.
PROCTOR: Noted.

> **Critical Criteria:**
> ❑ Did not take, or verbalize, body substance isolation (BSI) precautions when necessary

Scene Size-up

Scene Safety

Student: Is the scene safe?
PROCTOR: Yes.

Mechanism of Injury/Nature of Illness

Student: What is the nature of the illness?
PROCTOR: The patient is complaining of feeling like she could pass out.

Number of Patients

Student: How many patients are there?
PROCTOR: One.

Additional Resources

Student: I would call for advanced life support (ALS) assistance.
PROCTOR: Noted.

C-Spine Stabilization

Student: I would not stabilize the cervical spine (c-spine).
PROCTOR: Noted.

> **Critical Criteria:**
> ❑ Did not determine scene safety

Initial Assessment

General Impression

Student: My general impression is that the patient's condition is unstable.
PROCTOR: Noted.

Responsiveness/Level of Consciousness

Student: What is the patient's level of consciousness?
PROCTOR: Alert.

Chief Complaint/Apparent Life Threats

Student: What is the patient's chief complaint?
PROCTOR: The patient is complaining of feeling faint.

Assess the Airway and Breathing

Student: Is the airway open? Is the patient breathing?
PROCTOR: Yes, the airway is open and the patient is breathing.

▸ Assessment

Student: What are the rate and the quality of breathing?
PROCTOR: Rate: Tachypneic. Quality: Shallow.

▸ Provide Oxygen

Student: I am applying oxygen at 15 L/min via nonrebreathing mask.
PROCTOR: Noted.

▸ Ensure Adequate Ventilation

Student: The patient has adequate ventilations at this time.
PROCTOR: Noted.

Assess Circulation

Student: I am assessing the patient's circulation.
PROCTOR: Noted.

▸ Assess for and Control Major Bleeding

Student: Do I find any major bleeding?
PROCTOR: No.

▸ Assess the Pulse

Student: What are the rate and the quality of pulses?
PROCTOR: Rate: Tachycardic. Quality: Thready.

▸ Assess the Skin

Student: I am assessing the skin. What are the color, temperature, and condition of the skin?
PROCTOR: Color: Pale. Temperature: Cool. Condition: Diaphoretic.

Identify Priority Patients/Make Transport Decision

Student: The patient is a high priority and is a load-and-go. I will begin packaging and transport.
PROCTOR: Noted.

> **Critical Criteria:**
> ❑ Did not provide high concentration of oxygen
> ❑ Did not find or manage problems associated with airway, breathing, hemorrhage or shock (hypoperfusion)
> ❑ Did not differentiate patient's need for transportation versus continued assessment at the scene
> ❑ Did detailed or focused history/physical examination before assessing the airway, breathing and circulation

Focused History and Physical Examination/Rapid Assessment

Select the Appropriate Assessment (Focused or Rapid)

Student: I am selecting the focused assessment.
PROCTOR: Noted.

SAMPLE History

Student: At this time I will gather a SAMPLE history from the patient or family. What are the patient's signs and symptoms?
PROCTOR: Obstetrics/altered mental status.

Student: Are you pregnant?
PROCTOR: Yes.
Student: How long have you been pregnant?
PROCTOR: Maybe 3 months.
Student: Are you having pain or contractions?
PROCTOR: No.
Student: Are you having any bleeding or discharge?
PROCTOR: Yes, the bleeding is heavy.
Student: Do you feel the need to push?
PROCTOR: No.
Student: When was your last menstrual period?
PROCTOR: 4 months ago.
Student: I will begin asking questions regarding altered mental status. Can you describe the episode?
PROCTOR: She began bleeding and became light headed.
Student: What were you doing when this began?
PROCTOR: Sitting in her office.
Student: How long has this been going on?
PROCTOR: About 20 minutes.
Student: Do you have any other problems?
PROCTOR: Just the bleeding and feeling faint.
Student: Is there any evidence of trauma?
PROCTOR: No.
Student: Have you done anything to make this better?
PROCTOR: No.
Student: Did you have a seizure?
PROCTOR: No.
Student: Have you had a fever?
PROCTOR: No.

Student: Allergies?
PROCTOR: No allergies.

Student: Medications?
PROCTOR: No medications.
Student: Pertinent past medical history?
PROCTOR: No pertinent medical history.
Student: Last oral intake?
PROCTOR: 3 hours ago.
Student: Events leading up to the incident?
PROCTOR: The patient was at work in an office.

▼ Perform the Focused Physical Examination

Student: I am performing the focused physical examination.
PROCTOR: Noted.
Student: Have you seen a physician concerning your pregnancy?
PROCTOR: No.
Student: Have you passed any tissue other than blood?
PROCTOR: No.
Student: I am assessing the abdomen for DCAP-BTLS. This acronym stands for deformities, contusions, abrasions, punctures, penetrations, paradoxical motion in the chest, and burns, tenderness, lacerations, and swelling. I am assessing all four quadrants. Do I find any problems?
PROCTOR: No.
Student: I am assessing the genitalia/perineum as necessary for DCAP-BTLS.
PROCTOR: There is heavy bleeding noted but no fetal tissue is evident.
Student: I am applying a pad and treating for shock.
PROCTOR: Noted.
Student: I will check the blood glucose level.
PROCTOR: It is 104 mg/dL.

▼ Baseline Vital Signs

Student: What are the patient's baseline vital signs, including blood pressure, pulse, respirations, pulse oximetry, and level of consciousness?
PROCTOR: Blood pressure, 98/62 mm Hg; pulse rate, 122 beats/min; respirations, 28 breaths/min; pulse oximetry reading, 97%; and the patient is alert.

▼ Interventions

Student: I will continue to provide oxygen, position for shock, maintain temperature, and transport.
PROCTOR: Noted.
ALS Student: I will apply basic life support (BLS) interventions, plus the following: establish two large-bore IVs and maintain a blood pressure of 90 mm Hg.
ALS Proctor: Noted.

▼ Reevaluate Transport Decision

Student: The patient is a high priority and is a load-and-go.
PROCTOR: Noted.

▼ Detailed Physical Examination

Possible Answer #1
Student: I would not do a detailed physical exam.
PROCTOR: Noted. (Go to "Radio Report.")

Possible Answer #2
Student: I am conducting the detailed physical exam. I am looking for DCAP-BTLS.
PROCTOR: Noted. The detailed physical exam will be performed during transport.

► **Assess the Head**

Student: I am assessing the head. Do I find any DCAP-BTLS? Do I find any evidence of Battle's sign or raccoon eyes?
PROCTOR: No.

► **Inspect and Palpate the Head and Ears**

Student: I am assessing the head and ears.
PROCTOR: There are no obvious injuries.

► **Assess the Eyes**

Student: I am assessing the eyes. Are the pupils equal, round, and regular in size, and react properly to light (PEARRL)?
PROCTOR: They are PEARRL.

► **Assess the Facial Area Including Oral and Nasal Areas**

Student: I am assessing the face, nose, and mouth. Do I see any discharge or hear any obstructions?
PROCTOR: No.

► **Assess the Neck**

► **Inspect and Palpate the Neck**

Student: I am assessing the neck for DCAP-BTLS.
PROCTOR: There are no obvious injuries.

► **Assess for Jugular Vein Distention**

Student: Do I find any jugular vein distention (JVD)?
PROCTOR: No.

► **Assess for Tracheal Deviation**

Student: Do I see any tracheal deviation?
PROCTOR: No.

► **Assess the Chest**

Student: I am assessing the chest for DCAP-BTLS.
PROCTOR: Noted.

► **Inspect**

Student: What do I see when I look at the chest?
PROCTOR: There are no obvious injuries.
Student: Is the chest symmetric?
PROCTOR: Yes.

► **Palpate**

Student: When I touch the chest, do I feel crepitus or a flail segment?
PROCTOR: No.

► **Auscultate**

Student: Are lung sounds present in all fields?
PROCTOR: Yes.
Student: Do I hear any sucking sounds from the chest?
PROCTOR: No.

► **Assess the Abdomen/Pelvis**

► **Assess the Abdomen**

Student: I am assessing the abdomen for DCAP-BTLS. I am assessing all four quadrants. Do I find any problems?
PROCTOR: The patient has point tenderness in the lower middle abdomen.

► **Assess the Pelvis**

Student: I am assessing the pelvis for DCAP-BTLS. Is the pelvis stable?
PROCTOR: Yes.

► **Assess the Genitalia/Perineum as Needed (Verbalize in Training)**

Student: I am assessing the genitalia/perineum as necessary for DCAP-BTLS.
PROCTOR: There is heavy bleeding noted.
Student: I will add pads as necessary.
PROCTOR: Noted.

► **Assess the Extremities**

► **Inspect**

Student: I am assessing the lower and upper extremities for DCAP-BTLS. Do I find anything?
PROCTOR: No.

► **Palpate**

Student: Do I feel anything unusual?
PROCTOR: No.

► **Assess Motor, Sensory, and Circulatory Function**

Student: I am checking for DCAP-BTLS, motor and sensory function, and pulses. Right leg?
PROCTOR: Negative DCAP-BTLS. Motor and sensory functions are present. Pulses are present.

Student: Left leg?
PROCTOR: Negative DCAP-BTLS. Motor and sensory functions are present. Pulses are present.
Student: Right arm?
PROCTOR: Negative DCAP-BTLS. Motor and sensory functions are present. Pulses are present.
Student: Left arm?
PROCTOR: Negative DCAP-BTLS. Motor and sensory functions are present. Pulses are present.

Assess the Posterior

Student: We will not check the back.
PROCTOR: Noted.

Manage Secondary Injuries/Wounds

Student: I would direct my partner to monitor vital signs.
PROCTOR: Noted.

Reassess Interventions

Student: I will reassess my interventions: oxygen, treat for shock, and transport.
PROCTOR: Noted.
ALS Student: I will reassess BLS interventions, plus the following: two large-bore IVs flowing per local protocol.
ALS Proctor: Noted.

Critical Criteria:
- ❑ Did not obtain medical direction or verbalize standing orders for medical interventions
- ❑ Administered a dangerous or inappropriate intervention
- ❑ Did not ask questions about the present illness
- ❑ Did not differentiate patient's need for transportation versus continued assessment at the scene

Radio Report

(Provided by the student.)
PROCTOR: Noted.

Ongoing Assessment

Repeat the Initial Assessment

Student: I will repeat the initial assessment.
PROCTOR: Noted. (Reflected in "Repeat Vital Signs.")

Repeat Vital Signs

Student: I will reassess vital signs and mental status.
PROCTOR: Blood pressure, 94/60 mm Hg; pulse rate, 126 beats/min; respirations, 28 breaths/min; pulse oximetry reading, 98%; and the patient is alert.
Student: The vital signs have not changed significantly.
PROCTOR: Noted.

Check Interventions

Student: I will check my interventions: oxygen, check vital signs, and treat for shock.
PROCTOR: Noted.
ALS Student: I will check BLS interventions, plus the following: manage the two large-bore IVs.
ALS Proctor: Noted.

Repeat the Focused Assessment

Student: I will repeat the focused assessment.
PROCTOR: Noted.

Critical Criteria:
- ❑ Did not obtain medical direction or verbalize standing orders for medical interventions
- ❑ Administered a dangerous or inappropriate intervention

Handoff Report to Emergency Department Staff

Student: There was no change during transport.
PROCTOR: Noted.

Critical Criteria

(Inform the student of items missed, if any.)

❑ Pass ❑ Fail Date: ____________________

Proctor Comments: ____________________

Notes

CASE 109

Dispatch Information

PROCTOR: EMS 10, respond to a 4-year-old who has drunk a bottle of cold medicine. He is conscious and breathing.

Pre-Scene Action (BSI)

Student: I am wearing nonlatex gloves and safety glasses.
PROCTOR: Noted.

> **Critical Criteria:**
> ❑ Did not take, or verbalize, body substance isolation (BSI) precautions when necessary

Scene Size-up

Scene Safety

Student: Is the scene safe?
PROCTOR: Yes.

Mechanism of Injury/Nature of Illness

Student: What is the nature of the illness?
PROCTOR: Cold medication overdose.

Number of Patients

Student: How many patients are there?
PROCTOR: One.

Additional Resources

Student: I would call for advanced life support (ALS) assistance.
PROCTOR: Noted.

C-Spine Stabilization

Student: I would not stabilize the cervical spine (c-spine).
PROCTOR: Noted.

> **Critical Criteria:**
> ❑ Did not determine scene safety

Initial Assessment

General Impression

Student: My general impression is that the patient's condition is unstable.
PROCTOR: Noted.

Responsiveness/Level of Consciousness

Student: What is the patient's level of consciousness?
PROCTOR: Very tired.

Chief Complaint/Apparent Life Threats

Student: What is the patient's chief complaint?
PROCTOR: The patient is obviously drowsy.

Assess the Airway and Breathing

Student: Is the airway open? Is the patient breathing?
PROCTOR: Yes, the airway is open and the patient is breathing.

Assessment

Student: What are the rate and the quality of breathing?
PROCTOR: Rate: Tachypneic. Quality: Shallow.

Provide Oxygen

Student: I am applying oxygen at 15 L/min via pediatric nonrebreathing mask.
PROCTOR: Noted.

Ensure Adequate Ventilation

Student: The patient has adequate ventilations at this time.
PROCTOR: Noted.

Assess Circulation

Student: I am assessing the patient's circulation.
PROCTOR: Noted.

Assess for and Control Major Bleeding

Student: Do I find any major bleeding?
PROCTOR: No.

Assess the Pulse

Student: What are the rate and the quality of pulses?
PROCTOR: Rate: Tachycardic. Quality: Thready.

Assess the Skin

Student: I am assessing the skin. What are the color, temperature, and condition of the skin?
PROCTOR: Color: Normal. Temperature: Warm. Condition: Moist.

Identify Priority Patients/Make Transport Decision

Student: The patient is a high priority and is a load-and-go. I will begin packaging and transport.
PROCTOR: Noted.

> **Critical Criteria:**
> ❑ Did not provide high concentration of oxygen
> ❑ Did not find or manage problems associated with airway, breathing, hemorrhage or shock (hypoperfusion)
> ❑ Did not differentiate patient's need for transportation versus continued assessment at the scene
> ❑ Did detailed or focused history/physical examination before assessing the airway, breathing and circulation

Focused History and Physical Examination/Rapid Assessment

Select the Appropriate Assessment (Focused or Rapid)

Student: I am selecting the focused assessment.
PROCTOR: Noted.

SAMPLE History

Student: At this time I will gather a SAMPLE history from the patient or family. What are the patient's signs and symptoms?
PROCTOR: Poisoning/overdose.
 Student: What was the substance?
 PROCTOR: Vicks DayQuil® Cold and Flu Multi-symptom Relief, 10 fluid ounce bottle size.
 Student: When did the child ingest the medicine?
 PROCTOR: It was 30 minutes ago.
 Student: How much did the child ingest?
 PROCTOR: The bottle is just over half full (less than 5 fluid ounces).
 Student: Over what time period?
 PROCTOR: Over a few minutes.
 Student: Interventions: Have you done anything to make this better?
 PROCTOR: No, the babysitter called the mother.
 Student: What is the child's weight?
 PROCTOR: 45 pounds.
Student: Allergies?
PROCTOR: No allergies.
Student: Medications?
PROCTOR: No medications.
Student: Pertinent past medical history?
PROCTOR: No pertinent medical history.
Student: Last oral intake?
PROCTOR: 2 hours ago.
Student: Events leading up to the incident?
PROCTOR: The patient was playing when the babysitter went to use the restroom. The child went into another restroom and drank the cold medicine.

Perform the Focused Physical Examination

Student: I am performing the focused physical examination.
PROCTOR: Noted.

Student: I will bring the bottle of DayQuil® with the patient to the emergency department.
PROCTOR: Noted.
Student: What is his blood glucose level?
PROCTOR: 88 mg/dL.
Student: I will monitor the airway and be ready for vomiting.
PROCTOR: Noted.
Student: I will contact medical control and request a poison control consult for advice.
PROCTOR: Noted.

▼ Baseline Vital Signs

Student: What are the patient's baseline vital signs, including blood pressure, pulse, respirations, pulse oximetry, and level of consciousness?
PROCTOR: Blood pressure, N/A; pulse rate, 124 beats/min; respirations, 28 breaths/min; pulse oximetry reading, N/A; and the patient is very sleepy.

▼ Interventions

Student: I will apply oxygen, begin rapid transport, contact medical control, and follow poison control recommendations.
PROCTOR: Noted.
ALS Student: I will apply basic life support (BLS) interventions, plus the following: IV access, cardiac monitor, and local protocol/poison control recommendations.
ALS Proctor: Noted. The cardiac monitor shows sinus tachycardia.

▼ Reevaluate Transport Decision

Student: The patient is a high priority and is a load-and-go.
PROCTOR: Noted.

▼ Detailed Physical Examination

Possible Answer #1
Student: I would not do a detailed physical exam.
PROCTOR: Noted. (Go to "Radio Report.")

Possible Answer #2
Student: I am conducting the detailed physical exam. I am looking for DCAP-BTLS. This acronym stands for deformities, contusions, abrasions, punctures, penetrations, paradoxical motion in the chest, and burns, tenderness, lacerations, and swelling.
PROCTOR: Noted. The detailed physical exam will be performed during transport.

- **Assess the Head**

Student: I am assessing the head. Do I find any DCAP-BTLS? Do I find any evidence of Battle's sign or raccoon eyes?
PROCTOR: No.

  - **Inspect and Palpate the Head and Ears**

Student: I am assessing the head and ears.
PROCTOR: There are no obvious injuries.

  - **Assess the Eyes**

Student: I am assessing the eyes. Are the pupils equal, round, and regular in size, and react properly to light (PEARRL)?
PROCTOR: They are sluggish.

  - **Assess the Facial Area Including Oral and Nasal Areas**

Student: I am assessing the face, nose, and mouth. Do I see any discharge or hear any obstructions?
PROCTOR: No.

- **Assess the Neck**
  - **Inspect and Palpate the Neck**

Student: I am assessing the neck for DCAP-BTLS.
PROCTOR: There are no obvious injuries.

  - **Assess for Jugular Vein Distention**

Student: Do I find any jugular vein distention (JVD)?
PROCTOR: No.

  - **Assess for Tracheal Deviation**

Student: Do I see any tracheal deviation?
PROCTOR: No.

- **Assess the Chest**

Student: I am assessing the chest for DCAP-BTLS.
PROCTOR: Noted.

  - **Inspect**

Student: What do I see when I look at the chest?
PROCTOR: There are no obvious injuries.
Student: Is the chest symmetric?
PROCTOR: Yes.

  - **Palpate**

Student: When I touch the chest, do I feel crepitus or a flail segment?
PROCTOR: No.

  - **Auscultate**

Student: Are lung sounds present in all fields?
PROCTOR: Yes.
Student: Do I hear any sucking sounds from the chest?
PROCTOR: No.

- **Assess the Abdomen/Pelvis**
  - **Assess the Abdomen**

Student: I am assessing the abdomen for DCAP-BTLS. I am assessing all four quadrants. Do I find any problems?
PROCTOR: No.

  - **Assess the Pelvis**

Student: I am assessing the pelvis for DCAP-BTLS. Is the pelvis stable?
PROCTOR: Yes.

  - **Assess the Genitalia/Perineum as Needed (Verbalize in Training)**

Student: I am assessing the genitalia/perineum as necessary for DCAP-BTLS.
PROCTOR: The area is unremarkable.

- **Assess the Extremities**
  - **Inspect**

Student: I am assessing the lower and upper extremities for DCAP-BTLS. Do I find anything?
PROCTOR: No.

  - **Palpate**

Student: Do I feel anything unusual?
PROCTOR: No.

  - **Assess Motor, Sensory, and Circulatory Function**

Student: I am checking for DCAP-BTLS, motor and sensory function, and pulses. Right leg?
PROCTOR: Negative DCAP-BTLS. Motor and sensory functions are present. Pulses are present.
Student: Left leg?
PROCTOR: Negative DCAP-BTLS. Motor and sensory functions are present. Pulses are present.
Student: Right arm?
PROCTOR: Negative DCAP-BTLS. Motor and sensory functions are present. Pulses are present.
Student: Left arm?
PROCTOR: Negative DCAP-BTLS. Motor and sensory functions are present. Pulses are present.

- **Assess the Posterior**

Student: We will check the back.
PROCTOR: Noted.

  - **Assess the Thorax**

Student: I am assessing the thorax. Do I find injuries?
PROCTOR: No.

▸ **Assess the Lumbar Area**

Student: I am assessing the flanks and lumbar area. Do I find injuries?

PROCTOR: No.

▸ **Assess the Entire Backside**

Student: I am assessing the entire backside. Do I find injuries?

PROCTOR: No.

▸ **Manage Secondary Injuries/Wounds**

Student: I would direct my partner to monitor the airway.

PROCTOR: Noted.

▸ **Reassess Interventions**

Student: I will reassess my interventions: oxygen, monitor the airway, have suction ready, rapid transport, contact medical control, and carry out poison control recommendations.

PROCTOR: Noted.

ALS Student: I will reassess BLS interventions, plus the following: IVs, cardiac monitor, and poison control recommendations.

ALS Proctor: Noted. The cardiac monitor shows sinus tachycardia.

Critical Criteria:

- ❑ Did not obtain medical direction or verbalize standing orders for medical interventions
- ❑ Administered a dangerous or inappropriate intervention
- ❑ Did not ask questions about the present illness
- ❑ Did not differentiate patient's need for transportation versus continued assessment at the scene

Radio Report

(Provided by the student.)

PROCTOR: Noted.

Ongoing Assessment

Repeat the Initial Assessment

Student: I will repeat the initial assessment.

PROCTOR: Noted. (Reflected in "Repeat Vital Signs.")

Repeat Vital Signs

Student: I will reassess vital signs and mental status.

PROCTOR: Blood pressure, N/A; pulse rate, 124 beats/min; respirations, 28 breaths/min; pulse oximetry reading, N/A; and the patient is very sleepy.

Student: The vital signs have not significantly changed.

PROCTOR: Noted.

Check Interventions

Student: I will check my interventions: oxygen, monitor the airway, have suction ready, rapid transport, contact medical control, and poison control recommendations.

PROCTOR: Noted.

ALS Student: I will check BLS interventions, plus the following: IVs, cardiac monitor, and carry out poison control recommendations.

ALS Proctor: Noted. The cardiac monitor shows sinus tachycardia.

Repeat the Focused Assessment

Student: I will repeat the focused assessment.

PROCTOR: Noted.

Critical Criteria:

- ❑ Did not obtain medical direction or verbalize standing orders for medical interventions
- ❑ Administered a dangerous or inappropriate intervention

Handoff Report to Emergency Department Staff

Student: There was no change in the patient's condition during transport.

PROCTOR: Noted.

Critical Criteria

(Inform the student of items missed, if any.)

❑ Pass ❑ Fail Date: ____________________

Proctor Comments: ____________________

____

____

CASE 109

Notes

Dispatch Information

PROCTOR: EMS 10, respond to a 64-year-old male who is complaining of chest pain. He is conscious and breathing.

Pre-Scene Action (BSI)

Student: I am wearing nonlatex gloves and safety glasses.
PROCTOR: Noted.

Critical Criteria:
- ❑ Did not take, or verbalize, body substance isolation (BSI) precautions when necessary

Scene Size-up

Scene Safety

Student: Is the scene safe?
PROCTOR: Yes.

Mechanism of Injury/Nature of Illness

Student: What is the nature of the illness?
PROCTOR: Chest pain experienced when shoveling snow.

Number of Patients

Student: How many patients are there?
PROCTOR: One.

Additional Resources

Student: I would call for advanced life support (ALS) assistance.
PROCTOR: Noted.

C-Spine Stabilization

Student: I would not stabilize the cervical spine (c-spine).
PROCTOR: Noted.

Critical Criteria:
- ❑ Did not determine scene safety

Initial Assessment

General Impression

Student: My general impression is that the patient's condition is unstable.
PROCTOR: Noted.

Responsiveness/Level of Consciousness

Student: What is the patient's level of consciousness?
PROCTOR: Alert.

Chief Complaint/Apparent Life Threats

Student: What is the patient's chief complaint?
PROCTOR: The patient is complaining of chest pain.

Assess the Airway and Breathing

Student: Is the airway open? Is the patient breathing?
PROCTOR: Yes, the airway is open and the patient is breathing.

Assessment

Student: What are the rate and the quality of breathing?
PROCTOR: Rate: Within normal limits. Quality: Normal.

Provide Oxygen

Student: I am applying oxygen at 15 L/min via nonrebreathing mask.
PROCTOR: Noted.

Ensure Adequate Ventilation

Student: The patient has adequate ventilations at this time.
PROCTOR: Noted.

Assess Circulation

Student: I am assessing the patient's circulation.
PROCTOR: Noted.

Assess for and Control Major Bleeding

Student: Do I find any major bleeding?
PROCTOR: No.

Assess the Pulse

Student: What are the rate and the quality of pulses?
PROCTOR: Rate: Tachycardic. Quality: Thready.

Assess the Skin

Student: I am assessing the skin. What are the color, temperature, and condition of the skin?
PROCTOR: Color: Pale. Temperature: Cool. Condition: Moist.

Identify Priority Patients/Make Transport Decision

Student: The patient is a high priority and is a load-and-go. I will begin packaging and transport.
PROCTOR: Noted.

Critical Criteria:
- ❑ Did not provide high concentration of oxygen
- ❑ Did not find or manage problems associated with airway, breathing, hemorrhage or shock (hypoperfusion)
- ❑ Did not differentiate patient's need for transportation versus continued assessment at the scene
- ❑ Did detailed or focused history/physical examination before assessing the airway, breathing and circulation

Focused History and Physical Examination/Rapid Assessment

Select the Appropriate Assessment (Focused or Rapid)

Student: I am selecting the focused assessment.
PROCTOR: Noted.

SAMPLE History

Student: At this time I will gather a SAMPLE history from the patient or family. What are the patient's signs and symptoms?
PROCTOR: Cardiac.

> **Student:** Onset: What were you doing when this started?
> **PROCTOR:** Shoveling snow.
> **Student:** Provokes: What makes your condition worse or better?
> **PROCTOR:** Nitroglycerin and rest make it better.
> **Student:** Quality: Can you describe your pain?
> **PROCTOR:** Crushing.
> **Student:** Radiates: Do you have pain any where else?
> **PROCTOR:** No.
> **Student:** Severity: On a scale of 1 to 10 with 10 being the worst possible, how would you rate your pain?
> **PROCTOR:** 3 to 4.
> **Student:** Time: How long has this been going on?
> **PROCTOR:** 10 minutes.
> **Student:** Interventions: Have you done anything to make this better?
> **PROCTOR:** The patient has taken two nitroglycerin pills.

Student: Allergies?
PROCTOR: No allergies.
Student: Medications?
PROCTOR: Nitroglycerin.
Student: Pertinent past medical history?
PROCTOR: Angina, one previous attack a year ago. He felt scared this time but is getting relief.
Student: Last oral intake?
PROCTOR: 2 hours ago.
Student: Events leading up to the incident?
PROCTOR: The patient was shoveling snow.

Perform the Focused Physical Examination

Student: I am performing the focused physical examination.
PROCTOR: Noted.

Student: What are the patient's lung sounds?
PROCTOR: They are clear bilaterally.
Student: Does the patient have any edema evident in any extremity?
PROCTOR: No.

▼ Baseline Vital Signs

Student: What are the patient's baseline vital signs, including blood pressure, pulse, respirations, pulse oximetry, blood glucose level, and level of consciousness?
PROCTOR: Blood pressure, 130/80 mm Hg; pulse rate, 72 beats/min; respirations, 16 breaths/min; pulse oximetry reading, 96%; blood glucose level, 114 mg/dL; and the patient is alert.

▼ Interventions

Student: I will apply oxygen, loosen tight-fitting clothing, contact medical control for the third dose of nitroglycerin, transport the patient in the position of comfort, and give baby aspirin if permitted by local protocol.
PROCTOR: Noted.
ALS Student: I will apply basic life support (BLS) interventions, plus the following: IV access, cardiac monitor, 12-lead ECG, and advanced cardiac life support (ACLS) or local protocol.
ALS Proctor: Noted. The cardiac monitor shows normal sinus rhythm and there are no significant findings on the 12-lead ECG.

▼ Reevaluate Transport Decision

Student: The patient is a high priority and is a load-and-go.
PROCTOR: Noted.

▼ Detailed Physical Examination

Possible Answer #1
Student: I would not do a detailed physical exam.
PROCTOR: Noted. (Go to "Radio Report.")

Possible Answer #2
Student: I am conducting the detailed physical exam. I am looking for DCAP-BTLS. This acronym stands for deformities, contusions, abrasions, punctures, penetrations, paradoxical motion in the chest, and burns, tenderness, lacerations, and swelling.
PROCTOR: Noted. The detailed physical exam will be performed during transport.

► **Assess the Head**
Student: I am assessing the head. Do I find any DCAP-BTLS? Do I find any evidence of Battle's sign or raccoon eyes?
PROCTOR: No.

► **Inspect and Palpate the Head and Ears**
Student: I am assessing the head and ears.
PROCTOR: There are no obvious injuries.

► **Assess the Eyes**
Student: I am assessing the eyes. Are the pupils equal, round, and regular in size, and react properly to light (PEARRL)?
PROCTOR: They are PEARRL.

► **Assess the Facial Area Including Oral and Nasal Areas**
Student: I am assessing the face, nose, and mouth. Do I see any discharge or hear any obstructions?
PROCTOR: No.

► **Assess the Neck**

► **Inspect and Palpate the Neck**
Student: I am assessing the neck for DCAP-BTLS.
PROCTOR: There are no obvious injuries.

► **Assess for Jugular Vein Distention**
Student: Do I find any jugular vein distention (JVD)?
PROCTOR: No.

► **Assess for Tracheal Deviation**
Student: Do I see any tracheal deviation?
PROCTOR: No.

► **Assess the Chest**
Student: I am assessing the chest for DCAP-BTLS.
PROCTOR: Noted.

► **Inspect**
Student: What do I see when I look at the chest?
PROCTOR: There are no obvious injuries.
Student: Is the chest symmetric?
PROCTOR: Yes.

► **Palpate**
Student: When I touch the chest, do I feel crepitus or a flail segment?
PROCTOR: No.

► **Auscultate**
Student: Are lung sounds present in all fields?
PROCTOR: Yes.
Student: Do I hear any sucking sounds from the chest?
PROCTOR: No.

► **Assess the Abdomen/Pelvis**

► **Assess the Abdomen**
Student: I am assessing the abdomen for DCAP-BTLS. I am assessing all four quadrants. Do I find any problems?
PROCTOR: No.

► **Assess the Pelvis**
Student: I am assessing the pelvis for DCAP-BTLS. Is the pelvis stable?
PROCTOR: Yes.

► **Assess the Genitalia/Perineum as Needed (Verbalize in Training)**
Student: I am assessing the genitalia/perineum as necessary for DCAP-BTLS.
PROCTOR: The area is unremarkable.

► **Assess the Extremities**

► **Inspect**
Student: I am assessing the lower and upper extremities for DCAP-BTLS. Do I find anything?
PROCTOR: No.

► **Palpate**
Student: Do I feel anything unusual?
PROCTOR: No.

► **Assess Motor, Sensory, and Circulatory Function**
Student: I am checking for DCAP-BTLS, motor and sensory function, and pulses. Right leg?
PROCTOR: Negative DCAP-BTLS. Motor and sensory functions are present. Pulses are present.
Student: Left leg?
PROCTOR: Negative DCAP-BTLS. Motor and sensory functions are present. Pulses are present.
Student: Right arm?
PROCTOR: Negative DCAP-BTLS. Motor and sensory functions are present. Pulses are present.
Student: Left arm?
PROCTOR: Negative DCAP-BTLS. Motor and sensory functions are present. Pulses are present.

► **Assess the Posterior**
Student: We will check the back.
PROCTOR: Noted.

► **Assess the Thorax**
Student: I am assessing the thorax. Do I find injuries?
PROCTOR: No.

► **Assess the Lumbar Area**
Student: I am assessing the flanks and lumbar area. Do I find injuries?
PROCTOR: No.

► **Assess the Entire Backside**

Student: I am assessing the entire backside. Do I find injuries?

PROCTOR: No.

► **Manage Secondary Injuries/Wounds**

Student: I would direct my partner to continue providing oxygen and monitor the patient.

PROCTOR: Noted.

► **Reassess Interventions**

Student: I will reassess interventions: oxygen, loosen tight-fitting clothing, see if pain improved with nitroglycerin, and transport in the position of comfort.

PROCTOR: Noted.

ALS Student: I will reassess BLS interventions, plus the following: maintain IV access, cardiac monitor, 12-lead ECG, and ACLS or local protocol.

ALS Proctor: Noted. The cardiac monitor shows normal sinus rhythm and there are no significant findings on the 12-lead ECG.

Critical Criteria:

- ❑ Did not obtain medical direction or verbalize standing orders for medical interventions
- ❑ Administered a dangerous or inappropriate intervention
- ❑ Did not ask questions about the present illness
- ❑ Did not differentiate patient's need for transportation versus continued assessment at the scene

Radio Report

(Provided by the student.)

PROCTOR: Noted.

Ongoing Assessment

Repeat the Initial Assessment

Student: I will repeat the initial assessment.

PROCTOR: Noted. (Reflected in "Repeat Vital Signs.")

Repeat Vital Signs

Student: I will reassess vital signs and mental status.

PROCTOR: Blood pressure, 112/74 mm Hg; pulse rate, 68 beats/min; respirations, 16 breaths/min; pulse oximetry reading, 97%; blood glucose level, 114 mg/dL; and the patient is alert.

Student: The vital signs have not significantly changed.

PROCTOR: Noted.

Check Interventions

Student: I will check my interventions: oxygen, loosen tight-fitting clothing, and transport the patient in the position of comfort.

PROCTOR: Noted.

ALS Student: I will check BLS interventions, plus the following: maintain IV access, cardiac monitor, 12-lead ECG, and ACLS or local protocol.

ALS Proctor: Noted. The cardiac monitor shows normal sinus rhythm and there are no significant findings on the 12-lead-ECG.

Repeat the Focused Assessment

Student: I will repeat the focused assessment.

PROCTOR: Noted.

Critical Criteria:

- ❑ Did not obtain medical direction or verbalize standing orders for medical interventions
- ❑ Administered a dangerous or inappropriate intervention

Handoff Report to Emergency Department Staff

Student: There was no change in the patient's condition during transport.

PROCTOR: Noted.

Critical Criteria

(Inform the student of items missed, if any.)

❑ Pass ❑ Fail Date: ______________________

Proctor Comments: ______________________

____

____

Notes

Dispatch Information

PROCTOR: EMS 10, respond to an 8-year-old male who is complaining of being sick. He is conscious and breathing.

Pre-scene Action (BSI)

Student: I am wearing nonlatex gloves, mask, and safety glasses.
PROCTOR: Noted.

Critical Criteria:
- ❑ Did not take, or verbalize, body substance isolation (BSI) precautions when necessary

Scene Size-up

Scene Safety
Student: Is the scene safe?
PROCTOR: Yes.

Mechanism of Injury/Nature of Illness
Student: What is the nature of the illness?
PROCTOR: The patient has had a fever of 101.5°F (38.6°C) for 3 days. He has a productive cough and is feeling weak.

Number of Patients
Student: How many patients are there?
PROCTOR: One.

Additional Resources
Student: I would not call for advanced life support (ALS) assistance.
PROCTOR: Noted.

C-Spine Stabilization
Student: I would not stabilize the cervical spine (c-spine).
PROCTOR: Noted.

Critical Criteria:
- ❑ Did not determine scene safety

Initial Assessment

General Impression
Student: My general impression is that the patient's condition is stable.
PROCTOR: Noted.

Responsiveness/Level of Consciousness
Student: What is the patient's level of consciousness?
PROCTOR: Alert.

Chief Complaint/Apparent Life Threats
Student: What is the patient's chief complaint?
PROCTOR: The patient is complaining of a fever of 101.5°F (38.6°C), a productive cough, and feeling weak.

Assess the Airway and Breathing
Student: Is the airway open? Is the patient breathing?
PROCTOR: Yes, the airway is open and the patient is breathing.

Assessment
Student: What are the rate and the quality of breathing?
PROCTOR: Rate: Tachypneic. Quality: Labored.

Provide Oxygen
Student: I am applying oxygen at 15 L/min via pediatric nonrebreathing mask.
PROCTOR: Noted.

Ensure Adequate Ventilation
Student: The patient has adequate ventilations at this time.
PROCTOR: Noted.

Assess Circulation
Student: I am assessing the patient's circulation.
PROCTOR: Noted.

Assess for and Control Major Bleeding
Student: Do I find any major bleeding?
PROCTOR: No.

Assess the Pulse
Student: What are the rate and the quality of pulses?
PROCTOR: Rate: Tachycardic. Quality: Thready.

Assess the Skin
Student: I am assessing the skin. What are the color, temperature, and condition of the skin?
PROCTOR: Color: Pale. Temperature: Hot. Condition: Dry.

Identify Priority Patients/Make Transport Decision
Student: The patient is a high priority and is a load-and-go. I will begin packaging and transport.
PROCTOR: Noted.

Critical Criteria:
- ❑ Did not provide high concentration of oxygen
- ❑ Did not find or manage problems associated with airway, breathing, hemorrhage or shock (hypoperfusion)
- ❑ Did not differentiate patient's need for transportation versus continued assessment at the scene
- ❑ Did detailed or focused history/physical examination before assessing the airway, breathing and circulation

Focused History and Physical Examination/Rapid Assessment

Select the Appropriate Assessment (Focused or Rapid)
Student: I am selecting the focused assessment.
PROCTOR: Noted.

SAMPLE History
Student: At this time I will gather a SAMPLE history from the patient or family. What are the patient's signs and symptoms?
PROCTOR: Sick call/respiratory.

> Student: Onset: What were you doing when this started?
> **PROCTOR:** The condition has been getting worse for 3 days.
> Student: Provokes: What makes your condition worse or better?
> **PROCTOR:** The patient has not been eating or drinking, which is making the condition worse.
> Student: Quality: Can you describe your pain?
> **PROCTOR:** None, except when he coughs his muscles are sore.
> Student: Radiates: Do you have pain anywhere else?
> **PROCTOR:** No.
> Student: Severity: On a scale of 1 to 10 with 10 being the worst possible, how would you rate your distress?
> **PROCTOR:** 4.
> Student: Time: How long has this been going on?
> **PROCTOR:** 3 days.
> Student: Interventions: Have you done anything to make this better?
> **PROCTOR:** The patient has taken cold medications.

Student: Allergies?
PROCTOR: No allergies.
Student: Medications?
PROCTOR: Cold medications.
Student: Pertinent past medical history?
PROCTOR: No pertinent medical history.
Student: Last oral intake?
PROCTOR: 6 hours ago.
Student: Events leading up to the incident?
PROCTOR: The patient has been getting worse for 3 days.

Perform the Focused Physical Examination
Student: I am performing the focused physical examination.
PROCTOR: Noted.
Student: I will take his temperature.
PROCTOR: It is 100.3°F (37.9°C).

Student: What is the skin turgor?
PROCTOR: Normal.
Student: I will listen to the lung sounds.
PROCTOR: He has rhonchi.
Student: I will check his blood glucose level.
PROCTOR: It is 92 mg/dL.

▼ Baseline Vital Signs

Student: What are the patient's baseline vital signs, including blood pressure, pulse, respirations, pulse oximetry, and level of consciousness?
PROCTOR: Blood pressure, 90/50 mm Hg; pulse rate, 120 beats/min; respirations, 28 breaths/min; pulse oximetry reading, 97%; and the patient is alert.

▼ Interventions

Student: I will apply oxygen and transport the patient in the position of comfort.
PROCTOR: Noted.
ALS Student: I will apply basic life support (BLS) interventions, plus the following: establish IV access, perform cardiac monitoring, and follow the local protocol.
ALS Proctor: Noted. The cardiac monitor shows sinus tachycardia.

▼ Reevaluate Transport Decision

Student: The patient is a low priority and is not a load-and-go.
PROCTOR: Noted.

▼ Detailed Physical Examination

Possible Answer #1
Student: I would not do a detailed physical exam.
PROCTOR: Noted. (Go to "Radio Report.")

Possible Answer #2
Student: I am conducting the detailed physical exam. I am looking for DCAP-BTLS. This acronym stands for deformities, contusions, abrasions, punctures, penetrations, paradoxical motion in the chest, and burns, tenderness, lacerations, and swelling.
PROCTOR: Noted. The detailed physical exam will be performed during transport.

- **Assess the Head**

Student: I am assessing the head. Do I find any DCAP-BTLS? Do I find any evidence of Battle's sign or raccoon eyes?
PROCTOR: No.

- **Inspect and Palpate the Head and Ears**

Student: I am assessing the head and ears.
PROCTOR: There are no obvious injuries.

- **Assess the Eyes**

Student: I am assessing the eyes. Are the pupils equal, round, and regular in size, and react properly to light (PEARRL)?
PROCTOR: They are PEARRL.

- **Assess the Facial Area Including Oral and Nasal Areas**

Student: I am assessing the face, nose, and mouth. Do I see any discharge or hear any obstructions?
PROCTOR: No.

- **Assess the Neck**
- **Inspect and Palpate the Neck**

Student: I am assessing the neck for DCAP-BTLS.
PROCTOR: There are no obvious injuries.

- **Assess for Jugular Vein Distention**

Student: Do I find any jugular vein distention (JVD)?
PROCTOR: No.

- **Assess for Tracheal Deviation**

Student: Do I see any tracheal deviation?
PROCTOR: No.

- **Assess the Chest**

Student: I am assessing the chest for DCAP-BTLS.
PROCTOR: Noted.

- **Inspect**

Student: What do I see when I look at the chest?
PROCTOR: There are no obvious injuries.
Student: Is the chest symmetric?
PROCTOR: Yes.

- **Palpate**

Student: When I touch the chest, do I feel crepitus or a flail segment?
PROCTOR: No.

- **Auscultate**

Student: Are lung sounds present in all fields?
PROCTOR: Yes.
Student: Do I hear any sucking sounds from the chest?
PROCTOR: No.

- **Assess the Abdomen/Pelvis**
- **Assess the Abdomen**

Student: I am assessing the abdomen for DCAP-BTLS. I am assessing all four quadrants. Do I find any problems?
PROCTOR: No.

- **Assess the Pelvis**

Student: I am assessing the pelvis for DCAP-BTLS. Is the pelvis stable?
PROCTOR: Yes.

- **Assess the Genitalia/Perineum as Needed (Verbalize in Training)**

Student: I am assessing the genitalia/perineum as necessary for DCAP-BTLS.
PROCTOR: The area is unremarkable.

- **Assess the Extremities**
- **Inspect**

Student: I am assessing the lower and upper extremities for DCAP-BTLS. Do I find anything?
PROCTOR: No.

- **Palpate**

Student: Do I feel anything unusual?
PROCTOR: No.

- **Assess Motor, Sensory, and Circulatory Function**

Student: I am checking for DCAP-BTLS, motor and sensory function, and pulses. Right leg?
PROCTOR: Negative DCAP-BTLS. Motor and sensory functions are present. Pulses are present.
Student: Left leg?
PROCTOR: Negative DCAP-BTLS. Motor and sensory functions are present. Pulses are present.
Student: Right arm?
PROCTOR: Negative DCAP-BTLS. Motor and sensory functions are present. Pulses are present.
Student: Left arm?
PROCTOR: Negative DCAP-BTLS. Motor and sensory functions are present. Pulses are present.

- **Assess the Posterior**

Student: We will now check the back.
PROCTOR: Noted.

- **Assess the Thorax**

Student: I am assessing the thorax. Do I find injuries?
PROCTOR: No.

- **Assess the Lumbar Area**

Student: I am assessing the flanks and lumbar area. Do I find injuries?
PROCTOR: No.

- **Assess the Entire Backside**

Student: I am assessing the entire backside. Do I find injuries?
PROCTOR: No.

- **Manage Secondary Injuries/Wounds**

Student: I would direct my partner to reassure the patient.
PROCTOR: Noted.

▸ **Reassess Interventions**

Student: I will reassess my interventions: oxygen and transport the patient in the position of comfort.

PROCTOR: Noted.

ALS Student: I will reassess BLS interventions, plus the following: IVs, cardiac monitor, and local protocol.

ALS Proctor: Noted. The cardiac monitor shows sinus tachycardia.

Critical Criteria:
- ❑ Did not obtain medical direction or verbalize standing orders for medical interventions
- ❑ Administered a dangerous or inappropriate intervention
- ❑ Did not ask questions about the present illness
- ❑ Did not differentiate patient's need for transportation versus continued assessment at the scene

Radio Report

(Provided by the student.)

PROCTOR: Noted.

Ongoing Assessment

Repeat the Initial Assessment

Student: I will repeat the initial assessment.

PROCTOR: Noted. (Reflected in "Repeat Vital Signs.")

Repeat Vital Signs

Student: I will reassess vital signs and mental status.

PROCTOR: Blood pressure, 94/50 mm Hg; pulse rate, 122 beats/min; respirations, 26 breaths/min; pulse oximetry reading, 99%; and the patient is alert.

Student: The vital signs have not significantly changed.

PROCTOR: Noted.

Check Interventions

Student: I will check my interventions: oxygen and transport the patient in the position of comfort.

PROCTOR: Noted.

ALS Student: I will check BLS interventions, plus the following: IVs, cardiac monitor, and local protocol.

ALS Proctor: Noted. The cardiac monitor shows sinus tachycardia.

Repeat the Focused Assessment

Student: I will repeat the focused assessment.

PROCTOR: Noted.

Critical Criteria:
- ❑ Did not obtain medical direction or verbalize standing orders for medical interventions
- ❑ Administered a dangerous or inappropriate intervention

Handoff Report to Emergency Department Staff

Student: There was no change during transport.

PROCTOR: Noted.

Critical Criteria

(Inform the student of items missed, if any.)

❑ Pass ❑ Fail Date: ____________________

Proctor Comments: ____________________

Notes

Dispatch Information

PROCTOR: EMS 10, respond to a 27-year-old female who is full term with her pregnancy, with heavy bleeding and without contractions. She is conscious and breathing.

Pre-Scene Action (BSI)

Student: I am wearing nonlatex gloves, safety glasses, mask, and gown.
PROCTOR: Noted.

Critical Criteria:
- ❑ Did not take, or verbalize, body substance isolation (BSI) precautions when necessary

Scene Size-up

Scene Safety

Student: Is the scene safe?
PROCTOR: Yes.

Mechanism of Injury/Nature of Illness

Student: What is the nature of the illness?
PROCTOR: The patient is pregnant and complaining of heavy bleeding.

Number of Patients

Student: How many patients are there?
PROCTOR: One.

Additional Resources

Student: I would call for advanced life support (ALS) assistance.
PROCTOR: Noted.

C-Spine Stabilization

Student: I would not stabilize the cervical spine (c-spine).
PROCTOR: Noted.

Critical Criteria:
- ❑ Did not determine scene safety

Initial Assessment

General Impression

Student: My general impression is that the patient's condition is unstable.
PROCTOR: Noted.

Responsiveness/Level of Consciousness

Student: What is the patient's level of consciousness?
PROCTOR: Alert.

Chief Complaint/Apparent Life Threats

Student: What is the patient's chief complaint?
PROCTOR: The patient is complaining of heavy vaginal bleeding.

Assess the Airway and Breathing

Student: Is the airway open? Is the patient breathing?
PROCTOR: Yes, the airway is open and the patient is breathing.

Assessment

Student: What are the rate and the quality of breathing?
PROCTOR: Rate: Tachypneic. Quality: Deep.

Provide Oxygen

Student: I am applying oxygen at 15 L/min via nonrebreathing mask.
PROCTOR: Noted.

Ensure Adequate Ventilation

Student: The patient has adequate ventilations at this time.
PROCTOR: Noted.

Assess Circulation

Student: I am assessing the patient's circulation.
PROCTOR: Noted.

Assess for and Control Major Bleeding

Student: Do I find any major bleeding?
PROCTOR: Yes.
Student: I will position pads, treat for shock, and rapidly transport.
PROCTOR: Noted.

Assess the Pulse

Student: What is the rate and quality of pulses?
PROCTOR: Rate: Tachycardic. Quality: Thready.

Assess the Skin

Student: I am assessing the skin. What are the color, temperature, and condition of the skin?
PROCTOR: Color: Pale. Temperature: Cool. Condition: Diaphoretic.

Identify Priority Patients/Make Transport Decision

Student: The patient is a high priority and is a load-and-go. I will begin packaging and transport.
PROCTOR: Noted.

Critical Criteria:
- ❑ Did not provide high concentration of oxygen
- ❑ Did not find or manage problems associated with airway, breathing, hemorrhage or shock (hypoperfusion)
- ❑ Did not differentiate patient's need for transportation versus continued assessment at the scene
- ❑ Did detailed or focused history/physical examination before assessing the airway, breathing and circulation

Focused History and Physical Examination/Rapid Assessment

Select the Appropriate Assessment (Focused or Rapid)

Student: I am selecting the focused assessment.
PROCTOR: Noted.

SAMPLE History

Student: At this time I will gather a SAMPLE history from the patient or family. What are the patient's signs and symptoms?
PROCTOR: Obstetrics/full-term pregnancy with vaginal bleeding.
> **Student:** Are you pregnant?
> **PROCTOR:** Yes.
> **Student:** How long have you been pregnant?
> **PROCTOR:** 8½ months.
> **Student:** Are you having pain or contractions?
> **PROCTOR:** No.
> **Student:** Are you having any bleeding or discharge?
> **PROCTOR:** Yes, the bleeding is heavy.
> **Student:** Do you feel the need to push?
> **PROCTOR:** No.
> **Student:** When was your last menstrual period?
> **PROCTOR:** 9½ months ago.

Student: Allergies?
PROCTOR: No allergies.
Student: Medications?
PROCTOR: Prenatal vitamins.
Student: Pertinent past medical history?
PROCTOR: No pertinent medical history.
Student: Last oral intake?
PROCTOR: 3 hours ago.
Student: Events leading up to the incident?
PROCTOR: The patient was eating dinner.

▼ Perform the Focused Physical Examination

Student: I will perform the focused physical examination.

PROCTOR: Noted.

Student: I am assessing the abdomen for DCAP-BTLS. This acronym stands for deformities, contusions, abrasions, punctures, penetrations, paradoxical motion in the chest, and burns, tenderness, lacerations, and swelling. I am assessing all four quadrants. Do I find any problems?

PROCTOR: She has an obviously pregnant abdomen without pain.

Student: I am assessing the genitalia/perineum as necessary for DCAP-BTLS.

PROCTOR: There is no crowning, but she is bleeding heavily and the blood is bright red.

Student: I will place a pad over the vaginal area.

PROCTOR: Noted.

Student: Pregnancy-specific questions: Number of pregnancies?

PROCTOR: One.

Student: Number of live births?

PROCTOR: None.

Student: Prenatal care?

PROCTOR: Prenatal vitamins.

Student: Any problems during pregnancy?

PROCTOR: No. This is her first problem and first pregnancy.

Student: How many pads have you used?

PROCTOR: Two.

▼ Baseline Vital Signs

Student: What are the patient's baseline vital signs, including blood pressure, pulse, respirations, pulse oximetry, and level of consciousness?

PROCTOR: Blood pressure, 102/60 mm Hg; pulse rate, 122 beats/min; respirations, 28 breaths/min; pulse oximetry reading, 97%; and the patient is alert.

▼ Interventions

Student: I will apply oxygen and transport the patient in the left lateral position.

PROCTOR: Noted.

ALS Student: I will apply basic life support (BLS) interventions, plus the following: start two large-bore IVs.

ALS Proctor: Noted.

▼ Reevaluate Transport Decision

Student: The patient is a high priority and is a load-and-go.

PROCTOR: Noted.

▼ Detailed Physical Examination

Possible Answer #1

Student: I would not do a detailed physical exam.

PROCTOR: Noted. (Go to "Radio Report.")

Possible Answer #2

Student: I am conducting the detailed physical exam. I am looking for DCAP-BTLS.

PROCTOR: Noted. The detailed physical exam will be performed during transport.

► **Assess the Head**

Student: I am assessing the head. Do I find any DCAP-BTLS? Do I find any evidence of Battle's sign or raccoon eyes?

PROCTOR: No.

► **Inspect and Palpate the Head and Ears**

Student: I am assessing the head and ears.

PROCTOR: There are no obvious injuries.

► **Assess the Eyes**

Student: I am assessing the eyes. Are the pupils equal, round, and regular in size, and react properly to light (PEARRL)?

PROCTOR: They are PEARRL.

► **Assess the Facial Area Including Oral and Nasal Areas**

Student: I am assessing the face, nose, and mouth. Do I see any discharge or hear any obstructions?

PROCTOR: No.

► **Assess the Neck**

► **Inspect and Palpate the Neck**

Student: I am assessing the neck for DCAP-BTLS.

PROCTOR: There are no obvious injuries.

► **Assess for Jugular Vein Distention**

Student: Do I find any jugular vein distention (JVD)?

PROCTOR: No.

► **Assess for Tracheal Deviation**

Student: Do I see any tracheal deviation?

PROCTOR: No.

► **Assess the Chest**

Student: I am assessing the chest for DCAP-BTLS.

PROCTOR: Noted.

► **Inspect**

Student: What do I see when I look at the chest?

PROCTOR: There are no obvious injuries.

Student: Is the chest symmetric?

PROCTOR: Yes.

► **Palpate**

Student: When I touch the chest, do I feel crepitus or a flail segment?

PROCTOR: No.

► **Auscultate**

Student: Are lung sounds present in all fields?

PROCTOR: Yes.

Student: Do I hear any sucking sounds from the chest?

PROCTOR: No.

► **Assess the Abdomen/Pelvis**

► **Assess the Abdomen**

Student: I am assessing the abdomen for DCAP-BTLS. I am assessing all four quadrants. Do I find any problems?

PROCTOR: The patient has an obviously pregnant abdomen without pain.

► **Assess the Pelvis**

Student: I am assessing the pelvis for DCAP-BTLS. Is the pelvis stable?

PROCTOR: Yes.

► **Assess the Genitalia/Perineum as Needed (Verbalize in Training)**

Student: I am assessing the genitalia/perineum as necessary for DCAP-BTLS.

PROCTOR: There is no crowning, but she is bleeding heavily and the blood is bright red.

Student: How many pads has she used?

PROCTOR: Three.

Student: What is the color of the bleeding?

PROCTOR: Bright red.

► **Assess the Extremities**

► **Inspect**

Student: I am assessing the lower and upper extremities for DCAP-BTLS. Do I find anything?

PROCTOR: No.

► **Palpate**

Student: Do I feel anything unusual?

PROCTOR: No.

► **Assess Motor, Sensory, and Circulatory Function**

Student: I am checking for DCAP-BTLS, motor and sensory function, and pulses. Right leg?

PROCTOR: Negative DCAP-BTLS. Motor and sensory functions are present. Pulses are present.

Student: Left leg?

PROCTOR: Negative DCAP-BTLS. Motor and sensory functions are present. Pulses are present.

Student: Right arm?
PROCTOR: Negative DCAP-BTLS. Motor and sensory functions are present. Pulses are present.
Student: Left arm?
PROCTOR: Negative DCAP-BTLS. Motor and sensory functions are present. Pulses are present.

▸ Assess the Posterior

Student: We will not check the back.
PROCTOR: Noted.

▸ Manage Secondary Injuries/Wounds

Student: I would direct my partner to reassure the patient.
PROCTOR: Noted.

▸ Reassess Interventions

Student: I will reassess my interventions: apply oxygen and transport the patient in the left lateral recumbent position.
PROCTOR: Noted.
ALS Student: I will reassess BLS interventions, plus the following: two large-bore IVs.
ALS Proctor: Noted.

Critical Criteria:
- ❑ Did not obtain medical direction or verbalize standing orders for medical interventions
- ❑ Administered a dangerous or inappropriate intervention
- ❑ Did not ask questions about the present illness
- ❑ Did not differentiate patient's need for transportation versus continued assessment at the scene

Radio Report

(Provided by the student.)
PROCTOR: Noted.

Ongoing Assessment

Repeat the Initial Assessment

Student: I will repeat the initial assessment.
PROCTOR: Noted. (Reflected in "Repeat Vital Signs.")

Repeat Vital Signs

Student: I will reassess vital signs and mental status.
PROCTOR: Blood pressure, 104/62 mm Hg; pulse, 124 beats/min; respirations, 28 breaths/min; pulse oximetry reading, 98%; and the patient is alert.
Student: The vital signs have not significantly changed.
PROCTOR: Noted.

Check Interventions

Student: I will check my interventions: apply oxygen and transport the patient in the left lateral position.
PROCTOR: Noted.
ALS Student: I will check BLS interventions, plus the following: maintain two large-bore IVs.
ALS Proctor: Noted.

Repeat the Focused Assessment

Student: I will repeat the focused assessment.
PROCTOR: Noted.

Critical Criteria:
- ❑ Did not obtain medical direction or verbalize standing orders for medical interventions
- ❑ Administered a dangerous or inappropriate intervention

Handoff Report to Emergency Department Staff

Student: There was no change in the patient's condition during transport.
PROCTOR: Noted.

Critical Criteria

(Inform the student of items missed, if any.)

❑ Pass ❑ Fail Date: ______________________

Proctor Comments: ______________________

CASE 112

Notes

Dispatch Information

PROCTOR: EMS 10, respond to a 45-year-old male who was working on his car in the garage with the door shut. His wife believes he has carbon monoxide poisoning. He is conscious and breathing.

Pre-Scene Action (BSI)

Student: I am wearing nonlatex gloves and safety glasses.

Critical Criteria:
- ❑ Did not take, or verbalize, body substance isolation (BSI) precautions when necessary

Scene Size-up

Scene Safety

Student: Is the scene safe?
PROCTOR: Yes.

Mechanism of Injury/Nature of Illness

Student: What is the nature of the illness?
PROCTOR: The patient was working on his car while it was running in the garage. The garage door was closed.

Number of Patients

Student: How many patients are there?
PROCTOR: One.

Additional Resources

Student: I would call for advanced life support (ALS) assistance.
PROCTOR: Noted.

C-Spine Stabilization

Student: I would not stabilize the cervical spine (c-spine).
PROCTOR: Noted.

Critical Criteria:
- ❑ Did not determine scene safety

Initial Assessment

General Impression

Student: My general impression is that the patient's condition is unstable.
PROCTOR: Noted.

Responsiveness/Level of Consciousness

Student: What is the patient's level of consciousness?
PROCTOR: Alert.

Chief Complaint/Apparent Life Threats

Student: What is the patient's chief complaint?
PROCTOR: The patient is complaining of a headache, dizziness, and vomiting.

Assess the Airway and Breathing

Student: Is the airway open? Is the patient breathing?
PROCTOR: Yes, the airway is open and the patient is breathing.

Assessment

Student: What are the rate and the quality of breathing?
PROCTOR: Rate: Tachypneic. Quality: Labored.

Provide Oxygen

Student: I am applying oxygen at 15 L/min via nonrebreathing mask.
PROCTOR: Noted.

Ensure Adequate Ventilation

Student: The patient has adequate ventilations at this time.
PROCTOR: Noted.

Assess Circulation

Student: I am assessing the patient's circulation.
PROCTOR: Noted.

Assess for and Control Major Bleeding

Student: Do I find any major bleeding?
PROCTOR: No.

Assess the Pulse

Student: What are the rate and the quality of pulses?
PROCTOR: Rate: Tachycardic. Quality: Bounding.

Assess the Skin

Student: I am assessing the skin. What are the color, temperature, and condition of the skin?
PROCTOR: Color: Flushed. Temperature: Warm. Condition: Moist.

Identify Priority Patients/Make Transport Decision

Student: The patient is a high priority and is a load-and-go. I will begin packaging and transport to an appropriate facility (hyperbaric treatment center if available and per protocol).
PROCTOR: Noted.

Critical Criteria:
- ❑ Did not provide high concentration of oxygen
- ❑ Did not find or manage problems associated with airway, breathing, hemorrhage or shock (hypoperfusion)
- ❑ Did not differentiate patient's need for transportation versus continued assessment at the scene
- ❑ Did detailed or focused history/physical examination before assessing the airway, breathing and circulation

Focused History and Physical Examination/Rapid Assessment

Select the Appropriate Assessment (Focused or Rapid)

Student: I am selecting the focused assessment.
PROCTOR: Noted.

SAMPLE History

Student: At this time I will gather a SAMPLE history from the patient or family. What are the patient's signs and symptoms?
PROCTOR: Poisoning/overdose.

> **Student:** What was the substance?
> **PROCTOR:** Carbon monoxide.
> **Student:** When did you become exposed?
> **PROCTOR:** It was 15 minutes ago.
> **Student:** Over what time period?
> **PROCTOR:** Over 1 hour.
> **Student:** Interventions: Have you done anything to make this better?
> **PROCTOR:** He exited the structure and opened the garage door.
> **Student:** What is your weight?
> **PROCTOR:** 165 pounds.

Student: Allergies?
PROCTOR: No allergies.
Student: Medications?
PROCTOR: No medications.
Student: Pertinent past medical history?
PROCTOR: No pertinent medical history.
Student: Last oral intake?
PROCTOR: 4 hours ago.
Student: Events leading up to the incident?
PROCTOR: The patient was working on his car while it was running in the garage. The car was not running the entire time.

Perform the Focused Physical Examination

Student: I am performing the focused physical examination.
PROCTOR: Noted.
Student: What are his lung sounds?
PROCTOR: They are clear bilaterally.
Student: What is his level of consciousness?
PROCTOR: Alert.
Student: I will monitor his airway and prepare for vomiting.
PROCTOR: Noted.

▼ Baseline Vital Signs

Student: What are the patient's baseline vital signs, including blood pressure, pulse, respirations, pulse oximetry, and level of consciousness?

PROCTOR: Blood pressure, 140/84 mm Hg; pulse rate, 114 beats/min; respirations, 28 breaths/min; pulse oximetry reading, 100%; and the patient is alert.

▼ Interventions

Student: I will continue to provide oxygen and transport the patient to a hyperbaric center.

PROCTOR: Noted.

ALS Student: I will apply basic life support (BLS) interventions, plus the following: IV access, cardiac monitor, 12-lead ECG, and local protocol.

ALS Proctor: Noted. The cardiac monitor shows sinus tachycardia.

▼ Reevaluate Transport Decision

Student: The patient is a high priority and is a load-and-go due to the nature of the illness.

PROCTOR: Noted.

▼ Detailed Physical Examination

Possible Answer #1

Student: I would not do a detailed physical exam.

PROCTOR: Noted. (Go to "Radio Report.")

Possible Answer #2

Student: I am conducting the detailed physical exam. I am looking for DCAP-BTLS. This acronym stands for deformities, contusions, abrasions, punctures, penetrations, paradoxical motion in the chest, and burns, tenderness, lacerations, and swelling.

PROCTOR: Noted. The detailed exam will be performed during transport.

► **Assess the Head**

Student: I am assessing the head. Do I find any DCAP-BTLS? Do I find any evidence of Battle's sign or raccoon eyes?

PROCTOR: No.

► **Inspect and Palpate the Head and Ears**

Student: I am assessing the head and ears.

PROCTOR: There are no obvious injuries.

► **Assess the Eyes**

Student: I am assessing the eyes. Are the pupils equal, round, and regular in size, and react properly to light (PEARRL)?

Proctor: They are slow to react.

► **Assess the Facial Area Including Oral and Nasal Areas**

Student: I am assessing the face, nose, and mouth. Do I see any discharge or hear any obstructions?

PROCTOR: No.

► **Assess the Neck**

► **Inspect and Palpate the Neck**

Student: I am assessing the neck for DCAP-BTLS.

PROCTOR: There are no obvious injuries.

► **Assess for Jugular Vein Distention**

Student: Do I find any jugular vein distention (JVD)?

PROCTOR: No.

► **Assess for Tracheal Deviation**

Student: Do I see any tracheal deviation?

PROCTOR: No.

► **Assess the Chest**

Student: I am assessing the chest for DCAP-BTLS.

PROCTOR: Noted.

► **Inspect**

Student: What do I see when I look at the chest?

PROCTOR: There are no obvious injuries.

Student: Is the chest symmetric?

PROCTOR: Yes.

► **Palpate**

Student: When I touch the chest, do I feel crepitus or a flail segment?

PROCTOR: No.

► **Auscultate**

Student: Are lung sounds present in all fields?

PROCTOR: Yes.

Student: Do I hear any sucking sounds from the chest?

PROCTOR: No.

► **Assess the Abdomen/Pelvis**

► **Assess the Abdomen**

Student: I am assessing the abdomen for DCAP-BTLS. I am assessing all four quadrants. Do I find any problems?

PROCTOR: No.

► **Assess the Pelvis**

Student: I am assessing the pelvis for DCAP-BTLS. Is the pelvis stable?

PROCTOR: Yes.

► **Assess the Genitalia/Perineum as Needed (Verbalize in Training)**

Student: I am assessing the genitalia/perineum as necessary for DCAP-BTLS.

PROCTOR: The area is unremarkable.

► **Assess the Extremities**

► **Inspect**

Student: I am assessing the lower and upper extremities for DCAP-BTLS. Do I find anything?

PROCTOR: No.

► **Palpate**

Student: Do I feel anything unusual?

PROCTOR: No.

► **Assess Motor, Sensory, and Circulatory Function**

Student: I am checking for DCAP-BTLS, motor and sensory function, and pulses. Right leg?

PROCTOR: Negative DCAP-BTLS. Motor and sensory functions are present. Pulses are present.

Student: Left leg?

PROCTOR: Negative DCAP-BTLS. Motor and sensory functions are present. Pulses are present.

Student: Right arm?

PROCTOR: Negative DCAP-BTLS. Motor and sensory functions are present. Pulses are present.

Student: Left arm?

PROCTOR: Negative DCAP-BTLS. Motor and sensory functions are present. Pulses are present.

► **Assess the Posterior**

Student: We will check the back.

PROCTOR: Noted.

► **Assess the Thorax**

Student: I am assessing the thorax. Do I find injuries?

PROCTOR: No.

► **Assess the Lumbar Area**

Student: I am assessing the flanks and lumbar area. Do I find injuries?

PROCTOR: No.

► **Assess the Entire Backside**

Student: I am assessing the entire backside. Do I find injuries?

PROCTOR: No.

► **Manage Secondary Injuries/Wounds**

Student: I would direct my partner to monitor the airway.

PROCTOR: Noted.

► **Reassess Interventions**

Student: I will reassess my interventions: oxygen and transport the patient to a hyperbaric center.

PROCTOR: Noted.

ALS Student: I will reassess BLS interventions, plus the following: IV access, cardiac monitor, 12-lead ECG, and local protocol.

ALS Proctor: Noted. The cardiac monitor shows sinus tachycardia.

Critical Criteria:
- ❑ Did not obtain medical direction or verbalize standing orders for medical interventions
- ❑ Administered a dangerous or inappropriate intervention
- ❑ Did not ask questions about the present illness
- ❑ Did not differentiate patient's need for transportation versus continued assessment at the scene

Radio Report

(Provided by the student.)

PROCTOR: Noted.

Ongoing Assessment

Repeat the Initial Assessment

Student: I will repeat the initial assessment.

PROCTOR: (Reflected in "Repeat Vital Signs.")

Repeat Vital Signs

Student: I will reassess vital signs and mental status.

PROCTOR: Blood pressure, 136/80 mm Hg; pulse rate, 108 beats/min; respirations, 24 breaths/min; pulse oximetry reading, 100%; and the patient is alert.

Student: The vital signs have not significantly changed.

PROCTOR: Noted.

Check Interventions

Student: I will check my interventions: oxygen and transport the patient to a hyperbaric center.

PROCTOR: Noted.

ALS Student: I will check BLS interventions, plus the following: IV access, cardiac monitor, 12-lead ECG, and local protocol.

ALS Proctor: Noted. The cardiac monitor shows sinus tachycardia.

Repeat the Focused Assessment

Student: I will repeat the focused assessment.

PROCTOR: Noted.

Critical Criteria:
- ❑ Did not obtain medical direction or verbalize standing orders for medical interventions
- ❑ Administered a dangerous or inappropriate intervention

Handoff Report to Emergency Department Staff

Student: There was no change in the patient's condition during transport.

PROCTOR: Noted.

Critical Criteria

(Inform the student of items missed, if any.)

❑ Pass ❑ Fail Date: ______________________

Proctor Comments: ______________________

____

____

Notes

Dispatch Information

PROCTOR: EMS 10, respond to a 13-year-old female having a seizure. She is actively seizing at this time.

Pre-Scene Action (BSI)

Student: I am wearing nonlatex gloves and safety glasses.
PROCTOR: Noted.

Critical Criteria:
- ❑ Did not take, or verbalize, body substance isolation (BSI) precautions when necessary

Scene Size-up

Scene Safety

Student: Is the scene safe?
PROCTOR: Yes.

Mechanism of Injury/Nature of Illness

Student: What is the nature of the illness?
PROCTOR: The patient was having a seizure that affected her entire body. She was stiff and shaking (tonic-clonic).

Number of Patients

Student: How many patients are there?
PROCTOR: One.

Additional Resources

Student: I would call for advanced life support (ALS) assistance.
PROCTOR: Noted.

C-Spine Stabilization

Student: I would not stabilize the cervical spine (c-spine), but I will protect her from injury.
PROCTOR: Noted.

Critical Criteria:
- ❑ Did not determine scene safety

Initial Assessment

General Impression

Student: My general impression is that the patient's condition is stable.
PROCTOR: Noted.

Responsiveness/Level of Consciousness

Student: What is the patient's level of consciousness?
PROCTOR: Seizing.

Chief Complaint/Apparent Life Threats

Student: What is the patient's chief complaint?
PROCTOR: The patient was seizing.

Assess the Airway and Breathing

Student: Is the airway open? Is the patient breathing?
PROCTOR: She is snoring.
Student: I will open the airway with a head-tilt chin-lift if there is no evidence of trauma.
PROCTOR: Noted. The patient is breathing.

Assessment

Student: What are the rate and the quality of breathing?
PROCTOR: Rate: Slow. Quality: Shallow (consistent with a postictal state).

Provide Oxygen

Student: I am applying oxygen at 15 L/min via nonrebreathing mask.
PROCTOR: Noted.

Ensure Adequate Ventilation

Student: The patient has adequate ventilations at this time.
PROCTOR: Noted.

Assess Circulation

Student: I am assessing the patient's circulation.
PROCTOR: Noted.

Assess for and Control Major Bleeding

Student: Do I find any major bleeding?
PROCTOR: No.

Assess the Pulse

Student: What are the rate and the quality of pulses?
PROCTOR: Rate: Rapid. Quality: Thready.

Assess the Skin

Student: I am assessing the skin. What are the color, temperature, and condition of the skin?
PROCTOR: Color: Cyanotic. Temperature: Warm. Condition: Moist.

Identify Priority Patients/Make Transport Decision

Student: The patient is a low priority and does not require immediate transport.
PROCTOR: Noted.

Critical Criteria:
- ❑ Did not provide high concentration of oxygen
- ❑ Did not find or manage problems associated with airway, breathing, hemorrhage or shock (hypoperfusion)
- ❑ Did not differentiate patient's need for transportation versus continued assessment at the scene
- ❑ Did detailed or focused history/physical examination before assessing the airway, breathing and circulation

Focused History and Physical Examination/Rapid Assessment

Select the Appropriate Assessment (Focused or Rapid)

Student: I am selecting the focused assessment.
PROCTOR: Noted.

SAMPLE History

Student: At this time I will gather a SAMPLE history from the patient or family. What are the patient's signs and symptoms?
PROCTOR: Altered mental status.
> Student: Describe the episode.
> **PROCTOR:** The patient was at school when she had a seizure.
> Student: Onset: What was she doing when this started?
> **PROCTOR:** She was in class.
> Student: Duration: How long has this been going on?
> **PROCTOR:** 3 minutes and then it let up.
> Student: Are there any associated symptoms?
> **PROCTOR:** No.
> Student: Is there any evidence of trauma?
> **PROCTOR:** No.
> Student: Interventions: Has she done anything to make this better?
> **PROCTOR:** The patient has taken no actions.
> Student: Have there been any seizures?
> **PROCTOR:** Yes, just this one.
> Student: Has there been any fever?
> **PROCTOR:** No.

Student: Allergies?
PROCTOR: No allergies.
Student: Medications?
PROCTOR: Seizure medications.
Student: Pertinent past medical history?
PROCTOR: Epilepsy.
Student: Last oral intake?
PROCTOR: 2 hours ago.
Student: Events leading up to the incident?
PROCTOR: The patient was in class and began having a seizure.

Perform the Focused Physical Examination

Student: I am performing the focused physical examination.
PROCTOR: Noted.
Student: What is her level of consciousness at this time?
PROCTOR: She responds to verbal stimuli.
Student: Does she have any obvious injuries from the seizure?
PROCTOR: No.
Student: What is her blood glucose level?
PROCTOR: It is 114 mg/dL.

Baseline Vital Signs

Student: What are the patient's baseline vital signs, including blood pressure, pulse, respirations, pulse oximetry, and level of consciousness?
PROCTOR: Blood pressure, 112/72 mm Hg; pulse rate, 104 beats/min; respirations, 12 breaths/min; pulse oximetry reading, 94%; and the patient is tired.

Interventions

Student: I will apply my interventions: oxygen, recovery position, monitor the patient, and provide reassurance.
PROCTOR: Noted.
ALS Student: I will apply basic life support (BLS) interventions, plus the following: IV access and anticonvulsant per local protocol if seizure activity resumes.
ALS Proctor: Noted.

Reevaluate Transport Decision

Student: The patient is a low priority and does not require immediate transport.
PROCTOR: Noted.

Detailed Physical Examination

Possible Answer #1
Student: I would not do a detailed physical exam.
PROCTOR: Noted. (Go to "Radio Report.")

Possible Answer #2
Student: I am conducting the detailed physical exam. I am looking for DCAP-BTLS. This acronym stands for deformities, contusions, abrasions, punctures, penetrations, paradoxical motion in the chest, and burns, tenderness, lacerations, and swelling.
PROCTOR: Noted. The detailed physical exam will be performed during transport.

Assess the Head

Student: I am assessing the head. Do I find any DCAP-BTLS? Do I find any evidence of Battle's sign or raccoon eyes?
PROCTOR: No.

Inspect and Palpate the Head and Ears

Student: I am assessing the head and ears.
PROCTOR: There are no obvious injuries.

Assess the Eyes

Student: I am assessing the eyes. Are the pupils equal, round, and regular in size, and react properly to light (PEARRL)?
PROCTOR: They are PEARRL.

Assess the Facial Area Including Oral and Nasal Areas

Student: I am assessing the face, nose, and mouth. Do I see any discharge or hear any obstructions?
PROCTOR: No.

Assess the Neck

Inspect and Palpate the Neck

Student: I am assessing the neck for DCAP-BTLS.
PROCTOR: There are no obvious injuries.

Assess for Jugular Vein Distention

Student: Do I find any jugular vein distention (JVD)?
PROCTOR: No.

Assess for Tracheal Deviation

Student: Do I see any tracheal deviation?
PROCTOR: No.

Assess the Chest

Student: I am assessing the chest for DCAP-BTLS.
PROCTOR: Noted.

Inspect

Student: What do I see when I look at the chest?
PROCTOR: There are no obvious injuries.
Student: Is the chest symmetric?
PROCTOR: Yes.

Palpate

Student: When I touch the chest, do I feel crepitus or a flail segment?
PROCTOR: No.

Auscultate

Student: Are lung sounds present in all fields?
PROCTOR: Yes.
Student: Do I hear any sucking sounds from the chest?
PROCTOR: No.

Assess the Abdomen/Pelvis

Assess the Abdomen

Student: I am assessing the abdomen for DCAP-BTLS. I am assessing all four quadrants. Do I find any problems?
PROCTOR: No.

Assess the Pelvis

Student: I am assessing the pelvis for DCAP-BTLS. Is the pelvis stable?
PROCTOR: Yes.

Assess the Genitalia/Perineum as Needed (Verbalize in Training)

Student: I am assessing the genitalia/perineum as necessary for DCAP-BTLS.
PROCTOR: She is incontinent of urine.

Assess the Extremities

Inspect

Student: I am assessing the lower and upper extremities for DCAP-BTLS. Do I find anything?
PROCTOR: No.

Palpate

Student: Do I feel anything unusual?
PROCTOR: No.

Assess Motor, Sensory, and Circulatory Function

Student: I am checking for DCAP-BTLS, motor and sensory function, and pulses. Right leg?
PROCTOR: Negative DCAP-BTLS. Motor and sensory functions are present. Pulses are present.
Student: Left leg?
PROCTOR: Negative DCAP-BTLS. Motor and sensory functions are present. Pulses are present.
Student: Right arm?
PROCTOR: Negative DCAP-BTLS. Motor and sensory functions are present. Pulses are present.
Student: Left arm?
PROCTOR: Negative DCAP-BTLS. Motor and sensory functions are present. Pulses are present.

Assess the Posterior

Student: We will check the back.
PROCTOR: Noted.

Assess the Thorax

Student: I am assessing the thorax. Do I find injuries?
PROCTOR: No.

Assess the Lumbar Area

Student: I am assessing the flanks and lumbar area. Do I find injuries?
PROCTOR: No.

▸ **Assess the Entire Backside**

Student: I am assessing the entire backside. Do I find injuries?

PROCTOR: No.

▸ **Manage Secondary Injuries/Wounds**

Student: I would direct my partner to continue providing oxygen and monitor the patient.

PROCTOR: Noted.

▸ **Reassess Interventions**

Student: I will reassess my interventions: oxygen, recovery position, monitor the patient, and provide reassurance.

PROCTOR: Noted.

ALS Student: I will reassess BLS interventions, plus the following: IV access and anticonvulsant per local protocol if seizure activity resumes.

ALS Proctor: Noted.

Critical Criteria:
- ❑ Did not obtain medical direction or verbalize standing orders for medical interventions
- ❑ Administered a dangerous or inappropriate intervention
- ❑ Did not ask questions about the present illness
- ❑ Did not differentiate patient's need for transportation versus continued assessment at the scene

Radio Report

(Provided by the student.)

PROCTOR: Noted.

Ongoing Assessment

Repeat the Initial Assessment

Student: I will repeat the initial assessment.

PROCTOR: Noted. (Reflected in "Repeat Vital Signs.")

Repeat Vital Signs

Student: I will reassess vital signs and mental status.

PROCTOR: Blood pressure, 110/70 mm Hg; pulse rate, 96 beats/min; respirations, 16 breaths/min; pulse oximetry reading, 98%; and the patient is tired.

Student: The vital signs have not significantly changed.

PROCTOR: Noted.

Check Interventions

Student: I will check my interventions: oxygen, recovery position, monitor the patient, and provide reassurance.

PROCTOR: Noted.

ALS Student: I will check BLS interventions, plus the following: IV access and anticonvulsant per local protocol if seizure activity resumes.

ALS Proctor: Noted.

Repeat the Focused Assessment

Student: I will repeat the focused assessment.

PROCTOR: Noted.

Critical Criteria:
- ❑ Did not obtain medical direction or verbalize standing orders for medical interventions
- ❑ Administered a dangerous or inappropriate intervention

Handoff Report to Emergency Department Staff

Student: There was no change in the patient's condition during transport.

PROCTOR: Noted.

Critical Criteria

(Inform the student of items missed, if any.)

❑ Pass ❑ Fail Date: ____________________

Proctor Comments: ____________________

Notes

Dispatch Information

PROCTOR: EMS 10, respond to 17-year-old male who has a possible cold injury to his feet. He is conscious and breathing.

Pre-Scene Action (BSI)

Student: I am wearing clothing appropriate for the temperature, nonlatex gloves, and safety glasses.
PROCTOR: Noted.

Critical Criteria:
- ❑ Did not take, or verbalize, body substance isolation (BSI) precautions when necessary

Scene Size-up

Scene Safety

Student: Is the scene safe?
PROCTOR: Yes.

Mechanism of Injury/Nature of Illness

Student: What is the nature of the illness?
PROCTOR: Frost injury to the feet.

Number of Patients

Student: How many patients are there?
PROCTOR: One.

Additional Resources

Student: I would not call for advanced life support (ALS) assistance.
PROCTOR: Noted.

C-Spine Stabilization

Student: I would not stabilize the cervical spine (c-spine).
PROCTOR: Noted.

Critical Criteria:
- ❑ Did not determine scene safety

Initial Assessment

General Impression

Student: My general impression is that the patient's condition is stable.
PROCTOR: Noted.

Responsiveness/Level of Consciousness

Student: What is the patient's level of consciousness?
PROCTOR: Alert.

Chief Complaint/Apparent Life Threats

Student: What is the patient's chief complaint?
PROCTOR: The patient is complaining of frost injury to his feet.

Assess the Airway and Breathing

Student: Is the airway open? Is the patient breathing?
PROCTOR: Yes, the airway is open and the patient is breathing.

Assessment

Student: What are the rate and the quality of breathing?
PROCTOR: Rate: Tachypneic. Quality: Shallow.

Provide Oxygen

Student: I am applying oxygen at 15 L/min via nonrebreathing mask.
PROCTOR: Noted.

Ensure Adequate Ventilation

Student: The patient has adequate ventilations at this time.
PROCTOR: Noted.

Assess Circulation

Student: I am assessing the patient's circulation.
PROCTOR: Noted.

Assess for and Control Major Bleeding

Student: Do I find any major bleeding?
PROCTOR: No.

Assess the Pulse

Student: What are the rate and the quality of pulses?
PROCTOR: Rate: Tachycardic. Quality: Thready.

Assess the Skin

Student: I am assessing the skin. What are the color, temperature, and condition of the skin?
PROCTOR: Color: Pale, mottled to pasty-white on the feet. Temperature: Cool and cold on the feet. Condition: Moist.

Identify Priority Patients/Make Transport Decision

Student: The patient is a high priority and is a load-and-go. I will begin packaging and transport.
PROCTOR: Noted.

Critical Criteria:
- ❑ Did not provide high concentration of oxygen
- ❑ Did not find or manage problems associated with airway, breathing, hemorrhage or shock (hypoperfusion)
- ❑ Did not differentiate patient's need for transportation versus continued assessment at the scene
- ❑ Did detailed or focused history/physical examination before assessing the airway, breathing and circulation

Focused History and Physical Examination/Rapid Assessment

Select the Appropriate Assessment (Focused or Rapid)

Student: I am selecting the focused assessment.
PROCTOR: Noted.

SAMPLE History

Student: At this time I will gather a SAMPLE history from the patient or family. What are the patient's signs and symptoms?
PROCTOR: Environmental emergency.

> **Student:** What was the source?
> **PROCTOR:** It was snowing heavily and his shoes were wet from the previous day.
> **Student:** What was the environment?
> **PROCTOR:** It was 2°F.
> **Student:** What was the duration?
> **PROCTOR:** 45 to 55 minutes.
> **Student:** Was there any loss of consciousness?
> **PROCTOR:** No.
> **Student:** What were the effects—local or general?
> **PROCTOR:** Just to the toes.

Student: Allergies?
PROCTOR: No allergies.
Student: Medications?
PROCTOR: No medications.
Student: Pertinent past medical history?
PROCTOR: No pertinent medical history.
Student: Last oral intake?
PROCTOR: 3 hours ago.
Student: Events leading up to the incident?
PROCTOR: The patient had just walked to his girlfriend's house. It was 2°F and he was wearing wet shoes.

Perform the Focused Physical Examination

Student: I am performing the focused physical examination.
PROCTOR: Noted.
Student: I am checking for DCAP-BTLS. This acronym stands for deformities, contusions, abrasions, punctures, penetrations, paradoxical motion in the chest, and burns, tenderness, lacerations, and swelling. I am also checking motor and sensory function and pulses. Right leg?
PROCTOR: Frost injury noted to the toes. Motor and sensory functions are absent. Pulses are present.

Student: Left leg?

PROCTOR: Frost injury noted to the toes. Motor and sensory functions are absent. Pulses are present.

Student: I will dry the feet, dress them in a bulky dressing, and keep him warm.

PROCTOR: Noted.

▼ Baseline Vital Signs

Student: What are the patient's baseline vital signs, including blood pressure, pulse, respirations, pulse oximetry, and level of consciousness?

PROCTOR: Blood pressure, 134/78 mm Hg; pulse rate, 120 beats/min; respirations, 24 breaths/min; pulse oximetry reading, N/A; and the patient is alert.

▼ Interventions

Student: I will apply oxygen, remove wet clothing, place the patient in a warm environment, and prevent further injury.

PROCTOR: Noted.

ALS Student: I will apply basic life support (BLS) interventions, plus the following: IV access, cardiac monitor, and pain management per local protocol.

ALS Proctor: Noted. The cardiac monitor shows sinus tachycardia.

▼ Reevaluate Transport Decision

Student: The patient is a high priority and is a load-and-go.

PROCTOR: Noted.

▼ Detailed Physical Examination

Possible Answer #1

Student: I would not do a detailed physical exam.

PROCTOR: Noted. (Go to "Radio Report.")

Possible Answer #2

Student: I am conducting the detailed physical exam. I am looking for DCAP-BTLS.

PROCTOR: Noted. The detailed physical exam will be performed during transport.

- **Assess the Head**

Student: I am assessing the head. Do I find any DCAP-BTLS? Do I find any evidence of Battle's sign or raccoon eyes?

PROCTOR: No.

- **Inspect and Palpate the Head and Ears**

Student: I am assessing the head and ears.

PROCTOR: There are no obvious injuries.

- **Assess the Eyes**

Student: I am assessing the eyes. Are the pupils equal, round, and regular in size, and react properly to light (PEARRL)?

PROCTOR: They are PEARRL.

- **Assess the Facial Area Including Oral and Nasal Areas**

Student: I am assessing the face, nose, and mouth. Do I see any discharge or hear any obstructions?

PROCTOR: No.

- **Assess the Neck**
- **Inspect and Palpate the Neck**

Student: I am assessing the neck for DCAP-BTLS.

PROCTOR: There are no obvious injuries.

- **Assess for Jugular Vein Distention**

Student: Do I find any jugular vein distention (JVD)?

PROCTOR: No.

- **Assess for Tracheal Deviation**

Student: Do I see any tracheal deviation?

PROCTOR: No.

- **Assess the Chest**

Student: I am assessing the chest for DCAP-BTLS.

PROCTOR: Noted.

- **Inspect**

Student: What do I see when I look at the chest?

PROCTOR: There are no obvious injuries.

Student: Is the chest symmetric?

PROCTOR: Yes.

- **Palpate**

Student: When I touch the chest, do I feel crepitus or a flail segment?

PROCTOR: No.

- **Auscultate**

Student: Are lung sounds present in all fields?

PROCTOR: Yes.

Student: Do I hear any sucking sounds from the chest?

PROCTOR: No.

- **Assess the Abdomen/Pelvis**
- **Assess the Abdomen**

Student: I am assessing the abdomen for DCAP-BTLS. I am assessing all four quadrants. Do I find any problems?

PROCTOR: No.

- **Assess the Pelvis**

Student: I am assessing the pelvis for DCAP-BTLS. Is the pelvis stable?

PROCTOR: Yes.

- **Assess the Genitalia/Perineum as Needed (Verbalize in Training)**

Student: I am assessing the genitalia/perineum as necessary for DCAP-BTLS.

PROCTOR: The area is unremarkable.

- **Assess the Extremities**
- **Inspect**

Student: I am assessing the lower and upper extremities for DCAP-BTLS. Do I find anything?

PROCTOR: Yes, frostbite on both feet.

- **Palpate**

Student: Do I feel anything unusual?

PROCTOR: Yes. The feet feel hard to the touch.

- **Assess Motor, Sensory, and Circulatory Function**

Student: I am checking for DCAP-BTLS, motor and sensory function, and pulses. Right leg?

PROCTOR: Frost injury noted to the toes. Motor and sensory functions are absent. Pulses are present.

Student: Left leg?

PROCTOR: Frost injury noted to the toes. Motor and sensory functions are absent. Pulses are present.

Student: Right arm?

PROCTOR: Negative DCAP-BTLS. Motor and sensory functions are present. Pulses are present.

Student: Left arm?

PROCTOR: Negative DCAP-BTLS. Motor and sensory functions are present. Pulses are present.

- **Assess the Posterior**

Student: We will check the back.

PROCTOR: Noted.

- **Assess the Thorax**

Student: I am assessing the thorax. Do I find injuries?

PROCTOR: No.

- **Assess the Lumbar Area**

Student: I am assessing the flanks and lumbar area. Do I find injuries?

PROCTOR: No.

- **Assess the Entire Backside**

Student: I am assessing the entire backside. Do I find injuries?

PROCTOR: No.

- **Manage Secondary Injuries/Wounds**

Student: I would direct my partner to continue monitoring the patient.

PROCTOR: Noted.

▸ Reassess Interventions

Student: I will reassess oxygen, remove wet clothing, place the patient in a warm environment, and prevent further injury.

PROCTOR: Noted.

ALS Student: I will reassess BLS interventions, plus the following: maintain IV access, cardiac monitor, and pain management per local protocol.

ALS Proctor: Noted. The cardiac monitor shows sinus tachycardia.

Critical Criteria:
- ❑ Did not obtain medical direction or verbalize standing orders for medical interventions
- ❑ Administered a dangerous or inappropriate intervention
- ❑ Did not ask questions about the present illness
- ❑ Did not differentiate patient's need for transportation versus continued assessment at the scene

Radio Report

(Provided by the student.)

PROCTOR: Noted.

Ongoing Assessment

Repeat the Initial Assessment

Student: I will repeat the initial assessment.

PROCTOR: Noted. (Reflected in "Repeat Vital Signs.")

Repeat Vital Signs

Student: I will reassess vital signs and mental status.

PROCTOR: Blood pressure, 130/78 mm Hg; pulse rate, 116 beats/min; respirations, 20 breaths/min; pulse oximetry reading, N/A; and the patient is alert.

Student: The vital signs have not significantly changed.

PROCTOR: Noted.

Check Interventions

Student: I will check my interventions: oxygen, remove wet clothing, place the patient in a warm environment, and prevent further injury.

PROCTOR: Noted.

ALS Student: I will check BLS interventions, plus the following: maintain IV access, cardiac monitor, and pain management per local protocol.

ALS Proctor: Noted. The cardiac monitor shows sinus tachycardia.

Repeat the Focused Assessment

Student: I will repeat the focused assessment.

PROCTOR: Noted.

Critical Criteria:
- ❑ Did not obtain medical direction or verbalize standing orders for medical interventions
- ❑ Administered a dangerous or inappropriate intervention

Handoff Report to Emergency Department Staff

Student: There was no change in the patient's condition during transport.

PROCTOR: Noted.

Critical Criteria

(Inform the student of items missed, if any.)

❑ Pass ❑ Fail Date: ______________________

Proctor Comments: ______________________

____

____

Notes

Dispatch Information

PROCTOR: EMS 10, respond to a 79-year-old male who is complaining of a prolapsed rectum. He is conscious and breathing.

Pre-scene Action (BSI)

Student: I am wearing nonlatex gloves and safety glasses.
PROCTOR: Noted.

> **Critical Criteria:**
> ❑ Did not take, or verbalize, body substance isolation (BSI) precautions when necessary

Scene Size-up

Scene Safety

Student: Is the scene safe?
PROCTOR: Yes.

Mechanism of Injury/Nature of Illness

Student: What is the nature of the illness?
PROCTOR: Prolapsed rectum.

Number of Patients

Student: How many patients are there?
PROCTOR: One.

Additional Resources

Student: I would call for advanced life support (ALS) assistance.
PROCTOR: Noted.

C-Spine Stabilization

Student: I would not stabilize the cervical spine (c-spine).
PROCTOR: Noted.

> **Critical Criteria:**
> ❑ Did not determine scene safety

Initial Assessment

General Impression

Student: My general impression is that the patient's condition is stable.
PROCTOR: Noted.

Responsiveness/Level of Consciousness

Student: What is the patient's level of consciousness?
PROCTOR: Alert.

Chief Complaint/Apparent Life Threats

Student: What is the patient's chief complaint?
PROCTOR: The patient is complaining of a prolapsed rectum.

Assess the Airway and Breathing

Student: Is the airway open? Is the patient breathing?
PROCTOR: Yes, the airway is open and the patient is breathing.

Assessment

Student: What are the rate and the quality of breathing?
PROCTOR: Rate: Within normal limits. Quality: Normal.

Provide Oxygen

Student: I am applying oxygen at 15 L/min via nonrebreathing mask.
PROCTOR: Noted.

Ensure Adequate Ventilation

Student: The patient has adequate ventilations at this time.
PROCTOR: Noted.

Assess Circulation

Student: I am assessing the patient's circulation.
PROCTOR: Noted.

Assess for and Control Major Bleeding

Student: Do I find any major bleeding?
PROCTOR: No.

Assess the Pulse

Student: What are the rate and the quality of pulses?
PROCTOR: Rate: Within normal limits. Quality: Normal.

Assess the Skin

Student: I am assessing the skin. What are the color, temperature, and condition of the skin?
PROCTOR: Color: Flushed. Temperature: Warm. Condition: Diaphoretic.

Identify Priority Patients/Make Transport Decision

Student: The patient is a low priority and does not require immediate transport.
PROCTOR: Noted.

> **Critical Criteria:**
> ❑ Did not provide high concentration of oxygen
> ❑ Did not find or manage problems associated with airway, breathing, hemorrhage or shock (hypoperfusion)
> ❑ Did not differentiate patient's need for transportation versus continued assessment at the scene
> ❑ Did detailed or focused history/physical examination before assessing the airway, breathing and circulation

Focused History and Physical Examination/Rapid Assessment

Select the Appropriate Assessment (Focused or Rapid)

Student: I am selecting the focused assessment; I will focus on the patient complaint.
PROCTOR: Noted.

SAMPLE History

Student: At this time I will gather a SAMPLE history from the patient or family. What are the patient's signs and symptoms?
PROCTOR: Medical (pain and discomfort in his rectum).

Student: Onset: What were you doing when this started?
PROCTOR: Using the toilet.
Student: Provokes: What makes your condition worse or better?
PROCTOR: Nothing.
Student: Quality: Can you describe your pain?
PROCTOR: My pride is killing me.
Student: Radiates: Do you have pain anywhere else?
PROCTOR: No.
Student: Severity: On a scale of 1 to 10 with 10 being the worst possible, how would you rate your pain/distress?
PROCTOR: 10.
Student: Time: How long has this been going on?
PROCTOR: 10 minutes.
Student: Interventions: Have you done anything to make this better?
PROCTOR: The patient has taken no actions.

Student: Allergies?
PROCTOR: No allergies.
Student: Medications?
PROCTOR: Stool softeners, nitroglycerin, vitamins.
Student: Pertinent past medical history?
PROCTOR: Angina.
Student: Last oral intake?
PROCTOR: 5 hours ago.
Student: Events leading up to the incident?
PROCTOR: The patient was using the toilet and trying to pass stool after having been constipated.

▼ Perform the Focused Physical Examination

Student: I am performing the focused physical examination.
PROCTOR: Noted.
Student: I am assessing the genitalia/perineum as necessary for DCAP-BTLS. This acronym stands for deformities, contusions, abrasions, punctures, penetrations, paradoxical motion in the chest, burns, tenderness, lacerations, and swelling.
PROCTOR: The rectum is prolapsed.
Student: I will dress the organ with a moist sterile dressing per local protocol.
PROCTOR: Noted.

▼ Baseline Vital Signs

Student: What are the patient's baseline vital signs, including blood pressure, pulse, respirations, pulse oximetry, and level of consciousness?
PROCTOR: Blood pressure, 156/90 mm Hg; pulse rate, 96 beats/min; respirations, 16 breaths/min; pulse oximetry reading, 98%; and the patient is alert.

▼ Interventions

Student: I will apply oxygen, treat per local protocol, and transport the patient in the position of comfort.
PROCTOR: Noted.
ALS Student: I will apply basic life support (BLS) interventions, plus the following: IV access and local protocol.
ALS Proctor: Noted.

▼ Reevaluate Transport Decision

Student: The patient is a low priority and does not require immediate transport.
PROCTOR: Noted.

▼ Detailed Physical Examination

Possible Answer #1
Student: I would not do a detailed physical exam.
PROCTOR: Noted. (Go to "Radio Report.")

Possible Answer #2
Student: I am conducting the detailed physical exam. I am looking for DCAP-BTLS.
PROCTOR: Noted. The detailed physical exam will be performed during transport.

▸ Assess the Head

Student: I am assessing the head. Do I find any DCAP-BTLS? Do I find any evidence of Battle's sign or raccoon eyes?
PROCTOR: No.

▸ Inspect and Palpate the Head and Ears

Student: I am assessing the head and ears.
PROCTOR: There are no obvious injuries.

▸ Assess the Eyes

Student: I am assessing the eyes. Are the pupils equal, round, and regular in size, and react properly to light (PEARRL)?
PROCTOR: They are PEARRL.

▸ Assess the Facial Area Including Oral and Nasal Areas

Student: I am assessing the face, nose, and mouth. Do I see any discharge or hear any obstructions?
PROCTOR: No.

▸ Assess the Neck

▸ Inspect and Palpate the Neck

Student: I am assessing the neck for DCAP-BTLS.
PROCTOR: There are no obvious injuries.

▸ Assess for Jugular Vein Distention

Student: Do I find any jugular vein distention (JVD)?
PROCTOR: No.

▸ Assess for Tracheal Deviation

Student: Do I see any tracheal deviation?
PROCTOR: No.

▸ Assess the Chest

Student: I am assessing the chest for DCAP-BTLS.
PROCTOR: Noted.

▸ Inspect

Student: What do I see when I look at the chest?
PROCTOR: There are no obvious injuries.
Student: Is the chest symmetric?
PROCTOR: Yes.

▸ Palpate

Student: When I touch the chest, do I feel crepitus or a flail segment?
PROCTOR: No.

▸ Auscultate

Student: Are lung sounds present in all fields?
PROCTOR: Yes.
Student: Do I hear any sucking sounds from the chest?
PROCTOR: No.

▸ Assess the Abdomen/Pelvis

▸ Assess the Abdomen

Student: I am assessing the abdomen for DCAP-BTLS. I am assessing all four quadrants. Do I find any problems?
PROCTOR: No.

▸ Assess the Pelvis

Student: I am assessing the pelvis for DCAP-BTLS. Is the pelvis stable?
PROCTOR: Yes.

▸ Assess the Genitalia/Perineum as Needed (Verbalize in Training)

Student: I am assessing the genitalia/perineum as necessary for DCAP-BTLS.
PROCTOR: The rectum is prolapsed.
Student: I will check the dressing.
PROCTOR: Noted.

▸ Assess the Extremities

▸ Inspect

Student: I am assessing the lower and upper extremities for DCAP-BTLS. Do I find anything?
PROCTOR: No.

▸ Palpate

Student: Do I feel anything unusual?
PROCTOR: No.

▸ Assess Motor, Sensory, and Circulatory Function

Student: I am checking for DCAP-BTLS, motor and sensory function, and pulses. Right leg?
PROCTOR: Negative DCAP-BTLS. Motor and sensory functions are present. Pulses are present.
Student: Left leg?
PROCTOR: Negative DCAP-BTLS. Motor and sensory functions are present. Pulses are present.
Student: Right arm?
PROCTOR: Negative DCAP-BTLS. Motor and sensory functions are present. Pulses are present.
Student: Left arm?
PROCTOR: Negative DCAP-BTLS. Motor and sensory functions are present. Pulses are present.

▸ Assess the Posterior

Student: We will check the back.
PROCTOR: Noted.

▸ Assess the Thorax

Student: I am assessing the thorax. Do I find injuries?
PROCTOR: No.

Assess the Lumbar Area

Student: I am assessing the flanks and lumbar area. Do I find injuries?

PROCTOR: No.

Assess the Entire Backside

Student: I am assessing the entire backside. Do I find injuries?

PROCTOR: No.

Manage Secondary Injuries/Wounds

Student: I would direct my partner to continue providing oxygen and monitor the patient.

PROCTOR: Noted.

Reassess Interventions

Student: I will reassess interventions: oxygen, treat per local protocol, and transport the patient in the position of comfort.

PROCTOR: Noted.

ALS Student: I will reassess BLS interventions, plus the following: IVs and local protocol.

ALS Proctor: Noted.

Critical Criteria:
- ❑ Did not obtain medical direction or verbalize standing orders for medical interventions
- ❑ Administered a dangerous or inappropriate intervention
- ❑ Did not ask questions about the present illness
- ❑ Did not differentiate patient's need for transportation versus continued assessment at the scene

Radio Report

(Provided by the student.)

PROCTOR: Noted.

Ongoing Assessment

Repeat the Initial Assessment

Student: I will repeat the initial assessment.

PROCTOR: Noted. (Reflected in "Repeat Vital Signs.")

Repeat Vital Signs

Student: I will reassess vital signs and mental status.

PROCTOR: Blood pressure, 150/86 mm Hg; pulse rate, 96 beats/min; respirations, 16 breaths/min; pulse oximetry reading, 98%; and the patient is alert.

Student: The vital signs have not changed significantly.

PROCTOR: Noted.

Check Interventions

Student: I will reassess my interventions: oxygen and transport the patient in the position of comfort.

PROCTOR: Noted.

ALS Student: I will reassess BLS interventions, plus the following: IV access and local protocol.

ALS Proctor: Noted.

Repeat the Focused Assessment

Student: I will repeat the focused assessment.

PROCTOR: Noted.

Critical Criteria:
- ❑ Did not obtain medical direction or verbalize standing orders for medical interventions
- ❑ Administered a dangerous or inappropriate intervention

Handoff Report to Emergency Department Staff

Student: There was no change in the patient's condition during transport.

PROCTOR: Noted.

Critical Criteria

(Inform the student of items missed, if any.)

❑ Pass ❑ Fail Date: ____________________

Proctor Comments: ____________________

____

____

Notes

CASE 117

Dispatch Information

PROCTOR: EMS 10, respond to a 23-year-old male who has been sprayed with pepper spray by the police. He is conscious and breathing.

Pre-scene Action (BSI)

Student: I am wearing nonlatex gloves and safety glasses.
PROCTOR: Noted.

Critical Criteria:
- ❑ Did not take, or verbalize, body substance isolation (BSI) precautions when necessary

Scene Size-up

Scene Safety

Student: Is the scene safe?
PROCTOR: Yes.

Mechanism of Injury/Nature of Illness

Student: What is the nature of the illness?
PROCTOR: The patient was sprayed with pepper spray by the police. He is crying and coughing, and his skin and eyes are burning.

Number of Patients

Student: How many patients are there?
PROCTOR: One.

Additional Resources

Student: I would not call for advanced life support (ALS) assistance. I would thoroughly rinse the patient's eyes and skin with copious amounts of water prior to any assessment.
PROCTOR: Noted.

C-Spine Stabilization

Student: I would not stabilize the cervical spine (c-spine).
PROCTOR: Noted.

Critical Criteria:
- ❑ Did not determine scene safety

Initial Assessment

General Impression

Student: My general impression is that the patient's condition is stable.
PROCTOR: Noted.

Responsiveness/Level of Consciousness

Student: What is the patient's level of consciousness?
PROCTOR: Alert.

Chief Complaint/Apparent Life Threats

Student: What is the patient's chief complaint?
PROCTOR: The patient is complaining of coughing, and his skin and eyes are burning.

Assess the Airway and Breathing

Student: Is the airway open? Is the patient breathing?
PROCTOR: Yes, the airway is open and the patient is breathing.

Assessment

Student: What are the rate and the quality of breathing?
PROCTOR: Rate: Tachypneic. Quality: Crying.

Provide Oxygen

Student: I am applying oxygen at 15 L/min via nonrebreathing mask.
PROCTOR: Noted.

Ensure Adequate Ventilation

Student: The patient has adequate ventilations at this time.
PROCTOR: Noted.

Assess Circulation

Student: I am assessing the patient's circulation.
PROCTOR: Noted.

Assess for and Control Major Bleeding

Student: Do I find any major bleeding?
PROCTOR: No.

Assess the Pulse

Student: What are the rate and the quality of pulses?
PROCTOR: Rate: Tachycardic. Quality: Bounding.

Assess the Skin

Student: I am assessing the skin. What are the color, temperature, and condition of the skin?
PROCTOR: Color: Flushed. Temperature: Warm. Condition: Moist.

Identify Priority Patients/Make Transport Decision

Student: The patient is a low priority and does not require immediate transport.
PROCTOR: Noted.

Critical Criteria:
- ❑ Did not provide high concentration of oxygen
- ❑ Did not find or manage problems associated with airway, breathing, hemorrhage or shock (hypoperfusion)
- ❑ Did not differentiate patient's need for transportation versus continued assessment at the scene
- ❑ Did detailed or focused history/physical examination before assessing the airway, breathing and circulation

Focused History and Physical Examination/Rapid Assessment

Select the Appropriate Assessment (Focused or Rapid)

Student: I am selecting the focused assessment.
PROCTOR: Noted.

SAMPLE History

Student: At this time I will gather a SAMPLE history from the patient or family. What are the patient's signs and symptoms?
PROCTOR: Poisoning/overdose (burning to eyes and skin).

> **Student:** What was the substance?
> **PROCTOR:** Pepper spray.
> **Student:** When did you become exposed?
> **PROCTOR:** 10 minutes ago.
> **Student:** Over what time period?
> **PROCTOR:** Over 1 minute.
> **Student:** Interventions: Have you done anything to make this better?
> **PROCTOR:** The patient has been trying to wipe the substance from his eyes. There is a lot of tearing from his eyes.
> **Student:** What is your weight?
> **PROCTOR:** 220 pounds.

Student: Allergies?
PROCTOR: No allergies.
Student: Medications?
PROCTOR: No medications.
Student: Pertinent past medical history?
PROCTOR: No pertinent medical history.
Student: Last oral intake?
PROCTOR: 5 hours ago.
Student: Events leading up to the incident?
PROCTOR: The patient was resisting arrest when he was sprayed with pepper spray.

Perform the Focused Physical Examination

Student: I am performing the focused physical examination.
PROCTOR: Noted

Student: I am assessing the eyes. Are the pupils equal, round, and regular in size, and react properly to light (PEARRL)?
PROCTOR: They are bloodshot, burning, and producing a lot of tears.
Student: What are the lung sounds?
PROCTOR: They are clear bilaterally.

▼ Baseline Vital Signs

Student: What are the patient's baseline vital signs, including blood pressure, pulse, respirations, pulse oximetry, and level of consciousness?
PROCTOR: Blood pressure, 136/84 mm Hg; pulse rate, 112 beats/min; respirations, 24 breaths/min; pulse oximetry reading, 97%; and the patient is alert.

▼ Interventions

Student: I will flush the eyes and skin with water and apply oxygen.
PROCTOR: Noted.

▼ Reevaluate Transport Decision

Student: The patient is a low priority and does not require immediate transport.
PROCTOR: Noted.

▼ Detailed Physical Examination

Possible Answer #1
Student: I would not do a detailed physical exam.
PROCTOR: Noted. (Go to "Radio Report.")

Possible Answer #2
Student: I am conducting the detailed physical exam. I am looking for DCAP-BTLS. This acronym stands for deformities, contusions, abrasions, punctures, penetrations, paradoxical motion in the chest, and burns, tenderness, lacerations, and swelling.
PROCTOR: Noted. The detailed physical exam will be performed during transport.

▸ **Assess the Head**

Student: I am assessing the head. Do I find any DCAP-BTLS? Do I find any evidence of Battle's sign or raccoon eyes?
PROCTOR: No.

▸ **Inspect and Palpate the Head and Ears**

Student: I am assessing the head and ears.
PROCTOR: The skin on his face is irritated and red.

▸ **Assess the Eyes**

Student: I am assessing the eyes. Are the eyes PEARRL?
PROCTOR: They are bloodshot and burning and producing a lot of tears.

▸ **Assess the Facial Area Including Oral and Nasal Areas**

Student: I am assessing the face, nose, and mouth. Do I see any discharge or hear any obstructions?
PROCTOR: Yes, the patient is spitting and coughing.

▸ **Assess the Neck**

▸ **Inspect and Palpate the Neck**

Student: I am assessing the neck for DCAP-BTLS.
PROCTOR: The skin is irritated.

▸ **Assess for Jugular Vein Distention**

Student: Do I find any jugular vein distention (JVD)?
PROCTOR: No.

▸ **Assess for Tracheal Deviation**

Student: Do I see any tracheal deviation?
PROCTOR: No.

▸ **Assess the Chest**

Student: I am assessing the chest for DCAP-BTLS.
PROCTOR: Noted.

▸ **Inspect**

Student: What do I see when I look at the chest?
PROCTOR: The skin is irritated.
Student: Is the chest symmetric?
PROCTOR: Yes.

▸ **Palpate**

Student: When I touch the chest, do I feel crepitus or a flail segment?
PROCTOR: No.

▸ **Auscultate**

Student: Are lung sounds present in all fields?
PROCTOR: Yes.
Student: Do I hear any sucking sounds from the chest?
PROCTOR: No.

▸ **Assess the Abdomen/Pelvis**

▸ **Assess the Abdomen**

Student: I am assessing the abdomen for DCAP-BTLS. I am assessing all four quadrants. Do I find any problems?
PROCTOR: No.

▸ **Assess the Pelvis**

Student: I am assessing the pelvis for DCAP-BTLS. Is the pelvis stable?
PROCTOR: Yes.

▸ **Assess the Genitalia/Perineum as Needed (Verbalize in Training)**

Student: I am assessing the genitalia/perineum as necessary for DCAP-BTLS.
PROCTOR: The area is unremarkable.

▸ **Assess the Extremities**

▸ **Inspect**

Student: I am assessing the lower and upper extremities for DCAP-BTLS. Do I find anything?
PROCTOR: No.

▸ **Palpate**

Student: Do I feel anything unusual?
PROCTOR: No.

▸ **Assess Motor, Sensory, and Circulatory Function**

Student: I am checking for DCAP-BTLS, motor and sensory function, and pulses. Right leg?
PROCTOR: Negative DCAP-BTLS. Motor and sensory functions are present. Pulses are present.
Student: Left leg?
PROCTOR: Negative DCAP-BTLS. Motor and sensory functions are present. Pulses are present.
Student: Right arm?
PROCTOR: Negative DCAP-BTLS. Motor and sensory functions are present. Pulses are present.
Student: Left arm?
PROCTOR: Negative DCAP-BTLS. Motor and sensory functions are present. Pulses are present.

▸ **Assess the Posterior**

Student: We will check the back.
PROCTOR: Noted.

▸ **Assess the Thorax**

Student: I am assessing the thorax. Do I find injuries?
PROCTOR: No.

▸ **Assess the Lumbar Area**

Student: I am assessing the flanks and lumbar area. Do I find injuries?
PROCTOR: No.

▸ **Assess the Entire Backside**

Student: I am assessing the entire backside. Do I find injuries?
PROCTOR: No.

▸ **Manage Secondary Injuries/Wounds**

Student: I will direct my partner to flush the eyes and skin with water as needed and continue applying oxygen.
PROCTOR: Noted.

▸ Reassess Interventions

Student: I will reassess my interventions: flush the eyes and skin with water and apply oxygen.

PROCTOR: Noted.

Critical Criteria:

- ❑ Did not obtain medical direction or verbalize standing orders for medical interventions
- ❑ Administered a dangerous or inappropriate intervention
- ❑ Did not ask questions about the present illness
- ❑ Did not differentiate patient's need for transportation versus continued assessment at the scene

Radio Report

(Provided by the student.)

PROCTOR: Noted.

Ongoing Assessment

Repeat the Initial Assessment

Student: I will repeat the initial assessment.

PROCTOR: Noted. (Reflected in "Repeat Vital Signs.")

Repeat Vital Signs

Student: I will reassess vital signs and mental status.

PROCTOR: Blood pressure, 132/82 mm Hg; pulse rate, 108 beats/min; respirations, 20 breaths/min; pulse oximetry reading, 98%; and the patient is alert.

Student: The vital signs have not changed significantly.

PROCTOR: Noted.

Check Interventions

Student: I will check my interventions: flush the eyes and skin with water and apply oxygen.

PROCTOR: Noted.

Repeat the Focused Assessment

Student: I will repeat the focused assessment.

PROCTOR: Noted.

Critical Criteria:

- ❑ Did not obtain medical direction or verbalize standing orders for medical interventions
- ❑ Administered a dangerous or inappropriate intervention

Handoff Report to Emergency Department Staff

Student: There was no change in the patient's condition during transport.

PROCTOR: Noted.

Critical Criteria

(Inform the student of items missed, if any.)

❑ Pass ❑ Fail Date: ______________________

Proctor Comments: ______________________

____

____

Notes

Dispatch Information

PROCTOR: EMS 10, respond to a 60-year-old male who is complaining of shortness of breath and coughing. He is very weak. He is conscious and breathing.

Pre-scene Action (BSI)

Student: I am wearing nonlatex gloves and safety glasses.
PROCTOR: Noted.

Critical Criteria:
- ❑ Did not take, or verbalize, body substance isolation (BSI) precautions when necessary

Scene Size-up

Scene Safety

Student: Is the scene safe?
PROCTOR: Yes.

Mechanism of Injury/Nature of Illness

Student: What is the nature of the illness?
PROCTOR: Productive cough and shortness of breath.

Number of Patients

Student: How many patients are there?
PROCTOR: One.

Additional Resources

Student: I would not call for advanced life support (ALS) assistance.
PROCTOR: Noted.

C-Spine Stabilization

Student: I would not stabilize the cervical spine (c-spine).
PROCTOR: Noted.

Critical Criteria:
- ❑ Did not determine scene safety

Initial Assessment

General Impression

Student: My general impression is that the patient's condition is stable.
PROCTOR: Noted.

Responsiveness/Level of Consciousness

Student: What is the patient's level of consciousness?
PROCTOR: Alert.

Chief Complaint/Apparent Life Threats

Student: What is the patient's chief complaint?
PROCTOR: The patient is complaining of a productive cough, shortness of breath, and feeling weak.

Assess the Airway and Breathing

Student: Is the airway open? Is the patient breathing?
PROCTOR: Yes, the airway is open and the patient is breathing.

Assessment

Student: What are the rate and the quality of breathing?
PROCTOR: Rate: Tachypneic. Quality: Labored.

Provide Oxygen

Student: I am applying oxygen at 15 L/min via nonrebreathing mask.
PROCTOR: Noted.

Ensure Adequate Ventilation

Student: The patient has adequate ventilations at this time.
PROCTOR: Noted.

Assess Circulation

Student: I am assessing the patient's circulation.
PROCTOR: Noted.

Assess for and Control Major Bleeding

Student: Do I find any major bleeding?
PROCTOR: No.

Assess the Pulse

Student: What are the rate and the quality of pulses?
PROCTOR: Rate: Tachycardic. Quality: Thready.

Assess the Skin

Student: I am assessing the skin. What are the color, temperature, and condition of the skin?
PROCTOR: Color: Pale. Temperature: Hot. Condition: Dry.

Identify Priority Patients/Make Transport Decision

Student: The patient is a low priority and does not require immediate transport.
PROCTOR: Noted.

Critical Criteria:
- ❑ Did not provide high concentration of oxygen
- ❑ Did not find or manage problems associated with airway, breathing, hemorrhage or shock (hypoperfusion)
- ❑ Did not differentiate patient's need for transportation versus continued assessment at the scene
- ❑ Did detailed or focused history/physical examination before assessing the airway, breathing and circulation

Focused History and Physical Examination/Rapid Assessment

Select the Appropriate Assessment (Focused or Rapid)

Student: I am selecting the focused assessment.
PROCTOR: Noted.

SAMPLE History

Student: At this time I will gather a SAMPLE history from the patient or family. What are the patient's signs and symptoms?
PROCTOR: Respiratory (difficulty breathing with productive cough and weakness).

> **Student:** Onset: What were you doing when this started?
> **PROCTOR:** This has been going on for 2 or 3 days.
> **Student:** Provokes: What makes your condition worse or better?
> **PROCTOR:** Nothing.
> **Student:** Quality: Can you describe your pain?
> **PROCTOR:** The patient has rattling in his chest when he coughs.
> **Student:** Radiates: Do you have pain anywhere else?
> **PROCTOR:** No.
> **Student:** Severity: On a scale of 1 to 10 with 10 being the worst possible, how would you rate your distress?
> **PROCTOR:** 4.
> **Student:** Time: How long has this been going on?
> **PROCTOR:** 3 days.
> **Student:** Interventions: Have you done anything to make this better?
> **PROCTOR:** The patient has taken cold medications but has not been drinking fluids like he should. He has maxed out on his metered dose inhaler.

Student: Allergies?
PROCTOR: Penicillin (PCN).
Student: Medications?
PROCTOR: Asthma medications, inhaler, and other unknown medications.
Student: Pertinent past medical history?
PROCTOR: Asthma, bronchitis, and pneumonia.
Student: Last oral intake?
PROCTOR: 3 hours ago.
Student: Events leading up to the incident?
PROCTOR: The patient has been sick for 3 days.

Perform the Focused Physical Examination

Student: I am performing the focused physical examination.
PROCTOR: Noted.

Student: Are lung sounds present in all fields?
PROCTOR: Yes, they sound wet.
Student: Does he have any edema in his extremities?
PROCTOR: No.
Student: I will check his temperature.
PROCTOR: His temperature is 100.1°F (37.8°C).

▼ Baseline Vital Signs

Student: What are the patient's baseline vital signs, including blood pressure, pulse, respirations, pulse oximetry, and level of consciousness?
PROCTOR: Blood pressure, 118/68 mm Hg; pulse rate, 132 beats/min; respirations, 28 breaths/min; pulse oximetry reading, 96%; and the patient is alert.

▼ Interventions

Student: I will apply oxygen.
PROCTOR: Noted.
ALS Student: I will apply basic life support (BLS) interventions, plus the following: IV access, cardiac monitor, 12-lead ECG, and local protocol (breathing treatment).
ALS Proctor: Noted. The cardiac monitor shows sinus tachycardia.

▼ Reevaluate Transport Decision

Student: The patient is a low priority and does not require immediate transport.
PROCTOR: Noted.

▼ Detailed Physical Examination

Possible Answer #1
Student: I would not do a detailed physical exam.
PROCTOR: Noted. (Go to "Radio Report.")

Possible Answer #2
Student: I am conducting the detailed physical exam. I am looking for DCAP-BTLS. This acronym stands for deformities, contusions, abrasions, punctures, penetrations, paradoxical motion in the chest, and burns, tenderness, lacerations, and swelling.
PROCTOR: Noted. The detailed physical exam will be performed during transport.

► **Assess the Head**

Student: I am assessing the head. Do I find any DCAP-BTLS? Do I find any evidence of Battle's sign or raccoon eyes?
PROCTOR: No.

► **Inspect and Palpate the Head and Ears**

Student: I am assessing the head and ears.
PROCTOR: There are no obvious injuries.

► **Assess the Eyes**

Student: I am assessing the eyes. Are the pupils equal, round, and regular in size, and react properly to light (PEARRL)?
PROCTOR: They are PEARRL.

► **Assess the Facial Area Including Oral and Nasal Areas**

Student: I am assessing the face, nose, and mouth. Do I see any discharge or hear any obstructions?
PROCTOR: No.

► **Assess the Neck**

► **Inspect and Palpate the Neck**

Student: I am assessing the neck for DCAP-BTLS.
PROCTOR: There are no obvious injuries.

► **Assess for Jugular Vein Distention**

Student: Do I find any jugular vein distention (JVD)?
PROCTOR: No.

► **Assess for Tracheal Deviation**

Student: Do I see any tracheal deviation?
PROCTOR: No.

► **Assess the Chest**

Student: I am assessing the chest for DCAP-BTLS.
PROCTOR: Noted.

► **Inspect**

Student: What do I see when I look at the chest?
PROCTOR: There are no obvious injuries.
Student: Is the chest symmetric?
PROCTOR: Yes.

► **Palpate**

Student: When I touch the chest, do I feel crepitus or a flail segment?
PROCTOR: No.

► **Auscultate**

Student: Are lung sounds present in all fields?
PROCTOR: Yes, they sound wet.
Student: Do I hear any sucking sounds from the chest?
PROCTOR: No.

► **Assess the Abdomen/Pelvis**

► **Assess the Abdomen**

Student: I am assessing the abdomen for DCAP-BTLS. I am assessing all four quadrants. Do I find any problems?
PROCTOR: No.

► **Assess the Pelvis**

Student: I am assessing the pelvis for DCAP-BTLS. Is the pelvis stable?
PROCTOR: Yes.

► **Assess the Genitalia/Perineum as Needed (Verbalize in Training)**

Student: I am assessing the genitalia/perineum as necessary for DCAP-BTLS.
PROCTOR: The area is unremarkable.

► **Assess the Extremities**

► **Inspect**

Student: I am assessing the lower and upper extremities for DCAP-BTLS. Do I find anything?
PROCTOR: No.

► **Palpate**

Student: Do I feel anything unusual?
PROCTOR: No.

► **Assess Motor, Sensory, and Circulatory Function**

Student: I am checking for DCAP-BTLS, motor and sensory function, and pulses. Right leg?
PROCTOR: Negative DCAP-BTLS. Motor and sensory functions are present. Pulses are present.
Student: Left leg?
PROCTOR: Negative DCAP-BTLS. Motor and sensory functions are present. Pulses are present.
Student: Right arm?
PROCTOR: Poor skin turgor. Motor and sensory functions are present. Pulses are present.
Student: Left arm?
PROCTOR: Poor skin turgor. Motor and sensory functions are present. Pulses are present.

► **Assess the Posterior**

Student: We will check the back.
PROCTOR: Noted.

► **Assess the Thorax**

Student: I am assessing the thorax. Do I find injuries?
PROCTOR: No.

► **Assess the Lumbar Area**

Student: I am assessing the flanks and lumbar area. Do I find injuries?
PROCTOR: No.

► **Assess the Entire Backside**

Student: I am assessing the entire backside. Do I find injuries?
PROCTOR: No.

► **Manage Secondary Injuries/Wounds**

Student: I would direct my partner to continue providing oxygen.
PROCTOR: Noted.

▸ Reassess Interventions

Student: I will reassess my interventions: oxygen and transport the patient in the position of comfort.

PROCTOR: Noted.

ALS Student: I will reassess BLS interventions, plus the following: IVs, cardiac monitor, 12-lead ECG, and local protocol (breathing treatment).

ALS Proctor: Noted. The cardiac monitor shows sinus tachycardia.

Critical Criteria:

- ❑ Did not obtain medical direction or verbalize standing orders for medical interventions
- ❑ Administered a dangerous or inappropriate intervention
- ❑ Did not ask questions about the present illness
- ❑ Did not differentiate patient's need for transportation versus continued assessment at the scene

Radio Report

(Provided by the student.)

PROCTOR: Noted.

Ongoing Assessment

Repeat the Initial Assessment

Student: I will repeat the initial assessment.

PROCTOR: Noted. (Reflected in "Repeat Vital Signs.")

Repeat Vital Signs

Student: I will reassess vital signs and mental status.

PROCTOR: Blood pressure, 122/66 mm Hg; pulse rate, 122 beats/min; respirations, 24 breaths/min; pulse oximetry reading, 97%; and the patient is alert.

Student: The vital signs have not changed significantly.

PROCTOR: Noted.

Check Interventions

Student: I will reassess my interventions: oxygen and transport the patient in a position of comfort.

PROCTOR: Noted.

ALS Student: I will reassess BLS interventions, plus the following: IVs, cardiac monitor, 12-lead ECG, and local protocol (breathing treatment).

ALS Proctor: Noted. The cardiac monitor shows sinus tachycardia.

Repeat the Focused Assessment

Student: I will repeat the focused assessment.

PROCTOR: Noted.

Critical Criteria:

- ❑ Did not obtain medical direction or verbalize standing orders for medical interventions
- ❑ Administered a dangerous or inappropriate intervention

Handoff Report to Emergency Department Staff

Student: There was no change in the patient's condition during transport.

PROCTOR: Noted.

Critical Criteria

(Inform the student of items missed, if any.)

❑ Pass ❑ Fail Date: ______________________

Proctor Comments: ______________________

____

____

Notes

Dispatch Information

PROCTOR: EMS 10, respond to a 19-year-old pregnant female complaining of abdominal cramping. She is conscious and breathing.

Pre-scene Action (BSI)

Student: I am wearing nonlatex gloves and safety glasses.
PROCTOR: Noted.

Critical Criteria:
- ❑ Did not take, or verbalize, body substance isolation (BSI) precautions when necessary

Scene Size-up

Scene Safety

Student: Is the scene safe?
PROCTOR: Yes.

Mechanism of Injury/Nature of Illness

Student: What is the nature of the illness?
PROCTOR: Abdominal cramping.

Number of Patients

Student: How many patients are there?
PROCTOR: One.

Additional Resources

Student: I would call for advanced life support (ALS) assistance.
PROCTOR: Noted.

C-Spine Stabilization

Student: I would not stabilize the cervical spine (c-spine).
PROCTOR: Noted.

Critical Criteria:
- ❑ Did not determine scene safety

Initial Assessment

General Impression

Student: My general impression is that the patient's condition is unstable.
PROCTOR: Noted.

Responsiveness/Level of Consciousness

Student: What is the patient's level of consciousness?
PROCTOR: Alert.

Chief Complaint/Apparent Life Threats

Student: What is the patient's chief complaint?
PROCTOR: The patient is complaining of abdominal cramping.

Assess the Airway and Breathing

Student: Is the airway open?
PROCTOR: Yes.

Assessment

Student: What are the rate and the quality of breathing?
PROCTOR: Rate: Tachypneic. Quality: Shallow.

Provide Oxygen

Student: I am applying oxygen at 15 L/min via nonrebreathing mask.
PROCTOR: Noted.

Ensure Adequate Ventilation

Student: The patient has adequate ventilations at this time.
PROCTOR: Noted.

Assess Circulation

Student: I am assessing the patient's circulation.
PROCTOR: Noted.

Assess for and Control Major Bleeding

Student: Do I find any major bleeding?
PROCTOR: No.

Assess the Pulse

Student: What are the rate and the quality of pulses?
PROCTOR: Rate: Tachycardic. Quality: Bounding.

Assess the Skin

Student: I am assessing the skin. What are the color, temperature, and condition of the skin?
PROCTOR: Color: Normal. Temperature: Warm. Condition: Moist.

Identify Priority Patients/Make Transport Decision

Student: The patient is a high priority and is a load-and-go. I will begin packaging and transport.
PROCTOR: Noted.

Critical Criteria:
- ❑ Did not provide high concentration of oxygen
- ❑ Did not find or manage problems associated with airway, breathing, hemorrhage or shock (hypoperfusion)
- ❑ Did not differentiate patient's need for transportation versus continued assessment at the scene
- ❑ Did detailed or focused history/physical examination before assessing the airway, breathing and circulation

Focused History and Physical Examination/Rapid Assessment

Select the Appropriate Assessment (Focused or Rapid)

Student: I am selecting the focused assessment.
PROCTOR: Noted.

SAMPLE History

Student: At this time I will gather a SAMPLE history from the patient or family. What are the patient's signs and symptoms?
PROCTOR: Obstetrics (abdominal pain).

> **Student:** Are you pregnant?
> **PROCTOR:** Yes.
> **Student:** How long have you been pregnant?
> **PROCTOR:** 6 months.
> **Student:** Are you having pain or contractions?
> **PROCTOR:** Yes. Abdominal pain.
> **Student:** Are you having any bleeding or discharge?
> **PROCTOR:** No.
> **Student:** Do you feel the need to push?
> **PROCTOR:** No.
> **Student:** When was your last menstrual period?
> **PROCTOR:** 7 months ago.

Student: Allergies?
PROCTOR: No allergies.
Student: Medications?
PROCTOR: Vitamins.
Student: Pertinent past medical history?
PROCTOR: No pertinent medical history.
Student: Last oral intake?
PROCTOR: 4 hours ago.
Student: Events leading up to the incident?
PROCTOR: The patient was visiting family.

Perform the Focused Physical Examination

Student: I am performing the focused physical examination.
PROCTOR: Noted.
Student: I am assessing abdomen. What do I see?
PROCTOR: You see abdominal distention that is consistent with 6 months of pregnancy.

Student: I am assessing the abdomen for DCAP-BTLS. This acronym stands for deformities, contusions, abrasions, punctures, penetrations, paradoxical motion in the chest, and burns, tenderness, lacerations, and swelling. I am assessing all four quadrants. Do I find any problems?
PROCTOR: The patient has cramping in the lower left abdomen, and it is tender to palpation.
Student: I am assessing the pelvis for DCAP-BTLS. Is the pelvis stable?
PROCTOR: Yes.
Student: I am assessing the genitalia/perineum. Is there discharge or evidence of a miscarriage?
PROCTOR: There is no discharge or miscarriage present.

▼ Baseline Vital Signs

Student: What are the patient's baseline vital signs, including blood pressure, pulse, respirations, pulse oximetry, and level of consciousness?
PROCTOR: Blood pressure, 128/68 mm Hg; pulse rate, 126 beats/min; respirations, 28 breaths/min; pulse oximetry reading, 99%; and the patient is alert.

▼ Interventions

Student: I will apply oxygen and transport the patient on the left side.
PROCTOR: Noted.
ALS Student: I will apply basic life support (BLS) interventions, plus the following: establish two large-bore IVs and maintain a systolic blood pressure of 90 mm Hg.
ALS Proctor: Noted.

▼ Reevaluate Transport Decision

Student: The patient is a high priority and is a load-and-go.
PROCTOR: Noted.

▼ Detailed Physical Examination

Possible Answer #1
Student: I would not do a detailed physical exam.
PROCTOR: Noted. (Go to "Radio Report.")

Possible Answer #2
Student: I am conducting the detailed physical exam. I am looking for DCAP-BTLS.
PROCTOR: Noted. The detailed physical exam will be performed during transport.

▸ **Assess the Head**
Student: I am assessing the head. Do I find any DCAP-BTLS? Do I find any evidence of Battle's sign or raccoon eyes?
PROCTOR: No.

▸ **Inspect and Palpate the Head and Ears**
Student: I am assessing the head and ears.
PROCTOR: There are no obvious injuries.

▸ **Assess the Eyes**
Student: I am assessing the eyes. Are the pupils equal, round, and regular in size, and react properly to light (PEARRL)?
PROCTOR: They are PEARRL.

▸ **Assess the Facial Area Including Oral and Nasal Areas**
Student: I am assessing the face, nose, and mouth. Do I see any discharge or hear any obstructions?
PROCTOR: No.

▸ **Assess the Neck**

▸ **Inspect and Palpate the Neck**
Student: I am assessing the neck for DCAP-BTLS.
PROCTOR: There are no obvious injuries.

▸ **Assess for Jugular Vein Distention**
Student: Do I find any jugular vein distention (JVD)?
PROCTOR: No.

▸ **Assess for Tracheal Deviation**
Student: Do I see any tracheal deviation?
PROCTOR: No.

▸ **Assess the Chest**
Student: I am assessing the chest for DCAP-BTLS.
PROCTOR: Noted.

▸ **Inspect**
Student: What do I see when I look at the chest?
PROCTOR: There are no obvious injuries.
Student: Is the chest symmetric?
PROCTOR: Yes.

▸ **Palpate**
Student: When I touch the chest, do I feel crepitus or a flail segment?
PROCTOR: No.

▸ **Auscultate**
Student: Are lung sounds present in all fields?
PROCTOR: Yes.
Student: Do I hear any sucking sounds from the chest?
PROCTOR: No.

▸ **Assess the Abdomen/Pelvis**

▸ **Assess the Abdomen**
Student: I am assessing the abdomen for DCAP-BTLS. I am assessing all four quadrants. Do I find any problems?
PROCTOR: The patient has cramping in the lower left abdomen.

▸ **Assess the Pelvis**
Student: I am assessing the pelvis for DCAP-BTLS. Is the pelvis stable?
PROCTOR: Yes.

▸ **Assess the Genitalia/Perineum as Needed (Verbalize in Training)**
Student: I am assessing the genitalia/perineum as necessary for DCAP-BTLS.
PROCTOR: There is no discharge.

▸ **Assess the Extremities**

▸ **Inspect**
Student: I am assessing the lower and upper extremities for DCAP-BTLS. Do I find anything?
PROCTOR: No.

▸ **Palpate**
Student: Do I feel anything unusual?
PROCTOR: No.

▸ **Assess Motor, Sensory, and Circulatory Function**
Student: I am checking for DCAP-BTLS, motor and sensory function, and pulses. Right leg?
PROCTOR: Negative DCAP-BTLS. Motor and sensory functions are present. Pulses are present.
Student: Left leg?
PROCTOR: Negative DCAP-BTLS. Motor and sensory functions are present. Pulses are present.
Student: Right arm?
PROCTOR: Negative DCAP-BTLS. Motor and sensory functions are present. Pulses are present.
Student: Left arm?
PROCTOR: Negative DCAP-BTLS. Motor and sensory functions are present. Pulses are present.

▸ **Assess the Posterior**
Student: This is not necessary.
PROCTOR: Noted.

▸ **Manage Secondary Injuries/Wounds**
Student: I would reassure the patient.
PROCTOR: Noted.

▸ Reassess Interventions

Student: I will reassess my interventions: oxygen and transport the patient on the left side.

PROCTOR: Noted.

ALS Student: I will reassess BLS interventions, plus the following: IVs.

ALS Proctor: Noted.

Critical Criteria:
- ❑ Did not obtain medical direction or verbalize standing orders for medical interventions
- ❑ Administered a dangerous or inappropriate intervention
- ❑ Did not ask questions about the present illness
- ❑ Did not differentiate patient's need for transportation versus continued assessment at the scene

Radio Report

(Provided by the student.)

PROCTOR: Noted.

Ongoing Assessment

Repeat the Initial Assessment

Student: I will repeat the initial assessment.

PROCTOR: Noted. (Reflected in "Repeat Vital Signs.")

Repeat Vital Signs

Student: I will reassess vital signs and mental status.

PROCTOR: Blood pressure, 126/70 mm Hg; pulse rate, 122 beats/min; respirations, 24 breaths/min; pulse oximetry reading, 99%; and the patient is alert.

Student: The vital signs have not changed significantly.

PROCTOR: Noted.

Check Interventions

Student: I will reassess my interventions: oxygen and transport the patient on the left side.

PROCTOR: Noted.

ALS Student: I will reassess BLS interventions, plus the following: IVs.

ALS Proctor: Noted.

Repeat the Focused Assessment

Student: I will repeat the focused assessment.

PROCTOR: Noted.

Critical Criteria:
- ❑ Did not obtain medical direction or verbalize standing orders for medical interventions
- ❑ Administered a dangerous or inappropriate intervention

Handoff Report to Emergency Department Staff

Student: There was no change in the patient's condition during transport.

PROCTOR: Noted.

Critical Criteria

(Inform the student of items missed, if any.)

❑ Pass ❑ Fail Date: ______________________

Proctor Comments: ______________________

Notes

Dispatch Information

PROCTOR: EMS 10, respond to a 14-year-old male who has been huffing paint. He is having trouble breathing.

Pre-scene Action (BSI)

Student: I am wearing nonlatex gloves and safety glasses.
PROCTOR: Noted.

Critical Criteria:
- ❑ Did not take, or verbalize, body substance isolation (BSI) precautions when necessary

Scene Size-up

Scene Safety

Student: Is the scene safe?
PROCTOR: Yes.

Mechanism of Injury/Nature of Illness

Student: What is the nature of the illness?
PROCTOR: Huffing gold-colored aerosol paint.

Number of Patients

Student: How many patients are there?
PROCTOR: One.

Additional Resources

Student: I would call for advanced life support (ALS) assistance.
PROCTOR: Noted.

C-Spine Stabilization

Student: I would not stabilize the cervical spine (c-spine).
PROCTOR: Noted.

Critical Criteria:
- ❑ Did not determine scene safety

Initial Assessment

General Impression

Student: My general impression is that the patient's condition is unstable.
PROCTOR: Noted.

Responsiveness/Level of Consciousness

Student: What is the patient's level of consciousness?
PROCTOR: Alert.

Chief Complaint/Apparent Life Threats

Student: What is the patient's chief complaint?
PROCTOR: The patient is complaining of shortness of breath and chest pain.

Assess the Airway and Breathing

Student: Is the airway open?
PROCTOR: Yes.

Assessment

Student: What are the rate and the quality of breathing?
PROCTOR: Rate: Rapid. Quality: Labored.

Provide Oxygen

Student: I am applying oxygen at 15 L/min via nonrebreathing mask.
PROCTOR: Noted.

Ensure Adequate Ventilation

Student: The patient has adequate ventilations at this time.
PROCTOR: Noted.

Assess Circulation

Student: I am assessing the patient's circulation.
PROCTOR: Noted.

Assess for and Control Major Bleeding

Student: Do I find any major bleeding?
PROCTOR: No.

Assess the Pulse

Student: What are the rate and the quality of pulses?
PROCTOR: Rate: Tachycardic. Quality: Bounding.

Assess the Skin

Student: I am assessing the skin. What are the color, temperature, and condition of the skin?
PROCTOR: Color: Cyanotic. Temperature: Cool. Condition: Diaphoretic.

Identify Priority Patients/Make Transport Decision

Student: The patient is a high priority and is a load-and-go. I will begin packaging and transport.
PROCTOR: Noted.

Critical Criteria:
- ❑ Did not provide high concentration of oxygen
- ❑ Did not find or manage problems associated with airway, breathing, hemorrhage or shock (hypoperfusion)
- ❑ Did not differentiate patient's need for transportation versus continued assessment at the scene
- ❑ Did detailed or focused history/physical examination before assessing the airway, breathing and circulation

Focused History and Physical Examination/Rapid Assessment

Select the Appropriate Assessment (Focused or Rapid)

Student: I am selecting the focused assessment.
PROCTOR: Noted.

SAMPLE History

Student: At this time I will gather a SAMPLE history from the patient or family. What are the patient's signs and symptoms?
PROCTOR: Poisoning/overdose with difficulty breathing and chest pain.

> **Student:** What was the substance?
> **PROCTOR:** Gold spray paint.
> **Student:** When did you become exposed?
> **PROCTOR:** It was 15 minutes ago.
> **Student:** Over what time period?
> **PROCTOR:** Over 3 minutes.
> **Student:** What is your weight?
> **PROCTOR:** 115 pounds.
> **Student:** Onset: What were you doing when this began?
> **PROCTOR:** Huffing gold paint.
> **Student:** Provokes: What makes the condition worse?
> **PROCTOR:** Nothing.
> **Student:** Quality: Can you describe the pain?
> **PROCTOR:** He feels cold inside and it is hard to breathe.
> **Student:** Radiates: Do you have pain anywhere else?
> **PROCTOR:** No.
> **Student:** How long have you had the pain and trouble breathing?
> **PROCTOR:** About 15 minutes.
> **Student:** Interventions: Have you done anything to make this better?
> **PROCTOR:** Yes, he stopped huffing the paint.

Student: Allergies?
PROCTOR: No allergies.
Student: Medications?
PROCTOR: No medications.
Student: Pertinent past medical history?
PROCTOR: No pertinent medical history.
Student: Last oral intake?
PROCTOR: 3 hours ago.

Student: Events leading up to the incident?
PROCTOR: The patient was huffing paint with friends.

▼ Perform the Focused Physical Examination

Student: I am performing the focused physical examination.
PROCTOR: Noted.
Student: Do I see any cyanosis around the lips or elsewhere?
PROCTOR: Yes, he has some cyanosis around his lips, face, and fingertips that is improving with the oxygen.
Student: What are his lung sounds?
PROCTOR: His lungs are clear bilaterally.

▼ Baseline Vital Signs

Student: What are the patient's baseline vital signs, including blood pressure, pulse, respirations, pulse oximetry, and level of consciousness?
PROCTOR: Blood pressure, 128/82 mm Hg; pulse rate, 114 beats/min; respirations, 28 breaths/min; pulse oximetry reading, 92%; and the patient is alert.

▼ Interventions

Student: I will apply oxygen and contact medical control and poison control.
PROCTOR: Noted.
ALS Student: I will apply basic life support (BLS) interventions, plus the following: IV access, cardiac monitor, 12-lead ECG, and local protocol.
ALS Proctor: Noted. The cardiac monitor shows sinus tachycardia.

▼ Reevaluate Transport Decision

Student: The patient is a high priority and is a load-and-go.
PROCTOR: Noted.

▼ Detailed Physical Examination

Possible Answer #1
Student: I would not do a detailed physical exam.
PROCTOR: Noted. (Go to "Radio Report.")

Possible Answer #2
Student: I am conducting the detailed physical exam. I am looking for DCAP-BTLS. This acronym stands for deformities, contusions, abrasions, punctures, penetrations, paradoxical motion in the chest, and burns, tenderness, lacerations, and swelling.
PROCTOR: Noted. The detailed physical exam will be performed during transport.

▸ Assess the Head

Student: I am assessing the head. Do I find any DCAP-BTLS? Do I find any evidence of Battle's sign or raccoon eyes?
PROCTOR: No.

▸ Inspect and Palpate the Head and Ears

Student: I am assessing the head and ears.
PROCTOR: There are no obvious injuries.

▸ Assess the Eyes

Student: I am assessing the eyes. Are the pupils equal, round, and regular in size, and react properly to light (PEARRL)?
PROCTOR: They are sluggish.

▸ Assess the Facial Area Including Oral and Nasal Areas

Student: I am assessing the face, nose, and mouth. Do I see any discharge or hear any obstructions?
PROCTOR: No, but you do see evidence of gold paint around the lips.

▸ Assess the Neck

▸ Inspect and Palpate the Neck

Student: I am assessing the neck for DCAP-BTLS.
PROCTOR: There are no obvious injuries.

▸ Assess for Jugular Vein Distention

Student: Do I find any jugular vein distention (JVD)?
PROCTOR: No.

▸ Assess for Tracheal Deviation

Student: Do I see any tracheal deviation?
PROCTOR: No.

▸ Assess the Chest

Student: I am assessing the chest for DCAP-BTLS.
PROCTOR: Noted.

▸ Inspect

Student: What do I see when I look at the chest?
PROCTOR: There are no obvious injuries.
Student: Is the chest symmetric?
PROCTOR: Yes.

▸ Palpate

Student: When I touch the chest, do I feel crepitus or a flail segment?
PROCTOR: No.

▸ Auscultate

Student: Are lung sounds present in all fields?
PROCTOR: Yes.
Student: Do I hear any sucking sounds from the chest?
PROCTOR: No.

▸ Assess the Abdomen/Pelvis

▸ Assess the Abdomen

Student: I am assessing the abdomen for DCAP-BTLS. I am assessing all four quadrants. Do I find any problems?
PROCTOR: No.

▸ Assess the Pelvis

Student: I am assessing the pelvis for DCAP-BTLS. Is the pelvis stable?
PROCTOR: Yes.

▸ Assess the Genitalia/Perineum as Needed (Verbalize in Training)

Student: I am assessing the genitalia/perineum as necessary for DCAP-BTLS.
PROCTOR: The area is unremarkable.

▸ Assess the Extremities

▸ Inspect

Student: I am assessing the lower and upper extremities for DCAP-BTLS. Do I find anything?
PROCTOR: No.

▸ Palpate

Student: Do I feel anything unusual?
PROCTOR: No.

▸ Assess Motor, Sensory, and Circulatory Function

Student: I am checking for DCAP-BTLS, motor and sensory function, and pulses. Right leg?
PROCTOR: Negative DCAP-BTLS. Motor and sensory functions are present. Pulses are present.
Student: Left leg?
PROCTOR: Negative DCAP-BTLS. Motor and sensory functions are present. Pulses are present.
Student: Right arm?
PROCTOR: Negative DCAP-BTLS. Motor and sensory functions are present. Pulses are present.
Student: Left arm?
PROCTOR: Negative DCAP-BTLS. Motor and sensory functions are present. Pulses are present.

▸ Assess the Posterior

Student: We will check the back.
PROCTOR: Noted.

▸ Assess the Thorax

Student: I am assessing the thorax. Do I find injuries?
PROCTOR: No.

▸ Assess the Lumbar Area

Student: I am assessing the flanks and lumbar area. Do I find injuries?
PROCTOR: No.

Assess the Entire Backside

Student: I am assessing the entire backside. Do I find injuries?

PROCTOR: No.

Manage Secondary Injuries/Wounds

Student: I would direct my partner to continue providing oxygen.

PROCTOR: Noted.

Reassess Interventions

Student: I will reassess my interventions: oxygen and contact medical control.

PROCTOR: Noted.

ALS Student: I will reassess BLS interventions, plus the following: IV access, cardiac monitor, 12-lead ECG, and local protocol.

ALS Proctor: Noted. The cardiac monitor shows sinus tachycardia.

Critical Criteria:

- ❑ Did not obtain medical direction or verbalize standing orders for medical interventions
- ❑ Administered a dangerous or inappropriate intervention
- ❑ Did not ask questions about the present illness
- ❑ Did not differentiate patient's need for transportation versus continued assessment at the scene

Radio Report

(Provided by the student.)

PROCTOR: Noted.

Ongoing Assessment

Repeat the Initial Assessment

Student: I will repeat the initial assessment.

PROCTOR: Noted. (Reflected in "Repeat Vital Signs.")

Repeat Vital Signs

Student: I will reassess vital signs and mental status.

PROCTOR: Blood pressure, 124/78 mm Hg; pulse rate, 108 beats/min; respirations, 24 breaths/min; pulse oximetry reading, 95%; and the patient is alert.

Student: The vital signs have not changed significantly.

PROCTOR: Noted.

Check Interventions

Student: I will reassess my interventions: oxygen and contact medical control.

PROCTOR: Noted.

ALS Student: I will reassess BLS interventions, plus the following: IV access, cardiac monitor, 12-lead ECG, and local protocol.

ALS Proctor: Noted. The cardiac monitor shows sinus tachycardia.

Repeat the Focused Assessment

Student: I will repeat the focused assessment.

PROCTOR: Noted.

Critical Criteria:

- ❑ Did not obtain medical direction or verbalize standing orders for medical interventions
- ❑ Administered a dangerous or inappropriate intervention

Handoff Report to Emergency Department Staff

Student: There was no change in the patient's condition during transport.

PROCTOR: Noted.

Critical Criteria

(Inform the student of items missed, if any.)

❑ Pass ❑ Fail Date: ______________________________

Proctor Comments: ______________________________

____

____

Notes

Dispatch Information

PROCTOR: EMS 10, respond to a 36-year-old female who is complaining of difficulty breathing. She is conscious and breathing.

Pre-scene Action (BSI)

Student: I am wearing nonlatex gloves and safety glasses.
PROCTOR: Noted.

Critical Criteria:
- ❑ Did not take, or verbalize, body substance isolation (BSI) precautions when necessary

Scene Size-up

Scene Safety

Student: Is the scene safe?
PROCTOR: Yes.

Mechanism of Injury/Nature of Illness

Student: What is the nature of the illness?
PROCTOR: Hyperventilation. The patient's boyfriend just broke up with her and she started hyperventilating.

Number of Patients

Student: How many patients are there?
PROCTOR: One.

Additional Resources

Student: I would not call for advanced life support (ALS) assistance.
PROCTOR: Noted.

C-Spine Stabilization

Student: I would not stabilize the cervical spine (c-spine).
PROCTOR: Noted.

Critical Criteria:
- ❑ Did not determine scene safety

Initial Assessment

General Impression

Student: My general impression is that the patient's condition is stable.
PROCTOR: Noted.

Responsiveness/Level of Consciousness

Student: What is the patient's level of consciousness?
PROCTOR: Alert.

Chief Complaint/Apparent Life Threats

Student: What is the patient's chief complaint?
PROCTOR: The patient is complaining of difficulty breathing.

Assess the Airway and Breathing

Student: Is the airway open? Is the patient breathing?
PROCTOR: Yes, the airway is open and the patient is breathing.

Assessment

Student: What are the rate and the quality of breathing?
PROCTOR: Rate: Tachypneic. Quality: Crying.

Provide Oxygen

Student: I am applying oxygen per local protocol. I will try to coach the patient's breathing and provide reassurance.
PROCTOR: Noted.

Ensure Adequate Ventilation

Student: The patient has adequate ventilations at this time.
PROCTOR: Noted.

Assess Circulation

Student: I am assessing the patient's circulation.
PROCTOR: Noted.

Assess for and Control Major Bleeding

Student: Do I find any major bleeding?
PROCTOR: No.

Assess the Pulse

Student: What are the rate and the quality of pulses?
PROCTOR: Rate: Tachycardic. Quality: Strong.

Assess the Skin

Student: I am assessing the skin. What are the color, temperature, and condition of the skin?
PROCTOR: Color: Flushed. Temperature: Warm. Condition: Moist.

Identify Priority Patients/Make Transport Decision

Student: The patient is a low priority and does not require immediate transport.
PROCTOR: Noted.

Critical Criteria:
- ❑ Did not provide high concentration of oxygen
- ❑ Did not find or manage problems associated with airway, breathing, hemorrhage or shock (hypoperfusion)
- ❑ Did not differentiate patient's need for transportation versus continued assessment at the scene
- ❑ Did detailed or focused history/physical examination before assessing the airway, breathing and circulation

Focused History and Physical Examination/Rapid Assessment

Select the Appropriate Assessment (Focused or Rapid)

Student: I am selecting the focused assessment.
PROCTOR: Noted.

SAMPLE History

Student: At this time I will gather a SAMPLE history from the patient or family. What are the patient's signs and symptoms?
PROCTOR: Respiratory (difficulty breathing and shortness of breath).

> **Student:** Onset: What were you doing when this started?
> **PROCTOR:** The patient's boyfriend just broke up with her.
> **Student:** Provokes: What makes your condition worse or better?
> **PROCTOR:** Nothing.
> **Student:** Quality: Can you describe your pain?
> **PROCTOR:** None.
> **Student:** Radiates: Do you have pain anywhere else?
> **PROCTOR:** No.
> **Student:** Severity: On a scale of 1 to 10 with 10 being the worst possible, how would you rate your distress?
> **PROCTOR:** 8.
> **Student:** Time: How long has this been going on?
> **PROCTOR:** 15 minutes.
> **Student:** Interventions: Have you done anything to make this better?
> **PROCTOR:** The patient has taken no actions.

Student: Allergies?
PROCTOR: No allergies.
Student: Medications?
PROCTOR: No medications.
Student: Pertinent past medical history?
PROCTOR: No pertinent medical history.
Student: Last oral intake?
PROCTOR: 3 hours ago.
Student: Events leading up to the incident?
PROCTOR: Her boyfriend just broke up with her.

Perform the Focused Physical Examination

Student: I am performing the focused physical examination.
PROCTOR: Noted.
Student: Has she had previous anxiety attacks?
PROCTOR: Yes. She has them when she is afraid or upset.

Student: I am attempting to coach her to calm her down. Does this technique work?
PROCTOR: Yes, but she does occasionally begin to cry for a few seconds.

Baseline Vital Signs

Student: What are the patient's baseline vital signs, including blood pressure, pulse, respirations, pulse oximetry, and level of consciousness?
PROCTOR: Blood pressure, 136/74 mm Hg; pulse rate, 120 beats/min; respirations, 32 breaths/min; pulse oximetry reading, 99%; and the patient is alert.

Interventions

Student: I will apply oxygen, reassurance, and transport.
PROCTOR: Noted.

Reevaluate Transport Decision

Student: The patient is a low priority and does not require immediate transport.
PROCTOR: Noted.

Detailed Physical Examination

Possible Answer #1
Student: I would not do a detailed physical exam.
PROCTOR: Noted. (Go to "Radio Report.")

Possible Answer #2
Student: I am conducting the detailed physical exam. I am looking for DCAP-BTLS. This acronym stands for deformities, contusions, abrasions, punctures, penetrations, paradoxical motion in the chest, and burns, tenderness, lacerations, and swelling.
PROCTOR: Noted. The detailed physical exam will be performed during transport.

- **Assess the Head**

Student: I am assessing the head. Do I find any DCAP-BTLS? Do I find any evidence of Battle's sign or raccoon eyes?
PROCTOR: No.

- **Inspect and Palpate the Head and Ears**

Student: I am assessing the head and ears.
PROCTOR: There are no obvious injuries.

- **Assess the Eyes**

Student: I am assessing the eyes. Are the pupils equal, round, and regular in size, and react properly to light (PEARRL)?
PROCTOR: They are PEARRL.

- **Assess the Facial Area Including Oral and Nasal Areas**

Student: I am assessing the face, nose, and mouth. Do I see any discharge or hear any obstructions?
PROCTOR: No.

- **Assess the Neck**
- **Inspect and Palpate the Neck**

Student: I am assessing the neck for DCAP-BTLS.
PROCTOR: There are no obvious injuries.

- **Assess for Jugular Vein Distention**

Student: Do I find any jugular vein distention (JVD)?
PROCTOR: No.

- **Assess for Tracheal Deviation**

Student: Do I see any tracheal deviation?
PROCTOR: No.

- **Assess the Chest**

Student: I am assessing the chest for DCAP-BTLS.
PROCTOR: Noted.

- **Inspect**

Student: What do I see when I look at the chest?
PROCTOR: There are no obvious injuries.
Student: Is the chest symmetric?
PROCTOR: Yes.

- **Palpate**

Student: When I touch the chest, do I feel crepitus or a flail segment?
PROCTOR: No.

- **Auscultate**

Student: Are lung sounds present in all fields?
PROCTOR: Yes.
Student: Do I hear any sucking sounds from the chest?
PROCTOR: No.

- **Assess the Abdomen/Pelvis**
- **Assess the Abdomen**

Student: I am assessing the abdomen for DCAP-BTLS. I am assessing all four quadrants. Do I find any problems?
PROCTOR: No.

- **Assess the Pelvis**

Student: I am assessing the pelvis for DCAP-BTLS. Is the pelvis stable?
PROCTOR: Yes.

- **Assess the Genitalia/Perineum as Needed (Verbalize in Training)**

Student: I am assessing the genitalia/perineum as necessary for DCAP-BTLS.
PROCTOR: The area is unremarkable.

- **Assess the Extremities**
- **Inspect**

Student: I am assessing the lower and upper extremities for DCAP-BTLS. Do I find anything?
PROCTOR: No.

- **Palpate**

Student: Do I feel anything unusual?
PROCTOR: No.

- **Assess Motor, Sensory, and Circulatory Function**

Student: I am checking for DCAP-BTLS, motor and sensory function, and pulses. Right leg?
PROCTOR: Negative DCAP-BTLS. Motor and sensory functions are present. Pulses are present.
Student: Left leg?
PROCTOR: Negative DCAP-BTLS. Motor and sensory functions are present. Pulses are present.
Student: Right arm?
PROCTOR: Negative DCAP-BTLS. Motor and sensory functions are present. Pulses are present. She has a pins-and-needles sensation present.
Student: Left arm?
PROCTOR: Negative DCAP-BTLS. Motor and sensory functions are present. Pulses are present. She has a pins-and-needles sensation present.

- **Assess the Posterior**

Student: We will check the back.
PROCTOR: Noted.

- **Assess the Thorax**

Student: I am assessing the thorax. Do I find injuries?
PROCTOR: No.

- **Assess the Lumbar Area**

Student: I am assessing the flanks and lumbar area. Do I find injuries?
PROCTOR: No.

- **Assess the Entire Backside**

Student: I am assessing the entire backside. Do I find injuries?
PROCTOR: No.

- **Manage Secondary Injuries/Wounds**

Student: I would reassure the patient.
PROCTOR: Noted.

▸ **Reassess Interventions**

Student: I will reassess my interventions: oxygen, reassurance, and transport.

PROCTOR: Noted.

Critical Criteria:
- ❑ Did not obtain medical direction or verbalize standing orders for medical interventions
- ❑ Administered a dangerous or inappropriate intervention
- ❑ Did not ask questions about the present illness
- ❑ Did not differentiate patient's need for transportation versus continued assessment at the scene

Radio Report

(Provided by the student.)

PROCTOR: Noted.

Ongoing Assessment

Repeat the Initial Assessment

Student: I will repeat the initial assessment.

PROCTOR: Noted. (Reflected in "Repeat Vital Signs.")

Repeat Vital Signs

Student: I will reassess vital signs and mental status.

PROCTOR: Blood pressure, 130/70 mm Hg; pulse rate, 110 beats/min; respirations, 24 breaths/min; pulse oximetry reading, 99%; and the patient is alert.

Student: The vital signs have improved.

PROCTOR: Noted.

Check Interventions

Student: I will reassess my interventions: oxygen, reassurance, and transport.

PROCTOR: Noted.

Repeat the Focused Assessment

Student: I will repeat the focused assessment.

PROCTOR: Noted.

Critical Criteria:
- ❑ Did not obtain medical direction or verbalize standing orders for medical interventions
- ❑ Administered a dangerous or inappropriate intervention

Handoff Report to Emergency Department Staff

Student: The patient's condition improved during transport.

PROCTOR: Noted.

Critical Criteria

(Inform the student of items missed, if any.)

❑ Pass ❑ Fail Date: ______________________

Proctor Comments: ______________________

____

____

Notes

Dispatch Information

PROCTOR: EMS 10, respond to an 85-year-old male who is complaining of fever. He has a feeding tube. He is conscious and breathing.

Pre-scene Action (BSI)

Student: I am wearing nonlatex gloves and safety glasses.
PROCTOR: Noted.

> **Critical Criteria:**
> ❑ Did not take, or verbalize, body substance isolation (BSI) precautions when necessary

Scene Size-up

Scene Safety

Student: Is the scene safe?
PROCTOR: Yes.

Mechanism of Injury/Nature of Illness

Student: What is the nature of the illness?
PROCTOR: Fever of 102.5°F (39.2°C).

Number of Patients

Student: How many patients are there?
PROCTOR: One.

Additional Resources

Student: I would call for advanced life support (ALS) assistance.
PROCTOR: Noted.

C-Spine Stabilization

Student: I would not stabilize the cervical spine (c-spine).
PROCTOR: Noted.

> **Critical Criteria:**
> ❑ Did not determine scene safety

Initial Assessment

General Impression

Student: My general impression is that the patient's condition is stable.
PROCTOR: Noted.

Responsiveness/Level of Consciousness

Student: What is the patient's level of consciousness?
PROCTOR: Alert.

Chief Complaint/Apparent Life Threats

Student: What is the patient's chief complaint?
PROCTOR: The patient is complaining of a high temperature and weakness.

Assess the Airway and Breathing

Student: Is the airway open? Is the patient breathing?
PROCTOR: Yes, the airway is open and the patient is breathing.

▸ Assessment

Student: What are the rate and the quality of breathing?
PROCTOR: Rate: Within normal limits. Quality: Normal.

▸ Provide Oxygen

Student: I am applying oxygen at 15 L/min via nonrebreathing mask.
PROCTOR: Noted.

▸ Ensure Adequate Ventilation

Student: The patient has adequate ventilations at this time.
PROCTOR: Noted.

Assess Circulation

Student: I am assessing the patient's circulation.
PROCTOR: Noted.

▸ Assess for and Control Major Bleeding

Student: Do I find any major bleeding?
PROCTOR: No.

▸ Assess the Pulse

Student: What are the rate and the quality of pulses?
PROCTOR: Rate: Tachycardic. Quality: Thready.

▸ Assess the Skin

Student: I am assessing the skin. What are the color, temperature, and condition of the skin?
PROCTOR: Color: Jaundice. Temperature: Warm. Condition: Dry.

Identify Priority Patients/Make Transport Decision

Student: The patient is a low priority and does not require immediate transport.
PROCTOR: Noted.

> **Critical Criteria:**
> ❑ Did not provide high concentration of oxygen
> ❑ Did not find or manage problems associated with airway, breathing, hemorrhage or shock (hypoperfusion)
> ❑ Did not differentiate patient's need for transportation versus continued assessment at the scene
> ❑ Did detailed or focused history/physical examination before assessing the airway, breathing and circulation

Focused History and Physical Examination/Rapid Assessment

Select the Appropriate Assessment (Focused or Rapid)

Student: I am selecting the focused assessment.
PROCTOR: Noted.

SAMPLE History

Student: At this time I will gather a SAMPLE history from the patient or family. What are the patient's signs and symptoms?
PROCTOR: Fever and weakness (sick call).

> **Student:** Onset: What were you doing when this started?
> **PROCTOR:** Sleeping.
> **Student:** Provokes: What makes your condition worse or better?
> **PROCTOR:** He does not know.
> **Student:** Quality: Can you describe your pain?
> **PROCTOR:** None.
> **Student:** Radiates: Do you have pain anywhere else?
> **PROCTOR:** No.
> **Student:** Severity: On a scale of 1 to 10 with 10 being the worst possible, how would you rate your distress?
> **PROCTOR:** 2.
> **Student:** Time: How long has this been going on?
> **PROCTOR:** 12 hours.
> **Student:** Interventions: Have you done anything to make this better?
> **PROCTOR:** The patient has taken Tylenol. The Tylenol has helped with the temperature, which is now 100.5°F (38.1°C).

Student: Allergies?
PROCTOR: No allergies.
Student: Medications?
PROCTOR: Liver pills.
Student: Pertinent past medical history?
PROCTOR: The patient has hepatitis and a feeding tube. The feeding tube is disconnected from the pump at this time.
Student: Last oral intake?
PROCTOR: 2 hours ago.
Student: Events leading up to the incident?
PROCTOR: The patient had a fever for about 12 hours. His doctor is requesting that he be transported to the emergency room for treatment.

Perform the Focused Physical Examination

Student: I am performing the focused physical examination.
PROCTOR: Noted.
Student: What are the lung sounds?
PROCTOR: They are clear bilaterally.
Student: I am assessing the abdomen. I am assessing all four quadrants. Do I find any problems?
PROCTOR: No.

Baseline Vital Signs

Student: What are the patient's baseline vital signs, including blood pressure, pulse, respirations, pulse oximetry, and level of consciousness?
PROCTOR: Blood pressure, 148/88 mm Hg; pulse rate, 112 beats/min; respirations, 28 breaths/min; pulse oximetry reading, 97%; and the patient is alert.

Interventions

Student: I will apply oxygen and transport the patient.
PROCTOR: Noted.
ALS Student: I will apply basic life support (BLS) interventions, plus the following: IV access, cardiac monitor, and local protocol.
ALS Proctor: Noted. The cardiac monitor shows sinus tachycardia.

Reevaluate Transport Decision

Student: The patient is a low priority and does not require immediate transport.
PROCTOR: Noted.

Detailed Physical Examination

Possible Answer #1
Student: I would not do a detailed physical exam.
PROCTOR: Noted. (Go to "Radio Report.")

Possible Answer #2
Student: I am conducting the detailed physical exam. I am looking for DCAP-BTLS. This acronym stands for deformities, contusions, abrasions, punctures, penetrations, paradoxical motion in the chest, and burns, tenderness, lacerations, and swelling.
PROCTOR: Noted. The detailed physical exam will be performed during transport.

- **Assess the Head**

Student: I am assessing the head. Do I find any DCAP-BTLS? Do I find any evidence of Battle's sign or raccoon eyes?
PROCTOR: No.

- **Inspect and Palpate the Head and Ears**

Student: I am assessing the head and ears.
PROCTOR: There are no obvious injuries.

- **Assess the Eyes**

Student: I am assessing the eyes. Are the pupils equal, round, and regular in size, and react properly to light (PEARRL)?
PROCTOR: They are PEARRL.

- **Assess the Facial Area Including Oral and Nasal Areas**

Student: I am assessing the face, nose, and mouth. Do I see any discharge or hear any obstructions?
PROCTOR: No.

- **Assess the Neck**
- **Inspect and Palpate the Neck**

Student: I am assessing the neck for DCAP-BTLS.
PROCTOR: There are no obvious injuries.

- **Assess for Jugular Vein Distention**

Student: Do I find any jugular vein distention (JVD)?
PROCTOR: No.

- **Assess for Tracheal Deviation**

Student: Do I see any tracheal deviation?
PROCTOR: No.

- **Assess the Chest**

Student: I am assessing the chest for DCAP-BTLS.
PROCTOR: Noted.

- **Inspect**

Student: What do I see when I look at the chest?
PROCTOR: There are no obvious injuries.
Student: Is the chest symmetric?
PROCTOR: Yes.

- **Palpate**

Student: When I touch the chest, do I feel crepitus or a flail segment?
PROCTOR: No.

- **Auscultate**

Student: Are lung sounds present in all fields?
PROCTOR: Yes.
Student: Do I hear any sucking sounds from the chest?
PROCTOR: No.

- **Assess the Abdomen/Pelvis**
- **Assess the Abdomen**

Student: I am assessing the abdomen for DCAP-BTLS. I am assessing all four quadrants. Do I find any problems?
PROCTOR: No.

- **Assess the Pelvis**

Student: I am assessing the pelvis for DCAP-BTLS. Is the pelvis stable?
PROCTOR: Yes.

- **Assess the Genitalia/Perineum as Needed (Verbalize in Training)**

Student: I am assessing the genitalia/perineum as necessary for DCAP-BTLS.
PROCTOR: The area is unremarkable.

- **Assess the Extremities**
- **Inspect**

Student: I am assessing the lower and upper extremities for DCAP-BTLS. Do I find anything?
PROCTOR: No.

- **Palpate**

Student: Do I feel anything unusual?
PROCTOR: No.

- **Assess Motor, Sensory, and Circulatory Function**

Student: I am checking for DCAP-BTLS, motor and sensory function, and pulses. Right leg?
PROCTOR: Negative DCAP-BTLS. Motor and sensory functions are present. Pulses are present.
Student: Left leg?
PROCTOR: Negative DCAP-BTLS. Motor and sensory functions are present. Pulses are present.
Student: Right arm?
PROCTOR: Negative DCAP-BTLS. Motor and sensory functions are present. Pulses are present.
Student: Left arm?
PROCTOR: Negative DCAP-BTLS. Motor and sensory functions are present. Pulses are present.

- **Assess the Posterior**

Student: We will now check the back.
PROCTOR: Noted.

- **Assess the Thorax**

Student: I am assessing the thorax. Do I find injuries?
PROCTOR: No.

- **Assess the Lumbar Area**

Student: I am assessing the flanks and lumbar area. Do I find injuries?
PROCTOR: No.

- **Assess the Entire Backside**

Student: I am assessing the entire backside. Do I find injuries?
PROCTOR: No.

- **Manage Secondary Injuries/Wounds**

Student: I would direct my partner to continue providing oxygen.
PROCTOR: Noted.

▸ **Reassess Interventions**

Student: I will reassess my interventions: oxygen and transport the patient.

PROCTOR: Noted.

ALS Student: I will reassess BLS interventions, plus the following: IV access, cardiac monitor, 12-lead ECG, and local protocol.

ALS Proctor: Noted. The cardiac monitor shows sinus tachycardia.

Critical Criteria:
- ☐ Did not obtain medical direction or verbalize standing orders for medical interventions
- ☐ Administered a dangerous or inappropriate intervention
- ☐ Did not ask questions about the present illness
- ☐ Did not differentiate patient's need for transportation versus continued assessment at the scene

Radio Report

(Provided by the student.)

PROCTOR: Noted.

Ongoing Assessment

Repeat the Initial Assessment

Student: I will repeat the initial assessment.

PROCTOR: Noted. (Reflected in "Repeat Vital Signs.")

Repeat Vital Signs

Student: I will reassess vital signs and mental status.

PROCTOR: Blood pressure, 142/82 mm Hg; pulse rate, 102 beats/min; respirations, 24 breaths/min; pulse oximetry reading, 98%; and the patient is alert.

Student: The vital signs have not changed significantly.

PROCTOR: Noted.

Check Interventions

Student: I will reassess my interventions: oxygen and transport the patient.

PROCTOR: Noted.

ALS Student: I will reassess BLS interventions, plus the following: IVs, cardiac monitor, 12-lead ECG, and local protocol.

ALS Proctor: Noted. The cardiac monitor shows sinus tachycardia.

Repeat the Focused Assessment

Student: I will repeat the focused assessment.

PROCTOR: Noted.

Critical Criteria:
- ☐ Did not obtain medical direction or verbalize standing orders for medical interventions
- ☐ Administered a dangerous or inappropriate intervention

Handoff Report to Emergency Department Staff

Student: There was no change in the patient's condition during transport.

PROCTOR: Noted.

Critical Criteria

(Inform the student of items missed, if any.)

☐ Pass ☐ Fail Date: ____________________

Proctor Comments: ____________________

____

____

Notes

Dispatch Information

PROCTOR: EMS 10, respond to a 38-year-old male who is complaining of chest pain after shoveling snow. He is conscious and breathing.

Pre-scene Action (BSI)

Student: I am wearing nonlatex gloves and safety glasses.
PROCTOR: Noted.

Critical Criteria:
- ❑ Did not take, or verbalize, body substance isolation (BSI) precautions when necessary

Scene Size-up

Scene Safety

Student: Is the scene safe?
PROCTOR: Yes.

Mechanism of Injury/Nature of Illness

Student: What is the nature of the illness?
PROCTOR: The patient was shoveling snow when he began to have chest pain.

Number of Patients

Student: How many patients are there?
PROCTOR: One.

Additional Resources

Student: I would call for advanced life support (ALS) assistance.
PROCTOR: Noted.

C-Spine Stabilization

Student: I would not stabilize the cervical spine (c-spine).
PROCTOR: Noted.

Critical Criteria:
- ❑ Did not determine scene safety

Initial Assessment

General Impression

Student: My general impression is that the patient's condition is unstable.
PROCTOR: Noted.

Responsiveness/Level of Consciousness

Student: What is the patient's level of consciousness?
PROCTOR: Alert.

Chief Complaint/Apparent Life Threats

Student: What is the patient's chief complaint?
PROCTOR: The patient is complaining of right-sided chest pain.

Assess the Airway and Breathing

Student: Is the airway open? Is the patient breathing?
PROCTOR: Yes, the airway is open and the patient is breathing.

Assessment

Student: What are the rate and the quality of breathing?
PROCTOR: Rate: Within normal limits. Quality: Shallow. It hurts when he takes a deep breath.

Provide Oxygen

Student: I am applying oxygen at 15 L/min via nonrebreathing mask.
PROCTOR: Noted.

Ensure Adequate Ventilation

Student: The patient has adequate ventilations at this time.
PROCTOR: Noted.

Assess Circulation

Student: I am assessing the patient's circulation.
PROCTOR: Noted.

Assess for and Control Major Bleeding

Student: Do I find any major bleeding?
PROCTOR: No.

Assess the Pulse

Student: What are the rate and the quality of pulses?
PROCTOR: Rate: Within normal limits. Quality: Strong.

Assess the Skin

Student: I am assessing the skin. What are the color, temperature, and condition of the skin?
PROCTOR: Color: Normal. Temperature: Normal. Condition: Normal.

Identify Priority Patients/Make Transport Decision

Student: The patient is a low priority and does not require immediate transport.
PROCTOR: Noted.

Critical Criteria:
- ❑ Did not provide high concentration of oxygen
- ❑ Did not find or manage problems associated with airway, breathing, hemorrhage or shock (hypoperfusion)
- ❑ Did not differentiate patient's need for transportation versus continued assessment at the scene
- ❑ Did detailed or focused history/physical examination before assessing the airway, breathing and circulation

Focused History and Physical Examination/Rapid Assessment

Select the Appropriate Assessment (Focused or Rapid)

Student: I am selecting the focused assessment; I will focus on the isolated complaint.
PROCTOR: Noted.

SAMPLE History

Student: At this time I will gather a SAMPLE history from the patient or family. What are the patient's signs and symptoms?
PROCTOR: Respiratory/cardiac (right-sided chest pain).

> **Student:** Onset: What were you doing when this started?
> **PROCTOR:** Shoveling snow.
> **Student:** Provokes: What makes your condition worse or better?
> **PROCTOR:** Rotating the right shoulder downward makes the pain go away. Putting the shoulders back intensifies the pain.
> **Student:** Quality: Can you describe your pain?
> **PROCTOR:** It feels like a pulled muscle.
> **Student:** Radiates: Do you have pain anywhere else?
> **PROCTOR:** No.
> **Student:** Severity: On a scale of 1 to 10 with 10 being the worst possible, how would you rate your pain?
> **PROCTOR:** 4.
> **Student:** Time: How long has this been going on?
> **PROCTOR:** 15 minutes.
> **Student:** Interventions: Have you done anything to make this better?
> **PROCTOR:** The patient has taken no actions.

Student: Allergies?
PROCTOR: No allergies.
Student: Medications?
PROCTOR: No medications.
Student: Pertinent past medical history?
PROCTOR: No pertinent medical history.
Student: Last oral intake?
PROCTOR: 3 hours ago.
Student: Events leading up to the incident?
PROCTOR: The patient was quickly shoveling snow to prepare for guests who were coming over for dinner.

Perform the Focused Physical Examination

Student: I am performing the focused physical examination.
PROCTOR: Noted.

Student: I am assessing the chest for DCAP-BTLS. This acronym stands for deformities, contusions, abrasions, punctures, penetrations, paradoxical motion in the chest, and burns, tenderness, lacerations, and swelling.
PROCTOR: Noted.
Student: What do I see when I look at the chest?
PROCTOR: The position of comfort is having the right shoulder rotated forward.
Student: Is the chest symmetric?
PROCTOR: Yes.
Student: When I touch the chest, do I feel crepitus or a flail segment?
PROCTOR: No.
Student: Are lung sounds present in all fields?
PROCTOR: Yes.

▼ Baseline Vital Signs

Student: What are the patient's baseline vital signs, including blood pressure, pulse, respirations, pulse oximetry, and level of consciousness?
PROCTOR: Blood pressure, 138/82 mm Hg; pulse rate, 94 beats/min; respirations, 16 breaths/min; pulse oximetry reading, 99%; and the patient is alert.

▼ Interventions

Student: I will apply oxygen, loosen tight-fitting clothing, and transport the patient in the position of comfort.
PROCTOR: Noted.
ALS Student: I will apply basic life support (BLS) interventions, plus the following: IV access, cardiac monitor, 12-lead ECG, and advanced cardiac life support (ACLS) or local protocol.
ALS Proctor: Noted. The cardiac monitor shows normal sinus rhythm.

▼ Reevaluate Transport Decision

Student: The patient is a low priority and does not require immediate transport.
PROCTOR: Noted.

▼ Detailed Physical Examination

Possible Answer #1
Student: I would not do a detailed physical exam unless required to do so by local protocol.
PROCTOR: Noted. (Go to "Radio Report.")

Possible Answer #2
Student: I am conducting the detailed physical exam. I am looking for DCAP-BTLS.
PROCTOR: Noted. The detailed physical exam will be performed during transport.

▸ **Assess the Head**

Student: I am assessing the head. Do I find any DCAP-BTLS? Do I find any evidence of Battle's sign or raccoon eyes?
PROCTOR: No.

▸ **Inspect and Palpate the Head and Ears**

Student: I am assessing the head and ears.
PROCTOR: There are no obvious injuries.

▸ **Assess the Eyes**

Student: I am assessing the eyes. Are the pupils equal, round, and regular in size, and react properly to light (PEARRL)?
PROCTOR: They are PEARRL.

▸ **Assess the Facial Area Including Oral and Nasal Areas**

Student: I am assessing the face, nose, and mouth. Do I see any discharge or hear any obstructions?
PROCTOR: No.

▸ **Assess the Neck**

▸ **Inspect and Palpate the Neck**

Student: I am assessing the neck for DCAP-BTLS.
PROCTOR: There are no obvious injuries.

▸ **Assess for Jugular Vein Distention**

Student: Do I find any jugular vein distention (JVD)?
PROCTOR: No.

▸ **Assess for Tracheal Deviation**

Student: Do I see any tracheal deviation?
PROCTOR: No.

▸ **Assess the Chest**

Student: I am assessing the chest for DCAP-BTLS.
PROCTOR: Noted.

▸ **Inspect**

Student: What do I see when I look at the chest?
PROCTOR: The position of comfort is having the right shoulder rotated forward.
Student: Is the chest symmetric?
PROCTOR: Yes.

▸ **Palpate**

Student: When I touch the chest, do I feel crepitus or a flail segment?
PROCTOR: No.

▸ **Auscultate**

Student: Are lung sounds present in all fields?
PROCTOR: Yes.
Student: Do I hear any sucking sounds from the chest?
PROCTOR: No.

▸ **Assess the Abdomen/Pelvis**

▸ **Assess the Abdomen**

Student: I am assessing the abdomen for DCAP-BTLS. I am assessing all four quadrants. Do I find any problems?
PROCTOR: No.

▸ **Assess the Pelvis**

Student: I am assessing the pelvis for DCAP-BTLS. Is the pelvis stable?
PROCTOR: Yes.

▸ **Assess the Genitalia/Perineum as Needed (Verbalize in Training)**

Student: I am assessing the genitalia/perineum as necessary for DCAP-BTLS.
PROCTOR: The area is unremarkable.

▸ **Assess the Extremities**

▸ **Inspect**

Student: I am assessing the lower and upper extremities for DCAP-BTLS. Do I find anything?
PROCTOR: No.

▸ **Palpate**

Student: Do I feel anything unusual?
PROCTOR: No.

▸ **Assess Motor, Sensory, and Circulatory Function**

Student: I am checking for DCAP-BTLS, motor and sensory function, and pulses. Right leg?
PROCTOR: Negative DCAP-BTLS. Motor and sensory functions are present. Pulses are present.
Student: Left leg?
PROCTOR: Negative DCAP-BTLS. Motor and sensory functions are present. Pulses are present.
Student: Right arm?
PROCTOR: Negative DCAP-BTLS. Motor and sensory functions are present. Pulses are present.
Student: Left arm?
PROCTOR: Negative DCAP-BTLS. Motor and sensory functions are present. Pulses are present.

▸ **Assess the Posterior**

Student: We will check the back.
PROCTOR: Noted.

▸ **Assess the Thorax**

Student: I am assessing the thorax. Do I find injuries?
PROCTOR: No.

► **Assess the Lumbar Area**

Student: I am assessing the flanks and lumbar area. Do I find injuries?

PROCTOR: No.

► **Assess the Entire Backside**

Student: I am assessing the entire backside. Do I find injuries?

PROCTOR: No.

► **Reassess Interventions**

Student: I will reassess my interventions: oxygen, loosen tight-fitting clothing, and transport the patient in the position of comfort.

PROCTOR: Noted.

ALS Student: I will reassess BLS interventions, plus the following: IV access, cardiac monitor, 12-lead ECG, and ACLS or local protocol.

ALS Proctor: Noted. The cardiac monitor shows normal sinus rhythm.

Critical Criteria:
- ❑ Did not obtain medical direction or verbalize standing orders for medical interventions
- ❑ Administered a dangerous or inappropriate intervention
- ❑ Did not ask questions about the present illness
- ❑ Did not differentiate patient's need for transportation versus continued assessment at the scene

Radio Report

(Provided by the student.)

PROCTOR: Noted.

Ongoing Assessment

Repeat the Initial Assessment

Student: I will repeat the initial assessment.

PROCTOR: Noted. (Reflected in "Repeat Vital Signs.")

Repeat Vital Signs

Student: I will reassess vital signs and mental status.

PROCTOR: Blood pressure, 130/78 mm Hg; pulse rate, 86 beats/min; respirations, 16 breaths/min; pulse oximetry reading, 99%; and the patient is alert.

Student: The vital signs have not changed significantly.

PROCTOR: Noted.

Check Interventions

Student: I will check my interventions: oxygen, loosen tight-fitting clothing, and transport the patient in the position of comfort.

PROCTOR: Noted.

ALS Student: I will check BLS interventions, plus the following: IV access, cardiac monitor, 12-lead ECG, and ACLS or local protocol.

ALS Proctor: Noted. The cardiac monitor shows normal sinus rhythm.

Repeat the Focused Assessment

Student: I will repeat the focused assessment.

PROCTOR: Noted.

Critical Criteria:
- ❑ Did not obtain medical direction or verbalize standing orders for medical interventions
- ❑ Administered a dangerous or inappropriate intervention

Handoff Report to Emergency Department Staff

Student: There was no change in the patient's condition during transport.

PROCTOR: Noted.

Critical Criteria

(Inform the student of items missed, if any.)

❑ Pass ❑ Fail Date: ______________________

Proctor Comments: ______________________

____

____

Notes

Dispatch Information

PROCTOR: EMS 10, respond to a 24-year-old male who passed out at a party. He has been drinking. He is unconscious but breathing. Police officers are being sent to the scene.

Pre-scene Action (BSI)

Student: I am wearing nonlatex gloves and safety glasses.
PROCTOR: Noted.

Critical Criteria:
- ❑ Did not take, or verbalize, body substance isolation (BSI) precautions when necessary

Scene Size-up

Scene Safety

Student: Is the scene safe?
PROCTOR: Yes, police are on scene and you are given clearance to enter.

Mechanism of Injury/Nature of Illness

Student: What is the nature of the illness?
PROCTOR: The patient has been drinking heavily at a party. He has passed out and may have aspirated on his own vomit. He sounds as though he is choking. He did not fall.
Student: I will immediately clear the airway, suction, and place him in the recovery position.
PROCTOR: Noted.

Number of Patients

Student: How many patients are there?
PROCTOR: One.

Additional Resources

Student: I would call for advanced life support (ALS) assistance.
PROCTOR: Noted.

C-Spine Stabilization

Student: I would not stabilize the cervical spine (c-spine).
PROCTOR: Noted.

Critical Criteria:
- ❑ Did not determine scene safety

Initial Assessment

General Impression

Student: My general impression is that the patient's condition is unstable.
PROCTOR: Noted.

Responsiveness/Level of Consciousness

Student: What is the patient's level of consciousness?
PROCTOR: Unresponsive.

Chief Complaint/Apparent Life Threats

Student: What is the patient's chief complaint?
PROCTOR: The patient is unresponsive.

Assess the Airway and Breathing

Student: Is the airway open? Is the patient breathing?
PROCTOR: Yes, the airway is open and the patient is breathing.

▸ Assessment

Student: What are the rate and the quality of breathing?
PROCTOR: Rate: Normal (in the recovery position). Quality: Normal.
Student: I will suction and protect the airway.
PROCTOR: Noted.

▸ Provide Oxygen

Student: His breathing is now normal. I will keep him in the recovery position and provide blow-by oxygen in case he vomits again. I will be ready to suction if necessary.
PROCTOR: Noted.

▸ Ensure Adequate Ventilation

Student: Breathing is adequate in the recovery position.
PROCTOR: Noted.

Assess Circulation

Student: I am assessing the patient's circulation.
PROCTOR: Noted.

▸ Assess for and Control Major Bleeding

Student: Do I find any major bleeding?
PROCTOR: No.

▸ Assess the Pulse

Student: What are the rate and the quality of pulses?
PROCTOR: Rate: Tachycardic. Quality: Bounding.

▸ Assess the Skin

Student: I am assessing the skin. What are the color, temperature, and condition of the skin?
PROCTOR: Color: Flushed. Temperature: Warm. Condition: Moist.

Identify Priority Patients/Make Transport Decision

Student: The patient is a high priority and is a load-and-go. I will begin packaging and transport.
PROCTOR: Noted.

Critical Criteria:
- ❑ Did not provide high concentration of oxygen
- ❑ Did not find or manage problems associated with airway, breathing, hemorrhage or shock (hypoperfusion)
- ❑ Did not differentiate patient's need for transportation versus continued assessment at the scene
- ❑ Did detailed or focused history/physical examination before assessing the airway, breathing and circulation

Focused History and Physical Examination/Rapid Assessment

Select the Appropriate Assessment (Focused or Rapid)

Student: I am selecting the rapid physical exam. I am checking for DCAP-BTLS. This acronym stands for deformities, contusions, abrasions, punctures, penetrations, and paradoxical motion in the chest, and burns, tenderness, lacerations, and swelling.
PROCTOR: Noted.

▸ Head

Student: I am rapidly assessing the head.
PROCTOR: There are no obvious injuries.

▸ Neck

Student: I am rapidly assessing the neck.
PROCTOR: There are no obvious injuries.

▸ Chest

Student: I am rapidly assessing the chest. What are the lung sounds?
PROCTOR: There are no obvious injuries. They are clear bilaterally.

▸ Abdomen/Pelvis

Student: I am rapidly assessing the abdomen.
PROCTOR: There are no obvious injuries.
Student: I am rapidly assessing the pelvis.
PROCTOR: There are no obvious injuries.

▸ Extremities

Student: I am rapidly assessing the extremities.
PROCTOR: There are no obvious injuries.
Student: Do I feel anything unusual?
PROCTOR: No.

▸ Posterior

Student: I will rapidly assess the back.
PROCTOR: Noted.

▸ Assess the Thorax

Student: I am assessing the thorax. Do I find injuries?
PROCTOR: No.

▸ Assess the Lumbar Area

Student: I am assessing the flanks and lumbar area. Do I find injuries?
PROCTOR: No.

▸ Assess the Entire Backside

Student: I am assessing the entire backside. Do I find injuries?
PROCTOR: No.

▼ SAMPLE History

Student: At this time I will gather a SAMPLE history from the patient, family, or bystanders. What are the patient's signs and symptoms?
PROCTOR: Altered mental status.
Student: Describe the episode.
PROCTOR: The patient has been drinking all night. He passed out and may have choked on his vomit.
Student: Onset: What was he doing when this started?
PROCTOR: He was drinking beer.
Student: Duration: How long has this been going on?
PROCTOR: 10 minutes.
Student: Are there any associated symptoms?
PROCTOR: Yes, he has choked on his vomit.
Student: Is there any evidence of trauma?
PROCTOR: No.
Student: Interventions: Has he done anything to make this better?
PROCTOR: The patient has taken no actions.
Student: Have there been any seizures?
PROCTOR: No.
Student: Has there been any fever?
PROCTOR: No.
Student: Allergies?
PROCTOR: Unknown.
Student: Medications?
PROCTOR: Unknown.
Student: Pertinent past medical history?
PROCTOR: Unknown.
Student: Last oral intake?
PROCTOR: The patient has been drinking all night.
Student: Events leading up to the incident?
PROCTOR: He has been drinking all night. He passed out and choked on his vomit.

▼ Baseline Vital Signs

Student: What are the patient's baseline vital signs, including blood pressure, pulse, respirations, pulse oximetry, blood glucose level, and level of consciousness?
PROCTOR: Blood pressure, 144/90 mm Hg; pulse rate, 122 beats/min; respirations, 16 breaths/min; pulse oximetry reading, 95%; blood glucose level is 118 mg/dL; and the patient is unresponsive.

▼ Interventions

Student: I will keep him in the recovery position, apply suction as needed, provide blow-by oxygen and transport.
PROCTOR: Noted.
ALS Student: I will apply basic life support (BLS) interventions, plus the following: intubate (if necessary), IV access, cardiac monitor, and local protocol.
ALS Proctor: Noted. The cardiac monitor shows sinus tachycardia.

▼ Reevaluate Transport Decision

Student: The patient is a load-and-go due to unconsciousness.
PROCTOR: Noted.

▼ Detailed Physical Examination

Student: I am conducting the detailed physical exam. I am looking for DCAP-BTLS.
PROCTOR: Noted. The detailed physical exam will be performed during transport.

▸ Assess the Head

Student: I am assessing the head. Do I find any DCAP-BTLS? Do I find any evidence of Battle's sign or raccoon eyes?
PROCTOR: No.

▸ Inspect and Palpate the Head and Ears

Student: I am assessing the head and ears.
PROCTOR: There are no obvious injuries.

▸ Assess the Eyes

Student: I am assessing the eyes. Are the pupils equal, round, and regular in size, and react properly to light (PEARRL)?
PROCTOR: They are sluggish to respond.

▸ Assess the Facial Area Including Oral and Nasal Areas

Student: I am assessing the face, nose, and mouth. Do I see any discharge or hear any obstructions?
PROCTOR: Not at this time.
Student: I will have suction ready and keep the patient in the recovery position. If breathing problems arise, I will use a bag-valve device with the patient in the supine position.
PROCTOR: Noted.

▸ Assess the Neck

▸ Inspect and Palpate the Neck

Student: I am assessing the neck for DCAP-BTLS.
PROCTOR: There are no obvious injuries.

▸ Assess for Jugular Vein Distention

Student: Do I find any jugular vein distention (JVD)?
PROCTOR: No.

▸ Assess for Tracheal Deviation

Student: Do I see any tracheal deviation?
PROCTOR: No.

▸ Assess the Chest

Student: I am assessing the chest for DCAP-BTLS.
PROCTOR: Noted.

▸ Inspect

Student: What do I see when I look at the chest?
PROCTOR: There are no obvious injuries.
Student: Is the chest symmetric?
PROCTOR: Yes.

▸ Palpate

Student: When I touch the chest, do I feel crepitus or a flail segment?
PROCTOR: No.

▸ Auscultate

Student: Are lung sounds present in all fields?
PROCTOR: Yes, but you also hear some rales in the lungs.
Student: Do I hear any sucking sounds from the chest?
PROCTOR: No.

▸ Assess the Abdomen/Pelvis

▸ Assess the Abdomen

Student: I am assessing the abdomen for DCAP-BTLS. I am assessing all four quadrants. Do I find any problems?
PROCTOR: No.

▸ Assess the Pelvis

Student: I am assessing the pelvis for DCAP-BTLS. Is the pelvis stable?
PROCTOR: Yes.

▸ Assess the Genitalia/Perineum as Needed (Verbalize in Training)

Student: I am assessing the genitalia/perineum as necessary for DCAP-BTLS.
PROCTOR: The area is unremarkable.

- Assess the Extremities
  - Inspect

Student: I am assessing the lower and upper extremities for DCAP-BTLS. Do I find anything?
PROCTOR: No.

- Palpate

Student: Do I feel anything unusual?
PROCTOR: No.

- Assess Motor, Sensory, and Circulatory Function

Student: I am checking for DCAP-BTLS, motor and sensory function, and pulses. Right leg?
PROCTOR: Negative DCAP-BTLS. Motor and sensory functions are absent. Pulses are present.
Student: Left leg?
PROCTOR: Negative DCAP-BTLS. Motor and sensory functions are absent. Pulses are present.
Student: Right arm?
PROCTOR: Negative DCAP-BTLS. Motor and sensory functions are absent. Pulses are present.
Student: Left arm?
PROCTOR: Negative DCAP-BTLS. Motor and sensory functions are absent. Pulses are present.

- Assess the Posterior

Student: We will check the back.
PROCTOR: Noted.

- Assess the Thorax

Student: I am assessing the thorax. Do I find injuries?
PROCTOR: No.

- Assess the Lumbar Area

Student: I am assessing the flanks and lumbar area. Do I find injuries?
PROCTOR: No.

- Assess the Entire Backside

Student: I am assessing the entire backside. Do I find injuries?
PROCTOR: No.

- Manage Secondary Injuries/Wounds

Student: I would direct my partner to maintain the airway.
PROCTOR: Noted.

- Reassess Interventions

Student: I will reassess my interventions: suction as needed, keep him in the recovery position, oxygen, and transport.
PROCTOR: Noted.
ALS Student: I will reassess BLS interventions, plus the following: intubate (if necessary), IV access, cardiac monitor, and local protocol.
ALS Proctor: Noted. The cardiac monitor shows sinus tachycardia.

Critical Criteria:
- ❑ Did not obtain medical direction or verbalize standing orders for medical interventions
- ❑ Administered a dangerous or inappropriate intervention
- ❑ Did not ask questions about the present illness
- ❑ Did not differentiate patient's need for transportation versus continued assessment at the scene

Radio Report

(Provided by the student.)
PROCTOR: Noted.

Ongoing Assessment

Repeat the Initial Assessment

Student: I will repeat the initial assessment.
PROCTOR: Noted. (Reflected in "Repeat Vital Signs.")

Repeat Vital Signs

Student: I will reassess vital signs and mental status.
PROCTOR: Blood pressure, 140/86 mm Hg; pulse rate, 118 beats/min; respirations 16 per minute; pulse oximetry reading, 97%; and the patient is unresponsive.
Student: The vital signs have not changed significantly.
PROCTOR: Noted.

Check Interventions

Student: I will check my interventions: suction, keep him in the recovery position, oxygen, and transport.
PROCTOR: Noted.
ALS Student: I will check BLS interventions, plus the following: intubate (if necessary), IV access, cardiac monitor, and local protocol.
ALS Proctor: Noted. The cardiac monitor shows sinus tachycardia.

Repeat the Focused Assessment

Student: I will repeat the focused assessment.
PROCTOR: Noted.

Critical Criteria:
- ❑ Did not obtain medical direction or verbalize standing orders for medical interventions
- ❑ Administered a dangerous or inappropriate intervention

Handoff Report to Emergency Department Staff

Student: There was no change in the patient's condition during transport.
PROCTOR: Noted.

Critical Criteria

(Inform the student of items missed, if any.)

❑ Pass ❑ Fail Date: ____________________

Proctor Comments: ____________________

____

____

Notes

CASE 125

Dispatch Information

PROCTOR: EMS 10, respond to a 60-year-old male who is complaining of difficulty breathing. He is conscious and breathing.

Pre-scene Action (BSI)

Student: I am wearing nonlatex gloves and safety glasses.
PROCTOR: Noted.

Critical Criteria:
- ❑ Did not take, or verbalize, body substance isolation (BSI) precautions when necessary

Scene Size-up

Scene Safety

Student: Is the scene safe?
PROCTOR: Yes.

Mechanism of Injury/Nature of Illness

Student: What is the nature of the illness?
PROCTOR: The patient arrived in town a few minutes ago via airplane. He is in the United States visiting family members. He is a coal miner with a history of respiratory difficulties.

Number of Patients

Student: How many patients are there?
PROCTOR: One.

Additional Resources

Student: I would call for advanced life support (ALS) assistance.
PROCTOR: Noted.

C-Spine Stabilization

Student: I would not stabilize the cervical spine (c-spine).
PROCTOR: Noted.

Critical Criteria:
- ❑ Did not determine scene safety

Initial Assessment

General Impression

Student: My general impression is that the patient's condition is unstable.
PROCTOR: Noted.

Responsiveness/Level of Consciousness

Student: What is the patient's level of consciousness?
PROCTOR: Alert.

Chief Complaint/Apparent Life Threats

Student: What is the patient's chief complaint?
PROCTOR: The patient is complaining of difficulty breathing.

Assess the Airway and Breathing

Student: Is the airway open? Is the patient breathing?
PROCTOR: Yes, the airway is open and the patient is breathing.

▸ Assessment

Student: What are the rate and the quality of breathing?
PROCTOR: Rate: Within normal limits. Quality: Labored.

▸ Provide Oxygen

Student: I am applying oxygen at 15 L/min via nonrebreathing mask.
PROCTOR: Noted.

▸ Ensure Adequate Ventilation

Student: The patient has adequate ventilations at this time.
PROCTOR: Noted.

Assess Circulation

Student: I am assessing the patient's circulation.
PROCTOR: Noted.

▸ Assess for and Control Major Bleeding

Student: Do I find any major bleeding?
PROCTOR: No.

▸ Assess the Pulse

Student: What are the rate and the quality of pulses?
PROCTOR: Rate: Tachycardic. Quality: Bounding.

▸ Assess the Skin

Student: I am assessing the skin. What are the color, temperature, and condition of the skin?
PROCTOR: Color: Pale. Temperature: Cool. Condition: Moist.

Identify Priority Patients/Make Transport Decision

Student: The patient is a high priority and is a load-and-go. I will begin packaging and transport.
PROCTOR: Noted.

Critical Criteria:
- ❑ Did not provide high concentration of oxygen
- ❑ Did not find or manage problems associated with airway, breathing, hemorrhage or shock (hypoperfusion)
- ❑ Did not differentiate patient's need for transportation versus continued assessment at the scene
- ❑ Did detailed or focused history/physical examination before assessing the airway, breathing and circulation

Focused History and Physical Examination/Rapid Assessment

Select the Appropriate Assessment (Focused or Rapid)

Student: I am selecting the focused assessment.
PROCTOR: Noted.

SAMPLE History

Student: At this time I will gather a SAMPLE history from the patient or family. What are the patient's signs and symptoms?
PROCTOR: Respiratory (patient is complaining of difficulty breathing and feels short of breath).There is difficulty communicating with this patient due to a language barrier.

> Student: Onset: What were you doing when this started?
> **PROCTOR:** The patient got scared while in the airplane.
> Student: Provokes: What makes your condition worse or better?
> **PROCTOR:** He does not know.
> Student: Quality: Can you describe your pain?
> **PROCTOR:** None.
> Student: Radiates: Do you have pain or discomfort anywhere else?
> **PROCTOR:** No.
> Student: Severity: On a scale of 1 to 10 with 10 being the worst possible, how would you rate your distress?
> **PROCTOR:** 5.
> Student: Time: How long has this been going on?
> **PROCTOR:** 9 hours.
> Student: Interventions: Have you done anything to make this better?
> **PROCTOR:** The patient has taken no actions.

Student: Allergies?
PROCTOR: Unknown.
Student: Medications?
PROCTOR: Unknown.
Student: Pertinent past medical history?
PROCTOR: Possibly black lung disease.
Student: Last oral intake?
PROCTOR: Unknown.
Student: Events leading up to the incident?
PROCTOR: The patient became upset during his flight (he is afraid to fly).

Perform Focused Physical Examination

Student: I am performing the focused physical examination.
PROCTOR: Noted.

Student: What are his lung sounds?
PROCTOR: Rhonchi that produce coal-tinged sputum when he coughs.
Student: Does he have any edema in the extremities?
PROCTOR: No.
Student: I will loosen any tight-fitting clothing and transport him in the position of comfort.
PROCTOR: Noted.

▼ Baseline Vital Signs

Student: What are the patient's baseline vital signs, including blood pressure, pulse, respirations, pulse oximetry, blood glucose level, and level of consciousness?
PROCTOR: Blood pressure, 150/88 mm Hg; pulse, 110 beats/min; respirations, 16 breaths/min; pulse oximetry reading, 95%; blood glucose level, 114 mg/dL; and the patient is alert.

▼ Interventions

Student: I will apply oxygen.
PROCTOR: Noted.
ALS Student: I will apply basic life support (BLS) interventions, plus the following: establish IV access, perform cardiac monitoring, 12-lead ECG, a breathing treatment, and follow the local protocol.
ALS Proctor: Noted. The cardiac monitor shows sinus tachycardia.

▼ Reevaluate Transport Decision

Student: The patient is a high priority and is a load-and-go.
PROCTOR: Noted.

▼ Detailed Physical Examination

Possible Answer #1
Student: I would not do a detailed physical exam.
PROCTOR: Noted. (Go to "Radio Report.")

Possible Answer #2
Student: I am conducting the detailed physical exam. I am looking for DCAP-BTLS. This acronym stands for deformities, contusions, abrasions, punctures, penetrations, paradoxical motion in the chest, and burns, tenderness, lacerations, and swelling.
PROCTOR: Noted. The detailed physical exam will be performed during transport.

► **Assess the Head**

Student: I am assessing the head. Do I find any DCAP-BTLS? Do I find any evidence of Battle's sign or raccoon eyes?
PROCTOR: No.

► **Inspect and Palpate the Head and Ears**

Student: I am assessing the head and ears.
PROCTOR: There are no obvious injuries.

► **Assess the Eyes**

Student: I am assessing the eyes. Are the pupils equal, round, and regular in size, and react properly to light (PEARRL)?
PROCTOR: They are PEARRL.

► **Assess the Facial Area Including Oral and Nasal Areas**

Student: I am assessing the face, nose, and mouth. Do I see any discharge or hear any obstructions?
PROCTOR: No.

► **Assess the Neck**

► **Inspect and Palpate the Neck**

Student: I am assessing the neck for DCAP-BTLS.
PROCTOR: There are no obvious injuries.

► **Assess for Jugular Vein Distention**

Student: Do I find any jugular vein distention (JVD)?
PROCTOR: No.

► **Assess for Tracheal Deviation**

Student: Do I see any tracheal deviation?
PROCTOR: No.

► **Assess the Chest**

Student: I am assessing the chest for DCAP-BTLS.
PROCTOR: Noted.

► **Inspect**

Student: What do I see when I look at the chest?
PROCTOR: There are no obvious injuries.
Student: Is the chest symmetric?
PROCTOR: Yes.

► **Palpate**

Student: When I touch the chest, do I feel crepitus or a flail segment?
PROCTOR: No.

► **Auscultate**

Student: Are lung sounds present in all fields?
PROCTOR: Yes.
Student: Do I hear any sucking sounds from the chest?
PROCTOR: No.

► **Assess the Abdomen/Pelvis**

► **Assess the Abdomen**

Student: I am assessing the abdomen for DCAP-BTLS. I am assessing all four quadrants. Do I find any problems?
PROCTOR: No.

► **Assess the Pelvis**

Student: I am assessing the pelvis for DCAP-BTLS. Is the pelvis stable?
PROCTOR: Yes.

► **Assess the Genitalia/Perineum as Needed (Verbalize in Training)**

Student: I am assessing the genitalia/perineum as necessary for DCAP-BTLS.
PROCTOR: The area is unremarkable.

► **Assess the Extremities**

► **Inspect**

Student: I am assessing the lower and upper extremities for DCAP-BTLS. Do I find anything?
PROCTOR: No.

► **Palpate**

Student: Do I feel anything unusual?
PROCTOR: No.

► **Assess Motor, Sensory, and Circulatory Function**

Student: I am checking for DCAP-BTLS, motor and sensory function, and pulses. Right leg?
PROCTOR: Negative DCAP-BTLS. Motor and sensory functions are present. Pulses are present.
Student: Left leg?
PROCTOR: Negative DCAP-BTLS. Motor and sensory functions are present. Pulses are present.
Student: Right arm?
PROCTOR: Negative DCAP-BTLS. Motor and sensory functions are present. Pulses are present.
Student: Left arm?
PROCTOR: Negative DCAP-BTLS. Motor and sensory functions are present. Pulses are present.

► **Assess the Posterior**

Student: We will check the back.
PROCTOR: Noted.

► **Assess the Thorax**

Student: I am assessing the thorax. Do I find injuries?
PROCTOR: No.

► **Assess the Lumbar Area**

Student: I am assessing the flanks and lumbar area. Do I find injuries?
PROCTOR: No.

► **Assess the Entire Backside**

Student: I am assessing the entire backside. Do I find injuries?
PROCTOR: No.

► **Manage Secondary Injuries/Wounds**

Student: I would direct my partner to monitor the airway.
PROCTOR: Noted.

▸ Reassess Interventions

Student: I will reassess my interventions: oxygen and reassurance.

PROCTOR: Noted.

ALS Student: I will reassess BLS interventions, plus the following: IV, cardiac monitoring, 12-lead ECG, a breathing treatment, and local protocol.

ALS Proctor: Noted. The cardiac monitor shows sinus tachycardia.

Critical Criteria:

- ❑ Did not obtain medical direction or verbalize standing orders for medical interventions
- ❑ Administered a dangerous or inappropriate intervention
- ❑ Did not ask questions about the present illness
- ❑ Did not differentiate patient's need for transportation versus continued assessment at the scene

Radio Report

(Provided by the student.)

PROCTOR: Noted.

Ongoing Assessment

Repeat the Initial Assessment

Student: I will repeat the initial assessment.

PROCTOR: Noted. (Reflected in "Repeat Vital Signs.")

Repeat Vital Signs

Student: I will reassess vital signs and mental status.

PROCTOR: Blood pressure, 142/82 mm Hg; pulse, 108 beats/min; respirations, 16 breaths/min; pulse oximetry reading, 96%; and the patient is alert.

Student: The vital signs have not changed significantly.

PROCTOR: Noted.

Check Interventions

Student: I will check my interventions: oxygen and reassess pulse oximetry.

PROCTOR: Noted.

ALS Student: I will check BLS interventions, plus the following: IV access, cardiac monitor, 12-lead ECG, a breathing treatment, and local protocol.

ALS Proctor: Noted. The cardiac monitor shows sinus tachycardia.

Repeat the Focused Assessment

Student: I will repeat the focused assessment.

PROCTOR: Noted.

Critical Criteria:

- ❑ Did not obtain medical direction or verbalize standing orders for medical interventions
- ❑ Administered a dangerous or inappropriate intervention

Handoff Report to Emergency Department Staff

Student: There was no change in the patient's condition during transport.

PROCTOR: Noted.

Critical Criteria

(Inform the student of items missed, if any.)

❑ Pass ❑ Fail Date: ____________________

Proctor Comments: ____________________

____

____

CASE 125

Notes

Dispatch Information

PROCTOR: EMS 10, respond to a 26-year-old male who has been scuba diving and is now unconscious and not breathing.

Pre-scene Action (BSI)

Student: I am wearing nonlatex gloves and safety glasses.
PROCTOR: Noted.

Critical Criteria:
- ❑ Did not take, or verbalize, body substance isolation (BSI) precautions when necessary

Scene Size-up

Scene Safety

Student: Is the scene safe?
PROCTOR: Yes.

Mechanism of Injury/Nature of Illness

Student: What is the nature of the illness?
PROCTOR: The patient has been scuba diving and is now unresponsive.

Number of Patients

Student: How many patients are there?
PROCTOR: One.

Additional Resources

Student: I would call for advanced life support (ALS) assistance.
PROCTOR: Noted.

C-Spine Stabilization

Student: On the basis of the nature of the illness, I would stabilize the cervical spine (c-spine) in a neutral in-line position.
PROCTOR: Noted.

Critical Criteria:
- ❑ Did not determine scene safety

Initial Assessment

General Impression

Student: My general impression is that the patient's condition is unstable.
PROCTOR: Noted.

Responsiveness/Level of Consciousness

Student: What is the patient's level of consciousness?
PROCTOR: Unresponsive.

Chief Complaint/Apparent Life Threats

Student: What is the patient's chief complaint?
PROCTOR: The patient is unresponsive.

Assess the Airway and Breathing

Student: I will open the airway using the jaw-thrust maneuver. Is the patient breathing?
PROCTOR: You hear gurgling and see blood in the airway. The patient is not breathing.
Student: I will suction the airway.
PROCTOR: Noted.

▸ Assessment

Student: What are the rate and the quality of breathing?
PROCTOR: Rate: Absent. Quality: Absent. You hear gurgling and see blood.
Student: I will insert an oral/advanced airway and ventilate the patient with a bag-valve device.
PROCTOR: Noted.

▸ Provide Oxygen

Student: I will ventilate with a bag-valve device and 100% oxygen.
PROCTOR: Noted.

▸ Ensure Adequate Ventilation

Student: Bag-valve ventilations are adequate.
PROCTOR: Noted.

Assess Circulation

Student: I am assessing the patient's circulation.
PROCTOR: Noted.

▸ Assess for and Control Major Bleeding

Student: Do I find any major bleeding?
PROCTOR: No.

▸ Assess the Pulse

Student: What are the rate and the quality of pulses?
PROCTOR: Rate: Tachycardic. Quality: Bounding.

▸ Assess the Skin

Student: I am assessing the skin. What are the color, temperature, and condition of the skin?
PROCTOR: Color: Cyanotic. Temperature: Warm. Condition: Moist.

Identify Priority Patients/Make Transport Decision

Student: The patient is a high priority and is a load-and-go. I will begin packaging and transport.
PROCTOR: Noted.

Critical Criteria:
- ❑ Did not provide high concentration of oxygen
- ❑ Did not find or manage problems associated with airway, breathing, hemorrhage or shock (hypoperfusion)
- ❑ Did not differentiate patient's need for transportation versus continued assessment at the scene
- ❑ Did detailed or focused history/physical examination before assessing the airway, breathing and circulation

Focused History and Physical Examination/Rapid Assessment

Select the Appropriate Assessment (Focused or Rapid)

Student: I am selecting the rapid physical exam. I am checking for DCAP-BTLS. This acronym stands for deformities, contusions, abrasions, punctures, penetrations, paradoxical motion in the chest, and burns, tenderness, lacerations, and swelling.
PROCTOR: Noted.

▸ Head

Student: I am rapidly assessing the head.
PROCTOR: There are no obvious injuries.

▸ Neck

Student: I am rapidly assessing the neck.
PROCTOR: There are no obvious injuries.
Student: I will apply a cervical collar.
PROCTOR: Noted.

▸ Chest

Student: I am rapidly assessing the chest. What are the lung sounds?
PROCTOR: There are no obvious injuries. Lung sounds are clear bilaterally.

▸ Abdomen/Pelvis

Student: I am rapidly assessing the abdomen.
PROCTOR: There are no obvious injuries.
Student: I am rapidly assessing the pelvis.
PROCTOR: There are no obvious injuries.

▸ Extremities

Student: I am rapidly assessing the extremities.
PROCTOR: There are no obvious injuries.

▸ Assess Motor, Sensory, and Circulatory Function

Student: I am checking for DCAP-BTLS, motor and sensory function, and pulses. Right leg?
PROCTOR: Negative DCAP-BTLS. Motor and sensory functions are absent. Pulses are present.
Student: Left leg?
PROCTOR: Negative DCAP-BTLS. Motor and sensory functions are absent. Pulses are present.

Student: Right arm?
PROCTOR: Negative DCAP-BTLS. Motor and sensory functions are absent. Pulses are present.
Student: Left arm?
PROCTOR: Negative DCAP-BTLS. Motor and sensory functions are absent. Pulses are present.

▸ **Posterior**

Student: I will rapidly assess the back. We will now log roll the patient as a unit to check the back. The person at the head will count to three and we will roll the patient.
PROCTOR: Noted.

▸ **Assess the Thorax**

Student: I am assessing the thorax. Do I find injuries?
PROCTOR: No.

▸ **Assess the Lumbar Area**

Student: I am assessing the flanks and lumbar area. Do I find injuries?
PROCTOR: No.

▸ **Assess the Entire Backside**

Student: I am assessing the entire backside. Do I find injuries?
PROCTOR: No.

▸ **Manage Secondary Injuries/Wounds**

Student: We will apply a cervical collar and backboard with full immobilization per local protocol, if not yet done, at this time.
PROCTOR: Noted.
Student: Are there any changes in motor and sensory functions or pulses?
PROCTOR: No.

▸ **Reevaluate Transport Decision**

Student: The patient is a load-and-go due to respiratory arrest.
PROCTOR: Noted.

▼ Baseline Vital Signs

Student: What are the patient's baseline vital signs, including blood pressure, pulse, respirations, pulse oximetry, blood glucose level, and level of consciousness?
PROCTOR: Blood pressure, 134/80 mm Hg; pulse rate, 132 beats/min; respirations per bag-valve-mask; pulse oximetry reading, 85%; blood glucose level, 122 mg/dL, and the patient is unresponsive.

▼ SAMPLE History

Student: At this time I will gather a SAMPLE history from the patient or family. What are the patient's signs and symptoms?
PROCTOR: Environmental emergency.
Student: What was the source?
PROCTOR: He is a scuba diver and he held his breath to extend the dive.
Student: What was the environment?
PROCTOR: The ambient temperature is 92°F and the temperature of the surface water is 82°F.
Student: What was the duration of the dive?
PROCTOR: More than 26 minutes.
Student: Was there any loss of consciousness?
PROCTOR: Yes, for 5 minutes now.
Student: What were the effects—local or general?
PROCTOR: The whole body.
Student: Allergies?
PROCTOR: Unknown.
Student: Medications?
PROCTOR: Unknown.
Student: Pertinent past medical history?
PROCTOR: Unknown.
Student: Last oral intake?
PROCTOR: Unknown.
Student: Events leading up to the incident?
PROCTOR: The patient was scuba diving.
Student: Did he hit his head or hit the bottom?
PROCTOR: The dive buddy said the patient did not hit his head or the bottom.

▼ Interventions

Student: I will continue oxygen per bag-valve device, and rapid transport with the feet elevated to a hyperbaric center equipped hospital, if possible.
PROCTOR: Noted.
ALS Student: I will apply basic life support (BLS) interventions, plus the following: intubate, confirm end tidal CO_2 and lung sounds, establish IV access, provide cardiac monitoring, and follow the advanced cardiac life support (ACLS) and local protocol.
ALS Proctor: Noted. The cardiac monitor shows sinus tachycardia and end tidal CO_2 and lung sounds confirm placement of the endotracheal (ET) tube.

▼ Detailed Physical Examination

Student: I am conducting the detailed physical exam. I am looking for DCAP-BTLS.
PROCTOR: Noted. The detailed physical exam will be performed during transport.

▸ **Assess the Head**

Student: I am assessing the head. Do I find any DCAP-BTLS? Do I find any evidence of Battle's sign or raccoon eyes?
PROCTOR: No.

▸ **Inspect and Palpate the Head and Ears**

Student: I am assessing the head and ears.
PROCTOR: There are no obvious injuries.

▸ **Assess the Eyes**

Student: I am assessing the eyes. Are the pupils equal, round, and regular in size, and react properly to light (PEARRL)?
PROCTOR: They are nonreactive.

▸ **Assess the Facial Area Including Oral and Nasal Areas**

Student: I am assessing the face, nose, and mouth. Do I see any discharge or hear any obstructions?
PROCTOR: No.

▸ **Assess the Neck**

▸ **Inspect and Palpate the Neck**

Student: I am assessing the neck for DCAP-BTLS.
PROCTOR: There are no obvious injuries.

▸ **Assess for Jugular Vein Distention**

Student: Do I find any jugular vein distention (JVD)?
PROCTOR: No.

▸ **Assess for Tracheal Deviation**

Student: Do I see any tracheal deviation?
PROCTOR: No.

▸ **Assess the Chest**

Student: I am assessing the chest for DCAP-BTLS.
PROCTOR: Noted.

▸ **Inspect**

Student: What do I see when I look at the chest?
PROCTOR: There are no obvious injuries.
Student: Is the chest symmetric?
PROCTOR: Yes.

▸ **Palpate**

Student: When I touch the chest, do I feel crepitus or a flail segment?
PROCTOR: No.

▸ **Auscultate**

Student: Are lung sounds present in all fields?
PROCTOR: Yes.

Student: Do I hear any sucking sounds from the chest?
PROCTOR: No.

- Assess the Abdomen/Pelvis
  - Assess the Abdomen

Student: I am assessing the abdomen for DCAP-BTLS. I am assessing all four quadrants. Do I find any problems?
PROCTOR: No.

  - Assess the Pelvis

Student: I am assessing the pelvis for DCAP-BTLS. Is the pelvis stable?
PROCTOR: Yes.

  - Assess the Genitalia/Perineum as Needed (Verbalize in Training)

Student: I am assessing the genitalia/perineum as necessary for DCAP-BTLS.
PROCTOR: The area is unremarkable.

- Assess the Extremities
  - Inspect

Student: I am assessing the lower and upper extremities for DCAP-BTLS. Do I find anything?
PROCTOR: No.

  - Palpate

Student: Do I feel anything unusual?
PROCTOR: No.

  - Assess Motor, Sensory, and Circulatory Function

Student: I am checking for DCAP-BTLS, motor and sensory function, and pulses. Right leg?
PROCTOR: Negative DCAP-BTLS. Motor and sensory functions are absent. Pulses are present.
Student: Left leg?
PROCTOR: Negative DCAP-BTLS. Motor and sensory functions are absent. Pulses are present.
Student: Right arm?
PROCTOR: Negative DCAP-BTLS. Motor and sensory functions are absent. Pulses are present.
Student: Left arm?
PROCTOR: Negative DCAP-BTLS. Motor and sensory functions are absent. Pulses are present.

- Assess the Posterior

Note: This portion of the detailed physical exam would not be done if the patient were previously backboarded per local protocol.
Student: We will not check the back because it was previously checked and the patient is backboarded.
PROCTOR: Noted.

- Manage Secondary Injuries/Wounds

Student: I would direct my partner to maintain the airway.
PROCTOR: Noted.

- Reassess Interventions

Student: I will reassess my interventions: suction as necessary, monitor the oral/advanced airway, oxygen per bag-valve device, and full immobilization transporting with the feet elevated.
PROCTOR: Noted.
ALS Student: I will reassess BLS interventions, plus the following: confirm end tidal CO_2 and lung sounds, monitor IV access, cardiac monitoring, and follow the ACLS and local protocol (Narcan).
ALS Proctor: Noted. The cardiac monitor shows sinus tachycardia and end tidal CO_2 and lung sounds confirm placement of the ET tube.

Critical Criteria:

- ❑ Did not obtain medical direction or verbalize standing orders for medical interventions
- ❑ Administered a dangerous or inappropriate intervention
- ❑ Did not ask questions about the present illness
- ❑ Did not differentiate patient's need for transportation versus continued assessment at the scene

Radio Report

(Provided by the student.)
PROCTOR: Noted.

Ongoing Assessment

Repeat the Initial Assessment

Student: I will repeat the initial assessment.
PROCTOR: Noted. (Reflected in "Repeat Vital Signs.")

Repeat Vital Signs

Student: I will reassess vital signs and mental status.
PROCTOR: Blood pressure, 130/82 mm Hg; pulse rate, 126 beats/min; respirations per bag-valve; pulse oximetry reading, 92%; and the patient is unresponsive.
Student: The vital signs have not changed significantly.
PROCTOR: Noted.

Check Interventions

Student: I will check my interventions: suction as necessary, monitor the oral/advanced airway, oxygen per bag-valve, and full immobilization transporting with the feet elevated.
PROCTOR: Noted.
ALS Student: I will check BLS interventions, plus the following: intubate, confirm end-tidal CO_2 and lung sounds, establish IV access, cardiac monitoring, and follow the ACLS and local protocol.
ALS Proctor: Noted. The cardiac monitor shows sinus tachycardia and end-tidal CO_2 and lung sounds confirm placement of the ET tube.

Repeat the Focused Assessment

Student: I will repeat the focused assessment.
PROCTOR: Noted.

Critical Criteria:

- ❑ Did not obtain medical direction or verbalize standing orders for medical interventions
- ❑ Administered a dangerous or inappropriate intervention

Handoff Report to Emergency Department Staff

Student: There was no change in the patient's condition during transport.
PROCTOR: Noted.

Critical Criteria

(Inform the student of items missed, if any.)

❑ Pass ❑ Fail Date: ____________________

Proctor Comments: ____________________

Notes

Dispatch Information

PROCTOR: EMS 10, respond to a 36-year-old male who is complaining of kidney stones. He is conscious and breathing.

Pre-scene Action (BSI)

Student: I am wearing nonlatex gloves and safety glasses.
PROCTOR: Noted.

Critical Criteria:
- ❑ Did not take, or verbalize, body substance isolation (BSI) precautions when necessary

Scene Size-up

Scene Safety

Student: Is the scene safe?
PROCTOR: Yes.

Mechanism of Injury/Nature of Illness

Student: What is the nature of the illness?
PROCTOR: The patient has a history of kidney stones and believes he has one right now.

Number of Patients

Student: How many patients are there?
PROCTOR: One.

Additional Resources

Student: I would call for advanced life support (ALS) assistance.
PROCTOR: Noted.

C-Spine Stabilization

Student: I would not stabilize the cervical spine (c-spine).
PROCTOR: Noted.

Critical Criteria:
- ❑ Did not determine scene safety

Initial Assessment

General Impression

Student: My general impression is that the patient's condition is stable.
PROCTOR: Noted.

Responsiveness/Level of Consciousness

Student: What is the patient's level of consciousness?
PROCTOR: Alert.

Chief Complaint/Apparent Life Threats

Student: What is the patient's chief complaint?
PROCTOR: The patient is complaining of a kidney stone.

Assess the Airway and Breathing

Student: Is the airway open? Is the patient breathing?
PROCTOR: Yes, the airway is open and the patient is breathing.

Assessment

Student: What are the rate and the quality of breathing?
PROCTOR: Rate: Tachypneic. Quality: Shallow.

Provide Oxygen

Student: I am applying oxygen at 15 L/min via nonrebreathing mask.
PROCTOR: Noted.

Ensure Adequate Ventilation

Student: The patient has adequate ventilations at this time.
PROCTOR: Noted.

Assess Circulation

Student: I am assessing the patient's circulation.
PROCTOR: Noted.

Assess for and Control Major Bleeding

Student: Do I find any major bleeding?
PROCTOR: No.

Assess the Pulse

Student: What are the rate and the quality of pulses?
PROCTOR: Rate: Tachycardic. Quality: Bounding.

Assess the Skin

Student: I am assessing the skin. What are the color, temperature, and condition of the skin?
PROCTOR: Color: Normal. Temperature: Warm. Condition: Moist.

Identify Priority Patients/Make Transport Decision

Student: The patient is a low priority and does not require immediate transport.
PROCTOR: Noted.

Critical Criteria:
- ❑ Did not provide high concentration of oxygen
- ❑ Did not find or manage problems associated with airway, breathing, hemorrhage or shock (hypoperfusion)
- ❑ Did not differentiate patient's need for transportation versus continued assessment at the scene
- ❑ Did detailed or focused history/physical examination before assessing the airway, breathing and circulation

Focused History and Physical Examination/Rapid Assessment

Select the Appropriate Assessment (Focused or Rapid)

Student: I am selecting the focused assessment.
PROCTOR: Noted.

SAMPLE History

Student: At this time I will gather a SAMPLE history from the patient or family. What are the patient's signs and symptoms?
PROCTOR: Kidney stone.

> Student: Onset: What were you doing when this started?
> **PROCTOR:** Watching television.
> Student: Provokes: What makes your condition worse or better?
> **PROCTOR:** Nothing.
> Student: Quality: Can you describe your pain?
> **PROCTOR:** Stabbing.
> Student: Radiates: Do you have pain anywhere else?
> **PROCTOR:** No.
> Student: Severity: On a scale of 1 to 10 with 10 being the worst possible, how would you rate your pain?
> **PROCTOR:** 10.
> Student: Time: How long has this been going on?
> **PROCTOR:** 2 hours.
> Student: Interventions: Have you done anything to make this better?
> **PROCTOR:** The patient has taken no actions.

Student: Allergies?
PROCTOR: No allergies.
Student: Medications?
PROCTOR: Vitamins and supplements.
Student: Pertinent past medical history?
PROCTOR: Kidney stones.
Student: Last oral intake?
PROCTOR: 3 hours ago.
Student: Events leading up to the incident?
PROCTOR: The patient was just watching television. He has a history of kidney stones.

Perform the Focused Physical Examination

Student: I am performing the focused physical examination.
PROCTOR: Noted.

Student: I am assessing the abdomen for DCAP-BTLS. This acronym stands for deformities, contusions, abrasions, punctures, penetrations, paradoxical motion in the chest, and burns, tenderness, lacerations, and swelling. I am assessing all four quadrants. Do I find any problems?
PROCTOR: No.

▼ Baseline Vital Signs

Student: What are the patient's baseline vital signs, including blood pressure, pulse, respirations, pulse oximetry, and level of consciousness?
PROCTOR: Blood pressure, 144/84 mm Hg; pulse rate, 120 beats/min; respirations, 24 breaths/min; pulse oximetry reading, 99%; and the patient is alert.

▼ Interventions

Student: I will apply oxygen and transport the patient in the position of comfort.
PROCTOR: Noted.
ALS Student: I will apply basic life support (BLS) interventions, plus the following: IV access and pain management per local protocol.
ALS Proctor: Noted.

▼ Reevaluate Transport Decision

Student: The patient is a low priority and does not require immediate transport.
PROCTOR: Noted.

▼ Detailed Physical Examination

Possible Answer #1
Student: I would not do a detailed physical exam.
PROCTOR: Noted. (Go to "Radio Report.")

Possible Answer #2
Student: I am conducting the detailed physical exam. I am looking for DCAP-BTLS.
PROCTOR: Noted. The detailed physical exam will be performed during transport.

▸ **Assess the Head**

Student: I am assessing the head. Do I find any DCAP-BTLS? Do I find any evidence of Battle's sign or raccoon eyes?
PROCTOR: No.

▸ **Inspect and Palpate the Head and Ears**

Student: I am assessing the head and ears.
PROCTOR: There are no obvious injuries.

▸ **Assess the Eyes**

Student: I am assessing the eyes. Are the pupils equal, round, and regular in size, and react properly to light (PEARRL)?
PROCTOR: They are PEARRL.

▸ **Assess the Facial Area Including Oral and Nasal Areas**

Student: I am assessing the face, nose, and mouth. Do I see any discharge or hear any obstructions?
PROCTOR: No.

▸ **Assess the Neck**

▸ **Inspect and Palpate the Neck**

Student: I am assessing the neck for DCAP-BTLS.
PROCTOR: There are no obvious injuries.

▸ **Assess for Jugular Vein Distention**

Student: Do I find any jugular vein distention (JVD)?
PROCTOR: No.

▸ **Assess for Tracheal Deviation**

Student: Do I see any tracheal deviation?
PROCTOR: No.

▸ **Assess the Chest**

Student: I am assessing the chest for DCAP-BTLS.
PROCTOR: Noted.

▸ **Inspect**

Student: What do I see when I look at the chest?
PROCTOR: There are no obvious injuries.
Student: Is the chest symmetric?
PROCTOR: Yes.

▸ **Palpate**

Student: When I touch the chest, do I feel crepitus or a flail segment?
PROCTOR: No.

▸ **Auscultate**

Student: Are lung sounds present in all fields?
PROCTOR: Yes.
Student: Do I hear any sucking sounds from the chest?
PROCTOR: No.

▸ **Assess the Abdomen/Pelvis**

▸ **Assess the Abdomen**

Student: I am assessing the abdomen for DCAP-BTLS. I am assessing all four quadrants. Do I find any problems?
PROCTOR: No.

▸ **Assess the Pelvis**

Student: I am assessing the pelvis for DCAP-BTLS. Is the pelvis stable?
PROCTOR: Yes.

▸ **Assess the Genitalia/Perineum as Needed (Verbalize in Training)**

Student: I am assessing the genitalia/perineum as necessary for DCAP-BTLS.
PROCTOR: The area is unremarkable.

▸ **Assess the Extremities**

▸ **Inspect**

Student: I am assessing the lower and upper extremities for DCAP-BTLS. Do I find anything?
PROCTOR: No.

▸ **Palpate**

Student: Do I feel anything unusual?
PROCTOR: No.

▸ **Assess Motor, Sensory, and Circulatory Function**

Student: I am checking for DCAP-BTLS, motor and sensory function, and pulses. Right leg?
PROCTOR: Negative DCAP-BTLS. Motor and sensory functions are present. Pulses are present.
Student: Left leg?
PROCTOR: Negative DCAP-BTLS. Motor and sensory functions are present. Pulses are present.
Student: Right arm?
PROCTOR: Negative DCAP-BTLS. Motor and sensory functions are present. Pulses are present.
Student: Left arm?
PROCTOR: Negative DCAP-BTLS. Motor and sensory functions are present. Pulses are present.

▸ **Assess the Posterior**

Note: This portion of the detailed physical exam would not be done if the patient were previously backboarded per local protocol.
Student: We will check the back.
PROCTOR: Noted.

▸ **Assess the Thorax**

Student: I am assessing the thorax. Do I find injuries?
PROCTOR: No.

▸ **Assess the Lumbar Area**

Student: I am assessing the flanks and lumbar area. Do I find injuries?
PROCTOR: No.

▸ **Assess the Entire Backside**

Student: I am assessing the entire backside. Do I find injuries?
PROCTOR: No.

▸ **Manage Secondary Injuries/Wounds**

Student: I would direct my partner to reassure the patient.

PROCTOR: Noted.

▸ **Reassess Interventions**

Student: I will reassess my interventions: apply oxygen and transport the patient in the position of comfort.

PROCTOR: Noted.

ALS Student: I will reassess BLS interventions, plus the following: IV access and pain management per local protocol.

ALS Proctor: Noted.

Critical Criteria:

- ❑ Did not obtain medical direction or verbalize standing orders for medical interventions
- ❑ Administered a dangerous or inappropriate intervention
- ❑ Did not ask questions about the present illness
- ❑ Did not differentiate patient's need for transportation versus continued assessment at the scene

Radio Report

(Provided by the student.)

PROCTOR: Noted.

Ongoing Assessment

Repeat the Initial Assessment

Student: I will repeat the initial assessment.

PROCTOR: Noted. (Reflected in "Repeat Vital Signs.")

Repeat Vital Signs

Student: I will reassess vital signs and mental status.

PROCTOR: Blood pressure, 140/80 mm Hg; pulse rate, 112 beats/min; respirations, 24 breaths/min; pulse oximetry reading, 99%; and the patient is alert.

Student: The vital signs have not changed significantly.

PROCTOR: Noted.

Check Interventions

Student: I will check my interventions: apply oxygen and transport the patient in the position of comfort.

PROCTOR: Noted.

ALS Student: I will check BLS interventions, plus the following: IV access and pain management per local protocol.

ALS Proctor: Noted.

Repeat the Focused Assessment

Student: I will repeat the focused assessment.

PROCTOR: Noted.

Critical Criteria:

- ❑ Did not obtain medical direction or verbalize standing orders for medical interventions
- ❑ Administered a dangerous or inappropriate intervention

Handoff Report to Emergency Department Staff

Student: There was no change in the patient's condition during transport.

PROCTOR: Noted.

Critical Criteria

(Inform the student of items missed, if any.)

❑ Pass ❑ Fail Date: ______________________

Proctor Comments: ______________________

____

____

CASE 127

Notes

Dispatch Information

PROCTOR: EMS 10, respond to a 14-year-old female who has overdosed. She is conscious and breathing.

Pre-scene Action (BSI)

Student: I am wearing nonlatex gloves and safety glasses.
PROCTOR: Noted.

> **Critical Criteria:**
> ❑ Did not take, or verbalize, body substance isolation (BSI) precautions when necessary

Scene Size-up

Scene Safety

Student: Is the scene safe?
PROCTOR: Yes.

Mechanism of Injury/Nature of Illness

Student: What is the nature of the illness?
PROCTOR: The patient has overdosed on an entire bottle of acetaminophen (Tylenol®).

Number of Patients

Student: How many patients are there?
PROCTOR: One.

Additional Resources

Student: I would call for advanced life support (ALS) assistance.
PROCTOR: Noted.

C-Spine Stabilization

Student: I would not stabilize the cervical spine (c-spine).
PROCTOR: Noted.

> **Critical Criteria:**
> ❑ Did not determine scene safety

Initial Assessment

General Impression

Student: My general impression is that the patient's condition is stable.
PROCTOR: Noted.

Responsiveness/Level of Consciousness

Student: What is the patient's level of consciousness?
PROCTOR: Alert.

Chief Complaint/Apparent Life Threats

Student: What is the patient's chief complaint?
PROCTOR: The patient says she wants to kill herself.

Assess the Airway and Breathing

Student: Is the airway open? Is the patient breathing?
PROCTOR: Yes, the airway is open and the patient is breathing.

▸ Assessment

Student: What are the rate and the quality of breathing?
PROCTOR: Rate: Within normal limits. Quality: Normal.

▸ Provide Oxygen

Student: I am applying oxygen at 15 L/min via nonrebreathing mask.
PROCTOR: Noted.

▸ Ensure Adequate Ventilation

Student: The patient has adequate ventilations at this time.
PROCTOR: Noted.

Assess Circulation

Student: I am assessing the patient's circulation.
PROCTOR: Noted.

▸ Assess for and Control Major Bleeding

Student: Do I find any major bleeding?
PROCTOR: No.

▸ Assess the Pulse

Student: What are the rate and the quality of pulses?
PROCTOR: Rate: Within normal limits. Quality: Normal.

▸ Assess the Skin

Student: I am assessing the skin. What are the color, temperature, and condition of the skin?
PROCTOR: Color: Normal. Temperature: Normal. Condition: Normal.

Identify Priority Patients/Make Transport Decision

Student: The patient is a low priority and does not require immediate transport.
PROCTOR: Noted.

> **Critical Criteria:**
> ❑ Did not provide high concentration of oxygen
> ❑ Did not find or manage problems associated with airway, breathing, hemorrhage or shock (hypoperfusion)
> ❑ Did not differentiate patient's need for transportation versus continued assessment at the scene
> ❑ Did detailed or focused history/physical examination before assessing the airway, breathing and circulation

Focused History and Physical Examination/Rapid Assessment

Select the Appropriate Assessment (Focused or Rapid)

Student: I am selecting the focused assessment.
PROCTOR: Noted.

SAMPLE History

Student: At this time I will gather a SAMPLE history from the patient or family. What are the patient's signs and symptoms?
PROCTOR: Behavioral and poisoning/overdose.

- **Student:** How do you feel?
- **PROCTOR:** The patient wants to kill herself.
- **Student:** Do you want to hurt or kill yourself?
- **PROCTOR:** Yes.
- **Student:** Is the patient a threat to self or others? What do you think?
- **PROCTOR:** Yes.
- **Student:** Is there a medical problem?
- **PROCTOR:** Yes, overdose on acetaminophen.
- **Student:** Interventions: Have you done anything to make this better?
- **PROCTOR:** No.
- **Student:** What did you ingest?
- **PROCTOR:** Acetaminophen.
- **Student:** How much did you ingest?
- **PROCTOR:** 30 pills.
- **Student:** Over what time period?
- **PROCTOR:** 20 minutes ago.
- **Student:** Interventions: Have you done anything to make this better?
- **PROCTOR:** No.
- **Student:** How much do you weigh?
- **PROCTOR:** 92 lb (42 kg).

Student: Allergies?
PROCTOR: No allergies.
Student: Medications?
PROCTOR: No medications.
Student: Pertinent past medical history?
PROCTOR: No pertinent medical history.
Student: Last oral intake?
PROCTOR: 2 hours ago.

Student: Events leading up to the incident?
PROCTOR: The patient's boyfriend broke up with her.

▼ Perform the Focused Physical Examination

Student: I am performing the focused physical examination.
PROCTOR: Noted.
Student: Do you feel sick or nauseated?
PROCTOR: No.
Student: Will you tell me if you start to feel bad?
PROCTOR: Yes.
Student: Did you take anything else?
PROCTOR: No.
Student: I will take the bottle with me to the emergency department.
PROCTOR: Noted.
Student: I will notify medical control to contact poison control.
PROCTOR: Noted.

▼ Baseline Vital Signs

Student: What are the patient's baseline vital signs, including blood pressure, pulse, respirations, pulse oximetry, blood glucose level, and level of consciousness?
PROCTOR: Blood pressure, 114/62 mm Hg; pulse rate, 84 beats/min; respirations, 16 breaths/min; pulse oximetry reading, 100%; blood glucose level, 94 mg/dL; and the patient is alert.

▼ Interventions

Student: I will apply oxygen and administer activated charcoal per local protocol.
PROCTOR: Noted. The charcoal request has been granted.
ALS Student: I will apply basic life support (BLS) interventions, plus the following: IV access and cardiac monitor.
ALS Proctor: Noted. The cardiac monitor shows normal sinus rhythm.

▼ Reevaluate Transport Decision

Student: The patient is a low priority and does not require immediate transport.
PROCTOR: Noted.

▼ Detailed Physical Examination

Possible Answer #1
Student: I would not do a detailed physical exam.
PROCTOR: Noted. (Go to "Radio Report.")

Possible Answer #2
Student: I am conducting the detailed physical exam. I am looking for DCAP-BTLS. This acronym stands for deformities, contusions, abrasions, punctures, penetrations, paradoxical motion in the chest, and burns, tenderness, lacerations, and swelling.
PROCTOR: Noted. The detailed physical exam will be performed during transport.

▸ Assess the Head

Student: I am assessing the head. Do I find any DCAP-BTLS? Do I find any evidence of Battle's sign or raccoon eyes?
PROCTOR: No.

▸ Inspect and Palpate the Head and Ears

Student: I am assessing the head and ears.
PROCTOR: There are no obvious injuries.

▸ Assess the Eyes

Student: I am assessing the eyes. Are the pupils equal, round, and regular in size, and react properly to light (PEARRL)?
PROCTOR: They are PEARRL.

▸ Assess the Facial Area Including Oral and Nasal Areas

Student: I am assessing the face, nose, and mouth. Do I see any discharge or hear any obstructions?
PROCTOR: No.

▸ Assess the Neck

▸ Inspect and Palpate the Neck

Student: I am assessing the neck for DCAP-BTLS.
PROCTOR: There are no obvious injuries.

▸ Assess for Jugular Vein Distention

Student: Do I find any jugular vein distention (JVD)?
PROCTOR: No.

▸ Assess for Tracheal Deviation

Student: Do I see any tracheal deviation?
PROCTOR: No.

▸ Assess the Chest

Student: I am assessing the chest for DCAP-BTLS.
PROCTOR: Noted.

▸ Inspect

Student: What do I see when I look at the chest?
PROCTOR: There are no obvious injuries.
Student: Is the chest symmetric?
PROCTOR: Yes.

▸ Palpate

Student: When I touch the chest, do I feel crepitus or a flail segment?
PROCTOR: No.

▸ Auscultate

Student: Are lung sounds present in all fields?
PROCTOR: Yes.
Student: Do I hear any sucking sounds from the chest?
PROCTOR: No.

▸ Assess the Abdomen/Pelvis

▸ Assess the Abdomen

Student: I am assessing the abdomen for DCAP-BTLS. I am assessing all four quadrants. Do I find any problems?
PROCTOR: No.

▸ Assess the Pelvis

Student: I am assessing the pelvis for DCAP-BTLS. Is the pelvis stable?
PROCTOR: Yes.

▸ Assess the Genitalia/Perineum as Needed (Verbalize in Training)

Student: I am assessing the genitalia/perineum as necessary for DCAP-BTLS.
PROCTOR: The area is unremarkable.

▸ Assess the Extremities

▸ Inspect

Student: I am assessing the lower and upper extremities for DCAP-BTLS. Do I find anything?
PROCTOR: No.

▸ Palpate

Student: Do I feel anything unusual?
PROCTOR: No.

▸ Assess Motor, Sensory, and Circulatory Function

Student: I am checking for DCAP-BTLS, motor and sensory function, and pulses. Right leg?
PROCTOR: Negative DCAP-BTLS. Motor and sensory functions are present. Pulses are present.
Student: Left leg?
PROCTOR: Negative DCAP-BTLS. Motor and sensory functions are present. Pulses are present.
Student: Right arm?
PROCTOR: Negative DCAP-BTLS. Motor and sensory functions are present. Pulses are present.
Student: Left arm?
PROCTOR: Negative DCAP-BTLS. Motor and sensory functions are present. Pulses are present.

▸ Assess the Posterior

Student: We will check the back.

PROCTOR: Noted.

▸ Assess the Thorax

Student: I am assessing the thorax. Do I find injuries?

PROCTOR: No.

▸ Assess the Lumbar Area

Student: I am assessing the flanks and lumbar area. Do I find injuries?

PROCTOR: No.

▸ Assess the Entire Backside

Student: I am assessing the entire backside. Do I find injuries?

PROCTOR: No.

▸ Manage Secondary Injuries/Wounds

Student: I would direct my partner to monitor the airway.

PROCTOR: Noted.

▸ Reassess Interventions

Student: I will reassess my interventions: oxygen, reassurance, and activated charcoal.

PROCTOR: Noted. The activated charcoal is almost gone.

ALS Student: I will reassess BLS interventions, plus the following: IV access and cardiac monitor.

ALS Proctor: Noted. The cardiac monitor shows normal sinus rhythm.

Critical Criteria:
- ❑ Did not obtain medical direction or verbalize standing orders for medical interventions
- ❑ Administered a dangerous or inappropriate intervention
- ❑ Did not ask questions about the present illness
- ❑ Did not differentiate patient's need for transportation versus continued assessment at the scene

Radio Report

(Provided by the student.)

PROCTOR: Noted.

Ongoing Assessment

Repeat the Initial Assessment

Student: I will repeat the initial assessment.

PROCTOR: Noted. (Reflected in "Repeat Vital Signs.")

Repeat Vital Signs

Student: I will reassess vital signs and mental status.

PROCTOR: Blood pressure, 114/62 mm Hg; pulse rate, 84 beats/min; respirations, 16 breaths/min; pulse oximetry reading, 100%; and the patient is alert.

Student: The vital signs have not changed significantly.

PROCTOR: Noted.

Check Interventions

Student: I will check my interventions: oxygen, reassurance, and activated charcoal.

PROCTOR: Noted. The activated charcoal is gone.

ALS Student: I will check BLS interventions, plus the following: IV access and cardiac monitor.

ALS Proctor: Noted. The cardiac monitor shows normal sinus rhythm.

Repeat the Focused Assessment

Student: I will repeat the focused assessment.

PROCTOR: Noted.

Critical Criteria:
- ❑ Did not obtain medical direction or verbalize standing orders for medical interventions
- ❑ Administered a dangerous or inappropriate intervention

Handoff Report to Emergency Department Staff

Student: There was no change in the patient's condition during transport.

PROCTOR: Noted.

Critical Criteria

(Inform the student of items missed, if any.)

❑ Pass ❑ Fail Date: ______________________

Proctor Comments: ______________________

Notes

CASE 129

Dispatch Information

PROCTOR: EMS 10, respond to an 86-year-old male in the grocery store with slurred speech. He is conscious and breathing.

Pre-scene Action (BSI)

Student: I am wearing nonlatex gloves and safety glasses.
PROCTOR: Noted.

Critical Criteria:
- ❑ Did not take, or verbalize, body substance isolation (BSI) precautions when necessary

Scene Size-up

Scene Safety

Student: Is the scene safe?
PROCTOR: Yes.

Mechanism of Injury/Nature of Illness

Student: What is the nature of the illness?
PROCTOR: The patient was sitting on a display shelf when he was noticed by a stock boy.

Number of Patients

Student: How many patients are there?
PROCTOR: One.

Additional Resources

Student: I would call for advanced life support (ALS) assistance.
PROCTOR: Noted.

C-Spine Stabilization

Student: I would not stabilize the cervical spine (c-spine).
PROCTOR: Noted.

Critical Criteria:
- ❑ Did not determine scene safety

Initial Assessment

General Impression

Student: My general impression is that the patient's condition is unstable.
PROCTOR: Noted.

Responsiveness/Level of Consciousness

Student: What is the patient's level of consciousness?
PROCTOR: Awake but confused.

Chief Complaint/Apparent Life Threats

Student: What is the patient's chief complaint?
PROCTOR: The patient has slurred speech.

Assess the Airway and Breathing

Student: Is the airway open? Is the patient breathing?
PROCTOR: Yes, the airway is open and the patient is breathing.

Assessment

Student: What are the rate and the quality of breathing?
PROCTOR: Rate: Within normal limits. Quality: Normal.

Provide Oxygen

Student: I am applying oxygen at 15 L/min via nonrebreathing mask.
PROCTOR: Noted.

Ensure Adequate Ventilation

Student: The patient has adequate ventilations at this time.
PROCTOR: Noted.

Assess Circulation

Student: I am assessing the patient's circulation.
PROCTOR: Noted.

Assess for and Control Major Bleeding

Student: Do I find any major bleeding?
PROCTOR: No.

Assess the Pulse

Student: What are the rate and the quality of pulses?
PROCTOR: Rate: Within normal limits. Quality: Bounding.

Assess the Skin

Student: I am assessing the skin. What are the color, temperature, and condition of the skin?
PROCTOR: Color: Normal. Temperature: Warm. Condition: Moist.

Identify Priority Patients/Make Transport Decision

Student: The patient is a high priority and is a load-and-go. I will begin packaging and transport.
PROCTOR: Noted.

Critical Criteria:
- ❑ Did not provide high concentration of oxygen
- ❑ Did not find or manage problems associated with airway, breathing, hemorrhage or shock (hypoperfusion)
- ❑ Did not differentiate patient's need for transportation versus continued assessment at the scene
- ❑ Did detailed or focused history/physical examination before assessing the airway, breathing and circulation

Focused History and Physical Examination/Rapid Assessment

Select the Appropriate Assessment (Focused or Rapid)

Student: I am selecting the focused assessment.
PROCTOR: Noted.
Student: I will perform a Cincinnati stroke scale test (facial droop, arm drift, and speech test).
PROCTOR: Noted. His actions show evidence of a stroke including facial droop, slurred words, and right-sided weakness.
Student: I will transport the patient in the recovery position on the affected side, or other position per local protocol. I will transport to the appropriate hospital.
PROCTOR: Noted.

SAMPLE History

Student: At this time I will gather a SAMPLE history from the patient or family. What are the patient's signs and symptoms?
PROCTOR: Altered mental status.

> **Student:** Describe the episode.
> **PROCTOR:** The patient has slurred speech and right-sided weakness.
> **Student:** Onset: What was he doing when this started?
> **PROCTOR:** Shopping.
> **Student:** Duration: How long has this been going on?
> **PROCTOR:** 10 minutes.
> **Student:** Are there any associated symptoms?
> **PROCTOR:** Yes, he has slurred speech, facial drooping, and right-sided weakness.
> **Student:** Is there any evidence of trauma?
> **PROCTOR:** No.
> **Student:** Interventions: Has he done anything to make this better?
> **PROCTOR:** The patient has taken no actions.
> **Student:** Have there been any seizures?
> **PROCTOR:** No.
> **Student:** Has there been any fever?
> **PROCTOR:** No.

Student: Allergies?
PROCTOR: Unknown.
Student: Medications?
PROCTOR: Unknown.

Student: Pertinent past medical history?
PROCTOR: Unknown.
Student: Last oral intake?
PROCTOR: Unknown.
Student: Events leading up to the incident?
PROCTOR: The patient was shopping and sat down on a display.

▼ Perform the Focused Physical Examination

Student: I am performing the focused physical examination.
PROCTOR: Noted.
Student: I will perform a Cincinnati stroke scale test (facial droop, arm drift, and speech test) and transport in the recovery position on the affected side, or other position per local protocol. I will transport to the appropriate hospital.
PROCTOR: Noted. His actions show evidence of a stroke including facial droop, right-sided weakness, and slurred words.

▼ Baseline Vital Signs

Student: What are the patient's baseline vital signs, including blood pressure, pulse, respirations, pulse oximetry, blood glucose level, and level of consciousness?
PROCTOR: Blood pressure, 192/100 mm Hg; pulse rate, 98 beats/min; respirations, 20 breaths/min; pulse oximetry reading, 98%; blood glucose level, 114 mg/dL; and the patient is awake but confused.

▼ Interventions

Student: I will apply oxygen, be prepared to suction if necessary, and transport the patient in the recovery position on the affected side. I will transport him to the appropriate hospital.
PROCTOR: Noted.
ALS Student: I will apply basic life support (BLS) interventions, plus the following: IV access, cardiac monitor, and 12-lead ECG.
ALS Proctor: Noted. The cardiac monitor shows normal sinus rhythm.

▼ Reevaluate Transport Decision

Student: The patient is a load-and-go due to a possible stroke.
PROCTOR: Noted.

▼ Detailed Physical Examination

Possible Answer #1
Student: I would not do a detailed physical exam.
PROCTOR: Noted. (Go to "Radio Report.")

Possible Answer #2
Student: I am conducting the detailed physical exam. I am looking for DCAP-BTLS. This acronym stands for deformities, contusions, abrasions, punctures, penetrations, paradoxical motion in the chest, and burns, tenderness, lacerations, and swelling.
PROCTOR: Noted. The detailed physical exam will be performed during transport.

▸ Assess the Head

Student: I am assessing the head. Do I find any DCAP-BTLS? Do I find any evidence of Battle's sign or raccoon eyes?
PROCTOR: No.

▸ Inspect and Palpate the Head and Ears

Student: I am assessing the head and ears.
PROCTOR: There are no obvious injuries.

▸ Assess the Eyes

Student: I am assessing the eyes. Are the pupils equal, round, and regular in size, and react properly to light (PEARRL)?
PROCTOR: They are PEARRL.

▸ Assess the Facial Area Including Oral and Nasal Areas

Student: I am assessing the face, nose, and mouth. Do I see any discharge or hear any obstructions?
PROCTOR: No.

▸ Assess the Neck

▸ Inspect and Palpate the Neck

Student: I am assessing the neck for DCAP-BTLS.
PROCTOR: There are no obvious injuries.

▸ Assess for Jugular Vein Distention

Student: Do I find any jugular vein distention (JVD)?
PROCTOR: No.

▸ Assess for Tracheal Deviation

Student: Do I see any tracheal deviation?
PROCTOR: No.

▸ Assess the Chest

Student: I am assessing the chest for DCAP-BTLS.
PROCTOR: Noted.

▸ Inspect

Student: What do I see when I look at the chest?
PROCTOR: There are no obvious injuries.
Student: Is the chest symmetric?
PROCTOR: Yes.

▸ Palpate

Student: When I touch the chest, do I feel crepitus or a flail segment?
PROCTOR: No.

▸ Auscultate

Student: Are lung sounds present in all fields?
PROCTOR: Yes.
Student: Do I hear any sucking sounds from the chest?
PROCTOR: No.

▸ Assess the Abdomen/Pelvis

▸ Assess the Abdomen

Student: I am assessing the abdomen for DCAP-BTLS. I am assessing all four quadrants. Do I find any problems?
PROCTOR: No.

▸ Assess the Pelvis

Student: I am assessing the pelvis for DCAP-BTLS. Is the pelvis stable?
PROCTOR: Yes.

▸ Assess the Genitalia/Perineum as Needed (Verbalize in Training)

Student: I am assessing the genitalia/perineum as necessary for DCAP-BTLS.
PROCTOR: The area is unremarkable.

▸ Assess the Extremities

▸ Inspect

Student: I am assessing the lower and upper extremities for DCAP-BTLS. Do I find anything?
PROCTOR: No.

▸ Palpate

Student: Do I feel anything unusual?
PROCTOR: No.

▸ Assess Motor, Sensory, and Circulatory Function

Student: I am checking for DCAP-BTLS, motor and sensory function, and pulses. Right leg?
PROCTOR: Weakness. Motor and sensory functions are impaired. Pulses are present.
Student: Left leg?
PROCTOR: Negative DCAP-BTLS. Motor and sensory functions are present. Pulses are present.
Student: Right arm?
PROCTOR: Weakness. Motor and sensory functions are impaired. Pulses are present.
Student: Left arm?
PROCTOR: Negative DCAP-BTLS. Motor and sensory functions are present. Pulses are present.

▸ Assess the Posterior

Student: We will check the back.

PROCTOR: Noted.

▸ Assess the Thorax

Student: I am assessing the thorax. Do I find injuries?

PROCTOR: No.

▸ Assess the Lumbar Area

Student: I am assessing the flanks and lumbar area. Do I find injuries?

PROCTOR: No.

▸ Assess the Entire Backside

Student: I am assessing the entire backside. Do I find injuries?

PROCTOR: No.

▸ Manage Secondary Injuries/Wounds

Student: I would direct my partner to monitor the airway.

PROCTOR: Noted.

▸ Reassess Interventions

Student: I will reassess my interventions: oxygen and transport the patient in the recovery position on the affected side. I will transport him to the appropriate hospital.

PROCTOR: Noted. The patient's responses show evidence of a stroke.

ALS Student: I will reassess BLS interventions, plus the following: IV access, cardiac monitor, and 12-lead ECG.

ALS Proctor: Noted. The cardiac monitor shows normal sinus rhythm.

Critical Criteria:
- ❑ Did not obtain medical direction or verbalize standing orders for medical interventions
- ❑ Administered a dangerous or inappropriate intervention
- ❑ Did not ask questions about the present illness
- ❑ Did not differentiate patient's need for transportation versus continued assessment at the scene

Radio Report

(Provided by the student.)

PROCTOR: Noted.

Ongoing Assessment

Repeat the Initial Assessment

Student: I will repeat the initial assessment.

PROCTOR: Noted. (Reflected in "Repeat Vital Signs.")

Repeat Vital Signs

Student: I will reassess vital signs and mental status.

PROCTOR: Blood pressure, 186/94 mm Hg; pulse rate, 98 beats/min; respirations, 20 breaths/min; pulse oximetry reading, 98%; and the patient is awake but confused.

Student: The vital signs have not changed significantly.

PROCTOR: Noted.

Check Interventions

Student: I will check my interventions: oxygen and transport the patient in the recovery position on the affected side. I will transport him to the appropriate hospital.

PROCTOR: Noted. The patient's responses show evidence of a stroke.

ALS Student: I will check BLS interventions, plus the following: IV access, cardiac monitor, and 12-lead ECG.

ALS Proctor: Noted. The cardiac monitor shows normal sinus rhythm.

Repeat the Focused Assessment

Student: I will repeat the focused assessment.

PROCTOR: Noted.

Critical Criteria:
- ❑ Did not obtain medical direction or verbalize standing orders for medical interventions
- ❑ Administered a dangerous or inappropriate intervention

Handoff Report to Emergency Department Staff

Student: There was no change in the patient's condition during transport.

PROCTOR: Noted.

Critical Criteria:
- ❑ Did not obtain medical direction or verbalize standing orders for medical interventions
- ❑ Administered a dangerous or inappropriate intervention

Critical Criteria

(Inform the student of items missed, if any.)

❑ Pass ❑ Fail Date: ______________________

Proctor Comments: ______________________

Notes

Dispatch Information

PROCTOR: EMS 10, respond to a 26-year-old female who is giving birth. She is conscious and breathing.

Pre-scene Action (BSI)

Student: I am wearing nonlatex sterile gloves, mask, gown, and safety glasses.
PROCTOR: Noted.

Critical Criteria:
- ❑ Did not take, or verbalize, body substance isolation (BSI) precautions when necessary

Scene Size-up

Scene Safety

Student: Is the scene safe?
PROCTOR: Yes.

Mechanism of Injury/Nature of Illness

Student: What is the nature of the illness?
PROCTOR: The patient is in labor.

Number of Patients

Student: How many patients are there?
PROCTOR: One.

Additional Resources

Student: I would call for advanced life support (ALS) assistance.
PROCTOR: Noted.

C-Spine Stabilization

Student: I would not stabilize the cervical spine (c-spine).
PROCTOR: Noted.

Critical Criteria:
- ❑ Did not determine scene safety

Initial Assessment

General Impression

Student: My general impression is that the patient's condition is stable.
PROCTOR: Noted.

Responsiveness/Level of Consciousness

Student: What is the patient's level of consciousness?
PROCTOR: Alert.

Chief Complaint/Apparent Life Threats

Student: What is the patient's chief complaint?
PROCTOR: The patient is in labor.

Assess the Airway and Breathing

Student: Is the airway open? Is the patient breathing?
PROCTOR: Yes, the airway is open and the patient is breathing.

Assessment

Student: What are the rate and the quality of breathing?
PROCTOR: Rate: Tachypneic. Quality: Per her Lamaze class training.

Provide Oxygen

Student: I am applying oxygen at 15 L/min via nonrebreathing mask.
PROCTOR: Noted.

Ensure Adequate Ventilation

Student: The patient has adequate ventilations at this time.
PROCTOR: Noted.

Assess Circulation

Student: I am assessing the patient's circulation.
PROCTOR: Noted.

Assess for and Control Major Bleeding

Student: Do I find any major bleeding?
PROCTOR: Her bag of water has ruptured, but there is no major bleeding.

Assess the Pulse

Student: What are the rate and the quality of pulses?
PROCTOR: Rate: Tachycardic. Quality: Strong.

Assess the Skin

Student: I am assessing the skin. What are the color, temperature, and condition of the skin?
PROCTOR: Color: Normal. Temperature: Warm. Condition: Moist.

Identify Priority Patients/Make Transport Decision

Student: I do not yet have enough information for a transport decision.
PROCTOR: Noted.

Critical Criteria:
- ❑ Did not provide high concentration of oxygen
- ❑ Did not find or manage problems associated with airway, breathing, hemorrhage or shock (hypoperfusion)
- ❑ Did not differentiate patient's need for transportation versus continued assessment at the scene
- ❑ Did detailed or focused history/physical examination before assessing the airway, breathing and circulation

Focused History and Physical Examination/Rapid Assessment

Select the Appropriate Assessment (Focused or Rapid)

Student: I am selecting the focused assessment.
PROCTOR: Noted.

SAMPLE History

Student: At this time I will gather a SAMPLE history from the patient or family. What are the patient's signs and symptoms?
PROCTOR: Obstetrics.
Student: Are you pregnant?
PROCTOR: Yes.
Student: How long have you been pregnant?
PROCTOR: 9 months.
Student: Are you having pain or contractions?
PROCTOR: The contractions are less than 2 minutes apart.
Student: Are you having any bleeding or discharge?
PROCTOR: Yes, the bag of water has ruptured.
Student: Do you feel the need to push?
PROCTOR: Yes.
Student: When was your last menstrual period?
PROCTOR: 10 months ago.
Student: Allergies?
PROCTOR: No allergies.
Student: Medications?
PROCTOR: Prenatal vitamins.
Student: Pertinent past medical history?
PROCTOR: No pertinent medical history.
Student: Last oral intake?
PROCTOR: 3 hours ago.
Student: Events leading up to the incident?
PROCTOR: Her contractions started several hours ago. The patient was on the phone with her mother when her water broke.

Perform the Focused Physical Examination

Student: I am performing the focused physical examination.
PROCTOR: Noted.
Student: How many live births has she had?
PROCTOR: Four (this will make number five).

Student: How many times has she been pregnant?
PROCTOR: Five.
Student: I am assessing the abdomen. I am assessing all four quadrants. Do I find any problems?
PROCTOR: She has point tenderness in the lower middle abdomen.
Student: I am assessing for crowning. Do I see any crowning?
PROCTOR: Yes. The birth is taking place now. The head is presenting.

Baseline Vital Signs

Student: What are the patient's baseline vital signs, including blood pressure, pulse, respirations, pulse oximetry, and level of consciousness?
PROCTOR: Blood pressure, 132/68 mm Hg; pulse rate, 122 beats/min; respirations, 28 breaths/min; pulse oximetry reading, 98%; and the patient is alert.

Interventions

Student: I will provide reassurance, continue oxygen, and position the patient for the delivery (elevate the hips with towels and support the head and shoulders with blankets, towels, and pillows), prepare the delivery field with sterile items from the OB kit. I will assist the delivery and prevent an explosive delivery. As soon as the baby is born I will suction the mouth and then the nose of the baby using a bulb syringe while my partner dries and warms the baby. I will stimulate breathing and document the time. Is the baby breathing?
PROCTOR: Noted. Yes, the baby has a strong cry.
Student: I will keep the baby at the level of the vagina until the pulse stops in the cord. I will then clamp and cut the cord (per local protocol).
PROCTOR: Noted.
Student: I will perform an APGAR score on this baby, which includes checking the baby's appearance, pulse, grimace or irritability, activity or muscle tone, and respirations.
PROCTOR: Noted. The care of the newborn is in Case 131.
Student: I will allow for breastfeeding and perform a uterine massage. I will stay on scene (and wait for placenta delivery) or begin transport per local protocol.
PROCTOR: Noted.
ALS Student: I will apply basic life support (BLS) interventions, plus the following: IV access.
ALS Proctor: Noted.

Reevaluate Transport Decision

Student: The patient does not require immediate transport.
PROCTOR: Noted.

Detailed Physical Examination

Possible Answer #1
Student: I would not do a detailed physical exam.
PROCTOR: Noted. (Go to "Radio Report.")

Possible Answer #2
Student: I am conducting the detailed physical exam. I am looking for DCAP-BTLS. I am checking for DCAP-BTLS. This acronym stands for deformities, contusions, abrasions, punctures, penetrations, paradoxical motion in the chest, and burns, tenderness, lacerations, and swelling.
PROCTOR: Noted. The detailed physical exam will be performed during transport.

- **Assess the Head**

Student: I am assessing the head. Do I find any DCAP-BTLS? Do I find any evidence of Battle's sign or raccoon eyes?
PROCTOR: No.

- **Inspect and Palpate the Head and Ears**

Student: I am assessing the head and ears.
PROCTOR: There are no obvious injuries.

- **Assess the Eyes**

Student: I am assessing the eyes. Are the pupils equal, round, and regular in size, and react properly to light (PEARRL)?
PROCTOR: They are PEARRL.

- **Assess the Facial Area Including Oral and Nasal Areas**

Student: I am assessing the face, nose, and mouth. Do I see any discharge or hear any obstructions?
PROCTOR: No.

- **Assess the Neck**
- **Inspect and Palpate the Neck**

Student: I am assessing the neck for DCAP-BTLS.
PROCTOR: There are no obvious injuries.

- **Assess for Jugular Vein Distention**

Student: Do I find any jugular vein distention (JVD)?
PROCTOR: No.

- **Assess for Tracheal Deviation**

Student: Do I see any tracheal deviation?
PROCTOR: No.

- **Assess the Chest**

Student: I am assessing the chest for DCAP-BTLS.
PROCTOR: Noted.

- **Inspect**

Student: What do I see when I look at the chest?
PROCTOR: There are no obvious injuries.
Student: Is the chest symmetric?
PROCTOR: Yes.

- **Palpate**

Student: When I touch the chest, do I feel crepitus or a flail segment?
PROCTOR: No.

- **Auscultate**

Student: Are lung sounds present in all fields?
PROCTOR: Yes.
Student: Do I hear any sucking sounds from the chest?
PROCTOR: No.

- **Assess the Abdomen/Pelvis**
- **Assess the Abdomen**

Student: I am assessing the abdomen for DCAP-BTLS. I am assessing all four quadrants. Do I find any problems?
PROCTOR: The patient's abdomen is markedly smaller and the skin is wrinkled. The fundus is present in the abdomen.
Student: I will massage the fundus in a firm circular motion.
PROCTOR: Noted.

- **Assess the Pelvis**

Student: I am assessing the pelvis for DCAP-BTLS. Is the pelvis stable?
PROCTOR: Yes.

- **Assess the Genitalia/Perineum as Needed (Verbalize in Training)**

Student: I am assessing the genitalia/perineum as necessary for DCAP-BTLS.
PROCTOR: The birth has taken place and the cord is still protruding. The cord is not bleeding.
Student: I will continue the massage and assist with the delivery of the placenta. I will inspect and package the placenta using the bag provided in the OB kit. I will apply a pad from the OB kit over the vaginal opening.
PROCTOR: Noted.

- **Assess the Extremities**
- **Inspect**

Student: I am assessing the lower and upper extremities for DCAP-BTLS. Do I find anything?
PROCTOR: No.

▸ **Palpate**

Student: Do I feel anything unusual?

PROCTOR: No.

▸ **Assess Motor, Sensory, and Circulatory Function**

Student: I am checking for DCAP-BTLS, motor and sensory function, and pulses. Right leg?

PROCTOR: Negative DCAP-BTLS. Motor and sensory functions are present. Pulses are present.

Student: Left leg?

PROCTOR: Negative DCAP-BTLS. Motor and sensory functions are present. Pulses are present.

Student: Right arm?

PROCTOR: Negative DCAP-BTLS. Motor and sensory functions are present. Pulses are present.

Student: Left arm?

PROCTOR: Negative DCAP-BTLS. Motor and sensory functions are present. Pulses are present.

▸ **Assess the Posterior**

Student: We will check the back.

PROCTOR: Noted.

▸ **Assess the Thorax**

Student: I am assessing the thorax. Do I find injuries?

PROCTOR: No.

▸ **Assess the Lumbar Area**

Student: I am assessing the flanks and lumbar area. Do I find injuries?

PROCTOR: No.

▸ **Assess the Entire Backside**

Student: I am assessing the entire backside. Do I find injuries?

PROCTOR: No.

▸ **Manage Secondary Injuries/Wounds**

Student: I would direct my partner to provide reassurance and assist me in the care of the mother and baby.

PROCTOR: Noted.

▸ **Reassess Interventions**

Student: I will reassess my interventions: reassurance, apply oxygen, assist the delivery, transport the patient in the position of comfort, treat and transport the baby per local protocol.

PROCTOR: Noted.

ALS Student: I will reassess BLS interventions, plus the following: monitor the IV.

ALS Proctor: Noted.

Critical Criteria:

- ❑ Did not obtain medical direction or verbalize standing orders for medical interventions
- ❑ Administered a dangerous or inappropriate intervention
- ❑ Did not ask questions about the present illness
- ❑ Did not differentiate patient's need for transportation versus continued assessment at the scene

Radio Report

(Provided by the student.)

PROCTOR: Noted.

Ongoing Assessment

Repeat the Initial Assessment

Student: I will repeat the initial assessment.

PROCTOR: Noted. (Reflected in "Repeat Vital Signs.")

Repeat Vital Signs

Student: I will reassess vital signs and mental status.

PROCTOR: Blood pressure, 130/68 mm Hg; pulse rate, 120 beats/min; respirations, 28 breaths/min; pulse oximetry reading, 99%; and the patient is alert.

Student: The vital signs have not changed significantly.

PROCTOR: Noted.

Check Interventions

Student: I will check my interventions: reassurance, continue oxygen, monitor mother and baby.

PROCTOR: Noted.

ALS Student: I will check BLS interventions, plus the following: monitor the IV.

ALS Proctor: Noted.

Repeat the Focused Assessment

Student: I will repeat the focused assessment.

PROCTOR: Noted.

Critical Criteria:

- ❑ Did not obtain medical direction or verbalize standing orders for medical interventions
- ❑ Administered a dangerous or inappropriate intervention

Handoff Report to Emergency Department Staff

Student: There is now a second patient.

PROCTOR: Noted. Care of the newborn is covered in Case 131 of this book.

Critical Criteria

(Inform the student of items missed, if any.)

❑ Pass ❑ Fail Date: ____________________

Proctor Comments: ____________________

____

____

CASE 130

Notes

Dispatch Information

PROCTOR: EMS 10, respond to a female infant who has just been delivered.

Pre-scene Action (BSI)

Student: I am wearing nonlatex gloves, safety glasses, mask, and gown.
PROCTOR: Noted.

> **Critical Criteria:**
> ☐ Did not take, or verbalize, body substance isolation (BSI) precautions when necessary

Scene Size-up

Scene Safety

Student: Is the scene safe?
PROCTOR: Yes.

Mechanism of Injury/Nature of Illness

Student: What is the nature of the illness?
PROCTOR: The patient was just born.

Number of Patients

Student: How many patients are there?
PROCTOR: One.

Additional Resources

Student: I would call for advanced life support (ALS) assistance.
PROCTOR: Noted.

C-Spine Stabilization

Student: I would not stabilize the cervical spine (c-spine).
PROCTOR: Noted.

> **Critical Criteria:**
> ☐ Did not determine scene safety

Initial Assessment

General Impression

Student: My general impression is that the patient's condition is stable.
PROCTOR: Noted.

Responsiveness/Level of Consciousness

Student: What is the patient's level of consciousness?
PROCTOR: The patient is not yet crying.

Chief Complaint/Apparent Life Threats

Student: What is the patient's chief complaint?
PROCTOR: The patient is not yet crying.

Assess the Airway and Breathing

Student: I will suction the mouth first and then the nose. If necessary, I will stimulate breathing by tapping the sole of the foot or rubbing the back. Is the airway open?
PROCTOR: Yes.

Assessment

Student: What are the rate and the quality of breathing?
PROCTOR: Rate: Fast. Quality: Crying.

Provide Oxygen

Student: I am applying oxygen at 15 L/min via blow-by mask. I will be careful to protect the eyes from the flow of oxygen.
PROCTOR: Noted.

Ensure Adequate Ventilation

Student: The patient has adequate ventilations at this time.
PROCTOR: Noted.

Assess Circulation

Student: I am assessing the patient's circulation.
PROCTOR: Noted.

Assess for and Control Major Bleeding

Student: Do I find any major bleeding?
PROCTOR: No.

Assess the Pulse

Student: What are the rate and the quality of pulses?
PROCTOR: Rate: Tachycardic. Quality: Strong.

Assess the Skin

Student: I am assessing the skin. What are the color, temperature, and condition of the skin?
PROCTOR: Color: Pink to the head and trunk and cyanotic to the arms and legs. Temperature: Warm. Condition: Moist.

Identify Priority Patients/Make Transport Decision

Student: The patient does not require immediate transport. I will set the heat to a high setting in the ambulance and keep the baby warm.
PROCTOR: Noted.

> **Critical Criteria:**
> ☐ Did not provide high concentration of oxygen
> ☐ Did not find or manage problems associated with airway, breathing, hemorrhage or shock (hypoperfusion)
> ☐ Did not differentiate patient's need for transportation versus continued assessment at the scene
> ☐ Did detailed or focused history/physical examination before assessing the airway, breathing and circulation

Focused History and Physical Examination/Rapid Assessment

Select the Appropriate Assessment (Focused or Rapid)

Student: I am selecting the focused physical exam to identify and treat life threats.
PROCTOR: Noted.

SAMPLE History

Student: At this time I will gather a SAMPLE history from the patient or family. What are the patient's signs and symptoms?
PROCTOR: Newborn patient.

Student: Onset: What were you doing when this started?
PROCTOR: She was just born.
Student: Provokes: What makes your condition worse or better?
PROCTOR: N/A.
Student: Quality: Can you describe your pain?
PROCTOR: N/A.
Student: Radiates: Do you have pain anywhere else?
PROCTOR: N/A.
Student: Severity: On a scale of 1 to 10 with 10 being the worst possible, how would you rate your pain/distress?
PROCTOR: N/A.
Student: Time: How long has this been going on?
PROCTOR: 1 minute.
Student: Interventions: Have you done anything to make this better?
PROCTOR: N/A.

Student: Allergies?
PROCTOR: No allergies.
Student: Medications?
PROCTOR: No medications.
Student: Pertinent past medical history?
PROCTOR: No pertinent medical history.
Student: Last oral intake?
PROCTOR: Never.
Student: Events leading up to the incident?
PROCTOR: The patient was just born.

▼ Perform the Focused Physical Examination

Student: I am performing the focused physical examination for a newborn, which is the APGAR score. This includes checking the baby's appearance, pulse, grimace or irritablilty, activity or muscle tone, and respirations.

PROCTOR: Noted.

Student: What is the Appearance?

PROCTOR: The body is pink but the hands and feet are somewhat blue.

Student: What is the Pulse rate?

PROCTOR: The pulse rate is greater than 100 beats/min.

Student: What is the Grimace or irritability?

PROCTOR: She has a strong cry.

Student: What is the Activity or muscle tone?

PROCTOR: She makes some attempts to resist the straightening of the legs.

Student: What are the Respirations?

PROCTOR: She has rapid respirations.

Student: The APGAR score is an 8 at this time.

PROCTOR: Noted. The test score is as follows: Appearance [1], Pulse [2], Grimace [2], Activity [1], and Respiration [2].

▼ Baseline Vital Signs

Student: What are the patient's baseline vital signs, including blood pressure, pulse, respirations, pulse oximetry, and level of consciousness?

PROCTOR: Blood pressure, N/A; pulse rate, 156 beats/min; respirations, 42 breaths/min; pulse oximetry reading, N/A; and the patient is alert.

▼ Interventions

Student: I will apply suction to the mouth and then the nose as needed, continue oxygen, provide drying and warming measures, and obtain an APGAR score at 5 minutes.

PROCTOR: Noted.

▼ Reevaluate Transport Decision

Student: The patient does not require immediate transport.

PROCTOR: Noted.

▼ Detailed Physical Examination

Possible Answer #1

Student: I would not do a detailed physical exam.

PROCTOR: Noted. (Go to "Radio Report.")

Possible Answer #2

Student: I am conducting the detailed physical exam. I am looking for DCAP-BTLS. This acronym stands for deformities, contusions, abrasions, punctures, penetrations, paradoxical motion in the chest, and burns, tenderness, lacerations, and swelling.

PROCTOR: Noted. The detailed physical exam will be performed during transport.

▸ Assess the Head

Student: I am assessing the head. Do I find any DCAP-BTLS? Do I find any evidence of Battle's sign or raccoon eyes?

PROCTOR: No.

▸ Inspect and Palpate the Head and Ears

Student: I am assessing the head and ears.

PROCTOR: There are no obvious injuries.

▸ Assess the Eyes

Student: I am assessing the eyes. Are the pupils equal, round, and regular in size, and react properly to light (PEARRL)?

PROCTOR: They are PEARRL.

▸ Assess the Facial Area Including Oral and Nasal Areas

Student: I am assessing the face, nose, and mouth. Do I see any discharge or hear any obstructions?

PROCTOR: Gurgling sounds are present in the airway.

Student: I will suction the airway as needed.

PROCTOR: Noted.

▸ Assess the Neck

▸ Inspect and Palpate the Neck

Student: I am assessing the neck for DCAP-BTLS.

PROCTOR: There are no obvious injuries.

▸ Assess for Jugular Vein Distention

Student: Do I find any jugular vein distention (JVD)?

PROCTOR: No.

▸ Assess for Tracheal Deviation

Student: Do I see any tracheal deviation?

PROCTOR: No.

▸ Assess the Chest

Student: I am assessing the chest for DCAP-BTLS.

PROCTOR: Noted.

▸ Inspect

Student: What do I see when I look at the chest?

PROCTOR: There are no obvious injuries.

Student: Is the chest symmetric?

PROCTOR: Yes.

▸ Palpate

Student: When I touch the chest, do I feel crepitus or a flail segment?

PROCTOR: No.

▸ Auscultate

Student: Are lung sounds present in all fields?

PROCTOR: Yes.

Student: Do I hear any sucking sounds from the chest?

PROCTOR: No.

▸ Assess the Abdomen/Pelvis

▸ Assess the Abdomen

Student: I am assessing the abdomen for DCAP-BTLS. I am assessing all four quadrants. Do I find any problems?

PROCTOR: No.

▸ Assess the Pelvis

Student: I am assessing the pelvis for DCAP-BTLS. Is the pelvis stable?

PROCTOR: Yes.

▸ Assess the Genitalia/Perineum as Needed (Verbalize in Training)

Student: I am assessing the genitalia/perineum as necessary for DCAP-BTLS.

PROCTOR: The area is unremarkable.

▸ Assess the Extremities

▸ Inspect

Student: I am assessing the lower and upper extremities for DCAP-BTLS. Do I find anything?

PROCTOR: No.

▸ Palpate

Student: Do I feel anything unusual?

PROCTOR: No.

▸ Assess Motor, Sensory, and Circulatory Function

Student: I am checking for DCAP-BTLS, motor and sensory function, and pulses. Right leg?

PROCTOR: Color is improving. Motor and sensory functions are present. Pulses are present.

Student: Left leg?

PROCTOR: Color is improving. Motor and sensory functions are present. Pulses are present.

Student: Right arm?

PROCTOR: Color is improving. Motor and sensory functions are present. Pulses are present.

Student: Left arm?

PROCTOR: Color is improving. Motor and sensory functions are present. Pulses are present.

Assess the Posterior

Student: We will now check the back.

PROCTOR: Noted.

Assess the Thorax

Student: I am assessing the thorax. Do I find injuries?

PROCTOR: No.

Assess the Lumbar Area

Student: I am assessing the flanks and lumbar area. Do I find injuries?

PROCTOR: No.

Assess the Entire Backside

Student: I am assessing the entire backside. Do I find injuries?

PROCTOR: No.

Manage Secondary Injuries/Wounds

Student: I would continue suctioning the mouth and nose as necessary, continue oxygen, provide drying and warming measures, and obtain an APGAR score at 5 minutes.

PROCTOR: Noted.

Reassess Interventions

Student: I will reassess my interventions: apply suction to the mouth and then the nose, apply oxygen, provide drying and warming measures, and obtain an APGAR score.

PROCTOR: Noted.

Student: What is the Appearance?

PROCTOR: The entire body is pink.

Student: What is the Pulse rate?

PROCTOR: The pulse rate is greater than 100 beats/min.

Student: What is the Grimace or irritability?

PROCTOR: She has a strong cry.

Student: What is the Activity or muscle tone?

PROCTOR: She resists the straightening of the legs.

Student: What are the Respirations?

PROCTOR: She has rapid respirations.

Student: The APGAR score is a 10 at 5 minutes.

PROCTOR: Noted. The test score is as follows: Appearance [2], Pulse [2], Grimace [2], Activity [2], and Respiration [2].

Critical Criteria:

- ❑ Did not obtain medical direction or verbalize standing orders for medical interventions
- ❑ Administered a dangerous or inappropriate intervention
- ❑ Did not ask questions about the present illness
- ❑ Did not differentiate patient's need for transportation versus continued assessment at the scene

Radio Report

(Provided by the student.)

PROCTOR: Noted.

Ongoing Assessment

Repeat the Initial Assessment

Student: I will repeat the initial assessment.

PROCTOR: Noted. (Reflected in "Repeat Vital Signs.")

Repeat Vital Signs

Student: I will reassess vital signs and mental status.

PROCTOR: Blood pressure, N/A; pulse rate, 142 beats/min; respirations, 32 breaths/min; pulse oximetry reading, N/A; and the patient is alert.

Student: The vital signs and APGAR score have improved.

PROCTOR: Noted.

Check Interventions

Student: I will check my interventions: continue suction if needed, continue oxygen, provide drying and warming measures, and transport.

PROCTOR: Noted.

Repeat the Focused Assessment

Student: I will repeat the focused assessment.

PROCTOR: Noted.

Critical Criteria:

- ❑ Did not obtain medical direction or verbalize standing orders for medical interventions
- ❑ Administered a dangerous or inappropriate intervention

Handoff Report to Emergency Department Staff

Student: The patient's condition improved during transport.

PROCTOR: Noted.

Critical Criteria

(Inform the student of items missed, if any.)

❑ Pass ❑ Fail Date: ______________________

Proctor Comments: ______________________

____

____

Notes

Dispatch Information

PROCTOR: EMS 10, respond to a 23-year-old male who has ingested acid. He is conscious and breathing.

Pre-scene Action (BSI)

Student: I am wearing nonlatex gloves, safety glasses, a mask, and a gown.
PROCTOR: Noted.

Critical Criteria:
- ❑ Did not take, or verbalize, body substance isolation (BSI) precautions when necessary

Scene Size-up

Scene Safety

Student: Is the scene safe?
PROCTOR: Yes.

Mechanism of Injury/Nature of Illness

Student: What is the nature of the illness?
PROCTOR: The patient is upset about his girlfriend leaving him. He has consumed a large amount of an undetermined acid. He called his mother to say goodbye; his mother called 9-1-1.

Number of Patients

Student: How many patients are there?
PROCTOR: One.

Additional Resources

Student: I would call for advanced life support (ALS) assistance.
PROCTOR: Noted.

C-Spine Stabilization

Student: I would not stabilize the cervical spine (c-spine).
PROCTOR: Noted.

Critical Criteria:
- ❑ Did not determine scene safety

Initial Assessment

General Impression

Student: My general impression is that the patient's condition is unstable.
PROCTOR: Noted.

Responsiveness/Level of Consciousness

Student: What is the patient's level of consciousness?
PROCTOR: Conscious and alert.

Chief Complaint/Apparent Life Threats

Student: What is the patient's chief complaint?
PROCTOR: The patient is complaining of burning in his throat and stomach.

Assess the Airway and Breathing

Student: Is the airway open? Is the patient breathing?
PROCTOR: Yes, the airway is open and the patient is breathing.

Assessment

Student: What are the rate and the quality of breathing?
PROCTOR: Rate: Tachypneic. Quality: Labored.

Provide Oxygen

Student: I am applying oxygen at 15 L/min via nonrebreathing mask.
PROCTOR: Noted.

Ensure Adequate Ventilation

Student: The patient has adequate ventilations at this time.
PROCTOR: Noted.

Assess Circulation

Student: I am assessing the patient's circulation.
PROCTOR: Noted.

Assess for and Control Major Bleeding

Student: Do I find any major bleeding?
PROCTOR: No.

Assess the Pulse

Student: What are the rate and the quality of pulses?
PROCTOR: Rate: Tachycardic. Quality: Normal.

Assess the Skin

Student: I am assessing the skin. What are the color, temperature, and condition of the skin?
PROCTOR: Color: Pasty white. Temperature: Cold. Condition: Diaphoretic.

Identify Priority Patients/Make Transport Decision

Student: The patient is a high priority and is a load-and-go. I will begin packaging and transport.
PROCTOR: Noted.

Critical Criteria:
- ❑ Did not provide high concentration of oxygen
- ❑ Did not find or manage problems associated with airway, breathing, hemorrhage or shock (hypoperfusion)
- ❑ Did not differentiate patient's need for transportation versus continued assessment at the scene
- ❑ Did detailed or focused history/physical examination before assessing the airway, breathing and circulation

Focused History and Physical Examination/Rapid Assessment

Select the Appropriate Assessment (Focused or Rapid)

Student: I am selecting the focused assessment.
PROCTOR: Noted.

SAMPLE History

Student: At this time I will gather a SAMPLE history from the patient or family. What are the patient's signs and symptoms?
PROCTOR: Behavioral and poisoning/overdose.

Student: How do you feel?
PROCTOR: The patient suddenly begins to projectile vomit blood and cry for help.
Student: I will rapidly remove the nonrebreathing mask and allow the patient to vomit into a large emesis basin or emesis collection bag. I will continue oxygen administration by the blow-by method.
PROCTOR: Noted.
Student: Determine suicidal tendencies. Do you want to hurt or kill yourself?
PROCTOR: Yes.
Student: Is the patient a threat to self or others? What do you think?
PROCTOR: Yes.
Student: Is there a medical problem?
PROCTOR: Yes, he has an acid injury.
Student: Interventions: Have you done anything to make this better?
PROCTOR: No.
Student: What was the substance?
PROCTOR: It was an acid found in an old glass soda bottle with a handwritten label that said "Acid."
Student: When did you ingest this?
PROCTOR: Ten minutes ago.
Student: How much did you ingest?
PROCTOR: He drank about half of a 16-oz soda bottle (about 8 oz).

Student: Over what time period?
PROCTOR: He drank it as quick as he could swallow it down.
Student: Interventions: Have you done anything to make this better?
PROCTOR: No.
Student: How much do you weigh?
PROCTOR: He weighs 185 lb (84 kg).
Student: Allergies?
PROCTOR: No allergies.
Student: Medications?
PROCTOR: No medications.
Student: Pertinent past medical history?
PROCTOR: No pertinent medical history.
Student: Last oral intake?
PROCTOR: He ate a meal 3 hours ago. He drank the acid 5 minutes ago.
Student: Events leading up to the incident?
PROCTOR: The patient had an argument with his girlfriend and she left him.

▼ Perform the Focused Physical Examination

Student: I am performing the focused physical examination.
PROCTOR: Noted.
Student: I will contact medical control and have them contact poison control.
PROCTOR: Noted.
Student: I will transport the bottle safely in a plastic zip lock bag to the emergency room.
PROCTOR: Noted.
Student: Do I see evidence of acid ingestion?
PROCTOR: Yes. The projectile vomit has blood clots in it and the lips have blisters and scabs forming.
Student: What are his lung sounds?
PROCTOR: They are clear bilaterally at this time.
Student: I will monitor the airway and position the patient so that he can safely clear his own airway.
PROCTOR: Noted.

▼ Baseline Vital Signs

Student: What are the patient's baseline vital signs, including blood pressure, pulse, respirations, pulse oximetry, and level of consciousness?
PROCTOR: Blood pressure, 110/72 mm Hg; pulse rate, 140 beats/min; respirations, 24 breaths/min; pulse oximetry reading, 97%; and the patient is alert but becoming weak.

▼ Interventions

Student: I will apply oxygen, suction as needed, and contact medical control for a poison control consult.
PROCTOR: Noted.
ALS Student: I will apply basic life support (BLS) interventions, plus the following: I will establish two large-bore IVs en route to the hospital and administer a bolus of 20 mL/kg to maintain a systolic blood pressure of 90 mm Hg, perform cardiac monitoring, and local protocol.
ALS Proctor: Noted. The cardiac monitor shows sinus tachycardia.

▼ Reevaluate Transport Decision

Student: The patient is a high priority and is a load-and-go due to possible respiratory compromise and the effects of the acid.
PROCTOR: Noted.

▼ Detailed Physical Examination

Possible Answer #1
Student: I would not do a detailed physical exam.
PROCTOR: Noted. (Go to "Radio Report.")

Possible Answer #2
Student: I am conducting the detailed physical exam. I am looking for DCAP-BTLS. This acronym stands for deformities, contusions, abrasions, punctures, penetrations, paradoxical motion in the chest, and burns, tenderness, lacerations, and swelling.
PROCTOR: Noted. The detailed physical exam will be performed during transport.

▸ Assess the Head

Student: I am assessing the head. Do I find any DCAP-BTLS? Do I find any evidence of Battle's sign or raccoon eyes?
PROCTOR: No.

▸ Inspect and Palpate the Head and Ears

Student: I am assessing the head and ears.
PROCTOR: There are no obvious injuries.

▸ Assess the Eyes

Student: I am assessing the eyes. Are the pupils equal, round, and regular in size, and react properly to light (PEARRL)?
PROCTOR: They are PEARRL.

▸ Assess the Facial Area Including Oral and Nasal Areas

Student: I am assessing the face, nose, and mouth. Do I see any discharge or hear any obstructions?
PROCTOR: He occasionally projectile vomits.

▸ Assess the Neck

▸ Inspect and Palpate the Neck

Student: I am assessing the neck for DCAP-BTLS.
PROCTOR: There are no obvious injuries.

▸ Assess for Jugular Vein Distention

Student: Do I find any jugular vein distention (JVD)?
PROCTOR: No.

▸ Assess for Tracheal Deviation

Student: Do I see any tracheal deviation?
PROCTOR: No.

▸ Assess the Chest

Student: I am assessing the chest for DCAP-BTLS.
PROCTOR: Noted.

▸ Inspect

Student: What do I see when I look at the chest?
PROCTOR: There are no obvious injuries.
Student: Is the chest symmetric?
PROCTOR: Yes.

▸ Palpate

Student: When I touch the chest, do I feel crepitus or a flail segment?
PROCTOR: No.

▸ Auscultate

Student: Are lung sounds present in all fields?
PROCTOR: Yes.
Student: Do I hear any sucking sounds from the chest?
PROCTOR: No.

▸ Assess the Abdomen/Pelvis

▸ Assess the Abdomen

Student: I am assessing the abdomen for DCAP-BTLS. I am assessing all four quadrants. Do I find any problems?
PROCTOR: Yes. He has abdominal pain and is nauseated.

▸ Assess the Pelvis

Student: I am assessing the pelvis for DCAP-BTLS. Is the pelvis stable?
PROCTOR: Yes.

▸ Assess the Genitalia/Perineum as Needed (Verbalize in Training)

Student: I am assessing the genitalia/perineum as necessary for DCAP-BTLS.
PROCTOR: The area is unremarkable.

▸ Assess the Extremities

▸ Inspect

Student: I am assessing the lower and upper extremities for DCAP-BTLS. Do I find anything?

PROCTOR: No.

▸ Palpate

Student: Do I feel anything unusual?

PROCTOR: No.

▸ Assess Motor, Sensory, and Circulatory Function

Student: I am checking for DCAP-BTLS, motor and sensory function, and pulses. Right leg?

PROCTOR: Negative DCAP-BTLS. Motor and sensory functions are present. Pulses are present.

Student: Left leg?

PROCTOR: Negative DCAP-BTLS. Motor and sensory functions are present. Pulses are present.

Student: Right arm?

PROCTOR: Negative DCAP-BTLS. Motor and sensory functions are present. Pulses are present.

Student: Left arm?

PROCTOR: Negative DCAP-BTLS. Motor and sensory functions are present. Pulses are present.

▸ Assess the Posterior

Student: We will check the back.

PROCTOR: Noted.

▸ Assess the Thorax

Student: I am assessing the thorax. Do I find injuries?

PROCTOR: No.

▸ Assess the Lumbar Area

Student: I am assessing the flanks and lumbar area. Do I find injuries?

PROCTOR: No.

▸ Assess the Entire Backside

Student: I am assessing the entire backside. Do I find injuries?

PROCTOR: No.

▸ Reassess Interventions

Student: I will reassess my interventions: apply oxygen, suction as needed, and contact medical control for a poison control consult.

PROCTOR: Noted.

ALS Student: I will reassess BLS interventions, plus the following: IV access, cardiac monitor, and local protocol.

ALS Proctor: Noted. The cardiac monitor shows sinus tachycardia.

Critical Criteria:

- ❑ Did not obtain medical direction or verbalize standing orders for medical interventions
- ❑ Administered a dangerous or inappropriate intervention
- ❑ Did not ask questions about the present illness
- ❑ Did not differentiate patient's need for transportation versus continued assessment at the scene

Radio Report

(Provided by the student.)

PROCTOR: Noted.

Ongoing Assessment

Repeat the Initial Assessment

Student: I will repeat the initial assessment.

PROCTOR: Noted. (Reflected in "Repeat Vital Signs.")

Repeat Vital Signs

Student: I will reassess vital signs and mental status.

PROCTOR: Blood pressure, 100/60 mm Hg; pulse rate, 142 beats/min; respirations, 24 breaths/min; pulse oximetry reading, 94%; and the patient is becoming tired.

Student: The vital signs have deteriorated.

PROCTOR: Noted.

Check Interventions

Student: I will check my interventions: apply oxygen, suction as needed, and contact medical control.

PROCTOR: Noted.

ALS Student: I will check BLS interventions, plus the following: IV access, cardiac monitor, and local protocol.

ALS Proctor: Noted. The cardiac monitor shows sinus tachycardia.

Repeat the Focused Assessment

Student: I will repeat the focused assessment.

PROCTOR: Noted.

Critical Criteria:

- ❑ Did not obtain medical direction or verbalize standing orders for medical interventions
- ❑ Administered a dangerous or inappropriate intervention

Handoff Report to Emergency Department Staff

Student: The patient's condition deteriorated during transport.

PROCTOR: Noted.

Critical Criteria

(Inform the student of items missed, if any.)

❑ Pass ❑ Fail Date: ______________________

Proctor Comments: ______________________

____

____

Notes

CASE 133

Dispatch Information

PROCTOR: EMS 10, respond to an 87-year-old male who is complaining of tar-like stool. He is conscious and breathing.

Pre-scene Action (BSI)

Student: I am wearing nonlatex gloves and safety glasses.
PROCTOR: Noted.

Critical Criteria:
- ❑ Did not take, or verbalize, body substance isolation (BSI) precautions when necessary

Scene Size-up

Scene Safety

Student: Is the scene safe?
PROCTOR: Yes.

Mechanism of Injury/Nature of Illness

Student: What is the nature of the illness?
PROCTOR: The patient has not been feeling well for two days. Today he passed stool that has a tar-like appearance.

Number of Patients

Student: How many patients are there?
PROCTOR: One.

Additional Resources

Student: I would call for advanced life support (ALS) assistance.
PROCTOR: Noted.

C-Spine Stabilization

Student: I would not stabilize the cervical spine (c-spine).
PROCTOR: Noted.

Critical Criteria:
- ❑ Did not determine scene safety

Initial Assessment

General Impression

Student: My general impression is that the patient's condition is unstable.
PROCTOR: Noted.

Responsiveness/Level of Consciousness

Student: What is the patient's level of consciousness?
PROCTOR: Alert.

Chief Complaint/Apparent Life Threats

Student: What is the patient's chief complaint?
PROCTOR: The patient is complaining of tar-like stool.

Assess the Airway and Breathing

Student: Is the airway open? Is the patient breathing?
PROCTOR: Yes, the airway is open and the patient is breathing.

Assessment

Student: What are the rate and the quality of breathing?
PROCTOR: Rate: Tachypneic. Quality: Deep.

Provide Oxygen

Student: I am applying oxygen at 15 L/min via nonrebreathing mask.
PROCTOR: Noted.

Ensure Adequate Ventilation

Student: The patient has adequate ventilations at this time.
PROCTOR: Noted.

Assess Circulation

Student: I am assessing the patient's circulation.
PROCTOR: Noted.

Assess for and Control Major Bleeding

Student: Do I find any major bleeding?
PROCTOR: No.

Assess the Pulse

Student: What are the rate and the quality of pulses?
PROCTOR: Rate: Tachycardic. Quality: Bounding.

Assess the Skin

Student: I am assessing the skin. What are the color, temperature, and condition of the skin?
PROCTOR: Color: Flushed. Temperature: Warm. Condition: Dry.

Identify Priority Patients/Make Transport Decision

Student: The patient is a high priority and is a load-and-go. I will begin packaging and transport.
PROCTOR: Noted.

Critical Criteria:
- ❑ Did not provide high concentration of oxygen
- ❑ Did not find or manage problems associated with airway, breathing, hemorrhage or shock (hypoperfusion)
- ❑ Did not differentiate patient's need for transportation versus continued assessment at the scene
- ❑ Did detailed or focused history/physical examination before assessing the airway, breathing and circulation

Focused History and Physical Examination/Rapid Assessment

Select the Appropriate Assessment (Focused or Rapid)

Student: I am selecting the focused assessment.
PROCTOR: Noted.

SAMPLE History

Student: At this time I will gather a SAMPLE history from the patient or family. What are the patient's signs and symptoms?
PROCTOR: Gastrointestinal (GI) bleeding.

> **Student:** Onset: What were you doing when this started?
> **PROCTOR:** He has been sick for a few days.
> **Student:** Provokes: What makes your condition worse or better?
> **PROCTOR:** He does not know.
> **Student:** Quality: Can you describe your pain?
> **PROCTOR:** None.
> **Student:** Radiates: Do you have pain anywhere else?
> **PROCTOR:** No.
> **Student:** Severity: On a scale of 1 to 10 with 10 being the worst possible, how would you rate your distress?
> **PROCTOR:** 2.
> **Student:** Time: How long has this been going on?
> **PROCTOR:** 45 minutes.
> **Student:** Interventions: Have you done anything to make this better?
> **PROCTOR:** The patient has taken no actions.

Student: Allergies?
PROCTOR: Penicillin (PCN).
Student: Medications?
PROCTOR: No medications.
Student: Pertinent past medical history?
PROCTOR: No pertinent medical history.
Student: Last oral intake?
PROCTOR: 5 hours ago.
Student: Events leading up to the incident?
PROCTOR: The patient has not been feeling well for a few days.

Perform the Focused Physical Examination

Student: I am performing the focused physical examination.
PROCTOR: Noted.

Student: I am assessing the abdomen for DCAP-BTLS. This acronym stands for deformities, contusions, abrasions, punctures, penetrations, paradoxical motion in the chest, and burns, tenderness, lacerations, and swelling. I am assessing all four quadrants. Do I find any problems?

PROCTOR: Yes. He has abdominal pain in the area of the stomach and the lower left quadrant.

▼ Baseline Vital Signs

Student: What are the patient's baseline vital signs, including blood pressure, pulse, respirations, pulse oximetry, blood glucose level, and level of consciousness?

PROCTOR: Blood pressure, 148/90 mm Hg; pulse rate, 110 beats/min; respirations, 20 breaths/min; pulse oximetry reading, 97%; blood glucose level, 92 mg/dL; and the patient is alert.

▼ Interventions

Student: I will apply oxygen and transport the patient in the position of comfort.

PROCTOR: Noted.

ALS Student: I will apply basic life support (BLS) interventions, plus the following: IV access, cardiac monitor, 12-lead ECG, and local protocol.

ALS Proctor: Noted. The cardiac monitor shows sinus tachycardia.

▼ Reevaluate Transport Decision

Student: The patient is a high priority and is a load-and-go patient due to the GI bleeding.

PROCTOR: Noted.

▼ Detailed Physical Examination

Possible Answer #1

Student: I would not do a detailed physical exam.

PROCTOR: Noted. (Go to "Radio Report.")

Possible Answer #2

Student: I am conducting the detailed physical exam. I am looking for DCAP-BTLS.

PROCTOR: Noted. The detailed physical exam will be performed during transport.

- **Assess the Head**

Student: I am assessing the head. Do I find any DCAP-BTLS? Do I find any evidence of Battle's sign or raccoon eyes?

PROCTOR: No.

- **Inspect and Palpate the Head and Ears**

Student: I am assessing the head and ears.

PROCTOR: There are no obvious injuries.

- **Assess the Eyes**

Student: I am assessing the eyes. Are the pupils equal, round, and regular in size, and react properly to light (PEARRL)?

PROCTOR: They are PEARRL.

- **Assess the Facial Area Including Oral and Nasal Areas**

Student: I am assessing the face, nose, and mouth. Do I see any discharge or hear any obstructions?

PROCTOR: No.

- **Assess the Neck**

- **Inspect and Palpate the Neck**

Student: I am assessing the neck for DCAP-BTLS.

PROCTOR: There are no obvious injuries.

- **Assess for Jugular Vein Distention**

Student: Do I find any jugular vein distention (JVD)?

PROCTOR: No.

- **Assess for Tracheal Deviation**

Student: Do I see any tracheal deviation?

PROCTOR: No.

- **Assess the Chest**

Student: I am assessing the chest for DCAP-BTLS.

PROCTOR: Noted.

- **Inspect**

Student: What do I see when I look at the chest?

PROCTOR: There are no obvious injuries.

Student: Is the chest symmetric?

PROCTOR: Yes.

- **Palpate**

Student: When I touch the chest, do I feel crepitus or a flail segment?

PROCTOR: No.

- **Auscultate**

Student: Are lung sounds present in all fields?

PROCTOR: Yes.

Student: Do I hear any sucking sounds from the chest?

PROCTOR: No.

- **Assess the Abdomen/Pelvis**

- **Assess the Abdomen**

Student: I am assessing the abdomen for DCAP-BTLS. I am assessing all four quadrants. Do I find any problems?

PROCTOR: Yes. He has abdominal pain in the area of the stomach and the lower left quadrant.

- **Assess the Pelvis**

Student: I am assessing the pelvis for DCAP-BTLS. Is the pelvis stable?

PROCTOR: Yes.

- **Assess the Genitalia/Perineum as Needed (Verbalize in Training)**

Student: I am assessing the genitalia/perineum as necessary for DCAP-BTLS.

PROCTOR: The area is unremarkable.

- **Assess the Extremities**

- **Inspect**

Student: I am assessing the lower and upper extremities for DCAP-BTLS. Do I find anything?

PROCTOR: No.

- **Palpate**

Student: Do I feel anything unusual?

PROCTOR: No.

- **Assess Motor, Sensory, and Circulatory Function**

Student: I am checking for DCAP-BTLS, motor and sensory function, and pulses. Right leg?

PROCTOR: Negative DCAP-BTLS. Motor and sensory functions are present. Pulses are present.

Student: Left leg?

PROCTOR: Negative DCAP-BTLS. Motor and sensory functions are present. Pulses are present.

Student: Right arm?

PROCTOR: Negative DCAP-BTLS. Motor and sensory functions are present. Pulses are present.

Student: Left arm?

PROCTOR: Negative DCAP-BTLS. Motor and sensory functions are present. Pulses are present.

- **Assess the Posterior**

Student: We will check the back.

PROCTOR: Noted.

- **Assess the Thorax**

Student: I am assessing the thorax. Do I find injuries?

PROCTOR: No.

- **Assess the Lumbar Area**

Student: I am assessing the flanks and lumbar area. Do I find injuries?

PROCTOR: No.

- **Assess the Entire Backside**

Student: I am assessing the entire backside. Do I find injuries?

PROCTOR: No.

▸ Reassess Interventions

Student: I will reassess my interventions: oxygen and transport the patient in the position of comfort.

PROCTOR: Noted.

ALS Student: I will reassess BLS interventions, plus the following: IV access, cardiac monitor, 12-lead ECG, and local protocol.

ALS Proctor: Noted. The cardiac monitor shows sinus tachycardia.

Critical Criteria:
- ❑ Did not obtain medical direction or verbalize standing orders for medical interventions
- ❑ Administered a dangerous or inappropriate intervention
- ❑ Did not ask questions about the present illness
- ❑ Did not differentiate patient's need for transportation versus continued assessment at the scene

Radio Report

(Provided by the student.)

PROCTOR: Noted.

Ongoing Assessment

Repeat the Initial Assessment

Student: I will repeat the initial assessment.

PROCTOR: Noted. (Reflected in "Repeat Vital Signs.")

Repeat Vital Signs

Student: I will reassess vital signs and mental status.

PROCTOR: Blood pressure, 144/86 mm Hg; pulse rate, 102 beats/min; respirations, 20 breaths/min; pulse oximetry reading, 98%; and the patient is alert.

Student: The vital signs have not changed significantly.

PROCTOR: Noted.

Check Interventions

Student: I will check my interventions: oxygen and transport the patient in the position of comfort.

PROCTOR: Noted.

ALS Student: I will check BLS interventions, plus the following: IV access, cardiac monitor, 12-lead ECG, and local protocol.

ALS Proctor: Noted. The cardiac monitor shows sinus tachycardia.

Repeat the Focused Assessment

Student: I will repeat the focused assessment.

PROCTOR: Noted.

Critical Criteria:
- ❑ Did not obtain medical direction or verbalize standing orders for medical interventions
- ❑ Administered a dangerous or inappropriate intervention

Handoff Report to Emergency Department Staff

Student: There was no change in the patient's condition during transport.

PROCTOR: Noted.

Critical Criteria

(Inform the student of items missed, if any.)

❑ Pass ❑ Fail Date: ______________________________

Proctor Comments: ______________________________

____

____

CASE 133

Notes

CASE 134

Dispatch Information

PROCTOR: EMS 10, respond to a 17-year-old male who is complaining of difficulty breathing. He is conscious and breathing.

Pre-scene Action (BSI)

Student: I am wearing nonlatex gloves and safety glasses.
PROCTOR: Noted.

Critical Criteria:
- ❑ Did not take, or verbalize, body substance isolation (BSI) precautions when necessary

Scene Size-up

Scene Safety

Student: Is the scene safe?
PROCTOR: Yes.

Mechanism of Injury/Nature of Illness

Student: What is the nature of the illness?
PROCTOR: The patient was playing basketball when he felt a sudden onset of right-sided chest pain.

Number of Patients

Student: How many patients are there?
PROCTOR: One.

Additional Resources

Student: I would call for advanced life support (ALS) assistance.
PROCTOR: Noted.

C-Spine Stabilization

Student: I would not stabilize the cervical spine (c-spine).
PROCTOR: Noted.

Critical Criteria:
- ❑ Did not determine scene safety

Initial Assessment

General Impression

Student: My general impression is that the patient's condition is stable.
PROCTOR: Noted.

Responsiveness/Level of Consciousness

Student: What is the patient's level of consciousness?
PROCTOR: Alert.

Chief Complaint/Apparent Life Threats

Student: What is the patient's chief complaint?
PROCTOR: The patient is complaining of pain when he takes a deep breath.

Assess the Airway and Breathing

Student: Is the airway open? Is the patient breathing?
PROCTOR: Yes, the airway is open and the patient is breathing.

▸ Assessment

Student: What are the rate and the quality of breathing?
PROCTOR: Rate: Tachypneic. Quality: Shallow.

▸ Provide Oxygen

Student: I am applying oxygen at 15 L/min via nonrebreathing mask.
PROCTOR: Noted.

▸ Ensure Adequate Ventilation

Student: The patient has adequate ventilations at this time.
PROCTOR: Noted.

Assess Circulation

Student: I am assessing the patient's circulation.
PROCTOR: Noted.

▸ Assess for and Control Major Bleeding

Student: Do I find any major bleeding?
PROCTOR: No.

▸ Assess the Pulse

Student: What are the rate and the quality of pulses?
PROCTOR: Rate: Tachycardic. Quality: Strong.

▸ Assess the Skin

Student: I am assessing the skin. What are the color, temperature, and condition of the skin?
PROCTOR: Color: Flushed. Temperature: Warm. Condition: Moist.

Identify Priority Patients/Make Transport Decision

Student: The patient is a high priority and is a load-and-go. I will begin packaging and transport.
PROCTOR: Noted.

Critical Criteria:
- ❑ Did not provide high concentration of oxygen
- ❑ Did not find or manage problems associated with airway, breathing, hemorrhage or shock (hypoperfusion)
- ❑ Did not differentiate patient's need for transportation versus continued assessment at the scene
- ❑ Did detailed or focused history/physical examination before assessing the airway, breathing and circulation

Focused History and Physical Examination/Rapid Assessment

Select the Appropriate Assessment (Focused or Rapid)

Student: I am selecting the focused assessment.
PROCTOR: Noted.

SAMPLE History

Student: At this time I will gather a SAMPLE history from the patient or family. What are the patient's signs and symptoms?
PROCTOR: Respiratory.

> **Student:** Onset: What were you doing when this started?
> **PROCTOR:** Playing basketball.
> **Student:** Provokes: What makes your condition worse or better?
> **PROCTOR:** Sitting upright makes it better.
> **Student:** Quality: Can you describe your pain?
> **PROCTOR:** Stabbing.
> **Student:** Radiates: Do you have pain anywhere else?
> **PROCTOR:** No.
> **Student:** Severity: On a scale of 1 to 10 with 10 being the worst possible, how would you rate your pain?
> **PROCTOR:** 7.
> **Student:** Time: How long has this been going on?
> **PROCTOR:** 15 minutes.
> **Student:** Interventions: Have you done anything to make this better?
> **PROCTOR:** The patient has taken no actions.

Student: Allergies?
PROCTOR: No allergies.
Student: Medications?
PROCTOR: No medications.
Student: Pertinent past medical history?
PROCTOR: No pertinent medical history.
Student: Last oral intake?
PROCTOR: 3 hours ago.
Student: Events leading up to the incident?
PROCTOR: The patient was playing basketball when the problem started. He jumped up to rebound a ball and the pain came on all of a sudden.

Perform the Focused Physical Examination

Student: I am performing the focused physical examination.
PROCTOR: Noted.

Student: How tall is the patient?
PROCTOR: He is 6′ 5″ tall.
Student: How much does he weigh?
PROCTOR: He weighs 175 lb (79 kg).
Student: I am rapidly assessing the chest.
PROCTOR: There are no obvious injuries.
Student: I will assess the chest for tension pneumothorax by auscultation, and assessment (jugular vein distention [JVD], tracheal deviation, and decreased lung sounds).
PROCTOR: There are diminished lung sounds on the right side, jugular vein distension is not present, and the trachea is midline.
Student: Do I hear any sucking sounds from the chest?
PROCTOR: No.
ALS Student: I will assess the chest for hyperresonance to percussion.
ALS Proctor: Noted. There is no tension noted.
ALS Student: I will monitor the chest.
ALS Proctor: Noted.

▼ Baseline Vital Signs

Student: What are the patient's baseline vital signs, including blood pressure, pulse, respirations, pulse oximetry, and level of consciousness?
PROCTOR: Blood pressure, 136/82 mm Hg; pulse rate, 130 beats/min; respirations, 24 breaths/min; pulse oximetry reading, 99%; and the patient is alert.

▼ Interventions

Student: I will continue oxygen and transport in the position of comfort.
PROCTOR: Noted.
ALS Student: I will apply basic life support (BLS) interventions, plus the following: IV access, cardiac monitor, and 12-lead ECG.
ALS Proctor: Noted. The cardiac monitor shows sinus tachycardia.

▼ Reevaluate Transport Decision

Student: The patient is a high priority and is a load-and-go.
PROCTOR: Noted.

▼ Detailed Physical Examination

Possible Answer #1
Student: I would not do a detailed physical exam.
PROCTOR: Noted. (Go to "Radio Report.")

Possible Answer #2
Student: I am conducting the detailed physical exam. I am looking for DCAP-BTLS. This acronym stands for deformities, contusions, abrasions, punctures, penetrations, paradoxical motion in the chest, and burns, tenderness, lacerations, and swelling.
PROCTOR: Noted. The detailed physical exam will be performed during transport.

▶ Assess the Head

Student: I am assessing the head. Do I find any DCAP-BTLS? Do I find any evidence of Battle's sign or raccoon eyes?
PROCTOR: No.

▶ Inspect and Palpate the Head and Ears

Student: I am assessing the head and ears.
PROCTOR: There are no obvious injuries.

▶ Assess the Eyes

Student: I am assessing the eyes. Are the pupils equal, round, and regular in size, and react properly to light (PEARRL)?
PROCTOR: They are PEARRL.

▶ Assess the Facial Area Including Oral and Nasal Areas

Student: I am assessing the face, nose, and mouth. Do I see any discharge or hear any obstructions?
PROCTOR: No.

▶ Assess the Neck

▶ Inspect and Palpate the Neck

Student: I am assessing the neck for DCAP-BTLS.
PROCTOR: There are no obvious injuries.

▶ Assess for Jugular Vein Distention

Student: Do I find any jugular vein distention (JVD)?
PROCTOR: No.

▶ Assess for Tracheal Deviation

Student: Do I see any tracheal deviation?
PROCTOR: No.

▶ Assess the Chest

Student: I am assessing the chest for DCAP-BTLS.
PROCTOR: Noted.

▶ Inspect

Student: What do I see when I look at the chest?
PROCTOR: There are no obvious injuries.
Student: Is the chest symmetric?
PROCTOR: Yes.

▶ Palpate

Student: When I touch the chest, do I feel crepitus or a flail segment?
PROCTOR: No.

▶ Auscultate

Student: Are lung sounds present in all fields?
PROCTOR: The lung sounds appear diminished on the right side.
Student: Do I hear any sucking sounds from the chest?
PROCTOR: No.

▶ Assess the Abdomen/Pelvis

▶ Assess the Abdomen

Student: I am assessing the abdomen for DCAP-BTLS. I am assessing all four quadrants. Do I find any problems?
PROCTOR: No.

▶ Assess the Pelvis

Student: I am assessing the pelvis for DCAP-BTLS. Is the pelvis stable?
PROCTOR: Yes.

▶ Assess the Genitalia/Perineum as Needed (Verbalize in Training)

Student: I am assessing the genitalia/perineum as necessary for DCAP-BTLS.
PROCTOR: The area is unremarkable.

▶ Assess the Extremities

▶ Inspect

Student: I am assessing the lower and upper extremities for DCAP-BTLS. Do I find anything?
PROCTOR: No.

▶ Palpate

Student: Do I feel anything unusual?
PROCTOR: No.

▶ Assess Motor, Sensory, and Circulatory Function

Student: I am checking for DCAP-BTLS, motor and sensory function, and pulses. Right leg?
PROCTOR: Negative DCAP-BTLS. Motor and sensory functions are present. Pulses are present.
Student: Left leg?
PROCTOR: Negative DCAP-BTLS. Motor and sensory functions are present. Pulses are present.
Student: Right arm?
PROCTOR: Negative DCAP-BTLS. Motor and sensory functions are present. Pulses are present.
Student: Left arm?
PROCTOR: Negative DCAP-BTLS. Motor and sensory functions are present. Pulses are present.

▶ Assess the Posterior

Student: We will check the back.
PROCTOR: Noted.

▸ **Assess the Thorax**

Student: I am assessing the thorax. Do I find injuries?

PROCTOR: No.

▸ **Assess the Lumbar Area**

Student: I am assessing the flanks and lumbar area. Do I find injuries?

PROCTOR: No.

▸ **Assess the Entire Backside**

Student: I am assessing the entire backside. Do I find injuries?

PROCTOR: No.

▸ **Manage Secondary Injuries/Wounds**

Student: I would direct my partner to monitor for signs of tension in the chest.

PROCTOR: Noted.

▸ **Reassess Interventions**

Student: I will reassess my interventions: oxygen and position of comfort.

PROCTOR: Noted.

ALS Student: I will reassess BLS interventions, plus the following: IV access, cardiac monitor, 12-lead ECG, and continuously assess for tension pneumothorax.

ALS Proctor: Noted. The cardiac monitor shows sinus tachycardia. Tracheal deviation is not present. There is no JVD. Chest percussion is normal.

Critical Criteria:

- ❑ Did not obtain medical direction or verbalize standing orders for medical interventions
- ❑ Administered a dangerous or inappropriate intervention
- ❑ Did not ask questions about the present illness
- ❑ Did not differentiate patient's need for transportation versus continued assessment at the scene

Radio Report

(Provided by the student.)

PROCTOR: Noted.

Ongoing Assessment

Repeat the Initial Assessment

Student: I will repeat the initial assessment.

PROCTOR: Noted. (Reflected in "Repeat Vital Signs.")

Repeat Vital Signs

Student: I will reassess vital signs and mental status.

PROCTOR: Blood pressure, 128/78 mm Hg; pulse rate, 124 beats/min; respirations, 24 breaths/min; pulse oximetry reading, 99%; and the patient is alert.

Student: The vital signs have not changed significantly.

PROCTOR: Noted.

Check Interventions

Student: I will check my interventions: oxygen.

PROCTOR: Noted.

ALS Student: I will reassess BLS interventions, plus the following: IV access, cardiac monitor, 12-lead ECG, and continuously assess for tension pneumothorax.

ALS Proctor: Noted. The cardiac monitor shows sinus tachycardia. Tracheal deviation is not present. There is no JVD. Chest percussion is normal.

Repeat the Focused Assessment

Student: I will repeat the focused assessment.

PROCTOR: Noted.

Critical Criteria:

- ❑ Did not obtain medical direction or verbalize standing orders for medical interventions
- ❑ Administered a dangerous or inappropriate intervention

Handoff Report to Emergency Department Staff

Student: There was no change in the patient's condition during transport.

PROCTOR: Noted.

Critical Criteria

(Inform the student of items missed, if any.)

❑ Pass ❑ Fail Date: ______________________

Proctor Comments: ______________________

____

____

Notes

CASE 135

Dispatch Information

PROCTOR: EMS 10, respond to a 45-year-old female who is complaining of lower right abdominal pain. She is conscious and breathing.

Pre-scene Action (BSI)

Student: I am wearing nonlatex gloves and safety glasses.
PROCTOR: Noted.

Critical Criteria:
- ❑ Did not take, or verbalize, body substance isolation (BSI) precautions when necessary

Scene Size-up

Scene Safety

Student: Is the scene safe?
PROCTOR: Yes.

Mechanism of Injury/Nature of Illness

Student: What is the nature of the illness?
PROCTOR: The patient has lower right abdominal pain.

Number of Patients

Student: How many patients are there?
PROCTOR: One.

Additional Resources

Student: I would call for advanced life support (ALS) assistance.
PROCTOR: Noted.

C-Spine Stabilization

Student: I would not stabilize the cervical spine (c-spine).
PROCTOR: Noted.

Critical Criteria:
- ❑ Did not determine scene safety

Initial Assessment

General Impression

Student: My general impression is that the patient's condition is unstable.
PROCTOR: Noted.

Responsiveness/Level of Consciousness

Student: What is the patient's level of consciousness?
PROCTOR: Alert.

Chief Complaint/Apparent Life Threats

Student: What is the patient's chief complaint?
PROCTOR: The patient is complaining of lower right abdominal pain.

Assess the Airway and Breathing

Student: Is the airway open? Is the patient breathing?
PROCTOR: Yes, the airway is open and the patient is breathing.

Assessment

Student: What are the rate and the quality of breathing?
PROCTOR: Rate: Tachypneic. Quality: Shallow.

Provide Oxygen

Student: I am applying oxygen at 15 L/min via nonrebreathing mask.
PROCTOR: Noted.

Ensure Adequate Ventilation

Student: The patient has adequate ventilations at this time.
PROCTOR: Noted.

Assess Circulation

Student: I am assessing the patient's circulation.
PROCTOR: Noted.

Assess for and Control Major Bleeding

Student: Do I find any major bleeding?
PROCTOR: No.

Assess the Pulse

Student: What are the rate and the quality of pulses?
PROCTOR: Rate: Tachycardic. Quality: Thready.

Assess the Skin

Student: I am assessing the skin. What are the color, temperature, and condition of the skin?
PROCTOR: Color: Pale. Temperature: Cool. Condition: Diaphoretic.

Identify Priority Patients/Make Transport Decision

Student: The patient is a high priority and is a load-and-go. I will begin packaging and transport.
PROCTOR: Noted.

Critical Criteria:
- ❑ Did not provide high concentration of oxygen
- ❑ Did not find or manage problems associated with airway, breathing, hemorrhage or shock (hypoperfusion)
- ❑ Did not differentiate patient's need for transportation versus continued assessment at the scene
- ❑ Did detailed or focused history/physical examination before assessing the airway, breathing and circulation

Focused History and Physical Examination/Rapid Assessment

Select the Appropriate Assessment (Focused or Rapid)

Student: I am selecting the focused assessment.
PROCTOR: Noted.

SAMPLE History

Student: At this time I will gather a SAMPLE history from the patient or family. What are the patient's signs and symptoms?
PROCTOR: Abdominal pain.
Student: Onset: What were you doing when this started?
PROCTOR: Cleaning the house.
Student: Provokes: What makes your condition worse or better?
PROCTOR: Nothing.
Student: Quality: Can you describe your pain?
PROCTOR: Stabbing.
Student: Radiates: Do you have pain anywhere else?
PROCTOR: In the belly button.
Student: Severity: On a scale of 1 to 10 with 10 being the worst possible, how would you rate your pain?
PROCTOR: 10.
Student: Time: How long has this been going on?
PROCTOR: 2 hours.
Student: Interventions: Have you done anything to make this better?
PROCTOR: The patient has taken no actions.
Student: Allergies?
PROCTOR: No allergies.
Student: Medications?
PROCTOR: No medications.
Student: Pertinent past medical history?
PROCTOR: No pertinent medical history.
Student: Last oral intake?
PROCTOR: 4 hours ago.
Student: Events leading up to the incident?
PROCTOR: The patient was cleaning her house when the pain began.

Perform the Focused Physical Examination

Student: I am performing the focused physical examination.
PROCTOR: Noted.
Student: Is there any chance that you may be pregnant?
PROCTOR: No.

Student: When was your last menstrual period?
PROCTOR: 2 weeks ago.
Student: Was it unusual?
PROCTOR: No.
Student: I am assessing the abdomen for DCAP-BTLS. This acronym stands for deformities, contusions, abrasions, punctures, penetrations, paradoxical motion in the chest, and burns, tenderness, lacerations, and swelling. I am assessing all four quadrants. Do I find any problems?
PROCTOR: She has pain in the lower right quadrant upon palpation and in the area of the belly button as well.
Student: Does she have any pulsating masses noted?
PROCTOR: No.

▼ Baseline Vital Signs

Student: What are the patient's baseline vital signs, including blood pressure, pulse, respirations, pulse oximetry, and level of consciousness?
PROCTOR: Blood pressure, 118/68 mm Hg; pulse rate, 124 beats/min; respirations, 16 breaths/min; pulse oximetry reading, 98%; and the patient is alert.

▼ Interventions

Student: I will apply oxygen, treat for shock, and transport the patient.
PROCTOR: Noted.
ALS Student: I will apply basic life support (BLS) interventions, plus the following: IV access and local protocol.
ALS Proctor: Noted.

▼ Reevaluate Transport Decision

Student: The patient is a high priority and is a load-and-go patient due to the nature of the illness.
PROCTOR: Noted.

▼ Detailed Physical Examination

Possible Answer #1
Student: I would not do a detailed physical exam.
PROCTOR: Noted. (Go to "Radio Report.")

Possible Answer #2
Student: I am conducting the detailed physical exam. I am looking for DCAP-BTLS.
PROCTOR: Noted. The detailed physical exam will be performed during transport.

► **Assess the Head**

Student: I am assessing the head. Do I find any DCAP-BTLS? Do I find any evidence of Battle's sign or raccoon eyes?
PROCTOR: No.

► **Inspect and Palpate the Head and Ears**

Student: I am assessing the head and ears.
PROCTOR: There are no obvious injuries.

► **Assess the Eyes**

Student: I am assessing the eyes. Are the pupils equal, round, and regular in size, and react properly to light (PEARRL)?
PROCTOR: They are PEARRL.

► **Assess the Facial Area Including Oral and Nasal Areas**

Student: I am assessing the face, nose, and mouth. Do I see any discharge or hear any obstructions?
PROCTOR: No.

► **Assess the Neck**

► **Inspect and Palpate the Neck**

Student: I am assessing the neck for DCAP-BTLS.
PROCTOR: There are no obvious injuries.

► **Assess for Jugular Vein Distention**

Student: Do I find any jugular vein distention (JVD)?
PROCTOR: No.

► **Assess for Tracheal Deviation**

Student: Do I see any tracheal deviation?
PROCTOR: No.

► **Assess the Chest**

Student: I am assessing the chest for DCAP-BTLS.
PROCTOR: Noted.

► **Inspect**

Student: What do I see when I look at the chest?
PROCTOR: There are no obvious injuries.
Student: Is the chest symmetric?
PROCTOR: Yes.

► **Palpate**

Student: When I touch the chest, do I feel crepitus or a flail segment?
PROCTOR: No.

► **Auscultate**

Student: Are lung sounds present in all fields?
PROCTOR: Yes.
Student: Do I hear any sucking sounds from the chest?
PROCTOR: No.

► **Assess the Abdomen/Pelvis**

► **Assess the Abdomen**

Student: I am assessing the abdomen for DCAP-BTLS. I am assessing all four quadrants. Do I find any problems?
PROCTOR: She has pain in the lower right quadrant upon palpation and in the area of the belly button as well.

► **Assess the Pelvis**

Student: I am assessing the pelvis for DCAP-BTLS. Is the pelvis stable?
PROCTOR: Yes.

► **Assess the Genitalia/Perineum as Needed (Verbalize in Training)**

Student: I am assessing the genitalia/perineum as necessary for DCAP-BTLS.
PROCTOR: The area is unremarkable.

► **Assess the Extremities**

► **Inspect**

Student: I am assessing the lower and upper extremities for DCAP-BTLS. Do I find anything?
PROCTOR: No.

► **Palpate**

Student: Do I feel anything unusual?
PROCTOR: No.

► **Assess Motor, Sensory, and Circulatory Function**

Student: I am checking for DCAP-BTLS, motor and sensory function, and pulses. Right leg?
PROCTOR: Negative DCAP-BTLS. Motor and sensory functions are present. Pulses are present.
Student: Left leg?
PROCTOR: Negative DCAP-BTLS. Motor and sensory functions are present. Pulses are present.
Student: Right arm?
PROCTOR: Negative DCAP-BTLS. Motor and sensory functions are present. Pulses are present.
Student: Left arm?
PROCTOR: Negative DCAP-BTLS. Motor and sensory functions are present. Pulses are present.

► **Assess the Posterior**

Student: We will check the back.
PROCTOR: Noted.

► **Assess the Thorax**

Student: I am assessing the thorax. Do I find injuries?
PROCTOR: No.

▸ **Assess the Lumbar Area**

Student: I am assessing the flanks and lumbar area. Do I find injuries?

PROCTOR: No.

▸ **Assess the Entire Backside**

Student: I am assessing the entire backside. Do I find injuries?

PROCTOR: No.

▸ **Reassess Interventions**

Student: I will reassess my interventions: oxygen, treat for shock, and transport.

PROCTOR: Noted.

ALS Student: I will reassess BLS interventions, plus the following: IV access, cardiac monitor, 12-lead ECG, and local protocol.

ALS Proctor: Noted. The monitor shows sinus tachycardia.

Critical Criteria:

- ❑ Did not obtain medical direction or verbalize standing orders for medical interventions
- ❑ Administered a dangerous or inappropriate intervention
- ❑ Did not ask questions about the present illness
- ❑ Did not differentiate patient's need for transportation versus continued assessment at the scene

Radio Report

(Provided by the student.)

PROCTOR: Noted.

Ongoing Assessment

Repeat the Initial Assessment

Student: I will repeat the initial assessment.

PROCTOR: Noted. (Reflected in "Repeat Vital Signs.")

Repeat Vital Signs

Student: I will reassess vital signs and mental status.

PROCTOR: Blood pressure, 116/64 mm Hg; pulse rate, 122 beats/min; respirations, 16 breaths/min; pulse oximetry reading, 98%; and the patient is alert.

Student: The vital signs have not changed significantly.

PROCTOR: Noted.

Check Interventions

Student: I will reassess my interventions: oxygen, treat for shock, and transport.

PROCTOR: Noted.

ALS Student: I will reassess BLS interventions, plus the following: IV access, cardiac monitor, 12-lead ECG, and local protocol.

ALS Proctor: Noted. The monitor shows sinus tachycardia.

Repeat the Focused Assessment

Student: I will repeat the focused assessment.

PROCTOR: Noted.

Critical Criteria:

- ❑ Did not obtain medical direction or verbalize standing orders for medical interventions
- ❑ Administered a dangerous or inappropriate intervention

Handoff Report to Emergency Department Staff

Student: There was no change in the patient's condition during transport.

PROCTOR: Noted.

Critical Criteria

(Inform the student of items missed, if any.)

❑ Pass ❑ Fail Date: ______________________

Proctor Comments: ______________________

____

____

Notes

CASE 136

Dispatch Information

PROCTOR: EMS 10, respond to a possible mushroom poisoning. Two people have eaten home-picked mushrooms and are very sick. The patients are conscious and breathing.

Pre-scene Action (BSI)

Student: I am wearing nonlatex gloves and safety glasses.
PROCTOR: Noted.

Critical Criteria:
- ❑ Did not take, or verbalize, body substance isolation (BSI) precautions when necessary

Scene Size-up

Scene Safety

Student: Is the scene safe?
PROCTOR: Yes.

Mechanism of Injury/Nature of Illness

Student: What is the nature of the illness?
PROCTOR: The patients ate mushrooms that they picked themselves. Both are violently sick and vomiting.

Number of Patients

Student: How many patients are there?
PROCTOR: Two, but you will treat the 69-year-old male patient.

Additional Resources

Student: I would call for advanced life support (ALS) assistance.
PROCTOR: Noted.

C-Spine Stabilization

Student: I would not stabilize the cervical spine (c-spine).
PROCTOR: Noted.

Critical Criteria:
- ❑ Did not determine scene safety

Initial Assessment

General Impression

Student: My general impression is that the patient's condition is unstable.
PROCTOR: Noted.

Responsiveness/Level of Consciousness

Student: What is the patient's level of consciousness?
PROCTOR: Alert.

Chief Complaint/Apparent Life Threats

Student: What is the patient's chief complaint?
PROCTOR: The patient is vomiting and having difficulty breathing.

Assess the Airway and Breathing

Student: Is the airway open? Is the patient breathing?
PROCTOR: Yes. The airway is open and the patient is breathing.

Assessment

Student: What are the rate and the quality of breathing?
PROCTOR: Rate: Tachypneic. Quality: Shallow.

Provide Oxygen

Student: I am applying oxygen at 15 L/min via nonrebreathing mask.
PROCTOR: Noted.

Ensure Adequate Ventilation

Student: The patient has adequate ventilations at this time.
PROCTOR: Noted.

Assess Circulation

Student: I am assessing the patient's circulation.
PROCTOR: Noted.

Assess for and Control Major Bleeding

Student: Do I find any major bleeding?
PROCTOR: No.

Assess the Pulse

Student: What are the rate and the quality of pulses?
PROCTOR: Rate: Tachycardic. Quality: Bounding.

Assess the Skin

Student: I am assessing the skin. What are the color, temperature, and condition of the skin?
PROCTOR: Color: Pale. Temperature: Cool. Condition: Moist.

Identify Priority Patients/Make Transport Decision

Student: The patient is a high priority and is a load-and-go. I will begin packaging and transport.
PROCTOR: Noted.

Critical Criteria:
- ❑ Did not provide high concentration of oxygen
- ❑ Did not find or manage problems associated with airway, breathing, hemorrhage or shock (hypoperfusion)
- ❑ Did not differentiate patient's need for transportation versus continued assessment at the scene
- ❑ Did detailed or focused history/physical examination before assessing the airway, breathing and circulation

Focused History and Physical Examination/Rapid Assessment

Select the Appropriate Assessment (Focused or Rapid)

Student: I am selecting the focused assessment.
PROCTOR: Noted.

SAMPLE History

Student: At this time I will gather a SAMPLE history from the patient or family. What are the patient's signs and symptoms?
PROCTOR: Poisoning/overdose.
> **Student:** What was the substance?
> **PROCTOR:** Mushrooms.
> **Student:** When did you ingest/become exposed?
> **PROCTOR:** 20 minutes ago.
> **Student:** Over what time period?
> **PROCTOR:** Over 10 minutes.
> **Student:** Interventions: Have you done anything to make this better?
> **PROCTOR:** The patient has taken no actions.
> **Student:** What is your weight?
> **PROCTOR:** 165 pounds.

Student: Allergies?
PROCTOR: No allergies.
Student: Medications?
PROCTOR: No medications.
Student: Pertinent past medical history?
PROCTOR: No pertinent medical history.
Student: Last oral intake?
PROCTOR: 20 minutes ago.
Student: Events leading up to the incident?
PROCTOR: The patient was eating mushrooms that he had picked and cooked in a spaghetti sauce.

Perform the Focused Physical Examination

Student: I am performing the focused physical examination.
PROCTOR: Noted.

Student: I will bring the spaghetti sauce and mushrooms with the patient to the emergency department.
PROCTOR: Noted.
Student: I will notify medical control and relay information to a poison control center.
PROCTOR: Noted.

▼ Baseline Vital Signs

Student: What are the patient's baseline vital signs, including blood pressure, pulse, respirations, pulse oximetry, and level of consciousness?
PROCTOR: Blood pressure, 160/88 mm Hg; pulse rate, 134 beats/min; respirations, 28 breaths/min; pulse oximetry reading, 98%; and the patient is alert.

▼ Interventions

Student: I will apply oxygen, contact medical control, and consider an order for activated charcoal.
PROCTOR: Noted.
ALS Student: I will apply basic life support (BLS) interventions, plus the following: IV access, cardiac monitor, local protocol (nasogastric tube), and contact poison control.
ALS Proctor: Noted. The cardiac monitor shows sinus tachycardia.

▼ Reevaluate Transport Decision

Student: The patient is a high priority and is a load-and-go patient.
PROCTOR: Noted.

▼ Detailed Physical Examination

Possible Answer #1
Student: I would not do a detailed physical exam.
PROCTOR: Noted. (Go to "Radio Report.")

Possible Answer #2
Student: I am conducting the detailed physical exam. I am looking for DCAP-BTLS. This acronym stands for deformities, contusions, abrasions, punctures, penetrations, paradoxical motion in the chest, and burns, tenderness, lacerations, and swelling.
PROCTOR: Noted. The detailed physical exam will be performed during transport.

▸ **Assess the Head**

Student: I am assessing the head. Do I find any DCAP-BTLS? Do I find any evidence of Battle's sign or raccoon eyes?
PROCTOR: No.

▸ **Inspect and Palpate the Head and Ears**

Student: I am assessing the head and ears.
PROCTOR: There are no obvious injuries.

▸ **Assess the Eyes**

Student: I am assessing the eyes. Are the pupils equal, round, and regular in size, and react properly to light (PEARRL)?
PROCTOR: They are PEARRL.

▸ **Assess the Facial Area Including Oral and Nasal Areas**

Student: I am assessing the face, nose, and mouth. Do I see any discharge or hear any obstructions?
PROCTOR: No.

▸ **Assess the Neck**

▸ **Inspect and Palpate the Neck**

Student: I am assessing the neck for DCAP-BTLS.
PROCTOR: There are no obvious injuries.

▸ **Assess for Jugular Vein Distention**

Student: Do I find any jugular vein distention (JVD)?
PROCTOR: No.

▸ **Assess for Tracheal Deviation**

Student: Do I see any tracheal deviation?
PROCTOR: No.

▸ **Assess the Chest**

Student: I am assessing the chest for DCAP-BTLS.
PROCTOR: Noted.

▸ **Inspect**

Student: What do I see when I look at the chest?
PROCTOR: There are no obvious injuries.
Student: Is the chest symmetric?
PROCTOR: Yes.

▸ **Palpate**

Student: When I touch the chest, do I feel crepitus or a flail segment?
PROCTOR: No.

▸ **Auscultate**

Student: Are lung sounds present in all fields?
PROCTOR: Yes.
Student: Do I hear any sucking sounds from the chest?
PROCTOR: No.

▸ **Assess the Abdomen/Pelvis**

▸ **Assess the Abdomen**

Student: I am assessing the abdomen for DCAP-BTLS. I am assessing all four quadrants. Do I find any problems?
PROCTOR: The patient is very nauseated and has violent projectile vomiting.

▸ **Assess the Pelvis**

Student: I am assessing the pelvis for DCAP-BTLS. Is the pelvis stable?
PROCTOR: Yes.

▸ **Assess the Genitalia/Perineum as Needed (Verbalize in Training)**

Student: I am assessing the genitalia/perineum as necessary for DCAP-BTLS.
PROCTOR: The area is unremarkable.

▸ **Assess the Extremities**

▸ **Inspect**

Student: I am assessing the lower and upper extremities for DCAP-BTLS. Do I find anything?
PROCTOR: No.

▸ **Palpate**

Student: Do I feel anything unusual?
PROCTOR: No.

▸ **Assess Motor, Sensory, and Circulatory Function**

Student: I am checking for DCAP-BTLS, motor and sensory function, and pulses. Right leg?
PROCTOR: Negative DCAP-BTLS. Motor and sensory functions are present. Pulses are present.
Student: Left leg?
PROCTOR: Negative DCAP-BTLS. Motor and sensory functions are present. Pulses are present.
Student: Right arm?
PROCTOR: Negative DCAP-BTLS. Motor and sensory functions are present. Pulses are present.
Student: Left arm?
PROCTOR: Negative DCAP-BTLS. Motor and sensory functions are present. Pulses are present.

▸ **Assess the Posterior**

Student: We will check the back.
PROCTOR: Noted.

▸ **Assess the Thorax**

Student: I am assessing the thorax. Do I find injuries?
PROCTOR: No.

▸ **Assess the Lumbar Area**

Student: I am assessing the flanks and lumbar area. Do I find injuries?
PROCTOR: No.

▸ **Assess the Entire Backside**

Student: I am assessing the entire backside. Do I find injuries?
PROCTOR: No.

▸ **Reassess Interventions**

Student: I will reassess my interventions: apply oxygen, contact medical control, and follow the local protocol.

PROCTOR: Noted.

ALS Student: I will reassess BLS interventions, plus the following: IV access, cardiac monitor, local protocol (nasogastric tube), and poison control.

ALS Proctor: Noted. The cardiac monitor shows sinus tachycardia.

Critical Criteria:

- ❑ Did not obtain medical direction or verbalize standing orders for medical interventions
- ❑ Administered a dangerous or inappropriate intervention
- ❑ Did not ask questions about the present illness
- ❑ Did not differentiate patient's need for transportation versus continued assessment at the scene

Radio Report

(Provided by the student.)

PROCTOR: Noted.

Ongoing Assessment

Repeat the Initial Assessment

Student: I will repeat the initial assessment.

PROCTOR: Noted. (Reflected in "Repeat Vital Signs.")

Repeat Vital Signs

Student: I will reassess vital signs and mental status.

PROCTOR: Blood pressure, 156/82 mm Hg; pulse rate, 124 beats/min; respirations, 24 breaths/min; pulse oximetry reading, 99%; and the patient is alert.

Student: The vital signs have not changed significantly.

PROCTOR: Noted.

Check Interventions

Student: I will check my interventions: apply oxygen, contact medical control, and follow local protocols.

PROCTOR: Noted.

ALS Student: I will check BLS interventions, plus the following: IV access, cardiac monitor, and local protocol (nasogastric tube) and poison control consult.

ALS Proctor: Noted. The cardiac monitor shows sinus tachycardia.

Repeat the Focused Assessment

Student: I will repeat the focused assessment.

PROCTOR: Noted.

Critical Criteria:

- ❑ Did not obtain medical direction or verbalize standing orders for medical interventions
- ❑ Administered a dangerous or inappropriate intervention

Handoff Report to Emergency Department Staff

Student: There was no change in the patient's condition during transport.

PROCTOR: Noted.

Critical Criteria

(Inform the student of items missed, if any.)

❑ Pass ❑ Fail Date: ____________________

Proctor Comments: ____________________

____

____

Notes

Dispatch Information

PROCTOR: EMS 10, respond to a 24-year-old female who is giving birth. She is conscious and breathing.

Pre-scene Action (BSI)

Student: I am wearing nonlatex gloves, mask, gown, and safety glasses.
PROCTOR: Noted.

Critical Criteria:
- ❑ Did not take, or verbalize, body substance isolation (BSI) precautions when necessary

Scene Size-up

Scene Safety

Student: Is the scene safe?
PROCTOR: Yes.

Mechanism of Injury/Nature of Illness

Student: What is the nature of the illness?
PROCTOR: The patient is giving birth.

Number of Patients

Student: How many patients are there?
PROCTOR: One.

Additional Resources

Student: I would call for advanced life support (ALS) assistance.
PROCTOR: Noted.

C-Spine Stabilization

Student: I would not stabilize the cervical spine (c-spine).
PROCTOR: Noted.

Critical Criteria:
- ❑ Did not determine scene safety

Initial Assessment

General Impression

Student: My general impression is that the patient's condition is stable.
PROCTOR: Noted.

Responsiveness/Level of Consciousness

Student: What is the patient's level of consciousness?
PROCTOR: Alert.

Chief Complaint/Apparent Life Threats

Student: What is the patient's chief complaint?
PROCTOR: The patient is in labor.

Assess the Airway and Breathing

Student: Is the airway open? Is the patient breathing?
PROCTOR: Yes. The airway is open and the patient is breathing.

Assessment

Student: What are the rate and the quality of breathing?
PROCTOR: Rate: Tachypneic. Quality: Per her Lamaze training.

Provide Oxygen

Student: I am applying oxygen at 15 L/min via nonrebreathing mask.
PROCTOR: Noted.

Ensure Adequate Ventilation

Student: The patient has adequate ventilations at this time.
PROCTOR: Noted.

Assess Circulation

Student: I am assessing the patient's circulation.
PROCTOR: Noted.

Assess for and Control Major Bleeding

Student: Do I find any major bleeding?
PROCTOR: No.

Assess the Pulse

Student: What are the rate and the quality of pulses?
PROCTOR: Rate: Tachycardic. Quality: Bounding.

Assess the Skin

Student: I am assessing the skin. What are the color, temperature, and condition of the skin?
PROCTOR: Color: Pale. Temperature: Warm. Condition: Moist.

Identify Priority Patients/Make Transport Decision

Student: I do not have enough information to determine a transport decision.
PROCTOR: Noted.

Critical Criteria:
- ❑ Did not provide high concentration of oxygen
- ❑ Did not find or manage problems associated with airway, breathing, hemorrhage or shock (hypoperfusion)
- ❑ Did not differentiate patient's need for transportation versus continued assessment at the scene
- ❑ Did detailed or focused history/physical examination before assessing the airway, breathing and circulation

Focused History and Physical Examination/Rapid Assessment

Select the Appropriate Assessment (Focused or Rapid)

Student: I am selecting the focused assessment.
PROCTOR: Noted.

SAMPLE History

Student: At this time I will gather a SAMPLE history from the patient or family. What are the patient's signs and symptoms?
PROCTOR: Obstetrics.

> **Student:** Are you pregnant?
> **PROCTOR:** Yes.
> **Student:** How long have you been pregnant?
> **PROCTOR:** 9 months.
> **Student:** Are you having pain or contractions?
> **PROCTOR:** Yes, the contractions are 5 minutes apart.
> **Student:** Are you having any bleeding or discharge?
> **PROCTOR:** Yes, my bag of water has broken.
> **Student:** Do you feel the need to push?
> **PROCTOR:** Yes.
> **Student:** When was your last menstrual period?
> **PROCTOR:** 10 months ago.

Student: Allergies?
PROCTOR: No allergies.
Student: Medications?
PROCTOR: Vitamins.
Student: Pertinent past medical history?
PROCTOR: No pertinent medical history.
Student: Last oral intake?
PROCTOR: 2 hours ago.
Student: Events leading up to the incident?
PROCTOR: The patient was lying down.

▼ **Perform the Focused Physical Examination**

Student: I am assessing the abdomen. Do I find any abnormalities?
PROCTOR: Distention from the full-term pregnancy.
Student: I am assessing the pelvic area. Do I find any abnormalities?
PROCTOR: There is no crowning, but the cord is present.
Student: I will insert a gloved hand into the vagina to gently push the infant's head away from the cord and provide an airway. I will place a moist dressing over the cord. I will place the patient on a backboard in Trendelenburg position, or position her so that she is kneeling, bent forward, and face down, or place her in a position that is acceptable per local protocol.
PROCTOR: Noted.
Student: How many times has the patient been pregnant?
PROCTOR: Once.
Student: How many live births has the patient delivered?
PROCTOR: None.
Student: What type of prenatal care has the patient had?
PROCTOR: Prenatal vitamins.
Student: Have there been any problems during this pregnancy?
PROCTOR: No. This is her first problem and first pregnancy.

▼ **Baseline Vital Signs**

Student: What are the patient's baseline vital signs, including blood pressure, pulse, respirations, pulse oximetry, and level of consciousness?
PROCTOR: Blood pressure, 134/68 mm Hg; pulse rate, 126 beats/min; respirations, 28 breaths/min; pulse oximetry reading, 99%; and the patient is alert.

▼ **Interventions**

Student: I will apply oxygen and I will insert a gloved hand into the vagina to gently push the infant's head away from the cord and provide an airway and transport the patient in the approved position.
PROCTOR: Noted.
ALS Student: I will apply basic life support (BLS) interventions, plus the following: start one large-bore IV.
ALS Proctor: Noted.

▼ **Reevaluate Transport Decision**

Student: The patient is a load-and-go due to the prolapsed cord. I will check the dressing and ensure that the infant's head is kept away from the cord. I will provide early notification to the hospital and transport the patient.
PROCTOR: Noted.

Critical Criteria:
- ❑ Did not obtain medical direction or verbalize standing orders for medical interventions
- ❑ Administered a dangerous or inappropriate intervention
- ❑ Did not ask questions about the present illness
- ❑ Did not differentiate patient's need for transportation versus continued assessment at the scene

▼ Radio Report

(Provided by the student.)
PROCTOR: Noted.

▼ Ongoing Assessment

▼ **Repeat the Initial Assessment**

Student: I will repeat the initial assessment.
PROCTOR: Noted. (Reflected in "Repeat Vital Signs.")

▼ **Repeat Vital Signs**

Student: I will reassess vital signs and mental status.
PROCTOR: Blood pressure, 130/74 mm Hg; pulse rate, 118 beats/min; respirations, 24 breaths/min; pulse oximetry reading, 99%; and the patient is alert.
Student: The vital signs have not changed significantly.
PROCTOR: Noted.

▼ **Check Interventions**

Student: I will reassess my interventions: I will insert a gloved hand into the vagina to gently push the infant's head away from the cord, check the saline-moistened dressing, and provide an airway. I will apply oxygen, transport the patient on a backboard in the Trendelenburg position, or position her so that she is kneeling, bent forward, and face down, or place her in a position that is acceptable per local protocol.
PROCTOR: Noted.
ALS Student: I will reassess BLS interventions, plus the following: monitor large-bore IV.
ALS Proctor: Noted.

▼ **Repeat the Focused Assessment**

Student: I will repeat the focused assessment.
PROCTOR: Noted.

Critical Criteria:
- ❑ Did not obtain medical direction or verbalize standing orders for medical interventions
- ❑ Administered a dangerous or inappropriate intervention

▼ Handoff Report to Emergency Department Staff

Student: There was no change in the patient's condition during transport.
PROCTOR: Noted.

▼ Critical Criteria

(Inform the student of items missed, if any.)

❑ Pass ❑ Fail Date: ______________________________

Proctor Comments: ______________________________

____

____

Dispatch Information

PROCTOR: EMS 10, respond to a 29-year-old female who has threatened suicide. She has scratched her neck with her fingernail. She is not bleeding. She is conscious and breathing. Police officers are en route.

Pre-scene Action (BSI)

Student: I am wearing nonlatex gloves and safety glasses.
PROCTOR: Noted.

Critical Criteria:
- ❑ Did not take, or verbalize, body substance isolation (BSI) precautions when necessary

Scene Size-up

Scene Safety

Student: Is the scene safe?
PROCTOR: Yes, police are on scene and you are given clearance to enter.

Mechanism of Injury/Nature of Illness

Student: What is the nature of the illness?
PROCTOR: The patient threatened suicide and scratched her neck with her fingernail.

Number of Patients

Student: How many patients are there?
PROCTOR: One.

Additional Resources

Student: I would not call for additional resources.
PROCTOR: Noted.

C-Spine Stabilization

Student: I would not stabilize the cervical spine (c-spine).
PROCTOR: Noted.

Critical Criteria:
- ❑ Did not determine scene safety

Initial Assessment

General Impression

Student: My general impression is that the patient's condition is stable.
PROCTOR: Noted.

Responsiveness/Level of Consciousness

Student: What is the patient's level of consciousness?
PROCTOR: Alert.

Chief Complaint/Apparent Life Threats

Student: What is the patient's chief complaint?
PROCTOR: The patient is complaining that she wants to die.

Assess the Airway and Breathing

Student: Is the airway open? Is the patient breathing?
PROCTOR: Yes. The airway is open and the patient is breathing.

Assessment

Student: What are the rate and the quality of breathing?
PROCTOR: Rate: Within normal limits. Quality: Within normal limits.

Provide Oxygen

Student: I would not apply oxygen.
PROCTOR: Noted.

Ensure Adequate Ventilation

Student: The patient has adequate ventilations at this time.
PROCTOR: Noted.

Assess Circulation

Student: I am assessing the patient's circulation.
PROCTOR: Noted.

Assess for and Control Major Bleeding

Student: Do I find any major bleeding?
PROCTOR: No.

Assess the Pulse

Student: What are the rate and the quality of pulses?
PROCTOR: Rate: Within normal limits. Quality: Within normal limits.

Assess the Skin

Student: I am assessing the skin. What are the color, temperature, and condition of the skin?
PROCTOR: Color: Normal. Temperature: Normal. Condition: Normal.

Identify Priority Patients/Make Transport Decision

Student: The patient is a low priority and does not require immediate transport.
PROCTOR: Noted.

Critical Criteria:
- ❑ Did not provide high concentration of oxygen
- ❑ Did not find or manage problems associated with airway, breathing, hemorrhage or shock (hypoperfusion)
- ❑ Did not differentiate patient's need for transportation versus continued assessment at the scene
- ❑ Did detailed or focused history/physical examination before assessing the airway, breathing and circulation

Focused History and Physical Examination/Rapid Assessment

Select the Appropriate Assessment (Focused or Rapid)

Student: I am selecting the focused assessment.
PROCTOR: Noted.

SAMPLE History

Student: At this time I will gather a SAMPLE history from the patient or family. What are the patient's signs and symptoms?
PROCTOR: Behavioral.

> **Student:** How do you feel?
> **PROCTOR:** She says she wants to kill herself and you as well.
> **Student:** Do you want to hurt or kill yourself?
> **PROCTOR:** Yes.
> **Student:** Is the patient a threat to self or others? What do you think?
> **PROCTOR:** Yes.
> **Student:** Is there a medical problem?
> **PROCTOR:** No.
> **Student:** Interventions: Have you done anything to make this better?
> **PROCTOR:** No.

Student: Allergies?
PROCTOR: No allergies.
Student: Medications?
PROCTOR: No medications.
Student: Pertinent past medical history?
PROCTOR: No pertinent medical history.
Student: Last oral intake?
PROCTOR: 3 hours ago.
Student: Events leading up to the incident?
PROCTOR: The patient is depressed and no longer wants to be a wife or mother.
Student: I will have a police officer accompany the patient during transport.
PROCTOR: Noted.

▼ Perform the Focused Physical Examination

Student: I am performing the focused physical examination.
PROCTOR: Noted.
Student: Has the patient ever felt like this before?
PROCTOR: Several times over the last few months.
Student: Has she ever sought help for these feelings in the past?
PROCTOR: No.
Student: Will she allow the nurses and doctors to help her?
PROCTOR: Maybe.
Student: Has she attempted to kill herself before?
PROCTOR: No.

▼ Baseline Vital Signs

Student: What are the patient's baseline vital signs, including blood pressure, pulse, respirations, pulse oximetry, blood glucose level, and level of consciousness?
PROCTOR: Blood pressure, 122/70 mm Hg; pulse rate, 88 beats/min; respirations, 16 breaths/min; pulse oximetry reading, 99%; blood glucose level, 118 mg/dL; and the patient is alert.

▼ Interventions

Student: I will reassure the patient and transport in the position of comfort with a police officer onboard.
PROCTOR: Noted.

▼ Reevaluate Transport Decision

Student: The patient is a low priority and does not require immediate transport.
PROCTOR: Noted.

▼ Detailed Physical Examination

Possible Answer #1
Student: I would not do a detailed physical exam.
PROCTOR: Noted. (Go to "Radio Report.")

Possible Answer #2
Student: I am conducting the detailed physical exam. I am looking for DCAP-BTLS. This acronym stands for deformities, contusions, abrasions, punctures, penetrations, paradoxical motion in the chest, and burns, tenderness, lacerations, and swelling.
PROCTOR: Noted. The detailed physical exam will be performed during transport.

► Assess the Head

Student: I am assessing the head. Do I find any DCAP-BTLS? Do I find any evidence of Battle's sign or raccoon eyes?
PROCTOR: No.

► Inspect and Palpate the Head and Ears

Student: I am assessing the head and ears.
PROCTOR: There are no obvious injuries.

► Assess the Eyes

Student: I am assessing the eyes. Are the pupils equal, round, and regular in size, and react properly to light (PEARRL)?
PROCTOR: They are PEARRL.

► Assess the Facial Area Including Oral and Nasal Areas

Student: I am assessing the face, nose, and mouth. Do I see any discharge or hear any obstructions?
PROCTOR: No.

► Assess the Neck

► Inspect and Palpate the Neck

Student: I am assessing the neck for DCAP-BTLS.
PROCTOR: You see a few superficial fingernail marks on the skin.

► Assess for Jugular Vein Distention

Student: Do I find any jugular vein distention (JVD)?
PROCTOR: No.

► Assess for Tracheal Deviation

Student: Do I see any tracheal deviation?
PROCTOR: No.

► Assess the Chest

Student: I am assessing the chest for DCAP-BTLS.
PROCTOR: Noted.

► Inspect

Student: What do I see when I look at the chest?
PROCTOR: There are no obvious injuries.
Student: Is the chest symmetric?
PROCTOR: Yes.

► Palpate

Student: When I touch the chest, do I feel crepitus or a flail segment?
PROCTOR: No.

► Auscultate

Student: Are lung sounds present in all fields?
PROCTOR: Yes.
Student: Do I hear any sucking sounds from the chest?
PROCTOR: No.

► Assess the Abdomen/Pelvis

► Assess the Abdomen

Student: I am assessing the abdomen for DCAP-BTLS. I am assessing all four quadrants. Do I find any problems?
PROCTOR: No.

► Assess the Pelvis

Student: I am assessing the pelvis for DCAP-BTLS. Is the pelvis stable?
PROCTOR: Yes.

► Assess the Genitalia/Perineum as Needed (Verbalize in Training)

Student: I am assessing the genitalia/perineum as necessary for DCAP-BTLS.
PROCTOR: The area is unremarkable.

► Assess the Extremities

► Inspect

Student: I am assessing the lower and upper extremities for DCAP-BTLS. Do I find anything?
PROCTOR: No.

► Palpate

Student: Do I feel anything unusual?
PROCTOR: No.

► Assess Motor, Sensory, and Circulatory Function

Student: I am checking for DCAP-BTLS, motor and sensory function, and pulses. Right leg?
PROCTOR: Negative DCAP-BTLS. Motor and sensory functions are present. Pulses are present.
Student: Left leg?
PROCTOR: Negative DCAP-BTLS. Motor and sensory functions are present. Pulses are present.
Student: Right arm?
PROCTOR: Negative DCAP-BTLS. Motor and sensory functions are present. Pulses are present.
Student: Left arm?
PROCTOR: Negative DCAP-BTLS. Motor and sensory functions are present. Pulses are present.

► Assess the Posterior

Student: We will check the back.
PROCTOR: Noted.

► Assess the Thorax

Student: I am assessing the thorax. Do I find injuries?
PROCTOR: No.

► Assess the Lumbar Area

Student: I am assessing the flanks and lumbar area. Do I find injuries?
PROCTOR: No.

▸ **Assess the Entire Backside**

Student: I am assessing the entire backside. Do I find injuries?

PROCTOR: No.

▸ **Reassess Interventions**

Student: I will reassess my interventions: provide reassurance and transport the patient in the position of comfort.

PROCTOR: Noted.

Critical Criteria:
- ❑ Did not obtain medical direction or verbalize standing orders for medical interventions
- ❑ Administered a dangerous or inappropriate intervention
- ❑ Did not ask questions about the present illness
- ❑ Did not differentiate patient's need for transportation versus continued assessment at the scene

Radio Report

(Provided by the student.)

PROCTOR: Noted.

Ongoing Assessment

Repeat the Initial Assessment

Student: I will repeat the initial assessment.

PROCTOR: Noted. (Reflected in "Repeat Vital Signs.")

Repeat Vital Signs

Student: I will reassess vital signs and mental status.

PROCTOR: Blood pressure, 122/72 mm Hg; pulse rate, 86 beats/min; respirations, 16 breaths/min; pulse oximetry reading, 99%; and the patient is alert.

Student: The vital signs have not changed significantly.

PROCTOR: Noted.

Check Interventions

Student: I will check my interventions: provide reassurance and transport the patient in the position of comfort.

PROCTOR: Noted.

Repeat the Focused Assessment

Student: I will repeat the focused assessment.

PROCTOR: Noted.

Critical Criteria:
- ❑ Did not obtain medical direction or verbalize standing orders for medical interventions
- ❑ Administered a dangerous or inappropriate intervention

Handoff Report to Emergency Department Staff

Student: There was no change in the patient's condition during transport.

PROCTOR: Noted.

Critical Criteria

(Inform the student of items missed, if any.)

❑ Pass ❑ Fail Date: ______________________________

Proctor Comments: ______________________________

____

____

Notes

Dispatch Information

PROCTOR: EMS 10, respond to a 19-year-old female who has overdosed on heroin at a party. She is unresponsive and barely breathing.

Pre-scene Action (BSI)

Student: I am wearing nonlatex gloves and safety glasses.
PROCTOR: Noted.

Critical Criteria:
- ❑ Did not take, or verbalize, body substance isolation (BSI) precautions when necessary

Scene Size-up

Scene Safety

Student: Is the scene safe?
PROCTOR: Yes. Police are on the scene.

Mechanism of Injury/Nature of Illness

Student: What is the nature of the illness?
PROCTOR: The patient is unresponsive and barely breathing after using heroin.

Number of Patients

Student: How many patients are there?
PROCTOR: One.

Additional Resources

Student: I would call for advanced life support (ALS) assistance.
PROCTOR: Noted.

C-Spine Stabilization

Student: I would not stabilize the cervical spine (c-spine).
PROCTOR: Noted.

Critical Criteria:
- ❑ Did not determine scene safety

Initial Assessment

General Impression

Student: My general impression is that the patient's condition is unstable.
PROCTOR: Noted.

Responsiveness/Level of Consciousness

Student: What is the patient's level of consciousness?
PROCTOR: Unresponsive to painful stimuli.

Chief Complaint/Apparent Life Threats

Student: What is the patient's chief complaint?
PROCTOR: The patient is unresponsive and barely breathing after using heroin.

Assess the Airway and Breathing

Student: I will open the airway using a head-tilt chin-lift technique. Is she breathing?
PROCTOR: Barely.

Assessment

Student: What are the rate and the quality of breathing?
PROCTOR: Rate: Very slow. Quality: Shallow.

Provide Oxygen

Student: I will insert an oral airway and ventilate using 100% oxygen via bag-valve device.
PROCTOR: Noted.

Ensure Adequate Ventilation

Student: The patient is being ventilated by a bag-valve device at this time.
PROCTOR: Noted.

Assess Circulation

Student: I am assessing the patient's circulation.
PROCTOR: Noted.

Assess for and Control Major Bleeding

Student: Do I find any major bleeding?
PROCTOR: No.

Assess the Pulse

Student: What are the rate and the quality of pulses?
PROCTOR: Rate: Tachycardia. Quality: Normal.

Assess the Skin

Student: I am assessing the skin. What are the color, temperature, and condition of the skin?
PROCTOR: Color: Pale. Temperature: Cool. Condition: Diaphoretic.

Identify Priority Patients/Make Transport Decision

Student: The patient is a high priority and is a load-and-go. I will begin packaging and transport.
PROCTOR: Noted.

Critical Criteria:
- ❑ Did not provide high concentration of oxygen
- ❑ Did not find or manage problems associated with airway, breathing, hemorrhage or shock (hypoperfusion)
- ❑ Did not differentiate patient's need for transportation versus continued assessment at the scene
- ❑ Did detailed or focused history/physical examination before assessing the airway, breathing and circulation

Focused History and Physical Examination/ Rapid Assessment

Select the Appropriate Assessment (Focused or Rapid)

Student: I am selecting the focused assessment.
PROCTOR: Noted.

SAMPLE History

Student: At this time I will gather a SAMPLE history from the patient or family. What are the patient's signs and symptoms?
PROCTOR: Poisoning/overdose.
Student: What was the substance?
PROCTOR: Heroin.
Student: When did she take it?
PROCTOR: It was 10 minutes ago.
Student: How much did she take?
PROCTOR: Unknown.
Student: Over what time period?
PROCTOR: Quickly.
Student: Interventions: Has she done anything to make this better?
PROCTOR: No.
Student: What is her weight?
PROCTOR: 120 pounds.
Student: Allergies?
PROCTOR: No allergies.
Student: Medications?
PROCTOR: No medications.
Student: Pertinent past medical history?
PROCTOR: No pertinent medical history.
Student: Last oral intake?
PROCTOR: 2 hours ago.
Student: Events leading up to the incident?
PROCTOR: The patient was at a party and a friend offered her some heroin.

Perform the Focused Physical Examination

Student: I am performing the focused physical examination.
PROCTOR: Noted.

▼ Baseline Vital Signs

Student: What are the patient's baseline vital signs, including blood pressure, pulse, respirations, pulse oximetry, blood glucose level, and level of consciousness?

PROCTOR: Blood pressure, 112/78 mm Hg; pulse rate, 112 beats/min; respirations, per bag-valve device; pulse oximetry reading, 95%; blood glucose level, 108 mg/dL; and the patient is unresponsive.

▼ Interventions

Student: I will insert an oral/advanced airway and ventilate with 100% oxygen via bag-valve device, and transport on a long board.

PROCTOR: Noted.

ALS Student: I will apply basic life support (BLS) interventions, plus the following: IV access, naloxone (Narcan) per local dose, cardiac monitor and local protocol.

ALS Proctor: Noted. The naloxone (Narcan) worked. She is now awake and breathing at 16 breaths/min. The cardiac monitor shows sinus tachycardia.

▼ Reevaluate Transport Decision

Student: The patient is a high priority and is a load-and-go patient due to the overdose and respiratory effects.

PROCTOR: Noted.

ALS Student: The patient is now a low-priority transport.

ALS Proctor: Noted.

▼ Detailed Physical Examination

Possible Answer #1

Student: I would not do a detailed physical exam.

PROCTOR: Noted. (Go to "Radio Report.")

Possible Answer #2

Student: I am conducting the detailed physical exam. I am looking for DCAP-BTLS. This acronym stands for deformities, contusions, abrasions, punctures, penetrations, paradoxical motion in the chest, and burns, tenderness, lacerations, and swelling.

PROCTOR: Noted. The detailed physical exam will be performed during transport.

► Assess the Head

Student: I am assessing the head. Do I find any DCAP-BTLS? Do I find any evidence of Battle's sign or raccoon eyes?

PROCTOR: No.

► Inspect and Palpate the Head and Ears

Student: I am assessing the head and ears.

PROCTOR: There are no obvious injuries.

► Assess the Eyes

Student: I am assessing the eyes. Are the pupils equal, round, and regular in size, and react properly to light (PEARRL)?

PROCTOR: They are dilated.

► Assess the Facial Area Including Oral and Nasal Areas

Student: I am assessing the face, nose, and mouth. Do I see any discharge or hear any obstructions?

PROCTOR: No.

► Assess the Neck

► Inspect and Palpate the Neck

Student: I am assessing the neck for DCAP-BTLS.

PROCTOR: There are no obvious injuries.

► Assess for Jugular Vein Distention

Student: Do I find any jugular vein distention (JVD)?

PROCTOR: No.

► Assess for Tracheal Deviation

Student: Do I see any tracheal deviation?

PROCTOR: No.

► Assess the Chest

Student: I am assessing the chest for DCAP-BTLS.

PROCTOR: Noted.

► Inspect

Student: What do I see when I look at the chest?

PROCTOR: There are no obvious injuries.

Student: Is the chest symmetric?

PROCTOR: Yes.

► Palpate

Student: When I touch the chest, do I feel crepitus or a flail segment?

PROCTOR: No.

► Auscultate

Student: Are lung sounds present in all fields?

PROCTOR: Yes.

Student: Do I hear any sucking sounds from the chest?

PROCTOR: No.

► Assess the Abdomen/Pelvis

► Assess the Abdomen

Student: I am assessing the abdomen for DCAP-BTLS. I am assessing all four quadrants. Do I find any problems?

PROCTOR: No.

► Assess the Pelvis

Student: I am assessing the pelvis for DCAP-BTLS. Is the pelvis stable?

PROCTOR: Yes.

► Assess the Genitalia/Perineum as Needed (Verbalize in Training)

Student: I am assessing the genitalia/perineum as necessary for DCAP-BTLS.

PROCTOR: The area is unremarkable.

► Assess the Extremities

► Inspect

Student: I am assessing the lower and upper extremities for DCAP-BTLS. Do I find anything?

PROCTOR: No.

► Palpate

Student: Do I feel anything unusual?

PROCTOR: No.

► Assess Motor, Sensory, and Circulatory Function

Student: I am checking for DCAP-BTLS, motor and sensory function, and pulses. Right leg?

PROCTOR: Negative DCAP-BTLS. Motor and sensory functions are present. Pulses are present.

Student: Left leg?

PROCTOR: Negative DCAP-BTLS. Motor and sensory functions are present. Pulses are present.

Student: Right arm?

PROCTOR: Negative DCAP-BTLS. Motor and sensory functions are present. Pulses are present.

Student: Left arm?

PROCTOR: Negative DCAP-BTLS. Motor and sensory functions are present. Pulses are present.

► Assess the Posterior

Student: We will check the back.

PROCTOR: Noted.

► Assess the Thorax

Student: I am assessing the thorax. Do I find injuries?

PROCTOR: No.

► Assess the Lumbar Area

Student: I am assessing the flanks and lumbar area. Do I find injuries?

PROCTOR: No.

► Assess the Entire Backside

Student: I am assessing the entire backside. Do I find injuries?

PROCTOR: No.

▸ **Reassess Interventions**

Student: I will reassess my interventions: I will insert an oral/advanced airway and ventilate with 100% oxygen via bag-valve device, and transport on a long backboard.

PROCTOR: Noted.

ALS Student: I will reassess BLS interventions, plus the following: oxygen 15 L/min via nonrebreathing mask, monitor IV access, assess effects of naloxone (Narcan), and cardiac monitor.

ALS Proctor: Noted. The cardiac monitor shows sinus tachycardia.

Critical Criteria:
- ❑ Did not obtain medical direction or verbalize standing orders for medical interventions
- ❑ Administered a dangerous or inappropriate intervention
- ❑ Did not ask questions about the present illness
- ❑ Did not differentiate patient's need for transportation versus continued assessment at the scene

Radio Report

(Provided by the student.)

PROCTOR: Noted.

Ongoing Assessment

Repeat the Initial Assessment

Student: I will repeat the initial assessment.

PROCTOR: Noted. (Reflected in "Repeat Vital Signs.")

Repeat Vital Signs

Student: I will reassess vital signs and mental status.

PROCTOR: Blood pressure, 120/82 mm Hg; pulse rate, 104 beats/min; respirations, per bag-valve device; pulse oximetry reading, 97%; and the patient is unresponsive.

ALS Proctor: *Note*: If naloxone (Narcan) was administered, the patient will have the following vital signs instead: Blood pressure, 120/82 mm Hg; pulse rate, 104 beats/min; respirations, 16 breaths/min; pulse oximetry reading, 97%; and the patient is alert.

Student: The vital signs have improved.

PROCTOR: Noted.

Check Interventions

Student: I will check my interventions: continue 100% oxygen via bag-valve device and provide rapid transport on a longboard.

PROCTOR: Noted.

ALS Student: I will check BLS interventions, plus the following: oxygen 15 L/min via nonrebreathing mask, monitor IV access, assess effects of naloxone (Narcan), and cardiac monitor.

ALS Proctor: Noted. The cardiac monitor shows sinus tachycardia.

Repeat the Focused Assessment

Student: I will repeat the focused assessment.

PROCTOR: Noted.

Critical Criteria:
- ❑ Did not obtain medical direction or verbalize standing orders for medical interventions
- ❑ Administered a dangerous or inappropriate intervention

Handoff Report to Emergency Department Staff

Student: The patient's condition improved during transport.

PROCTOR: Noted.

Critical Criteria

(Inform the student of items missed, if any.)

❑ Pass ❑ Fail Date: ______________________

Proctor Comments: ______________________

____

____

Notes

CASE 140

Dispatch Information

PROCTOR: EMS 10, respond to a 62-year-old male who has a history of congestive heart failure (CHF) and is complaining of shortness of breath. He is conscious and breathing.

Pre-scene Action (BSI)

Student: I am wearing nonlatex gloves and safety glasses.
PROCTOR: Noted.

Critical Criteria:
- ❑ Did not take, or verbalize, body substance isolation (BSI) precautions when necessary

Scene Size-up

Scene Safety

Student: Is the scene safe?
PROCTOR: Yes.

Mechanism of Injury/Nature of Illness

Student: What is the nature of the illness?
PROCTOR: The patient has been out of his medications for about a week and cannot afford to buy them. He has congestive heart failure and is complaining of shortness of breath.

Number of Patients

Student: How many patients are there?
PROCTOR: One.

Additional Resources

Student: I would call for advanced life support (ALS) assistance.
PROCTOR: Noted.

C-Spine Stabilization

Student: I would not stabilize the cervical spine (c-spine).
PROCTOR: Noted.

Critical Criteria:
- ❑ Did not determine scene safety

Initial Assessment

General Impression

Student: My general impression is that the patient's condition is unstable.
PROCTOR: Noted.

Responsiveness/Level of Consciousness

Student: What is the patient's level of consciousness?
PROCTOR: Alert.

Chief Complaint/Apparent Life Threats

Student: What is the patient's chief complaint?
PROCTOR: The patient is complaining of shortness of breath.

Assess the Airway and Breathing

Student: Is the airway open? Is the patient breathing?
PROCTOR: Yes. The airway is open and the patient is breathing.

Assessment

Student: What are the rate and the quality of breathing?
PROCTOR: Rate: Tachypneic. Quality: Labored.

Provide Oxygen

Student: I am applying oxygen at 15 L/min via nonrebreathing mask (continuous positive airway pressure [CPAP] or other local treatment may be administered per local protocol).
PROCTOR: Noted.

Ensure Adequate Ventilation

Student: The patient has adequate ventilations at this time.
PROCTOR: Noted.

Assess Circulation

Student: I am assessing the patient's circulation.
PROCTOR: Noted.

Assess for and Control Major Bleeding

Student: Do I find any major bleeding?
PROCTOR: No.

Assess the Pulse

Student: What are the rate and the quality of pulses?
PROCTOR: Rate: Fast. Quality: Thready.

Assess the Skin

Student: I am assessing the skin. What are the color, temperature, and condition of the skin?
PROCTOR: Color: Pale. Temperature: Cool. Condition: Moist.

Identify Priority Patients/Make Transport Decision

Student: The patient is a high priority and is a load-and-go. I will begin packaging and transport.
PROCTOR: Noted.

Critical Criteria:
- ❑ Did not provide high concentration of oxygen
- ❑ Did not find or manage problems associated with airway, breathing, hemorrhage or shock (hypoperfusion)
- ❑ Did not differentiate patient's need for transportation versus continued assessment at the scene
- ❑ Did detailed or focused history/physical examination before assessing the airway, breathing and circulation

Focused History and Physical Examination/ Rapid Assessment

Select the Appropriate Assessment (Focused or Rapid)

Student: I am selecting the focused assessment.
PROCTOR: Noted.

SAMPLE History

Student: At this time I will gather a SAMPLE history from the patient or family. What are the patient's signs and symptoms?
PROCTOR: Respiratory/cardiac.

> Student: Onset: What were you doing when this started?
> **PROCTOR:** The patient has not been able to buy his medications in a week.
> Student: Provokes: What makes your condition worse or better?
> **PROCTOR:** Lasix makes it better.
> Student: Quality: Can you describe your pain?
> **PROCTOR:** None.
> Student: Radiates: Do you have pain anywhere else?
> **PROCTOR:** Swelling to the feet.
> Student: Severity: On a scale of 1 to 10 with 10 being the worst possible, how would you rate your distress?
> **PROCTOR:** 8½.
> Student: Time: How long has this been going on?
> **PROCTOR:** 1 week.
> Student: Interventions: Have you done anything to make this better?
> **PROCTOR:** The patient has taken no actions.

Student: Allergies?
PROCTOR: No allergies.
Student: Medications?
PROCTOR: Lasix 40 mg. He has been without his medications for about a week.
Student: Pertinent past medical history?
PROCTOR: Congestive heart failure.
Student: Last oral intake?
PROCTOR: 4 hours ago.

Student: Events leading up to the incident?
PROCTOR: The patient ran out of Lasix a week ago and his condition has worsened over the week.

▼ Perform the Focused Physical Examination

Student: I am performing the focused physical examination.
PROCTOR: Noted.
Student: What do I see when I look at the chest?
PROCTOR: There are no obvious injuries.
Student: Are lung sounds present in all fields?
PROCTOR: Yes. He has rales (crackles) noted.
Student: Is pedal edema found?
PROCTOR: Yes. Pedal edema is noted.

▼ Baseline Vital Signs

Student: What are the patient's baseline vital signs, including blood pressure, pulse, respirations, pulse oximetry, blood glucose level, and level of consciousness?
PROCTOR: Blood pressure, 150/92 mm Hg; pulse rate, 140 beats/min; respirations, 28 breaths/min; pulse oximetry reading, 94%; blood glucose level, 136 mg/dL; and the patient is alert.

▼ Interventions

Student: I will apply oxygen, loosen tight-fitting clothing, and transport the patient in the position of comfort.
PROCTOR: Noted.
ALS Student: I will apply basic life support (BLS) interventions, plus the following: IV access, cardiac monitor, 12-lead ECG, and advanced cardiac life support (ACLS) or local protocol (CPAP, nitroglycerin, furosemide [Lasix], and morphine).
ALS Proctor: Noted. The cardiac monitor shows sinus tachycardia.

▼ Reevaluate Transport Decision

Student: The patient is a high priority and is a load-and-go patient.
PROCTOR: Noted.

▼ Detailed Physical Examination

Possible Answer #1
Student: I would not do a detailed physical exam.
PROCTOR: Noted. (Go to "Radio Report.")

Possible Answer #2
Student: I am conducting the detailed physical exam. I am looking for DCAP-BTLS. This acronym stands for deformities, contusions, abrasions, punctures, penetrations, paradoxical motion in the chest, and burns, tenderness, lacerations, and swelling.
PROCTOR: Noted. The detailed physical exam will be performed during transport.

► Assess the Head

Student: I am assessing the head. Do I find any DCAP-BTLS? Do I find any evidence of Battle's sign or raccoon eyes?
PROCTOR: No.

► Inspect and Palpate the Head and Ears

Student: I am assessing the head and ears.
PROCTOR: There are no obvious injuries.

► Assess the Eyes

Student: I am assessing the eyes. Are the pupils equal, round, and regular in size, and react properly to light (PEARRL)?
PROCTOR: They are PEARRL.

► Assess the Facial Area Including Oral and Nasal Areas

Student: I am assessing the face, nose, and mouth. Do I see any discharge or hear any obstructions?
PROCTOR: No.

► Assess the Neck

► Inspect and Palpate the Neck

Student: I am assessing the neck for DCAP-BTLS.
PROCTOR: There are no obvious injuries.

► Assess for Jugular Vein Distention

Student: Do I find any jugular vein distention (JVD)?
PROCTOR: No.

► Assess for Tracheal Deviation

Student: Do I see any tracheal deviation?
PROCTOR: No.

► Assess the Chest

Student: I am assessing the chest for DCAP-BTLS.
PROCTOR: Noted.

► Inspect

Student: What do I see when I look at the chest?
PROCTOR: There are no obvious injuries.
Student: Is the chest symmetric?
PROCTOR: Yes.

► Palpate

Student: When I touch the chest, do I feel crepitus or a flail segment?
PROCTOR: No.

► Auscultate

Student: Are lung sounds present in all fields?
PROCTOR: Yes. He has rales (crackles) noted.
Student: Do I hear any sucking sounds from the chest?
PROCTOR: No.

► Assess the Abdomen/Pelvis

► Assess the Abdomen

Student: I am assessing the abdomen for DCAP-BTLS. I am assessing all four quadrants. Do I find any problems?
PROCTOR: No.

► Assess the Pelvis

Student: I am assessing the pelvis for DCAP-BTLS. Is the pelvis stable?
PROCTOR: Yes.

► Assess the Genitalia/Perineum as Needed (Verbalize in Training)

Student: I am assessing the genitalia/perineum as necessary for DCAP-BTLS.
PROCTOR: The area is unremarkable.

► Assess the Extremities

► Inspect

Student: I am assessing the lower and upper extremities for DCAP-BTLS. Do I find anything?
PROCTOR: Yes. Pedal edema is noted.

► Palpate

Student: Do I feel anything unusual?
PROCTOR: Yes, swelling of the feet.

► Assess Motor, Sensory, and Circulatory Function

Student: I am checking for DCAP-BTLS, motor and sensory function, and pulses. Right leg?
PROCTOR: Negative DCAP-BTLS. Motor and sensory functions are present. Pulses are present.
Student: Left leg?
PROCTOR: Negative DCAP-BTLS. Motor and sensory functions are present. Pulses are present.
Student: Right arm?
PROCTOR: Negative DCAP-BTLS. Motor and sensory functions are present. Pulses are present.
Student: Left arm?
PROCTOR: Negative DCAP-BTLS. Motor and sensory functions are present. Pulses are present.

► Assess the Posterior

Student: We will check the back.
PROCTOR: Noted.

▸ **Assess the Thorax**

Student: I am assessing the thorax. Do I find injuries?

PROCTOR: No.

▸ **Assess the Lumbar Area**

Student: I am assessing the flanks and lumbar area. Do I find injuries?

PROCTOR: No.

▸ **Assess the Entire Backside**

Student: I am assessing the entire backside. Do I find injuries?

PROCTOR: No.

▸ **Reassess Interventions**

Student: I will reassess my interventions: oxygen, loosen tight-fitting clothing, and transport the patient in the position of comfort.

PROCTOR: Noted.

ALS Student: I will reassess BLS interventions, plus the following: IV access, cardiac monitor, 12-lead ECG, and ACLS or local protocol (CPAP, nitroglycerin, furosemide [Lasix], and morphine).

ALS Proctor: Noted. The cardiac monitor shows sinus tachycardia.

Critical Criteria:

- ❑ Did not obtain medical direction or verbalize standing orders for medical interventions
- ❑ Administered a dangerous or inappropriate intervention
- ❑ Did not ask questions about the present illness
- ❑ Did not differentiate patient's need for transportation versus continued assessment at the scene

Radio Report

(Provided by the student.)

PROCTOR: Noted.

Ongoing Assessment

Repeat the Initial Assessment

Student: I will repeat the initial assessment.

PROCTOR: Noted. (Reflected in "Repeat Vital Signs.")

Repeat Vital Signs

Student: I will reassess vital signs and mental status.

PROCTOR: Blood pressure, 146/84 mm Hg; pulse rate, 130 beats/min; respirations, 24 breaths/min; pulse oximetry reading, 95%; and the patient is alert.

ALS Proctor: Note: If ALS medications were administered, the patient will have the following vital signs instead: Blood pressure, 138/78 mm Hg; pulse rate, 118 beats/min; respirations, 16 breaths/min; pulse oximetry reading, 97%; and the patient is alert.

Student: The vital signs have not changed significantly.

PROCTOR: Noted.

Check Interventions

Student: I will check my interventions: oxygen, loosen tight-fitting clothing, and transport the patient in the position of comfort.

PROCTOR: Noted.

ALS Student: I will check BLS interventions, plus the following: monitor IV access, cardiac monitor, 12-lead ECG, and ACLS or local protocol (CPAP, nitroglycerin, furosemide [Lasix], and morphine).

ALS Proctor: Noted. The cardiac monitor shows sinus tachycardia.

Repeat the Focused Assessment

Student: I will repeat the focused assessment.

PROCTOR: Noted.

Critical Criteria:

- ❑ Did not obtain medical direction or verbalize standing orders for medical interventions
- ❑ Administered a dangerous or inappropriate intervention

Handoff Report to Emergency Department Staff

Student: There was no change in the patient's condition during transport.

ALS Student: The patient's condition improved during transport.

PROCTOR: Noted.

Critical Criteria

(Inform the student of items missed, if any.)

❑ Pass ❑ Fail Date: ____________________

Proctor Comments: ____________________

____

____

Notes

CASE 141

Dispatch Information

PROCTOR: EMS 10, respond to an 89-year-old female who is vomiting stool. She is conscious and breathing.

Pre-scene Action (BSI)

Student: I am wearing nonlatex gloves and safety glasses.
PROCTOR: Noted.

Critical Criteria:
- ❑ Did not take, or verbalize, body substance isolation (BSI) precautions when necessary

Scene Size-up

Scene Safety

Student: Is the scene safe?
PROCTOR: Yes.

Mechanism of Injury/Nature of Illness

Student: What is the nature of the illness?
PROCTOR: The patient has been ill for a few days and is now vomiting stool.

Number of Patients

Student: How many patients are there?
PROCTOR: One.

Additional Resources

Student: I would call for advanced life support (ALS) assistance.
PROCTOR: Noted.

C-Spine Stabilization

Student: I would not stabilize the cervical spine (c-spine).
PROCTOR: Noted.

Critical Criteria:
- ❑ Did not determine scene safety

Initial Assessment

General Impression

Student: My general impression is that the patient's condition is unstable.
PROCTOR: Noted.

Responsiveness/Level of Consciousness

Student: What is the patient's level of consciousness?
PROCTOR: Alert.

Chief Complaint/Apparent Life Threats

Student: What is the patient's chief complaint?
PROCTOR: The patient is complaining of vomiting stool.

Assess the Airway and Breathing

Student: Is the airway open? Is the patient breathing?
PROCTOR: Yes. The airway is open and the patient is breathing.

Assessment

Student: What are the rate and the quality of breathing?
PROCTOR: Rate: Tachypneic. Quality: Labored.

Provide Oxygen

Student: I am applying oxygen at 15 L/min via nonrebreathing mask.
PROCTOR: Noted.

Ensure Adequate Ventilation

Student: The patient has adequate ventilations at this time.
PROCTOR: Noted.

Assess Circulation

Student: I am assessing the patient's circulation.
PROCTOR: Noted.

Assess for and Control Major Bleeding

Student: Do I find any major bleeding?
PROCTOR: No.

Assess the Pulse

Student: What are the rate and the quality of pulses?
PROCTOR: Rate: Slow. Quality: Thready and irregular.

Assess the Skin

Student: I am assessing the skin. What are the color, temperature, and condition of the skin?
PROCTOR: Color: Pale. Temperature: Warm. Condition: Dry.

Identify Priority Patients/Make Transport Decision

Student: The patient is a low priority and does not require immediate transport.
PROCTOR: Noted.

Critical Criteria:
- ❑ Did not provide high concentration of oxygen
- ❑ Did not find or manage problems associated with airway, breathing, hemorrhage or shock (hypoperfusion)
- ❑ Did not differentiate patient's need for transportation versus continued assessment at the scene
- ❑ Did detailed or focused history/physical examination before assessing the airway, breathing and circulation

Focused History and Physical Examination/ Rapid Assessment

Select the Appropriate Assessment (Focused or Rapid)

Student: I am selecting the focused assessment.
PROCTOR: Noted.

SAMPLE History

Student: At this time I will gather a SAMPLE history from the patient or family. What are the patient's signs and symptoms?
PROCTOR: Respiratory/cardiac/other.

> Student: Onset: What were you doing when this started?
> **PROCTOR:** Sleeping.
> Student: Provokes: What makes your condition worse or better?
> **PROCTOR:** Unknown.
> Student: Quality: Can you describe your pain?
> **PROCTOR:** None.
> Student: Radiates: Do you have pain anywhere else?
> **PROCTOR:** No.
> Student: Severity: On a scale of 1 to 10 with 10 being the worst possible, how would you rate your distress?
> **PROCTOR:** 10.
> Student: Time: How long has this been going on?
> **PROCTOR:** 15 minutes.
> Student: Interventions: Have you done anything to make this better?
> **PROCTOR:** The patient has taken no actions.

Student: Allergies?
PROCTOR: No allergies.
Student: Medications?
PROCTOR: Blood pressure medications (Atenolol, which is a beta-blocker), stool softeners (she has been without them for a few weeks), and Nyquil®.
Student: Pertinent past medical history?
PROCTOR: High blood pressure and bowel obstructions.
Student: Last oral intake?
PROCTOR: 5 hours ago.
Student: Events leading up to the incident?
PROCTOR: The patient was sleeping when she began to vomit stool.

Perform the Focused Physical Examination

Student: I am performing the focused physical examination.
PROCTOR: Noted.

Student: Can the patient describe the sickness that she has had the last few days?
PROCTOR: Yes, she has had a nonproductive cough, a low-grade temperature, restlessness, and chills.

▼ Baseline Vital Signs
Student: What are the patient's baseline vital signs, including blood pressure, pulse, respirations, pulse oximetry, blood glucose level, and level of consciousness?
PROCTOR: Blood pressure, 104/62 mm Hg; pulse rate, 56 beats/min; respirations, 28 breaths/min; pulse oximetry reading, 97%; blood glucose level, 102 mg/dL; and the patient is alert.

▼ Interventions
Student: I will apply oxygen and transport the patient in the recovery position.
PROCTOR: Noted.
ALS Student: I will apply basic life support (BLS) interventions, plus the following: IV access, cardiac monitor, 12-lead ECG, and local protocol.
ALS Proctor: Noted. The cardiac monitor shows sinus bradycardia.

▼ Reevaluate Transport Decision
Student: The patient is a low priority and does not require immediate transport.
PROCTOR: Noted.

▼ Detailed Physical Examination
Possible Answer #1
Student: I would not do a detailed physical exam.
PROCTOR: Noted. (Go to "Radio Report.")

Possible Answer #2
Student: I am conducting the detailed physical exam. I am looking for DCAP-BTLS. This acronym stands for deformities, contusions, abrasions, punctures, penetrations, paradoxical motion in the chest, and burns, tenderness, lacerations, and swelling.
PROCTOR: Noted. The detailed physical exam will be performed during transport.

▸ **Assess the Head**
Student: I am assessing the head. Do I find any DCAP-BTLS? Do I find any evidence of Battle's sign or raccoon eyes?
PROCTOR: No.

▸ **Inspect and Palpate the Head and Ears**
Student: I am assessing the head and ears.
PROCTOR: There are no obvious injuries.

▸ **Assess the Eyes**
Student: I am assessing the eyes. Are the pupils equal, round, and regular in size, and react properly to light (PEARRL)?
PROCTOR: They are PEARRL.

▸ **Assess the Facial Area Including Oral and Nasal Areas**
Student: I am assessing the face, nose, and mouth. Do I see any discharge or hear any obstructions?
PROCTOR: No.

▸ **Assess the Neck**

▸ **Inspect and Palpate the Neck**
Student: I am assessing the neck for DCAP-BTLS.
PROCTOR: There are no obvious injuries.

▸ **Assess for Jugular Vein Distention**
Student: Do I find any jugular vein distention (JVD)?
PROCTOR: No.

▸ **Assess for Tracheal Deviation**
Student: Do I see any tracheal deviation?
PROCTOR: No.

▸ **Assess the Chest**
Student: I am assessing the chest for DCAP-BTLS.
PROCTOR: Noted.

▸ **Inspect**
Student: What do I see when I look at the chest?
PROCTOR: There are no obvious injuries.
Student: Is the chest symmetric?
PROCTOR: Yes.

▸ **Palpate**
Student: When I touch the chest, do I feel crepitus or a flail segment?
PROCTOR: No.

▸ **Auscultate**
Student: Are lung sounds present in all fields?
PROCTOR: Yes.
Student: Do I hear any sucking sounds from the chest?
PROCTOR: No.

▸ **Assess the Abdomen/Pelvis**

▸ **Assess the Abdomen**
Student: I am assessing the abdomen for DCAP-BTLS. I am assessing all four quadrants. Do I find any problems?
PROCTOR: There is some point tenderness to the right lower quadrant.

▸ **Assess the Pelvis**
Student: I am assessing the pelvis for DCAP-BTLS. Is the pelvis stable?
PROCTOR: Yes.

▸ **Assess the Genitalia/Perineum as Needed (Verbalize in Training)**
Student: I am assessing the genitalia/perineum as necessary for DCAP-BTLS.
PROCTOR: The area is unremarkable.

▸ **Assess the Extremities**

▸ **Inspect**
Student: I am assessing the lower and upper extremities for DCAP-BTLS. Do I find anything?
PROCTOR: No.

▸ **Palpate**
Student: Do I feel anything unusual?
PROCTOR: No.

▸ **Assess Motor, Sensory, and Circulatory Function**
Student: I am checking for DCAP-BTLS, motor and sensory function, and pulses. Right leg?
PROCTOR: Negative DCAP-BTLS. Motor and sensory functions are present. Pulses are present.
Student: Left leg?
PROCTOR: Negative DCAP-BTLS. Motor and sensory functions are present. Pulses are present.
Student: Right arm?
PROCTOR: Negative DCAP-BTLS. Motor and sensory functions are present. Pulses are present.
Student: Left arm?
PROCTOR: Negative DCAP-BTLS. Motor and sensory functions are present. Pulses are present.

▸ **Assess the Posterior**
Student: We will check the back.
PROCTOR: Noted.

▸ **Assess the Thorax**
Student: I am assessing the thorax. Do I find injuries?
PROCTOR: No.

▸ **Assess the Lumbar Area**
Student: I am assessing the flanks and lumbar area. Do I find injuries?
PROCTOR: No.

▸ **Assess the Entire Backside**
Student: I am assessing the entire backside. Do I find injuries?
PROCTOR: No.

▸ **Reassess Interventions**

Student: I will reassess my interventions: apply oxygen and transport the patient in the recovery position or position of comfort.

PROCTOR: Noted.

ALS Student: I will reassess BLS interventions, plus the following: IV access, cardiac monitor, 12-lead ECG, and local protocol.

ALS Proctor: Noted. The cardiac monitor shows sinus bradycardia.

Critical Criteria:
- ❑ Did not obtain medical direction or verbalize standing orders for medical interventions
- ❑ Administered a dangerous or inappropriate intervention
- ❑ Did not ask questions about the present illness
- ❑ Did not differentiate patient's need for transportation versus continued assessment at the scene

Radio Report

(Provided by the student.)

PROCTOR: Noted.

Ongoing Assessment

Repeat the Initial Assessment

Student: I will repeat the initial assessment.

PROCTOR: Noted. (Reflected in "Repeat Vital Signs.")

Repeat Vital Signs

Student: I will reassess vital signs and mental status.

PROCTOR: Blood pressure, 108/64 mm Hg; pulse rate, 54 beats/min; respirations, 24 breaths/min; pulse oximetry reading, 98%; and the patient is alert.

Student: The vital signs have not changed significantly.

PROCTOR: Noted.

Check Interventions

Student: I will check my interventions: apply oxygen and transport the patient in the recovery position or position of comfort.

PROCTOR: Noted.

ALS Student: I will check BLS interventions, plus the following: IV access, cardiac monitor, 12-lead ECG, and local protocol.

ALS Proctor: Noted. The cardiac monitor shows sinus bradycardia.

Repeat the Focused Assessment

Student: I will repeat the focused assessment.

PROCTOR: Noted.

Critical Criteria:
- ❑ Did not obtain medical direction or verbalize standing orders for medical interventions
- ❑ Administered a dangerous or inappropriate intervention

Handoff Report to Emergency Department Staff

Student: There was no change in the patient's condition during transport.

PROCTOR: Noted.

Critical Criteria

(Inform the student of items missed, if any.)

❑ Pass ❑ Fail Date: ______________________

Proctor Comments: ______________________

____

____

CASE 141

Notes

Dispatch Information

PROCTOR: EMS 10, respond to a 76-year-old female with stroke-like symptoms. She is conscious and breathing.

Pre-scene Action (BSI)

Student: I am wearing nonlatex gloves and safety glasses.
PROCTOR: Noted.

> **Critical Criteria:**
> ❑ Did not take, or verbalize, body substance isolation (BSI) precautions when necessary

Scene Size-up

Scene Safety

Student: Is the scene safe?
PROCTOR: Yes.

Mechanism of Injury/Nature of Illness

Student: What is the nature of the illness?
PROCTOR: The patient is having right-sided weakness and slurred speech.

Number of Patients

Student: How many patients are there?
PROCTOR: One.

Additional Resources

Student: I would call for advanced life support (ALS) assistance.
PROCTOR: Noted.

C-Spine Stabilization

Student: I would not stabilize the cervical spine (c-spine).
PROCTOR: Noted.

> **Critical Criteria:**
> ❑ Did not determine scene safety

Initial Assessment

General Impression

Student: My general impression is that the patient's condition is unstable.
PROCTOR: Noted.

Responsiveness/Level of Consciousness

Student: What is the patient's level of consciousness?
PROCTOR: Alert.

Chief Complaint/Apparent Life Threats

Student: What is the patient's chief complaint?
PROCTOR: The patient is complaining of stroke-like symptoms.

Assess the Airway and Breathing

Student: Is the airway open? Is the patient breathing?
PROCTOR: Yes. The airway is open and the patient is breathing.

Assessment

Student: What are the rate and the quality of breathing?
PROCTOR: Rate: Within normal limits. Quality: Normal.

Provide Oxygen

Student: I am applying oxygen at 15 L/min via nonrebreathing mask.
PROCTOR: Noted.

Ensure Adequate Ventilation

Student: The patient has adequate ventilations at this time.
PROCTOR: Noted.

Assess Circulation

Student: I am assessing the patient's circulation.
PROCTOR: Noted.

Assess for and Control Major Bleeding

Student: Do I find any major bleeding?
PROCTOR: No.

Assess the Pulse

Student: What are the rate and the quality of pulses?
PROCTOR: Rate: Within normal limits. Quality: Bounding.

Assess the Skin

Student: I am assessing the skin. What are the color, temperature, and condition of the skin?
PROCTOR: Color: Normal. Temperature: Warm. Condition: Moist.

Identify Priority Patients/Make Transport Decision

Student: The patient is a high priority and requires immediate transport.
PROCTOR: Noted.

> **Critical Criteria:**
> ❑ Did not provide high concentration of oxygen
> ❑ Did not find or manage problems associated with airway, breathing, hemorrhage or shock (hypoperfusion)
> ❑ Did not differentiate patient's need for transportation versus continued assessment at the scene
> ❑ Did detailed or focused history/physical examination before assessing the airway, breathing and circulation

Focused History and Physical Examination/ Rapid Assessment

Select the Appropriate Assessment (Focused or Rapid)

Student: I am selecting the focused assessment.
PROCTOR: Noted.

SAMPLE History

Student: At this time I will gather a SAMPLE history from the patient or family. What are the patient's signs and symptoms?
PROCTOR: Altered mental status.
  Student: Describe the episode.
  PROCTOR: The patient has had right-sided weakness and slurred speech.
  Student: Onset: What she doing when this started?
  PROCTOR: Making dinner.
  Student: Duration: How long has this been going on?
  PROCTOR: 2 hours.
  Student: Are there any associated symptoms?
  PROCTOR: Yes, drooling.
  Student: Is there any evidence of trauma?
  PROCTOR: No.
  Student: Interventions: Has she done anything to make this better?
  PROCTOR: The patient has taken no actions.
  Student: Have there been any seizures?
  PROCTOR: No.
  Student: Has there been any fever?
  PROCTOR: No.
Student: Allergies?
PROCTOR: No allergies.
Student: Medications?
PROCTOR: No medications.
Student: Pertinent past medical history?
PROCTOR: No pertinent medical history.
Student: Last oral intake?
PROCTOR: 1 hour ago.
Student: Events leading up to the incident?
PROCTOR: The patient was cooking when she noticed the problems.

Perform the Focused Physical Examination

Student: I am performing the focused physical examination.
PROCTOR: Noted.

Student: I will perform a Cincinnati prehospital stroke scale assessment. I will ask the patient to show her teeth or smile. Does she have any facial droop?
PROCTOR: She has some facial drooping.
Student: I will ask the patient to hold both of her arms out with her palms up. Does she have any arm drift?
PROCTOR: Yes, arm drift is noted in the right arm.
Student: I will ask the patient to say, "The sky is blue in Cincinnati." Does she have any speech difficulties?
PROCTOR: She has some slurring of words.
Student: I will have the patient squeeze my fingers with her hand to determine unequal strength.
PROCTOR: The right side is obviously weaker. She is showing evidence of stroke.
Student: I am assessing the lower and upper extremities for DCAP-BTLS. This acronym stands for deformities, contusions, abrasions, punctures, penetrations, paradoxical motion in the chest, and burns, tenderness, lacerations, and swelling. Do I find anything?
PROCTOR: Yes. The right side is weak.
Student: Do I feel anything unusual?
PROCTOR: No.

▸ **Assess Motor, Sensory, and Circulatory Function**

Student: I am checking for DCAP-BTLS, motor and sensory function, and pulses. Right leg?
PROCTOR: Negative DCAP-BTLS. Motor and sensory functions are present. Weakness is noted. Pulses are present.
Student: Left leg?
PROCTOR: Negative DCAP-BTLS. Motor and sensory functions are present. Pulses are present.
Student: Right arm?
PROCTOR: Negative DCAP-BTLS. Motor and sensory functions are present. Weakness is noted. Pulses are present.
Student: Left arm?
PROCTOR: Negative DCAP-BTLS. Motor and sensory functions are present. Pulses are present.

▾ Baseline Vital Signs

Student: What are the patient's baseline vital signs, including blood pressure, pulse, respirations, pulse oximetry, blood glucose level, and level of consciousness?
PROCTOR: Blood pressure, 156/92 mm Hg; pulse rate, 94 beats/min; respirations, 16 breaths/min; pulse oximetry reading, 98%; blood glucose level, 132 mg/dL; and the patient is alert.

▾ Interventions

Student: I will apply oxygen, check blood glucose level (132 mg/dL), and notify the hospital that signs and symptoms began 2 hours ago.
PROCTOR: Noted.
ALS Student: I will apply basic life support (BLS) interventions, plus the following: establish IV access, perform cardiac monitoring, 12-lead ECG, and follow local protocol.
ALS Proctor: Noted. The cardiac monitor shows normal sinus rhythm.

▾ Reevaluate Transport Decision

Student: The patient is a high priority and requires immediate transport.
PROCTOR: Noted.

▾ Detailed Physical Examination

Possible Answer #1
Student: I would not do a detailed physical exam.
PROCTOR: Noted. (Go to "Radio Report.")

Possible Answer #2
Student: I am conducting the detailed physical exam. I am looking for DCAP-BTLS.
PROCTOR: Noted. The detailed physical exam will be performed during transport.

▸ **Assess the Head**

Student: I am assessing the head. Do I find any DCAP-BTLS? Do I find any evidence of Battle's sign or raccoon eyes?
PROCTOR: No.

▸ **Inspect and Palpate the Head and Ears**

Student: I am assessing the head and ears.
PROCTOR: There are no obvious injuries.

▸ **Assess the Eyes**

Student: I am assessing the eyes. Are the pupils equal, round, and regular in size, and react properly to light (PEARRL)?
PROCTOR: They are PEARRL.

▸ **Assess the Facial Area Including Oral and Nasal Areas**

Student: I am assessing the face, nose, and mouth. Do I see any discharge or hear any obstructions?
PROCTOR: She has some facial drooping.

▸ **Assess the Neck**

▸ **Inspect and Palpate the Neck**

Student: I am assessing the neck for DCAP-BTLS.
PROCTOR: There are no obvious injuries.

▸ **Assess for Jugular Vein Distention**

Student: Do I find any jugular vein distention (JVD)?
PROCTOR: No.

▸ **Assess for Tracheal Deviation**

Student: Do I see any tracheal deviation?
PROCTOR: No.

▸ **Assess the Chest**

Student: I am assessing the chest for DCAP-BTLS.
PROCTOR: Noted.

▸ **Inspect**

Student: What do I see when I look at the chest?
PROCTOR: There are no obvious injuries.
Student: Is the chest symmetric?
PROCTOR: Yes.

▸ **Palpate**

Student: When I touch the chest, do I feel crepitus or a flail segment?
PROCTOR: No.

▸ **Auscultate**

Student: Are lung sounds present in all fields?
PROCTOR: Yes.
Student: Do I hear any sucking sounds from the chest?
PROCTOR: No.

▸ **Assess the Abdomen/Pelvis**

▸ **Assess the Abdomen**

Student: I am assessing the abdomen for DCAP-BTLS. I am assessing all four quadrants. Do I find any problems?
PROCTOR: No.

▸ **Assess the Pelvis**

Student: I am assessing the pelvis for DCAP-BTLS. Is the pelvis stable?
PROCTOR: Yes.

▸ **Assess the Genitalia/Perineum as Needed (Verbalize in Training)**

Student: I am assessing the genitalia/perineum as necessary for DCAP-BTLS.
PROCTOR: The area is unremarkable.

▸ **Assess the Extremities**

▸ **Inspect**

Student: I am assessing the lower and upper extremities for DCAP-BTLS. Do I find anything?

PROCTOR: Yes. The right side is weak.

▸ **Palpate**

Student: Do I feel anything unusual?

PROCTOR: No.

▸ **Assess Motor, Sensory, and Circulatory Function**

Student: I am checking for DCAP-BTLS, motor and sensory function, and pulses. Right leg?

PROCTOR: Negative DCAP-BTLS. Motor and sensory functions are present. Weakness is noted. Pulses are present.

Student: Left leg?

PROCTOR: Negative DCAP-BTLS. Motor and sensory functions are present. Pulses are present.

Student: Right arm?

PROCTOR: Negative DCAP-BTLS. Motor and sensory functions are present. Weakness is noted. Pulses are present.

Student: Left arm?

PROCTOR: Negative DCAP-BTLS. Motor and sensory functions are present. Pulses are present.

▸ **Assess the Posterior**

Student: We will check the back.

PROCTOR: Noted.

▸ **Assess the Thorax**

Student: I am assessing the thorax. Do I find injuries?

PROCTOR: No.

▸ **Assess the Lumbar Area**

Student: I am assessing the flanks and lumbar area. Do I find injuries?

PROCTOR: No.

▸ **Assess the Entire Backside**

Student: I am assessing the entire backside. Do I find injuries?

PROCTOR: No.

▸ **Reassess Interventions**

Student: I will reassess my interventions: apply oxygen, monitor the airway, and transport in the recovery position or other locally approved position.

PROCTOR: Noted.

ALS Student: I will reassess BLS interventions, plus the following: IV access, cardiac monitor, 12–lead ECG, and local protocol.

ALS Proctor: Noted. The cardiac monitor shows normal sinus rhythm.

Critical Criteria:

- ❑ Did not obtain medical direction or verbalize standing orders for medical interventions
- ❑ Administered a dangerous or inappropriate intervention
- ❑ Did not ask questions about the present illness
- ❑ Did not differentiate patient's need for transportation versus continued assessment at the scene

Radio Report

(Provided by the student.)

PROCTOR: Noted.

Ongoing Assessment

Repeat the Initial Assessment

Student: I will repeat the initial assessment.

PROCTOR: Noted. (Reflected in "Repeat Vital Signs.")

Repeat Vital Signs

Student: I will reassess vital signs and mental status.

PROCTOR: Blood pressure, 152/90 mm Hg; pulse rate, 90 beats/min; respirations, 16 breaths/min; pulse oximetry reading, 98%; and the patient is alert.

Student: The vital signs have not changed significantly.

PROCTOR: Noted.

Check Interventions

Student: I will check my interventions: oxygen, monitor the airway, and transport in the recovery position or other locally approved position.

PROCTOR: Noted. She is showing evidence of a stroke.

ALS Student: I will check BLS interventions, plus the following: IV access, cardiac monitor, 12-lead ECG, and local protocol.

ALS Proctor: Noted. The cardiac monitor shows normal sinus rhythm.

Repeat the Focused Assessment

Student: I will repeat the focused assessment.

PROCTOR: Noted.

Critical Criteria:

- ❑ Did not obtain medical direction or verbalize standing orders for medical interventions
- ❑ Administered a dangerous or inappropriate intervention

Handoff Report to Emergency Department Staff

Student: There was no change in the patient's condition during transport.

PROCTOR: Noted.

Critical Criteria

(Inform the student of items missed, if any.)

❑ Pass ❑ Fail Date: ______________________

Proctor Comments: ______________________

____

____

Notes

Dispatch Information

PROCTOR: EMS 10, respond to a 46-year-old banker who has received a white powdery substance in the mail. He is conscious and alert.

Pre-scene Action (BSI)

Student: I am wearing nonlatex gloves and safety glasses.
PROCTOR: Noted.

Critical Criteria:
- ❑ Did not take, or verbalize, body substance isolation (BSI) precautions when necessary

Scene Size-up

Scene Safety

Student: Is the scene safe?
PROCTOR: No, not until the patient has been decontaminated.

Mechanism of Injury/Nature of Illness

Student: What is the nature of the illness?
PROCTOR: The patient has received a package in the mail containing a death threat and a white powdery substance.

Number of Patients

Student: How many patients are there?
PROCTOR: One.

Additional Resources

Student: I would call for police, fire/rescue, and hazardous materials. I will allow fire/rescue and hazardous materials responders to decontaminate the patient before I make contact with him.
PROCTOR: Noted. The hazardous materials team has decontaminated the patient and now states that the material is not dangerous.

C-Spine Stabilization

Student: I would not stabilize the cervical spine (c-spine).
PROCTOR: Noted.

Critical Criteria:
- ❑ Did not determine scene safety

Initial Assessment

General Impression

Student: My general impression is that the patient's condition is stable.
PROCTOR: Noted.

Responsiveness/Level of Consciousness

Student: What is the patient's level of consciousness?
PROCTOR: Alert.

Chief Complaint/Apparent Life Threats

Student: What is the patient's chief complaint?
PROCTOR: The patient is very upset.

Assess the Airway and Breathing

Student: Is the airway open?
PROCTOR: Yes.

Assessment

Student: What are the rate and the quality of breathing?
PROCTOR: Rate: Tachypneic. Quality: Normal.

Provide Oxygen

Student: I will provide oxygen per local protocol.
PROCTOR: Noted.

Ensure Adequate Ventilation

Student: The patient has adequate ventilations at this time.
PROCTOR: Noted.

Assess Circulation

Student: I am assessing the patient's circulation.
PROCTOR: Noted.

Assess for and Control Major Bleeding

Student: Do I find any major bleeding?
PROCTOR: No.

Assess the Pulse

Student: What are the rate and the quality of pulses?
PROCTOR: Rate: Tachycardic. Quality: Strong.

Assess the Skin

Student: I am assessing the skin. What are the color, temperature, and condition of the skin?
PROCTOR: Color: Flushed. Temperature: Warm. Condition: Moist.

Identify Priority Patients/Make Transport Decision

Student: The patient is a low priority and does not require immediate transport.
PROCTOR: Noted.

Critical Criteria:
- ❑ Did not provide high concentration of oxygen
- ❑ Did not find or manage problems associated with airway, breathing, hemorrhage or shock (hypoperfusion)
- ❑ Did not differentiate patient's need for transportation versus continued assessment at the scene
- ❑ Did detailed or focused history/physical examination before assessing the airway, breathing and circulation

Focused History and Physical Examination/Rapid Assessment

Select the Appropriate Assessment (Focused or Rapid)

Student: I am selecting the focused assessment.
PROCTOR: Noted.

SAMPLE History

Student: At this time I will gather a SAMPLE history from the patient or family. What are the patient's signs and symptoms?
PROCTOR: Poisoning/overdose.

> Student: What was the substance?
> **PROCTOR:** The hazardous materials team has determined that the substance was flour.
> Student: When did you become exposed?
> **PROCTOR:** It was 40 minutes ago. (The patient had to be decontaminated.)
> Student: Over what time period?
> **PROCTOR:** Over 2 minutes.
> Student: Interventions: Have you done anything to make this better?
> **PROCTOR:** Yes. He washed his hands with soap and water. He was also decontaminated by the hazmat team.
> Student: What is your weight?
> **PROCTOR:** 260 pounds.

Student: Allergies?
PROCTOR: No allergies.
Student: Medications?
PROCTOR: No medications.
Student: Pertinent past medical history?
PROCTOR: No pertinent medical history.
Student: Last oral intake?
PROCTOR: 3 hours ago.
Student: Events leading up to the incident?
PROCTOR: The patient opened the package with the white powder in it.

Perform the Focused Physical Examination

Student: I am performing the focused physical examination.
PROCTOR: Noted.
Student: Did the patient come into direct contact with the powder?
PROCTOR: When he opened the letter, the powder got on his hands and fingers. He washed his hands with soap and water.
Student: Does he have any localized effects from the powder?
PROCTOR: No.

Baseline Vital Signs

Student: What are the patient's baseline vital signs, including blood pressure, pulse, respirations, pulse oximetry, and level of consciousness?
PROCTOR: Blood pressure, 160/84 mm Hg; pulse rate, 112 beats/min; respirations, 24 breaths/min; pulse oximetry reading, 99%; and the patient is alert.

Interventions

Student: I will reassure the patient and transport him in the position of comfort.
PROCTOR: Noted.

Reevaluate Transport Decision

Student: The patient is a low priority and does not require immediate transport.
PROCTOR: Noted.

Detailed Physical Examination

Possible Answer #1
Student: I would not do a detailed physical exam.
PROCTOR: Noted. (Go to "Radio Report.")

Possible Answer #2
Student: I am conducting the detailed physical exam. I am looking for DCAP-BTLS. This acronym stands for deformities, contusions, abrasions, punctures, penetrations, paradoxical motion in the chest, and burns, tenderness, lacerations, and swelling.
PROCTOR: Noted. The detailed physical exam will be performed during transport.

Assess the Head

Student: I am assessing the head. Do I find any DCAP-BTLS? Do I find any evidence of Battle's sign or raccoon eyes?
PROCTOR: No.

Inspect and Palpate the Head and Ears

Student: I am assessing the head and ears.
PROCTOR: There are no obvious injuries.

Assess the Eyes

Student: I am assessing the eyes. Are the pupils equal, round, and regular in size, and react properly to light (PEARRL)?
PROCTOR: They are PEARRL.

Assess the Facial Area Including Oral and Nasal Areas

Student: I am assessing the face, nose, and mouth. Do I see any discharge or hear any obstructions?
PROCTOR: No.

Assess the Neck

Inspect and Palpate the Neck

Student: I am assessing the neck for DCAP-BTLS.
PROCTOR: There are no obvious injuries.

Assess for Jugular Vein Distention

Student: Do I find any jugular vein distention (JVD)?
PROCTOR: No.

Assess for Tracheal Deviation

Student: Do I see any tracheal deviation?
PROCTOR: No.

Assess the Chest

Student: I am assessing the chest for DCAP-BTLS.
PROCTOR: Noted.

Inspect

Student: What do I see when I look at the chest?
PROCTOR: There are no obvious injuries.
Student: Is the chest symmetric?
PROCTOR: Yes.

Palpate

Student: When I touch the chest, do I feel crepitus or a flail segment?
PROCTOR: No.

Auscultate

Student: Are lung sounds present in all fields?
PROCTOR: Yes.
Student: Do I hear any sucking sounds from the chest?
PROCTOR: No.

Assess the Abdomen/Pelvis

Assess the Abdomen

Student: I am assessing the abdomen for DCAP-BTLS. I am assessing all four quadrants. Do I find any problems?
PROCTOR: No.

Assess the Pelvis

Student: I am assessing the pelvis for DCAP-BTLS. Is the pelvis stable?
PROCTOR: Yes.

Assess the Genitalia/Perineum as Needed (Verbalize in Training)

Student: I am assessing the genitalia/perineum as necessary for DCAP-BTLS.
PROCTOR: The area is unremarkable.

Assess the Extremities

Inspect

Student: I am assessing the lower and upper extremities for DCAP-BTLS. Do I find anything?
PROCTOR: No.

Palpate

Student: Do I feel anything unusual?
PROCTOR: No.

Assess Motor, Sensory, and Circulatory Function

Student: I am checking for DCAP-BTLS, motor and sensory function, and pulses. Right leg?
PROCTOR: Negative DCAP-BTLS. Motor and sensory functions are present. Pulses are present.
Student: Left leg?
PROCTOR: Negative DCAP-BTLS. Motor and sensory functions are present. Pulses are present.
Student: Right arm?
PROCTOR: Negative DCAP-BTLS. Motor and sensory functions are present. Pulses are present.
Student: Left arm?
PROCTOR: Negative DCAP-BTLS. Motor and sensory functions are present. Pulses are present.

Assess the Posterior

Student: We will check the back.
PROCTOR: Noted.

Assess the Thorax

Student: I am assessing the thorax. Do I find injuries?
PROCTOR: No.

Assess the Lumbar Area

Student: I am assessing the flanks and lumbar area. Do I find injuries?
PROCTOR: No.

Assess the Entire Backside

Student: I am assessing the entire backside. Do I find injuries?
PROCTOR: No.

▸ **Reassess Interventions**

Student: I will reassess my interventions: provide reassurance and transport the patient in the position of comfort.
PROCTOR: Noted.

Critical Criteria:
- ❑ Did not obtain medical direction or verbalize standing orders for medical interventions
- ❑ Administered a dangerous or inappropriate intervention
- ❑ Did not ask questions about the present illness
- ❑ Did not differentiate patient's need for transportation versus continued assessment at the scene

Radio Report

(Provided by the student.)
PROCTOR: Noted.

Ongoing Assessment

Repeat the Initial Assessment

Student: I will repeat the initial assessment.
PROCTOR: Noted. (Reflected in "Repeat Vital Signs.")

Repeat Vital Signs

Student: I will reassess vital signs and mental status.
PROCTOR: Blood pressure, 148/80 mm Hg; pulse rate, 108 beats/min; respirations, 20 breaths/min; pulse oximetry reading, 99%; and the patient is alert.
Student: The vital signs have improved.
PROCTOR: Noted.

Check Interventions

Student: I will check my interventions: provide reassurance and transport the patient in the position of comfort.
PROCTOR: Noted.

Repeat the Focused Assessment

Student: I will repeat the focused assessment.
PROCTOR: Noted.

Critical Criteria:
- ❑ Did not obtain medical direction or verbalize standing orders for medical interventions
- ❑ Administered a dangerous or inappropriate intervention

Handoff Report to Emergency Department Staff

Student: There was some improvement in the patient's condition during transport.
PROCTOR: Noted.

Critical Criteria

(Inform the student of items missed, if any.)

❑ Pass ❑ Fail Date: ______________________

Proctor Comments: ______________________

CASE 143

Notes

Dispatch Information

PROCTOR: EMS 10, respond to a 72-year-old female who is complaining of chest pain. She is conscious and breathing.

Pre-scene Action (BSI)

Student: I am wearing nonlatex gloves and safety glasses.
PROCTOR: Noted.

Critical Criteria:
- ❑ Did not take, or verbalize, body substance isolation (BSI) precautions when necessary

Scene Size-up

Scene Safety

Student: Is the scene safe?
PROCTOR: Yes.

Mechanism of Injury/Nature of Illness

Student: What is the nature of the illness?
PROCTOR: The patient was working in her yard when her chest pain began.

Number of Patients

Student: How many patients are there?
PROCTOR: One.

Additional Resources

Student: I would call for advanced life support (ALS) assistance.
PROCTOR: Noted.

C-Spine Stabilization

Student: I would not stabilize the cervical spine (c-spine).
PROCTOR: Noted.

Critical Criteria:
- ❑ Did not determine scene safety

Initial Assessment

General Impression

Student: My general impression is that the patient's condition is unstable.
PROCTOR: Noted.

Responsiveness/Level of Consciousness

Student: What is the patient's level of consciousness?
PROCTOR: Alert.

Chief Complaint/Apparent Life Threats

Student: What is the patient's chief complaint?
PROCTOR: The patient is complaining of chest pain.

Assess the Airway and Breathing

Student: Is the airway open? Is the patient breathing?
PROCTOR: Yes. The airway is open and the patient is breathing.

Assessment

Student: What are the rate and the quality of breathing?
PROCTOR: Rate: Tachypneic. Quality: Normal.

Provide Oxygen

Student: I am applying oxygen at 15 L/min via nonrebreathing mask.
PROCTOR: Noted.

Ensure Adequate Ventilation

Student: The patient has adequate ventilations at this time.
PROCTOR: Noted.

Assess Circulation

Student: I am assessing the patient's circulation.
PROCTOR: Noted.

Assess for and Control Major Bleeding

Student: Do I find any major bleeding?
PROCTOR: No.

Assess the Pulse

Student: What are the rate and the quality of pulses?
PROCTOR: Rate: Tachycardic. Quality: Bounding.

Assess the Skin

Student: I am assessing the skin. What are the color, temperature, and condition of the skin?
PROCTOR: Color: Flushed. Temperature: Warm. Condition: Moist.

Identify Priority Patients/Make Transport Decision

Student: The patient is a high priority and is a load-and-go. I will begin packaging and transport.
PROCTOR: Noted.

Critical Criteria:
- ❑ Did not provide high concentration of oxygen
- ❑ Did not find or manage problems associated with airway, breathing, hemorrhage or shock (hypoperfusion)
- ❑ Did not differentiate patient's need for transportation versus continued assessment at the scene
- ❑ Did detailed or focused history/physical examination before assessing the airway, breathing and circulation

Focused History and Physical Examination/ Rapid Assessment

Select the Appropriate Assessment (Focused or Rapid)

Student: I am selecting the focused assessment.
PROCTOR: Noted.

SAMPLE History

Student: At this time I will gather a SAMPLE history from the patient or family. What are the patient's signs and symptoms?
PROCTOR: Cardiac.

> **Student:** Onset: What were you doing when this started?
> **PROCTOR:** Working in the yard.
> **Student:** Provokes: What makes your condition worse or better?
> **PROCTOR:** She does not know.
> **Student:** Quality: Can you describe your pain?
> **PROCTOR:** Dull pressure.
> **Student:** Radiates: Do you have pain anywhere else?
> **PROCTOR:** No.
> **Student:** Severity: On a scale of 1 to 10 with 10 being the worst possible, how would you rate your pain/distress?
> **PROCTOR:** 5.
> **Student:** Time: How long has this been going on?
> **PROCTOR:** 8 minutes.
> **Student:** Interventions: Have you done anything to make this better?
> **PROCTOR:** The patient has taken no actions.

Student: Allergies?
PROCTOR: No allergies.
Student: Medications?
PROCTOR: Nitroglycerin.
Student: Pertinent past medical history?
PROCTOR: Angina.
Student: Last oral intake?
PROCTOR: 3 hours ago.
Student: Events leading up to the incident?
PROCTOR: The patient was working in the yard when the pain began.

Perform the Focused Physical Examination

Student: I am performing the focused physical examination.
PROCTOR: Noted.

Student: I will listen to lung sounds.
PROCTOR: Noted.
Student: Are lung sounds present in all fields?
PROCTOR: Yes.

Baseline Vital Signs

Student: What are the patient's baseline vital signs, including blood pressure, pulse, respirations, pulse oximetry, blood glucose level, and level of consciousness?
PROCTOR: Blood pressure, 148/90 mm Hg; pulse rate, 110 beats/min; respirations, 24 breaths/min; pulse oximetry reading, 97%; blood glucose level, 108 mg/dL; and the patient is alert.

Interventions

Student: I will apply oxygen and contact medical control for permission to assist with nitroglycerin administration. I will loosen tight-fitting clothing, and transport the patient in the position of comfort.
PROCTOR: Noted.
ALS Student: I will apply basic life support (BLS) interventions, plus the following: establish IV access, begin cardiac monitoring, 12-lead ECG, and follow advanced cardiac life support (ACLS) or local protocol (nitroglycerin tablet or spray up to three times pending blood pressure over 10 minutes, aspirin, and morphine for pain relief per local protocol).
ALS Proctor: Noted. The cardiac monitor shows sinus tachycardia.

Reevaluate Transport Decision

Student: The patient is a high priority and is a load-and-go due to chest pain.
PROCTOR: Noted.

Detailed Physical Examination

Possible Answer #1
Student: I would not do a detailed physical exam.
PROCTOR: Noted. (Go to "Radio Report.")

Possible Answer #2
Student: I am conducting the detailed physical exam. I am looking for DCAP-BTLS. This acronym stands for deformities, contusions, abrasions, punctures, penetrations, paradoxical motion in the chest, and burns, tenderness, lacerations, and swelling.
PROCTOR: Noted. The detailed physical exam will be performed during transport.

Assess the Head

Student: I am assessing the head. Do I find any DCAP-BTLS? Do I find any evidence of Battle's sign or raccoon eyes?
PROCTOR: No.

Inspect and Palpate the Head and Ears

Student: I am assessing the head and ears.
PROCTOR: There are no obvious injuries.

Assess the Eyes

Student: I am assessing the eyes. Are the pupils equal, round, and regular in size, and react properly to light (PEARRL)?
PROCTOR: They are PEARRL.

Assess the Facial Area Including Oral and Nasal Areas

Student: I am assessing the face, nose, and mouth. Do I see any discharge or hear any obstructions?
PROCTOR: No.

Assess the Neck

Inspect and Palpate the Neck

Student: I am assessing the neck for DCAP-BTLS.
PROCTOR: There are no obvious injuries.

Assess for Jugular Vein Distention

Student: Do I find any jugular vein distention (JVD)?
PROCTOR: No.

Assess for Tracheal Deviation

Student: Do I see any tracheal deviation?
PROCTOR: No.

Assess the Chest

Student: I am assessing the chest for DCAP-BTLS.
PROCTOR: Noted.

Inspect

Student: What do I see when I look at the chest?
PROCTOR: There are no obvious injuries.
Student: Is the chest symmetric?
PROCTOR: Yes.

Palpate

Student: When I touch the chest, do I feel crepitus or a flail segment?
PROCTOR: No.

Auscultate

Student: Are lung sounds present in all fields?
PROCTOR: Yes.
Student: Do I hear any sucking sounds from the chest?
PROCTOR: No.

Assess the Abdomen/Pelvis

Assess the Abdomen

Student: I am assessing the abdomen for DCAP-BTLS. I am assessing all four quadrants. Do I find any problems?
PROCTOR: No.

Assess the Pelvis

Student: I am assessing the pelvis for DCAP-BTLS. Is the pelvis stable?
PROCTOR: Yes.

Assess the Genitalia/Perineum as Needed (Verbalize in Training)

Student: I am assessing the genitalia/perineum as necessary for DCAP-BTLS.
PROCTOR: The area is unremarkable.

Assess the Extremities

Inspect

Student: I am assessing the lower and upper extremities for DCAP-BTLS. Do I find anything?
PROCTOR: No.

Palpate

Student: Do I feel anything unusual?
PROCTOR: No.

Assess Motor, Sensory, and Circulatory Function

Student: I am checking for DCAP-BTLS, motor and sensory function, and pulses. Right leg?
PROCTOR: Negative DCAP-BTLS. Motor and sensory functions are present. Pulses are present.
Student: Left leg?
PROCTOR: Negative DCAP-BTLS. Motor and sensory functions are present. Pulses are present.
Student: Right arm?
PROCTOR: Negative DCAP-BTLS. Motor and sensory functions are present. Pulses are present.
Student: Left arm?
PROCTOR: Negative DCAP-BTLS. Motor and sensory functions are present. Pulses are present.

Assess the Posterior

Student: We will check the back.
PROCTOR: Noted.

Assess the Thorax

Student: I am assessing the thorax. Do I find injuries?
PROCTOR: No.

Assess the Lumbar Area

Student: I am assessing the flanks and lumbar area. Do I find injuries?

PROCTOR: No.

Assess the Entire Backside

Student: I am assessing the entire backside. Do I find injuries?

PROCTOR: No.

Reassess Interventions

Student: I will reassess my interventions: oxygen, contact medical control for permission to assist with nitroglycerin administration, I will loosen tight-fitting clothing, and transport the patient in the position of comfort.

PROCTOR: Noted.

ALS Student: I will reassess BLS interventions, plus the following: establish IV access, cardiac monitor, 12-lead ECG, and ACLS or local protocol (nitroglycerin tablet or spray up to three times pending blood pressure over 10 minutes, aspirin, and morphine for pain relief per local protocol) and assess the effectiveness of treatments.

ALS Proctor: Noted. The cardiac monitor shows sinus tachycardia. Her chest pain has diminished to a 3 on a scale of 10.

Critical Criteria:

- ❑ Did not obtain medical direction or verbalize standing orders for medical interventions
- ❑ Administered a dangerous or inappropriate intervention
- ❑ Did not ask questions about the present illness
- ❑ Did not differentiate patient's need for transportation versus continued assessment at the scene

Radio Report

(Provided by the student.)

PROCTOR: Noted.

Ongoing Assessment

Repeat the Initial Assessment

Student: I will repeat the initial assessment.

PROCTOR: Noted. (Reflected in "Repeat Vital Signs.")

Repeat Vital Signs

Student: I will reassess vital signs and mental status.

PROCTOR: Blood pressure, 128/70 mm Hg; pulse rate, 96 beats/min; respirations, 16 breaths/min; pulse oximetry reading, 98%; and the patient is alert with pain relief.

Student: The vital signs have improved.

PROCTOR: Noted.

Check Interventions

Student: I will check my interventions: oxygen, assess the effectiveness of the nitroglycerin, and transport the patient in the position of comfort.

PROCTOR: Noted.

ALS Student: I will check BLS interventions, plus the following: monitor IV access, cardiac monitor, 12-lead ECG, and ACLS or local protocol, and assess the effectiveness of treatments.

ALS Proctor: Noted. The cardiac monitor shows sinus tachycardia. Her chest pain has diminished to a 1 on a scale of 10.

Repeat the Focused Assessment

Student: I will repeat the focused assessment.

PROCTOR: Noted.

Critical Criteria:

- ❑ Did not obtain medical direction or verbalize standing orders for medical interventions
- ❑ Administered a dangerous or inappropriate intervention

Handoff Report to Emergency Department Staff

Student: The patient's condition improved during transport.

PROCTOR: Noted.

Critical Criteria

(Inform the student of items missed, if any.)

❑ Pass ❑ Fail Date: ____________________

Proctor Comments: ____________________

____

____

CASE 144

Notes

CASE 145

Dispatch Information

PROCTOR: EMS 10, respond to a 15-year-old male who is complaining of a pain crisis from sickle cell anemia. He is conscious and breathing.

Pre-scene Action (BSI)

Student: I am wearing nonlatex gloves and safety glasses.
PROCTOR: Noted.

Critical Criteria:
❑ Did not take, or verbalize, body substance isolation (BSI) precautions when necessary

Scene Size-up

Scene Safety

Student: Is the scene safe?
PROCTOR: Yes.

Mechanism of Injury/Nature of Illness

Student: What is the nature of the illness?
PROCTOR: The patient has pain in the chest, stomach, arms, and legs from sickle cell anemia.

Number of Patients

Student: How many patients are there?
PROCTOR: One.

Additional Resources

Student: I would call for advanced life support (ALS) assistance.
PROCTOR: Noted.

C-Spine Stabilization

Student: I would not stabilize the cervical spine (c-spine).
PROCTOR: Noted.

Critical Criteria:
❑ Did not determine scene safety

Initial Assessment

General Impression

Student: My general impression is that the patient's condition is unstable.
PROCTOR: Noted.

Responsiveness/Level of Consciousness

Student: What is the patient's level of consciousness?
PROCTOR: Alert.

Chief Complaint/Apparent Life Threats

Student: What is the patient's chief complaint?
PROCTOR: The patient is complaining of pain in the chest, stomach, arms, and legs from sickle cell anemia.

Assess the Airway and Breathing

Student: Is the airway open? Is the patient breathing?
PROCTOR: Yes. The airway is open and the patient is breathing.

Assessment

Student: What are the rate and the quality of breathing?
PROCTOR: Rate: Within normal limits. Quality: Normal.

Provide Oxygen

Student: I am applying oxygen at 15 L/min via nonrebreathing mask.
PROCTOR: Noted.

Ensure Adequate Ventilation

Student: The patient has adequate ventilations at this time.
PROCTOR: Noted.

Assess Circulation

Student: I am assessing the patient's circulation.
PROCTOR: Noted.

Assess for and Control Major Bleeding

Student: Do I find any major bleeding?
PROCTOR: No.

Assess the Pulse

Student: What are the rate and the quality of pulses?
PROCTOR: Rate: Tachycardic. Quality: Normal.

Assess the Skin

Student: I am assessing the skin. What are the color, temperature, and condition of the skin?
PROCTOR: Color: Normal. Temperature: Warm. Condition: Moist.

Identify Priority Patients/Make Transport Decision

Student: The patient is a high priority and requires immediate transport.
PROCTOR: Noted.

Critical Criteria:
❑ Did not provide high concentration of oxygen
❑ Did not find or manage problems associated with airway, breathing, hemorrhage or shock (hypoperfusion)
❑ Did not differentiate patient's need for transportation versus continued assessment at the scene
❑ Did detailed or focused history/physical examination before assessing the airway, breathing and circulation

Focused History and Physical Examination/Rapid Assessment

Select the Appropriate Assessment (Focused or Rapid)

Student: I am selecting the focused assessment.
PROCTOR: Noted.

SAMPLE History

Student: At this time I will gather a SAMPLE history from the patient or family. What are the patient's signs and symptoms?
PROCTOR: Respiratory/cardiac.

Student: Onset: What were you doing when this started?
PROCTOR: This has progressed over the last few days.
Student: Provokes: What makes your condition worse or better?
PROCTOR: Blood transfusions make this better.
Student: Quality: Can you describe your pain?
PROCTOR: Aching.
Student: Radiates: Do you have pain anywhere else?
PROCTOR: Chest, stomach, arms, and legs.
Student: Severity: On a scale of 1 to 10 with 10 being the worst possible, how would you rate your pain?
PROCTOR: 7.
Student: Time: How long has this been going on?
PROCTOR: 3 days.
Student: Interventions: Have you done anything to make this better?
PROCTOR: The patient has taken no actions.

Student: Allergies?
PROCTOR: No allergies.
Student: Medications?
PROCTOR: Folic acid and penicillin.
Student: Pertinent past medical history?
PROCTOR: Sickle cell anemia.
Student: Last oral intake?
PROCTOR: 3 hours ago.
Student: Events leading up to the incident?
PROCTOR: The patient has sickle cell anemia and is having a painful crisis episode.

▼ Perform the Focused Physical Examination

Student: I am performing the focused physical examination.
PROCTOR: Noted.
Student: Have you had similar episodes in the past?
PROCTOR: Yes.
Student: Do the blood transfusions help?
PROCTOR: Yes.

▼ Baseline Vital Signs

Student: What are the patient's baseline vital signs, including blood pressure, pulse, respirations, pulse oximetry, blood glucose level, and level of consciousness?
PROCTOR: Blood pressure, 112/68 mm Hg; pulse rate, 96 beats/min; respirations, 28 breaths/min; pulse oximetry reading, 98%; blood glucose level, 114 mg/dL; and the patient is alert.

▼ Interventions

Student: I will apply oxygen, loosen tight-fitting clothing, and transport the patient.
PROCTOR: Noted.
ALS Student: I will apply basic life support (BLS) interventions, plus the following: IV access, cardiac monitor, and pain management per local protocol.
ALS Proctor: Noted. The cardiac monitor shows normal sinus rhythm.

▼ Reevaluate Transport Decision

Student: The patient is a high priority and requires immediate transport.
PROCTOR: Noted.

▼ Detailed Physical Examination

Possible Answer #1
Student: I would not do a detailed physical exam.
PROCTOR: Noted. (Go to "Radio Report.")

Possible Answer #2
Student: I am conducting the detailed physical exam. I am looking for DCAP-BTLS. This acronym stands for deformities, contusions, abrasions, punctures, penetrations, paradoxical motion in the chest, and burns, tenderness, lacerations, and swelling.
PROCTOR: Noted. The detailed physical exam will be performed during transport.

▸ Assess the Head

Student: I am assessing the head. Do I find any DCAP-BTLS? Do I find any evidence of Battle's sign or raccoon eyes?
PROCTOR: No.

▸ Inspect and Palpate the Head and Ears

Student: I am assessing the head and ears.
PROCTOR: There are no obvious injuries.

▸ Assess the Eyes

Student: I am assessing the eyes. Are the pupils equal, round, and regular in size, and react properly to light (PEARRL)?
PROCTOR: They are PEARRL.

▸ Assess the Facial Area Including Oral and Nasal Areas

Student: I am assessing the face, nose, and mouth. Do I see any discharge or hear any obstructions?
PROCTOR: No.

▸ Assess the Neck

▸ Inspect and Palpate the Neck

Student: I am assessing the neck for DCAP-BTLS.
PROCTOR: There are no obvious injuries.

▸ Assess for Jugular Vein Distention

Student: Do I find any jugular vein distention (JVD)?
PROCTOR: No.

▸ Assess for Tracheal Deviation

Student: Do I see any tracheal deviation?
PROCTOR: No.

▸ Assess the Chest

Student: I am assessing the chest for DCAP-BTLS.
PROCTOR: Noted.

▸ Inspect

Student: What do I see when I look at the chest?
PROCTOR: There are no obvious injuries.
Student: Is the chest symmetric?
PROCTOR: Yes.

▸ Palpate

Student: When I touch the chest, do I feel crepitus or a flail segment?
PROCTOR: No.

▸ Auscultate

Student: Are lung sounds present in all fields?
PROCTOR: Yes.
Student: Do I hear any sucking sounds from the chest?
PROCTOR: No.

▸ Assess the Abdomen/Pelvis

▸ Assess the Abdomen

Student: I am assessing the abdomen for DCAP-BTLS. I am assessing all four quadrants. Do I find any problems?
PROCTOR: No.

▸ Assess the Pelvis

Student: I am assessing the pelvis for DCAP-BTLS. Is the pelvis stable?
PROCTOR: Yes.

▸ Assess the Genitalia/Perineum as Needed (Verbalize in Training)

Student: I am assessing the genitalia/perineum as necessary for DCAP-BTLS.
PROCTOR: The area is unremarkable.

▸ Assess the Extremities

▸ Inspect

Student: I am assessing the lower and upper extremities for DCAP-BTLS. Do I find anything?
PROCTOR: No.

▸ Palpate

Student: Do I feel anything unusual?
PROCTOR: No.

▸ Assess Motor, Sensory, and Circulatory Function

Student: I am checking for DCAP-BTLS, motor and sensory function, and pulses. Right leg?
PROCTOR: Negative DCAP-BTLS. Motor and sensory functions are present. Pulses are present.
Student: Left leg?
PROCTOR: Negative DCAP-BTLS. Motor and sensory functions are present. Pulses are present.
Student: Right arm?
PROCTOR: Negative DCAP-BTLS. Motor and sensory functions are present. Pulses are present.
Student: Left arm?
PROCTOR: Negative DCAP-BTLS. Motor and sensory functions are present. Pulses are present.

▸ Assess the Posterior

Student: We will check the back.
PROCTOR: Noted.

▸ Assess the Thorax

Student: I am assessing the thorax. Do I find injuries?
PROCTOR: No.

▸ Assess the Lumbar Area

Student: I am assessing the flanks and lumbar area. Do I find injuries?
PROCTOR: No.

▸ Assess the Entire Backside

Student: I am assessing the entire backside. Do I find injuries?
PROCTOR: No.

▸ **Reassess Interventions**

Student: I will reassess my interventions: apply oxygen, loosen tight-fitting clothing, and transport the patient.

PROCTOR: Noted.

ALS Student: I will reassess BLS interventions, plus the following: IV access, cardiac monitor, and pain management per local protocol.

ALS Proctor: Noted. The cardiac monitor shows normal sinus rhythm.

Critical Criteria:
- ❑ Did not obtain medical direction or verbalize standing orders for medical interventions
- ❑ Administered a dangerous or inappropriate intervention
- ❑ Did not ask questions about the present illness
- ❑ Did not differentiate patient's need for transportation versus continued assessment at the scene

Radio Report

(Provided by the student.)

PROCTOR: Noted.

Ongoing Assessment

Repeat the Initial Assessment

Student: I will repeat the initial assessment.

PROCTOR: Noted. (Reflected in "Repeat Vital Signs.")

Repeat Vital Signs

Student: I will reassess vital signs and mental status.

PROCTOR: Blood pressure, 110/64 mm Hg; pulse rate, 90 beats/min; respirations, 24 breaths/min; pulse oximetry reading, 98%; and the patient is alert.

Student: The vital signs have not changed significantly.

PROCTOR: Noted.

Check Interventions

Student: I will check my interventions: oxygen, loosen tight-fitting clothing, and transport the patient.

PROCTOR: Noted.

ALS Student: I will check BLS interventions, plus the following: IV access, cardiac monitor, and pain management per local protocol.

ALS Proctor: Noted. The cardiac monitor shows normal sinus rhythm.

Repeat the Focused Assessment

Student: I will repeat the focused assessment.

PROCTOR: Noted.

Critical Criteria:
- ❑ Did not obtain medical direction or verbalize standing orders for medical interventions
- ❑ Administered a dangerous or inappropriate intervention

Handoff Report to Emergency Department Staff

Student: There was no change in the patient's condition during transport.

PROCTOR: Noted.

Critical Criteria

(Inform the student of items missed, if any.)

❑ Pass ❑ Fail Date: ____________________

Proctor Comments: ____________________

____

____

Notes

Dispatch Information

PROCTOR: EMS 10, respond to a 50-year-old farmer who has possible organophosphate poisoning. He is unresponsive.

Pre-scene Action (BSI)

Student: I am wearing nonlatex gloves, safety glasses, mask, and gown.
PROCTOR: Noted.

Critical Criteria:
- ❑ Did not take, or verbalize, body substance isolation (BSI) precautions when necessary

Scene Size-up

Scene Safety

Student: Is the scene safe?
PROCTOR: Yes, after the patient has been decontaminated by fire/rescue and hazardous materials responders.

Mechanism of Injury/Nature of Illness

Student: What is the nature of the illness?
PROCTOR: The patient was working on a farm when he was overcome by contact with an organophosphate cloud.

Number of Patients

Student: How many patients are there?
PROCTOR: One.

Additional Resources

Student: I would call for advanced life support (ALS) assistance and additional resources: fire/rescue and hazardous materials responders.
PROCTOR: Noted.
Student: I will allow fire/rescue and hazardous materials crews to decontaminate the patient before I make contact. I will refer to the Emergency Response Guidebook and other resources (three sources minimum).
PROCTOR: Noted.

C-Spine Stabilization

Student: I would not stabilize the cervical spine (c-spine).
PROCTOR: Noted.

Critical Criteria:
- ❑ Did not determine scene safety

Initial Assessment

General Impression

Student: My general impression is that the patient's condition is unstable.
PROCTOR: Noted.

Responsiveness/Level of Consciousness

Student: What is the patient's level of consciousness?
PROCTOR: Unresponsive.

Chief Complaint/Apparent Life Threats

Student: What is the patient's chief complaint?
PROCTOR: The patient is unresponsive.

Assess the Airway and Breathing

Student: Is the airway open? Is the patient breathing?
PROCTOR: Yes, the airway is open and the patient is breathing. He is drooling heavily and has vomited several times.
Student: I will suction as needed.
PROCTOR: Noted.

Assessment

Student: What are the rate and the quality of breathing?
PROCTOR: Rate: Tachypneic. Quality: Shallow.

Provide Oxygen

Student: I will insert an oral airway and assist ventilations with a bag-valve device with 100% oxygen.
PROCTOR: Noted.

Ensure Adequate Ventilation

Student: As noted earlier, I am assisting ventilation with a bag-valve device.
PROCTOR: Noted.

Assess Circulation

Student: I am assessing the patient's circulation.
PROCTOR: Noted.

Assess for and Control Major Bleeding

Student: Do I find any major bleeding?
PROCTOR: No.

Assess the Pulse

Student: What are the rate and the quality of pulses?
PROCTOR: Rate: Bradycardic. Quality: Bounding.

Assess the Skin

Student: I am assessing the skin. What are the color, temperature, and condition of the skin?
PROCTOR: Color: Cyanotic. Temperature: Cool. Condition: Diaphoretic.

Identify Priority Patients/Make Transport Decision

Student: The patient is a high priority and is a load-and-go. I will begin packaging and transport.
PROCTOR: Noted.

Critical Criteria:
- ❑ Did not provide high concentration of oxygen
- ❑ Did not find or manage problems associated with airway, breathing, hemorrhage or shock (hypoperfusion)
- ❑ Did not differentiate patient's need for transportation versus continued assessment at the scene
- ❑ Did detailed or focused history/physical examination before assessing the airway, breathing and circulation

Focused History and Physical Examination/Rapid Assessment

Select the Appropriate Assessment (Focused or Rapid)

Student: I am selecting the rapid physical exam to identify and treat life threats.
PROCTOR: Noted.
Student: I am checking for DCAP-BTLS. This acronym stands for deformities, contusions, abrasions, punctures, penetrations, paradoxical motion in the chest, and burns, tenderness, lacerations, and swelling. I am also checking for motor and sensory function and pulses.
PROCTOR: Noted.

Head

Student: I am rapidly assessing the head.
PROCTOR: His pupils are pinpoint. He is diaphoretic and has vomit all over his face.
Student: I will suction as needed.
PROCTOR: Noted.

Neck

Student: I am rapidly assessing the neck.
PROCTOR: He is very sweaty.

▸ **Chest**

Student: I am rapidly assessing the chest.
PROCTOR: He is very sweaty.
Student: Are there lung sounds present?
PROCTOR: You hear wheezes bilaterally.

▸ **Abdomen/Pelvis**

Student: I am rapidly assessing the abdomen.
PROCTOR: There are no obvious injuries.
Student: I am rapidly assessing the pelvis.
PROCTOR: The patient is incontinent of urine and stool.

▸ **Extremities**

Student: I am rapidly assessing the extremities.
PROCTOR: There are no obvious injuries.

▸ **Assess Motor, Sensory, and Circulatory Function**

Student: I am checking for DCAP-BTLS. Right leg?
PROCTOR: Negative DCAP-BTLS. Motor and sensory functions are absent. Pulses are present.
Student: Left leg?
PROCTOR: Negative DCAP-BTLS. Motor and sensory functions are absent. Pulses are present.
Student: Right arm?
PROCTOR: Negative DCAP-BTLS. Motor and sensory functions are absent. Pulses are present.
Student: Left arm?
PROCTOR: Negative DCAP-BTLS. Motor and sensory functions are absent. Pulses are present.

▸ **Posterior**

Student: I will rapidly assess the back.
PROCTOR: Noted.

▸ **Assess the Thorax**

Student: I am assessing the thorax. Do I find injuries?
PROCTOR: No.

▸ **Assess the Lumbar Area**

Student: I am assessing the flanks and lumbar area. Do I find injuries?
PROCTOR: No.

▸ **Assess the Entire Backside**

Student: I am assessing the entire backside. Do I find injuries?
PROCTOR: No.

▸ **Reevaluate Transport Decision**

Student: The patient is a high priority and is a load-and-go due to the nature of the illness.
PROCTOR: Noted.

▾ SAMPLE History

Student: At this time I will gather a SAMPLE history from the patient or family. What are the patient's signs and symptoms?
PROCTOR: Poisoning/overdose.
Student: What was the substance?
PROCTOR: An organophosphate.
Student: When did the patient become exposed to the material?
PROCTOR: 15 minutes ago.
Student: How much did he ingest?
PROCTOR: None.
Student: Over what time period?
PROCTOR: Over 5 minutes.
Student: Interventions: Has he done anything to make this better?
PROCTOR: No. But he has been decontaminated by the hazardous materials team.
Student: What is the patient's weight?
PROCTOR: 175 pounds.
Student: Allergies?
PROCTOR: Unknown.
Student: Medications?
PROCTOR: Unknown.
Student: Pertinent past medical history?
PROCTOR: Unknown.
Student: Last oral intake?
PROCTOR: Unknown.
Student: Events leading up to the incident?
PROCTOR: The patient was working on the farm when he walked into a cloud of organophosphate.
Student: Are SLUDGEM (The SLUDGEM mnemonic stands for Salivation, Sweating, Seizures; Lacrimation [tearing]; Urination; Defecation, Drooling, Diarrhea; Gastric upset and cramps; Emesis; and Muscle twitching) or DUMBELS present (The DUMBELS mnemonic stands for Diarrhea; Urination; Miosis [pinpoint pupils]; Bradycardia, Bronchospasm; Emesis; Lacrimation [tearing]; and Seizures, Salivation, Sweating.)?
PROCTOR: Yes. He is drooling heavily and vomiting. He is incontinent of urine and stool with diarrhea. He is sweating profusely and has muscle twitching. His pupils are pinpoint. His heart rate is bradycardic.

▾ Interventions

Student: I will apply suction, insert an oral/advanced airway, and apply oxygen with a bag-valve device. I will transport on a backboard.
PROCTOR: Noted.
ALS Student: I will apply basic life support (BLS) interventions, plus the following: intubation confirmed with end tidal CO_2 and lung sounds, IV access with two large-bore IVs, cardiac monitor, advanced cardiac life support (ACLS) and local protocol (Mark I Kits and possible diazepam).
ALS Proctor: Noted. The cardiac monitor shows sinus bradycardia.

▾ Baseline Vital Signs

Student: What are the patient's baseline vital signs, including blood pressure, pulse, respirations, pulse oximetry, blood glucose level, and level of consciousness?
PROCTOR: Blood pressure, 140/90 mm Hg; pulse rate, 56 beats/min; respirations per bag-valve-mask; pulse oximetry reading, N/A; blood glucose level, 104 mg/dL and the patient is unresponsive.

▾ Detailed Physical Examination

Possible Answer #1
Student: I would not do a detailed physical exam.
PROCTOR: Noted. (Go to "Radio Report.")

Possible Answer #2
Student: I am conducting the detailed physical exam. I am looking for DCAP-BTLS.
PROCTOR: Noted. The detailed physical exam will be performed during transport.

▸ **Assess the Head**

Student: I am assessing the head. Do I find any DCAP-BTLS? Do I find any evidence of Battle's sign or raccoon eyes?
PROCTOR: No.

▸ **Inspect and Palpate the Head and Ears**

Student: I am assessing the head and ears.
PROCTOR: He is very sweaty.

▸ **Assess the Eyes**

Student: I am assessing the eyes. Are the pupils equal, round, and regular in size, and react properly to light (PEARRL)?
PROCTOR: They are pinpoint.

▸ **Assess the Facial Area Including Oral and Nasal Areas**

Student: I am assessing the face, nose, and mouth. Do I see any discharge or hear any obstructions?
PROCTOR: Yes, he is drooling.

Student: I will suction the airway as needed.
PROCTOR: Noted.
ALS Student: I will confirm endotracheal (ET) tube placement with lung sounds and end tidal CO_2.
ALS Proctor: Lung sounds and end tidal CO_2 confirm tube placement.

- **Assess the Neck**
  - **Inspect and Palpate the Neck**

Student: I am assessing the neck for DCAP-BTLS.
PROCTOR: There are no obvious injuries.

- **Assess for Jugular Vein Distention**

Student: Do I find any jugular vein distention (JVD)?
PROCTOR: No.

- **Assess for Tracheal Deviation**

Student: Do I see any tracheal deviation?
PROCTOR: No.

- **Assess the Chest**

Student: I am assessing the chest for DCAP-BTLS.
PROCTOR: He is very sweaty.

- **Inspect**

Student: What do I see when I look at the chest?
PROCTOR: There are no obvious injuries.
Student: Is the chest symmetric?
PROCTOR: Yes.

- **Palpate**

Student: When I touch the chest, do I feel crepitus or a flail segment?
PROCTOR: No.

- **Auscultate**

Student: Are lung sounds present in all fields?
PROCTOR: There is wheezing present.
Student: Do I hear any sucking sounds from the chest?
PROCTOR: No.

- **Assess the Abdomen/Pelvis**
  - **Assess the Abdomen**

Student: I am assessing the abdomen for DCAP-BTLS. I am assessing all four quadrants. Do I find any problems?
PROCTOR: No.

- **Assess the Pelvis**

Student: I am assessing the pelvis for DCAP-BTLS. Is the pelvis stable?
PROCTOR: Yes.

- **Assess the Genitalia/Perineum as Needed (Verbalize in Training)**

Student: I am assessing the genitalia/perineum as necessary for DCAP-BTLS.
PROCTOR: The patient is incontinent of urine and stool.

- **Assess the Extremities**
  - **Inspect**

Student: I am assessing the lower and upper extremities for DCAP-BTLS. Do I find anything?
PROCTOR: No.

- **Palpate**

Student: Do I feel anything unusual?
PROCTOR: No.

- **Assess Motor, Sensory, and Circulatory Function**

Student: I am checking for DCAP-BTLS, motor and sensory function, and pulses. Right leg?
PROCTOR: Negative DCAP-BTLS. Motor and sensory functions are absent. Pulses are present.
Student: Left leg?
PROCTOR: Negative DCAP-BTLS. Motor and sensory functions are absent. Pulses are present.
Student: Right arm?
PROCTOR: Negative DCAP-BTLS. Motor and sensory functions are absent. Pulses are present.
Student: Left arm?
PROCTOR: Negative DCAP-BTLS. Motor and sensory functions are absent. Pulses are present.

- **Assess the Posterior**

Student: We will check the back.
PROCTOR: Noted.

- **Assess the Thorax**

Student: I am assessing the thorax. Do I find injuries?
PROCTOR: No.

- **Assess the Lumbar Area**

Student: I am assessing the flanks and lumbar area. Do I find injuries?
PROCTOR: No.

- **Assess the Entire Backside**

Student: I am assessing the entire backside. Do I find injuries?
PROCTOR: No.

- **Reassess Interventions**

Student: I will reassess my interventions: apply suction as needed, insert an oral/advanced airway, and apply oxygen using a bag-valve device, and transport on a backboard.
PROCTOR: Noted.
ALS Student: I will reassess BLS interventions, plus the following: intubation confirmed with end tidal CO_2 and lung sounds, IV access, cardiac monitor, 12-lead ECG, ACLS and local protocol (Mark I Kits and possible diazepam).
ALS Proctor: Noted. The cardiac monitor shows sinus bradycardia.

Critical Criteria:
- ❑ Did not obtain medical direction or verbalize standing orders for medical interventions
- ❑ Administered a dangerous or inappropriate intervention
- ❑ Did not ask questions about the present illness
- ❑ Did not differentiate patient's need for transportation versus continued assessment at the scene

Radio Report

(Provided by the student.)
PROCTOR: Noted.

Ongoing Assessment

Repeat the Initial Assessment

Student: I will repeat the initial assessment.
PROCTOR: Noted. (Reflected in "Repeat Vital Signs.")

Repeat Vital Signs

Student: I will reassess vital signs and mental status.
PROCTOR: Blood pressure, 146/90 mm Hg; pulse rate, 50 beats/min; respirations per bag-valve-mask; pulse oximetry reading, N/A; and the patient is unresponsive.
Student: The vital signs have not changed significantly.
PROCTOR: Noted.

▼ Check Interventions

Student: I will check my interventions: apply suction as needed, insert an oral/advanced airway, and apply oxygen using a bag-valve device, and transport on a backboard.

PROCTOR: Noted.

ALS Student: I will check BLS interventions, plus the following: intubation confirmed with end tidal CO_2 and lung sounds, IV access, cardiac monitor, 12-lead ECG, ACLS, and local protocol (Mark I Kits and possible diazepam).

ALS Proctor: Noted. The cardiac monitor shows sinus bradycardia.

Critical Criteria:
- ❑ Did not obtain medical direction or verbalize standing orders for medical interventions
- ❑ Administered a dangerous or inappropriate intervention

▼ Handoff Report to Emergency Department Staff

Student: There was no change in the patient's condition during transport.

PROCTOR: Noted.

▼ Critical Criteria

(Inform the student of items missed, if any.)

❑ Pass ❑ Fail Date: ____________________

Proctor Comments: ____________________

____

____

Dispatch Information

PROCTOR: EMS 10, respond to a church where a 30-year-old female has passed out. She is conscious and breathing.

Pre-scene Action (BSI)

Student: I am wearing nonlatex gloves and safety glasses.
PROCTOR: Noted.

Critical Criteria:
- ❑ Did not take, or verbalize, body substance isolation (BSI) precautions when necessary

Scene Size-up

Scene Safety

Student: Is the scene safe?
PROCTOR: Yes.

Mechanism of Injury/Nature of Illness

Student: What is the nature of the illness?
PROCTOR: The patient was singing a solo in church and passed out.

Number of Patients

Student: How many patients are there?
PROCTOR: One.

Additional Resources

Student: I would call for advanced life support (ALS) assistance.
PROCTOR: Noted.

C-Spine Stabilization

Student: On the basis of the nature of the illness, I would stabilize the cervical spine (c-spine) in a neutral in-line position.
PROCTOR: Noted.

Critical Criteria:
- ❑ Did not determine scene safety

Initial Assessment

Student: As I perform midline c-spine stabilization, I identify myself and ask the patient not to move.
PROCTOR: Noted.

General Impression

Student: My general impression is that the patient's condition is stable.
PROCTOR: Noted.

Responsiveness/Level of Consciousness

Student: What is the patient's level of consciousness?
PROCTOR: Alert.

Chief Complaint/Apparent Life Threats

Student: What is the patient's chief complaint?
PROCTOR: The patient has pain in the neck and back.

Assess the Airway and Breathing

Student: Is the airway open? Is the patient breathing?
PROCTOR: Yes, the airway is open and the patient is breathing.

Assessment

Student: What are the rate and the quality of breathing?
PROCTOR: Rate: Within normal limits. Quality: Normal.

Provide Oxygen

Student: I am applying oxygen at 15 L/min via nonrebreathing mask.
PROCTOR: Noted.

Ensure Adequate Ventilation

Student: The patient has adequate ventilations at this time.
PROCTOR: Noted.

Assess Circulation

Student: I am assessing the patient's circulation.
PROCTOR: Noted.

Assess for and Control Major Bleeding

Student: Do I find any major bleeding?
PROCTOR: No.

Assess the Pulse

Student: What are the rate and the quality of pulses?
PROCTOR: Rate: Within normal limits. Quality: Normal.

Assess the Skin

Student: I am assessing the skin. What are the color, temperature, and condition of the skin?
PROCTOR: Color: Flushed. Temperature: Warm. Condition: Moist.

Identify Priority Patients/Make Transport Decision

Student: The patient is a low priority and does not require immediate transport.
PROCTOR: Noted.

Critical Criteria:
- ❑ Did not provide high concentration of oxygen
- ❑ Did not find or manage problems associated with airway, breathing, hemorrhage or shock (hypoperfusion)
- ❑ Did not differentiate patient's need for transportation versus continued assessment at the scene
- ❑ Did detailed or focused history/physical examination before assessing the airway, breathing and circulation

Focused History and Physical Examination/Rapid Assessment

Select the Appropriate Assessment (Focused or Rapid)

Student: I am selecting the rapid assessment.
PROCTOR: Noted.
Student: I am checking for DCAP-BTLS. This acronym stands for deformities, contusions, abrasions, punctures, penetrations, paradoxical motion in the chest, and burns, tenderness, lacerations, and swelling. I am also checking for motor and sensory function and pulses.
PROCTOR: Noted.

Head

Student: I am rapidly assessing the head.
PROCTOR: There are no obvious injuries.

Neck

Student: I am rapidly assessing the neck.
PROCTOR: She is complaining of neck pain.
Student: I will apply a cervical collar.
PROCTOR: Noted.

Chest

Student: I am rapidly inspecting and palpating the chest.
PROCTOR: There are no obvious injuries.
Student: Are there lung sounds present?
PROCTOR: They are clear bilaterally.

Abdomen

Student: I am rapidly assessing the abdomen.
PROCTOR: There are no obvious injuries.

Pelvis

Student: I am rapidly assessing the pelvis.
PROCTOR: There are no obvious injuries.

Extremities

Student: I am rapidly assessing the extremities.
PROCTOR: There are no obvious injuries.

Assess Motor, Sensory, and Circulatory Function

Student: I am checking for DCAP-BTLS. Right leg?
PROCTOR: Negative DCAP-BTLS. Motor and sensory functions are present. Pulses are present.

Student: Left leg?
PROCTOR: Negative DCAP-BTLS. Motor and sensory functions are present. Pulses are present.
Student: Right arm?
PROCTOR: Negative DCAP-BTLS. Motor and sensory functions are present. Pulses are present.
Student: Left arm?
PROCTOR: Negative DCAP-BTLS. Motor and sensory functions are present. Pulses are present.

▶ **Posterior**

Student: I am rapidly assessing the back. We will now log roll the patient as a unit to check the back. The person at the head will count to three and we will roll the patient.
PROCTOR: Noted.

▶ **Assess the Thorax**

Student: I am assessing the thorax. Do I find injuries?
PROCTOR: Yes, she has a bruise to her upper middle back.

▶ **Assess the Lumbar Area**

Student: I am assessing the flanks and lumbar area. Do I find injuries?
PROCTOR: No.

▶ **Assess the Entire Backside**

Student: I am assessing the entire backside. Do I find injuries?
PROCTOR: No.

▶ **Manage Secondary Injuries/Wounds**

Student: We will apply a cervical collar and backboard with full immobilization per local protocol, if not yet done, at this time.
PROCTOR: Noted.
Student: Are there any changes in motor and sensory functions and pulses?
PROCTOR: No.

▶ **Reevaluate Transport Decision**

Student: The patient is a low priority and does not require immediate transport.
PROCTOR: Noted.

▼ Baseline Vital Signs

Student: What are the patient's baseline vital signs, including blood pressure, pulse, respirations, pulse oximetry, blood glucose level, and level of consciousness?
PROCTOR: Blood pressure, 118/68 mm Hg; pulse rate, 62 beats/min; respirations, 16 breaths/min; pulse oximetry reading, 98%; blood glucose level, 116 mg/dL; and the patient is alert.

▼ SAMPLE History

Student: At this time I will gather a SAMPLE history from the patient or family. What are the patient's signs and symptoms?
PROCTOR: Altered mental status.
Student: Describe the episode.
PROCTOR: The patient was singing a solo for the first time when she passed out and fell off the stage.
Student: Onset: What was she doing when this started?
PROCTOR: Singing a solo.
Student: Duration: How long has this been going on?
PROCTOR: 2 minutes.
Student: Are there any associated symptoms?
PROCTOR: Yes, she has pain in the neck and back.
Student: Is there any evidence of trauma?
PROCTOR: Yes, she has a bruise to her upper middle back.
Student: Interventions: Has she done anything to make this better?
PROCTOR: The patient has taken no actions.
Student: Have there been any seizures?
PROCTOR: No.
Student: Has there been any fever?
PROCTOR: No.
Student: Allergies?
PROCTOR: No allergies.
Student: Medications?
PROCTOR: No medications.
Student: Pertinent past medical history?
PROCTOR: No pertinent medical history.
Student: Last oral intake?
PROCTOR: 2 hours ago.
Student: Events leading up to the incident?
PROCTOR: The patient was singing and passed out.

▼ Interventions

Student: I will continue oxygen at 15 L/min via nonrebreathing mask. I will check her blood glucose level, and transport her fully immobilized.
PROCTOR: Noted. Her blood glucose level is 116 mg/dL.
ALS Student: I will apply basic life support (BLS) interventions, plus the following: IV access and cardiac monitor.
ALS Proctor: Noted. The cardiac monitor shows normal sinus rhythm.

▼ Detailed Physical Examination

Possible Answer #1
Student: I would not do a detailed physical exam.
PROCTOR: Noted. (Go to "Radio Report.")

Possible Answer #2
Student: I am conducting the detailed physical exam. I am looking for DCAP-BTLS.
PROCTOR: Noted. The detailed physical exam will be performed during transport.

▶ **Assess the Head**

Student: I am assessing the head. Do I find any DCAP-BTLS? Do I find any evidence of Battle's sign or raccoon eyes?
PROCTOR: No.

▶ **Inspect and Palpate the Head and Ears**

Student: I am assessing the head and ears.
PROCTOR: There are no obvious injuries.

▶ **Assess the Eyes**

Student: I am assessing the eyes. Are the pupils equal, round, and regular in size, and react properly to light (PEARRL)?
PROCTOR: They are PEARRL.

▶ **Assess the Facial Area Including Oral and Nasal Areas**

Student: I am assessing the face, nose, and mouth. Do I see any discharge or hear any obstructions?
PROCTOR: No.

▶ **Assess the Neck**

▶ **Inspect and Palpate the Neck**

Student: I am assessing the neck for DCAP-BTLS.
PROCTOR: The patient has pain.

▶ **Assess for Jugular Vein Distention**

Student: Do I find any jugular vein distention (JVD)?
PROCTOR: No.

▶ **Assess for Tracheal Deviation**

Student: Do I see any tracheal deviation?
PROCTOR: No.

▶ **Assess the Chest**

Student: I am assessing the chest for DCAP-BTLS.
PROCTOR: Noted.

▶ **Inspect**

Student: What do I see when I look at the chest?
PROCTOR: There are no obvious injuries.
Student: Is the chest symmetric?
PROCTOR: Yes.

▸ **Palpate**

Student: When I touch the chest, do I feel crepitus or a flail segment?

PROCTOR: No.

▸ **Auscultate**

Student: Are lung sounds present in all fields?

PROCTOR: Yes.

Student: Do I hear any sucking sounds from the chest?

PROCTOR: No.

▸ **Assess the Abdomen/Pelvis**

▸ **Assess the Abdomen**

Student: I am assessing the abdomen for DCAP-BTLS. I am assessing all four quadrants. Do I find any problems?

PROCTOR: No.

▸ **Assess the Pelvis**

Student: I am assessing the pelvis for DCAP-BTLS. Is the pelvis stable?

PROCTOR: Yes.

▸ **Assess the Genitalia/Perineum as Needed (Verbalize in Training)**

Student: I am assessing the genitalia/perineum as necessary for DCAP-BTLS.

PROCTOR: The area is unremarkable.

▸ **Assess the Extremities**

▸ **Inspect**

Student: I am assessing the lower and upper extremities for DCAP-BTLS. Do I find anything?

PROCTOR: No.

▸ **Palpate**

Student: Do I feel anything unusual?

PROCTOR: No.

▸ **Assess Motor, Sensory, and Circulatory Function**

Student: I am checking for DCAP-BTLS, motor and sensory function, and pulses. Right leg?

PROCTOR: Negative DCAP-BTLS. Motor and sensory functions are present. Pulses are present.

Student: Left leg?

PROCTOR: Negative DCAP-BTLS. Motor and sensory functions are present. Pulses are present.

Student: Right arm?

PROCTOR: Negative DCAP-BTLS. Motor and sensory functions are present. Pulses are present.

Student: Left arm?

PROCTOR: Negative DCAP-BTLS. Motor and sensory functions are present. Pulses are present.

▸ **Assess the Posterior**

Note: This portion of the detailed physical exam would not be done if the patient were previously backboarded per local protocol.

Student: We will not check the back because it was previously checked and the patient is backboarded.

PROCTOR: Noted.

▸ **Reassess Interventions**

Student: I will reassess my interventions: oxygen, immobilization, and straps.

PROCTOR: Noted.

ALS Student: I will reassess BLS interventions, plus the following: IV access and cardiac monitor.

ALS Proctor: Noted. The cardiac monitor shows normal sinus rhythm.

Critical Criteria:

- ❑ Did not obtain medical direction or verbalize standing orders for medical interventions
- ❑ Administered a dangerous or inappropriate intervention
- ❑ Did not ask questions about the present illness
- ❑ Did not differentiate patient's need for transportation versus continued assessment at the scene

Radio Report

(Provided by the student.)

PROCTOR: Noted.

Ongoing Assessment

Repeat the Initial Assessment

Student: I will repeat the initial assessment.

PROCTOR: Noted. (Reflected in "Repeat Vital Signs.")

Repeat Vital Signs

Student: I will reassess vital signs and mental status.

PROCTOR: Blood pressure, 124/72 mm Hg; pulse rate, 66 beats/min; respirations, 16 breaths/min; pulse oximetry reading, 98%; and the patient is alert.

Student: The vital signs have not changed significantly.

PROCTOR: Noted.

Check Interventions

Student: I will check my interventions: oxygen, immobilization, and straps.

PROCTOR: Noted.

ALS Student: I will check BLS interventions, plus the following: IV access and cardiac monitor.

ALS Proctor: Noted. The cardiac monitor shows normal sinus rhythm.

Repeat the Focused Assessment

Student: I will repeat the focused assessment.

PROCTOR: Noted.

Critical Criteria:

- ❑ Did not obtain medical direction or verbalize standing orders for medical interventions
- ❑ Administered a dangerous or inappropriate intervention

Handoff Report to Emergency Department Staff

Student: There was no change in the patient's condition during transport.

PROCTOR: Noted.

Critical Criteria

(Inform the student of items missed, if any.)

❑ Pass ❑ Fail Date: ______________________

Proctor Comments: ______________________

Notes

CASE 148

Dispatch Information

PROCTOR: EMS 10, respond to a 15-year-old female who is complaining of a possible asthma attack. She is conscious and breathing.

Pre-scene Action (BSI)

Student: I am wearing nonlatex gloves and safety glasses.
PROCTOR: Noted.

Critical Criteria:
- ❑ Did not take, or verbalize, body substance isolation (BSI) precautions when necessary

Scene Size-up

Scene Safety

Student: Is the scene safe?
PROCTOR: Yes.

Mechanism of Injury/Nature of Illness

Student: What is the nature of the illness?
PROCTOR: The patient was participating in a school nature hike and is having a possible asthma attack.

Number of Patients

Student: How many patients are there?
PROCTOR: One.

Additional Resources

Student: I would call for advanced life support (ALS) assistance.
PROCTOR: Noted.

C-Spine Stabilization

Student: I would not stabilize the cervical spine (c-spine).
PROCTOR: Noted.

Critical Criteria:
- ❑ Did not determine scene safety

Initial Assessment

General Impression

Student: My general impression is that the patient's condition is unstable.
PROCTOR: Noted.

Responsiveness/Level of Consciousness

Student: What is the patient's level of consciousness?
PROCTOR: Alert.

Chief Complaint/Apparent Life Threats

Student: What is the patient's chief complaint?
PROCTOR: The patient is complaining of difficulty breathing.

Assess the Airway and Breathing

Student: Is the airway open? Is the patient breathing?
PROCTOR: Yes, the airway is open and the patient is breathing.

Assessment

Student: What are the rate and the quality of breathing?
PROCTOR: Rate: Tachypneic. Quality: Shallow with wheezes during exhalation.

Provide Oxygen

Student: I am applying oxygen at 15 L/min via nonrebreathing mask.
PROCTOR: Noted.

Ensure Adequate Ventilation

Student: The patient has adequate ventilations at this time.
PROCTOR: Noted.

Assess Circulation

Student: I am assessing the patient's circulation.
PROCTOR: Noted.

Assess for and Control Major Bleeding

Student: Do I find any major bleeding?
PROCTOR: No.

Assess the Pulse

Student: What are the rate and the quality of pulses?
PROCTOR: Rate: Tachycardic. Quality: Bounding.

Assess the Skin

Student: I am assessing the skin. What are the color, temperature, and condition of the skin?
PROCTOR: Color: Pale. Temperature: Cool. Condition: Moist.

Identify Priority Patients/Make Transport Decision

Student: The patient is a high priority and is a load-and-go. I will begin packaging and transport.
PROCTOR: Noted.

Critical Criteria:
- ❑ Did not provide high concentration of oxygen
- ❑ Did not find or manage problems associated with airway, breathing, hemorrhage or shock (hypoperfusion)
- ❑ Did not differentiate patient's need for transportation versus continued assessment at the scene
- ❑ Did detailed or focused history/physical examination before assessing the airway, breathing and circulation

Focused History and Physical Examination/Rapid Assessment

Select the Appropriate Assessment (Focused or Rapid)

Student: I am selecting the focused assessment.
PROCTOR: Noted.

SAMPLE History

Student: At this time I will gather a SAMPLE history from the patient or family. What are the patient's signs and symptoms?
PROCTOR: Respiratory (difficulty breathing).

> **Student:** Onset: What were you doing when this started?
> **PROCTOR:** The patient was on a nature hike.
> **Student:** Provokes: What makes your condition worse or better?
> **PROCTOR:** Nothing has made it better.
> **Student:** Quality: Can you describe your pain?
> **PROCTOR:** None.
> **Student:** Radiates: Do you have pain anywhere else?
> **PROCTOR:** No.
> **Student:** Severity: On a scale of 1 to 10 with 10 being the worst possible, how would you rate your distress?
> **PROCTOR:** 9.
> **Student:** Time: How long has this been going on?
> **PROCTOR:** 15 minutes.
> **Student:** Interventions: Have you done anything to make this better?
> **PROCTOR:** The patient has taken no actions.

Student: Allergies?
PROCTOR: No allergies.
Student: Medications?
PROCTOR: No medications.
Student: Pertinent past medical history?
PROCTOR: No pertinent medical history.
Student: Last oral intake?
PROCTOR: 4 hours ago.
Student: Events leading up to the incident?
PROCTOR: The patient was on a nature hike.

▼ Perform the Focused Physical Examination

Student: I am performing the focused physical examination.
PROCTOR: Noted.
Student: Are there lung sounds present?
PROCTOR: There are wheezes on exhalation bilaterally.

▼ Baseline Vital Signs

Student: What are the patient's baseline vital signs, including blood pressure, pulse, respirations, pulse oximetry, and level of consciousness?
PROCTOR: Blood pressure, 120/76 mm Hg; pulse rate, 120 beats/min; respirations, 28 breaths/min; pulse oximetry reading, 96%; and the patient is anxious.

▼ Interventions

Student: I will apply oxygen, basic life support (BLS) breathing treatment (if permitted by local protocol), and reassurance.
PROCTOR: Noted.
ALS Student: I will apply BLS interventions, plus the following: IV access, cardiac monitor, and local protocol (breathing treatment).
ALS Proctor: Noted. The cardiac monitor shows sinus tachycardia.

▼ Reevaluate Transport Decision

Student: The patient is a high priority and a load-and-go if I am unable to provide breathing treatment.
PROCTOR: Noted.

▼ Detailed Physical Examination

Possible Answer #1
Student: I would not do a detailed physical exam.
PROCTOR: Noted. (Go to "Radio Report.")

Possible Answer #2
Student: I am conducting the detailed physical exam. I am looking for DCAP-BTLS. This acronym stands for deformities, contusions, abrasions, punctures, penetrations, paradoxical motion in the chest, and burns, tenderness, lacerations, and swelling.
PROCTOR: Noted. The detailed physical exam will be performed during transport.

▶ **Assess the Head**

Student: I am assessing the head. Do I find any DCAP-BTLS? Do I find any evidence of Battle's sign or raccoon eyes?
PROCTOR: No.

▶ **Inspect and Palpate the Head and Ears**

Student: I am assessing the head and ears.
PROCTOR: There are no obvious injuries.

▶ **Assess the Eyes**

Student: I am assessing the eyes. Are the pupils equal, round, and regular in size, and react properly to light (PEARRL)?
PROCTOR: They are PEARRL.

▶ **Assess the Facial Area Including Oral and Nasal Areas**

Student: I am assessing the face, nose, and mouth. Do I see any discharge or hear any obstructions?
PROCTOR: No.

▶ **Assess the Neck**

▶ **Inspect and Palpate the Neck**

Student: I am assessing the neck for DCAP-BTLS.
PROCTOR: There are no obvious injuries.

▶ **Assess for Jugular Vein Distention**

Student: Do I find any jugular vein distention (JVD)?
PROCTOR: No.

▶ **Assess for Tracheal Deviation**

Student: Do I see any tracheal deviation?
PROCTOR: No.

▶ **Assess the Chest**

Student: I am assessing the chest for DCAP-BTLS.
PROCTOR: Noted.

▶ **Inspect**

Student: What do I see when I look at the chest?
PROCTOR: There are no obvious injuries.
Student: Is the chest symmetric?
PROCTOR: Yes.

▶ **Palpate**

Student: When I touch the chest, do I feel crepitus or a flail segment?
PROCTOR: No.

▶ **Auscultate**

Student: Are lung sounds present in all fields?
PROCTOR: Yes. She has wheezes on exhalation bilaterally.
Student: Do I hear any sucking sounds from the chest?
PROCTOR: No.

▶ **Assess the Abdomen/Pelvis**

▶ **Assess the Abdomen**

Student: I am assessing the abdomen for DCAP-BTLS. I am assessing all four quadrants. Do I find any problems?
PROCTOR: No.

▶ **Assess the Pelvis**

Student: I am assessing the pelvis for DCAP-BTLS. Is the pelvis stable?
PROCTOR: Yes.

▶ **Assess the Genitalia/Perineum as Needed (Verbalize in Training)**

Student: I am assessing the genitalia/perineum as necessary for DCAP-BTLS.
PROCTOR: The area is unremarkable.

▶ **Assess the Extremities**

▶ **Inspect**

Student: I am assessing the lower and upper extremities for DCAP-BTLS. Do I find anything?
PROCTOR: No.

▶ **Palpate**

Student: Do I feel anything unusual?
PROCTOR: No.

▶ **Assess Motor, Sensory, and Circulatory Function**

Student: I am checking for DCAP-BTLS, motor and sensory function, and pulses. Right leg?
PROCTOR: Negative DCAP-BTLS. Motor and sensory functions are present. Pulses are present.
Student: Left leg?
PROCTOR: Negative DCAP-BTLS. Motor and sensory functions are present. Pulses are present.
Student: Right arm?
PROCTOR: Negative DCAP-BTLS. Motor and sensory functions are present. Pulses are present.
Student: Left arm?
PROCTOR: Negative DCAP-BTLS. Motor and sensory functions are present. Pulses are present.

▶ **Assess the Posterior**

Student: We will check the back.
PROCTOR: Noted.

▶ **Assess the Thorax**

Student: I am assessing the thorax. Do I find injuries?
PROCTOR: No.

▶ **Assess the Lumbar Area**

Student: I am assessing the flanks and lumbar area. Do I find injuries?
PROCTOR: No.

▶ **Assess the Entire Backside**

Student: I am assessing the entire backside. Do I find injuries?
PROCTOR: No.

▸ **Reassess Interventions**

Student: I will reassess my interventions: oxygen, BLS breathing treatment (if permitted), and reassurance.

PROCTOR: Noted. Breathing improved with treatment if given.

ALS Student: I will reassess BLS interventions, plus the following: IV access, cardiac monitor, and local protocol (breathing treatment).

ALS Proctor: Noted. The cardiac monitor shows sinus tachycardia. Breathing improved with treatment.

Critical Criteria:
- ❑ Did not obtain medical direction or verbalize standing orders for medical interventions
- ❑ Administered a dangerous or inappropriate intervention
- ❑ Did not ask questions about the present illness
- ❑ Did not differentiate patient's need for transportation versus continued assessment at the scene

Radio Report

(Provided by the student.)

PROCTOR: Noted.

Ongoing Assessment

Repeat the Initial Assessment

Student: I will repeat the initial assessment.

PROCTOR: Noted. (Reflected in "Repeat Vital Signs.")

Repeat Vital Signs

Student: I will reassess vital signs and mental status.

PROCTOR: Blood pressure, 118/70 mm Hg; pulse rate, 114 beats/min; respirations, 22 breaths/min; pulse oximetry reading, 97%; and the patient is anxious.

Student: The vital signs have not changed significantly.

PROCTOR: Noted.

Check Interventions

Student: I will check my interventions: oxygen, BLS breathing treatment (if permitted), and reassurance.

PROCTOR: Noted. Breathing improved with treatment if given.

ALS Student: I will check BLS interventions, plus the following: IV access, cardiac monitor, and local protocol (breathing treatment).

ALS Proctor: Noted. The cardiac monitor shows sinus tachycardia. Breathing improved with treatment.

Repeat the Focused Assessment

Student: I will repeat the focused assessment.

PROCTOR: Noted.

Critical Criteria:
- ❑ Did not obtain medical direction or verbalize standing orders for medical interventions
- ❑ Administered a dangerous or inappropriate intervention

Handoff Report to Emergency Department Staff

Student: There was no change in the patient's condition during transport.

PROCTOR: Noted.

Critical Criteria

(Inform the student of items missed, if any.)

❑ Pass ❑ Fail Date: ______________________

Proctor Comments: ______________________

____

____

CASE 148

Notes

CASE 149

Dispatch Information

PROCTOR: EMS 10, respond to a 51-year-old male patient who is unresponsive in his car on the interstate. He is breathing very rapidly. There is no evidence of damage to the car.

Pre-scene Action (BSI)

Student: I am wearing an appropriate high-visibility vest, nonlatex gloves, safety glasses, and a mask.
PROCTOR: Noted.

Critical Criteria:
- ❑ Did not take, or verbalize, body substance isolation (BSI) precautions when necessary

Scene Size-up

Scene Safety

Student: Is the scene safe?
PROCTOR: Yes.

Mechanism of Injury/Nature of Illness

Student: What is the nature of the illness?
PROCTOR: The patient was discovered on the highway in his car. He is unresponsive.

Number of Patients

Student: How many patients are there?
PROCTOR: One.

Additional Resources

Student: I would call for advanced life support (ALS) assistance.
PROCTOR: Noted.

C-Spine Stabilization

Student: I would not stabilize the cervical spine (c-spine).
PROCTOR: Noted.

Critical Criteria:
- ❑ Did not determine scene safety

Initial Assessment

General Impression

Student: My general impression is that the patient's condition is unstable.
PROCTOR: Noted.

Responsiveness/Level of Consciousness

Student: What is the patient's level of consciousness?
PROCTOR: Unresponsive.

Chief Complaint/Apparent Life Threats

Student: What is the patient's chief complaint?
PROCTOR: The patient is unresponsive.

Assess the Airway and Breathing

Student: Is the airway open? Is the patient breathing?
PROCTOR: He is snoring.
Student: I will open the airway with the head tilt–chin lift maneuver. Does that eliminate the snoring?
PROCTOR: Yes, snoring is relieved. He has a strong acetone odor on his breath.

Assessment

Student: What are the rate and the quality of breathing?
PROCTOR: Rate: Rapid. Quality: Deep (Kussmaul respirations).

Provide Oxygen

Student: I am applying oxygen at 15 L/min via nonrebreathing mask.
PROCTOR: Noted.

Ensure Adequate Ventilation

Student: The patient has adequate ventilations at this time.
PROCTOR: Noted.

Assess Circulation

Student: I am assessing the patient's circulation.
PROCTOR: Noted.

Assess for and Control Major Bleeding

Student: Do I find any major bleeding?
PROCTOR: No.

Assess the Pulse

Student: What are the rate and the quality of pulses?
PROCTOR: Rate: Tachycardic. Quality: Thready.

Assess the Skin

Student: I am assessing the skin. What are the color, temperature, and condition of the skin?
PROCTOR: Color: Flushed. Temperature: Warm. Condition: Dry.

Identify Priority Patients/Make Transport Decision

Student: The patient is a high priority and is a load-and-go. I will begin packaging and transport.
PROCTOR: Noted.

Critical Criteria:
- ❑ Did not provide high concentration of oxygen
- ❑ Did not find or manage problems associated with airway, breathing, hemorrhage or shock (hypoperfusion)
- ❑ Did not differentiate patient's need for transportation versus continued assessment at the scene
- ❑ Did detailed or focused history/physical examination before assessing the airway, breathing and circulation

Focused History and Physical Examination/Rapid Assessment

Select the Appropriate Assessment (Focused or Rapid)

Student: I am selecting the rapid assessment.
PROCTOR: Noted.
Student: I am checking for DCAP-BTLS. This acronym stands for deformities, contusions, abrasions, punctures, penetrations, paradoxical motion in the chest, and burns, tenderness, lacerations, and swelling. I am also checking for motor and sensory function and pulses.
PROCTOR: Noted.

Head

Student: I am rapidly assessing the head.
PROCTOR: There are no obvious injuries. He has a strong acetone odor on his breath.

Neck

Student: I am rapidly assessing the neck.
PROCTOR: There are no obvious injuries.

Chest

Student: I am rapidly inspecting and palpating the chest.
PROCTOR: There are no obvious injuries.
Student: Are there lung sounds present?
PROCTOR: They are clear bilaterally.

Abdomen

Student: I am rapidly assessing the abdomen.
PROCTOR: There are no obvious injuries.

Pelvis

Student: I am rapidly assessing the pelvis.
PROCTOR: There are no obvious injuries.

Extremities

Student: I am rapidly assessing the extremities.
PROCTOR: There are no obvious injuries.

▸ Posterior

Student: I am rapidly assessing the back.
PROCTOR: Noted.

▸ Assess the Thorax

Student: I am assessing the thorax. Do I find injuries?
PROCTOR: No.

▸ Assess the Lumbar Area

Student: I am assessing the flanks and lumbar area. Do I find injuries?
PROCTOR: No.

▸ Assess the Entire Backside

Student: I am assessing the entire backside. Do I find injuries?
PROCTOR: No.

▸ Reevaluate Transport Decision

Student: The patient is a high priority and is a load-and-go.
PROCTOR: Noted.

▾ Baseline Vital Signs

Student: What are the patient's baseline vital signs, including blood pressure, pulse, respirations, pulse oximetry, blood glucose level, and level of consciousness?
PROCTOR: Blood pressure, 122/84 mm Hg; pulse, 124 beats/min; respirations, 36 breaths/min; pulse oximetry reading, 95%; blood glucose level, HIGH; and the patient is unresponsive (to painful stimuli).

▾ SAMPLE History

Student: At this time I will gather a SAMPLE history from the patient or family. What are the patient's signs and symptoms?
PROCTOR: Altered mental status.

Student: Describe the episode.
PROCTOR: The patient is unresponsive.
Student: Onset: What was he doing when this started?
PROCTOR: It appears that he had been driving.
Student: Duration: How long has this been going on?
PROCTOR: Unknown.
Student: Are there any associated symptoms?
PROCTOR: He has a medic alert bracelet indicating that he has diabetes. He also has a strong acetone odor on his breath.
Student: Is there any evidence of trauma?
PROCTOR: No.
Student: Interventions: Has he done anything to make this better?
PROCTOR: Unknown.
Student: Has there been a seizure?
PROCTOR: Unknown.
Student: Has there been any fever?
PROCTOR: He does feel hot to the touch.

Student: Allergies?
PROCTOR: Unknown.
Student: Medications?
PROCTOR: Insulin is indicated on the medic alert bracelet.
Student: Pertinent past medical history?
PROCTOR: Diabetes per the medic alert bracelet.
Student: Last oral intake?
PROCTOR: Unknown.
Student: Events leading up to the incident?
PROCTOR: Unknown.

▾ Interventions

Student: I will apply oxygen and check the blood glucose level.
PROCTOR: Noted. The blood glucose level indicated on the meter is HIGH.
ALS Student: I will apply basic life support (BLS) interventions, plus the following: establish IV access, perform cardiac monitoring, and obtain a 12-lead ECG.
ALS Proctor: Noted. The cardiac monitor shows sinus tachycardia.

▾ Detailed Physical Examination

Possible Answer #1
Student: I would not do a detailed physical exam.
PROCTOR: Noted. (Go to "Radio Report.")

Possible Answer #2
Student: I am conducting the detailed physical exam.
PROCTOR: Noted. The detailed physical exam will be performed during transport.

▾ Assess the Head

Student: I am assessing the head. Do I find any DCAP-BTLS? Do I find any evidence of Battle's sign or raccoon eyes?
PROCTOR: No.

▸ Inspect and Palpate the Head and Ears

Student: I am assessing the head and ears.
PROCTOR: There are no obvious injuries.

▸ Assess the Eyes

Student: I am assessing the eyes. Are the pupils equal, round, and regular in size, and react properly to light (PEARRL)?
PROCTOR: They are nonreactive.

▸ Assess the Facial Area Including Oral and Nasal Areas

Student: I am assessing the face, nose, and mouth. Do I see any discharge or hear any obstructions?
PROCTOR: No, but you smell an acetone odor on his breath (like very strong Juicy Fruit gum).

▾ Assess the Neck

▸ Inspect and Palpate the Neck

Student: I am assessing the neck for DCAP-BTLS.
PROCTOR: There are no obvious injuries.

▸ Assess for Jugular Vein Distention

Student: Do I find any jugular vein distention (JVD)?
PROCTOR: No.

▸ Assess for Tracheal Deviation

Student: Do I see any tracheal deviation?
PROCTOR: No.

▾ Assess the Chest

Student: I am assessing the chest for DCAP-BTLS.
PROCTOR: Noted.

▸ Inspect

Student: What do I see when I look at the chest?
PROCTOR: There are no obvious injuries.
Student: Is the chest symmetric?
PROCTOR: Yes.

▸ Palpate

Student: When I touch the chest, do I feel crepitus or a flail segment?
PROCTOR: No.

▸ Auscultate

Student: Are lung sounds present in all fields?
PROCTOR: Yes.
Student: Do I hear any sucking sounds from the chest?
PROCTOR: No.

▾ Assess the Abdomen/Pelvis

▸ Assess the Abdomen

Student: I am assessing the abdomen for DCAP-BTLS. I am assessing all four quadrants. Do I find any problems?
PROCTOR: No.

▸ Assess the Pelvis

Student: I am assessing the pelvis for DCAP-BTLS. Is the pelvis stable?
PROCTOR: Yes.

- Assess the Genitalia/Perineum as Needed (Verbalize in Training)

Student: I am assessing the genitalia/perineum as necessary for DCAP-BTLS.
PROCTOR: The area is unremarkable.

Assess the Extremities

- Inspect

Student: I am assessing the lower and upper extremities for DCAP-BTLS. Do I find anything?
PROCTOR: No.

- Palpate

Student: Do I feel anything unusual?
PROCTOR: No.

- Assess Motor, Sensory, and Circulatory Function

Student: I am checking for DCAP-BTLS, motor and sensory function, and pulses. Right leg?
PROCTOR: Negative DCAP-BTLS. Motor and sensory functions are absent. Pulses are present.
Student: Left leg?
PROCTOR: Negative DCAP-BTLS. Motor and sensory functions are absent. Pulses are present.
Student: Right arm?
PROCTOR: Negative DCAP-BTLS. Motor and sensory functions are absent. Pulses are present.
Student: Left arm?
PROCTOR: Negative DCAP-BTLS. Motor and sensory functions are absent. Pulses are present.

Assess the Posterior

Student: We will check the back.
PROCTOR: Noted.

- Assess the Thorax

Student: I am assessing the thorax. Do I find injuries?
PROCTOR: No.

- Assess the Lumbar Area

Student: I am assessing the flanks and lumbar area. Do I find injuries?
PROCTOR: No.

- Assess the Entire Backside

Student: I am assessing the entire backside. Do I find injuries?
PROCTOR: No.

- Manage Secondary Injuries/Wounds

Student: I would direct my partner to monitor the airway.
PROCTOR: Noted.

- Reassess Interventions

Student: I will reassess my interventions: oxygen and maintain the airway.
PROCTOR: Noted.
ALS Student: I will reassess BLS interventions, plus the following: airway per local protocol, IV access, cardiac monitor, and 12-lead ECG.
ALS Proctor: Noted. The cardiac monitor shows sinus tachycardia.

Critical Criteria:
- ❑ Did not obtain medical direction or verbalize standing orders for medical interventions
- ❑ Administered a dangerous or inappropriate intervention
- ❑ Did not ask questions about the present illness
- ❑ Did not differentiate patient's need for transportation versus continued assessment at the scene

Radio Report

(Provided by the student.)
PROCTOR: Noted.

Ongoing Assessment

Repeat the Initial Assessment

Student: I will repeat the initial assessment.
PROCTOR: Noted. (Reflected in "Repeat Vital Signs.")

Repeat Vital Signs

Student: I will reassess vital signs and mental status.
PROCTOR: Blood pressure, 120/80 mm Hg; pulse, 128 beats/min; respirations, 36 breaths/min; pulse oximetry reading, 95%; and the patient is unresponsive.
Student: The vital signs have not changed significantly.
PROCTOR: Noted.

Check Interventions

Student: I will check my interventions: oxygen and maintain the airway.
PROCTOR: Noted.
ALS Student: I will check BLS interventions, plus the following: airway per local protocol, IV access, cardiac monitor, and 12-lead ECG.
ALS Proctor: Noted. The cardiac monitor shows sinus tachycardia.

Repeat the Focused Assessment

Student: I will repeat the focused assessment.
PROCTOR: Noted.

Critical Criteria:
- ❑ Did not obtain medical direction or verbalize standing orders for medical interventions
- ❑ Administered a dangerous or inappropriate intervention

Handoff Report to Emergency Department Staff

Student: There was no change in the patient's condition during transport.
PROCTOR: Noted.

Critical Criteria

(Inform the student of items missed, if any.)

❑ Pass ❑ Fail Date: ______________________

Proctor Comments: ______________________

CASE 149

Notes

Dispatch Information

PROCTOR: EMS 10, respond to a 20-year-old female who is combative. She is conscious and breathing.

Pre-scene Action (BSI)

Student: I am wearing nonlatex gloves and safety glasses.
PROCTOR: Noted.

Critical Criteria:
❑ Did not take, or verbalize, body substance isolation (BSI) precautions when necessary

Scene Size-up

Scene Safety
Student: Is the scene safe?
PROCTOR: No. I will call for law enforcement and enter the scene once police have given clearance.

Mechanism of Injury/Nature of Illness
Student: What is the nature of the illness?
PROCTOR: The patient was with new friends from college and began acting strangely. She is combative.

Number of Patients
Student: How many patients are there?
PROCTOR: One.

Additional Resources
Student: I would call for advanced life support (ALS) assistance.
PROCTOR: Noted.

C-Spine Stabilization
Student: I would not stabilize the cervical spine (c-spine).
PROCTOR: Noted.

Critical Criteria:
❑ Did not determine scene safety

Initial Assessment

General Impression
Student: My general impression is that the patient's condition is unstable.
PROCTOR: Noted.

Responsiveness/Level of Consciousness
Student: What is the patient's level of consciousness?
PROCTOR: Alert.

Chief Complaint/Apparent Life Threats
Student: What is the patient's chief complaint?
PROCTOR: The patient is combative.

Assess the Airway and Breathing
Student: Is the airway open? Is the patient breathing?
PROCTOR: Yes, the airway is open and the patient is breathing.

Assessment
Student: What are the rate and the quality of breathing?
PROCTOR: Rate: Rapid. Quality: Normal.

Provide Oxygen
Student: I am applying oxygen at 15 L/min via nonrebreathing mask.
PROCTOR: Noted. She refuses to wear the mask.

Ensure Adequate Ventilation
Student: The patient has adequate ventilations at this time.
PROCTOR: Noted.

Assess Circulation
Student: I am assessing the patient's circulation.
PROCTOR: Noted.

Assess for and Control Major Bleeding
Student: Do I find any major bleeding?
PROCTOR: No.

Assess the Pulse
Student: What are the rate and the quality of pulses?
PROCTOR: Rate: Tachycardic. Quality: Bounding.

Assess the Skin
Student: I am assessing the skin. What are the color, temperature, and condition of the skin?
PROCTOR: Color: Normal. Temperature: Cool. Condition: Moist.

Identify Priority Patients/Make Transport Decision
Student: The patient is a high priority and is a load-and-go. I will begin packaging and transport.
PROCTOR: Noted.

Critical Criteria:
❑ Did not provide high concentration of oxygen
❑ Did not find or manage problems associated with airway, breathing, hemorrhage or shock (hypoperfusion)
❑ Did not differentiate patient's need for transportation versus continued assessment at the scene
❑ Did detailed or focused history/physical examination before assessing the airway, breathing and circulation

Focused History and Physical Examination/Rapid Assessment

Select the Appropriate Assessment (Focused or Rapid)
Student: I am selecting the focused assessment.
PROCTOR: Noted.

SAMPLE History
Student: At this time I will gather a SAMPLE history from the patient or family. What are the patient's signs and symptoms?
PROCTOR: Altered mental status.

Student: Describe the episode.
PROCTOR: The patient has not been acting right. She suddenly became combative.
Student: Onset: What she doing when this started?
PROCTOR: She was with new friends from college.
Student: Duration: How long has this been going on?
PROCTOR: 25 minutes.
Student: Are there any associated symptoms?
PROCTOR: Yes, she is confused.
Student: Is there any evidence of trauma?
PROCTOR: No.
Student: Interventions: Has she done anything to make this better?
PROCTOR: The patient has taken no actions.
Student: Have there been any seizures?
PROCTOR: No.
Student: Has there been any fever?
PROCTOR: No.

Student: Allergies?
PROCTOR: Unknown.
Student: Medications?
PROCTOR: Unknown.
Student: Pertinent past medical history?
PROCTOR: Unknown.
Student: Last oral intake?
PROCTOR: Unknown.
Student: Events leading up to the incident?
PROCTOR: The patient was with some new friends from college. She suddenly became combative.

▼ Perform the Focused Physical Examination

Student: I am performing the focused physical examination.
PROCTOR: Noted.
Student: I will check the blood glucose level.
PROCTOR: Noted. The blood glucose level is 37 mg/dL.

▼ Baseline Vital Signs

Student: What are the patient's baseline vital signs, including blood pressure, pulse, respirations, pulse oximetry, blood glucose level, and level of consciousness?
PROCTOR: Blood pressure, 150/92 mm Hg; pulse, 132 beats/min; respirations, 32 breaths/min; pulse oximetry reading, 98%; blood glucose level, 37 mg/dL; and the patient is confused.

▼ Interventions

Student: I will ascertain if she can swallow and maintain her own airway. If she can swallow and maintain her own airway, I will apply one tube of oral glucose to a tongue depressor, and apply it to the inner cheek per medical control order.
PROCTOR: Noted. She is able to swallow and maintain her own airway.
Student: Do I see improvement in the patient following administration of the oral glucose?
PROCTOR: Yes. She is no longer combative and is somewhat embarrassed.
ALS Student: I will apply basic life support (BLS) interventions, plus the following: establish IV access, perform cardiac monitoring, and follow the local protocol (D_{50} IV [rather than oral glucose]).
ALS Proctor: Noted. The cardiac monitor shows sinus tachycardia.
ALS Student: Do I see improvement in the patient following administration of the D_{50} or oral glucose?
ALS Proctor: Yes. She is no longer combative and is somewhat embarrassed.

▼ Reevaluate Transport Decision

Student: The patient is now a low priority.
PROCTOR: Noted.

▼ Detailed Physical Examination

Possible Answer #1
Student: I would not do a detailed physical exam.
PROCTOR: Noted. (Go to "Radio Report.")

Possible Answer #2
Student: I am conducting the detailed physical exam. I am looking for DCAP-BTLS. This acronym stands for deformities, contusions, abrasions, punctures, penetrations, paradoxical motion in the chest, and burns, tenderness, lacerations, and swelling.
PROCTOR: Noted. The detailed physical exam will be performed during transport.

► **Assess the Head**

Student: I am assessing the head. Do I find any DCAP-BTLS? Do I find any evidence of Battle's sign or raccoon eyes?
PROCTOR: No.

► **Inspect and Palpate the Head and Ears**

Student: I am assessing the head and ears.
PROCTOR: There are no obvious injuries.

► **Assess the Eyes**

Student: I am assessing the eyes. Are the pupils equal, round, and regular in size, and react properly to light (PEARRL)?
PROCTOR: They are dilated.

► **Assess the Facial Area Including Oral and Nasal Areas**

Student: I am assessing the face, nose, and mouth. Do I see any discharge or hear any obstructions?
PROCTOR: No.

► **Assess the Neck**

► **Inspect and Palpate the Neck**

Student: I am assessing the neck for DCAP-BTLS.
PROCTOR: There are no obvious injuries.

► **Assess for Jugular Vein Distention**

Student: Do I find any jugular vein distention (JVD)?
PROCTOR: No.

► **Assess for Tracheal Deviation**

Student: Do I see any tracheal deviation?
PROCTOR: No.

► **Assess the Chest**

Student: I am assessing the chest for DCAP-BTLS.
PROCTOR: Noted.
Student: Are there lung sounds present?
PROCTOR: They are clear bilaterally.

► **Inspect**

Student: What do I see when I look at the chest?
PROCTOR: There are no obvious injuries.
Student: Is the chest symmetric?
PROCTOR: Yes.

► **Palpate**

Student: When I touch the chest, do I feel crepitus or a flail segment?
PROCTOR: No.

► **Auscultate**

Student: Are lung sounds present in all fields?
PROCTOR: Yes.
Student: Do I hear any sucking sounds from the chest?
PROCTOR: No.

► **Assess the Abdomen/Pelvis**

► **Assess the Abdomen**

Student: I am assessing the abdomen for DCAP-BTLS. I am assessing all four quadrants. Do I find any problems?
PROCTOR: No.

► **Assess the Pelvis**

Student: I am assessing the pelvis for DCAP-BTLS. Is the pelvis stable?
PROCTOR: Yes.

► **Assess the Genitalia/Perineum as Needed (Verbalize in Training)**

Student: I am assessing the genitalia/perineum as necessary for DCAP-BTLS.
PROCTOR: The area is unremarkable.

► **Assess the Extremities**

► **Inspect**

Student: I am assessing the lower and upper extremities for DCAP-BTLS. Do I find anything?
PROCTOR: No.

► **Palpate**

Student: Do I feel anything unusual?
PROCTOR: No.

► **Assess Motor, Sensory, and Circulatory Function**

Student: I am checking for DCAP-BTLS, motor and sensory function, and pulses. Right leg?
PROCTOR: Negative DCAP-BTLS. Motor and sensory functions are present. Pulses are present.
Student: Left leg?
PROCTOR: Negative DCAP-BTLS. Motor and sensory functions are present. Pulses are present.
Student: Right arm?

PROCTOR: Negative DCAP-BTLS. Motor and sensory functions are present. Pulses are present.
Student: Left arm?
PROCTOR: Negative DCAP-BTLS. Motor and sensory functions are present. Pulses are present.

▸ **Assess the Posterior**

Student: We will check the back.
PROCTOR: Noted.

▸ **Assess the Thorax**

Student: I am assessing the thorax. Do I find injuries?
PROCTOR: No.

▸ **Assess the Lumbar Area**

Student: I am assessing the flanks and lumbar area. Do I find injuries?
PROCTOR: No.

▸ **Assess the Entire Backside**

Student: I am assessing the entire backside. Do I find injuries?
PROCTOR: No.

▸ **Manage Secondary Injuries/Wounds**

Student: I would direct my partner to monitor the patient's level of consciousness.
PROCTOR: Noted.

▸ **Reassess Interventions**

Student: I will reassess my interventions: apply oxygen and monitor the blood glucose level.
PROCTOR: Noted. The blood glucose level is now 134 mg/dL.
ALS Student: I will reassess BLS interventions, plus the following: IVs, cardiac monitoring, and local protocol.
ALS Proctor: Noted. The cardiac monitor shows sinus tachycardia.

Critical Criteria:
- ❑ Did not obtain medical direction or verbalize standing orders for medical interventions
- ❑ Administered a dangerous or inappropriate intervention
- ❑ Did not ask questions about the present illness
- ❑ Did not differentiate patient's need for transportation versus continued assessment at the scene

Radio Report

(Provided by the student.)
PROCTOR: Noted.

Ongoing Assessment

Repeat the Initial Assessment

Student: I will repeat the initial assessment.
PROCTOR: Noted. (Reflected in "Repeat Vital Signs.")

Repeat Vital Signs

Student: I will reassess vital signs and mental status.
PROCTOR: Blood pressure, 144/86 mm Hg; pulse, 122 beats/min; respirations, 28 breaths/min; pulse oximetry reading, 99%; blood glucose level, 134 mg/dL; and the patient is alert and oriented.
Student: The vital signs have not changed significantly.
PROCTOR: Noted.

Check Interventions

Student: I will check my interventions: apply oxygen and monitor the blood glucose level.
PROCTOR: The blood glucose level is 134 mg/dL.
ALS Student: I will check BLS interventions plus the following: IVs, cardiac monitoring, and local protocol.
ALS Proctor: Noted. The cardiac monitor shows sinus tachycardia.

Repeat the Focused Assessment

Student: I will repeat the focused assessment.
PROCTOR: Noted.

Critical Criteria:
- ❑ Did not obtain medical direction or verbalize standing orders for medical interventions
- ❑ Administered a dangerous or inappropriate intervention

Handoff Report to Emergency Department Staff

Student: The patient's condition improved during transport.
PROCTOR: Noted.

Critical Criteria

(Inform the student of items missed, if any.)

❑ Pass ❑ Fail Date: ______________________________

Proctor Comments: ______________________________

____

____

CASE 150

Notes

Key of Cases

Cases by Topic

Abdominal

Allergic Reaction

Altered Mental Status

Bariatric

Behavioral

Burns

Cardiovascular

Chest Injury

Crush Injury

Diabetic

Electrical

▼ Multiple Injuries

▼ Musculoskeletal

▼ Neonatal

▼ Obstetric

▼ Paralysis

▼ Pediatric

Cases in Numeric Order

Medical